MANUAL OF EQUINE REPRODUCTION

SECOND EDITION

MANUAL OF EQUINE REPRODUCTION

SECOND EDITION

Terry L. Blanchard
DVM, MS, Dipl ACT
Professor of Theriogenology
Department of Large Animal Medicine and Surgery
Texas A&M University, College Station, Texas

Charles C. Love
DVM, PhD, Dipl ACT
Research Scientist
Department of Large Animal Medicine and Surgery
Texas A&M University, College Station, Texas

Dickson D. Varner
DVM, MS, Dipl ACT
Professor and Chief of Theriogenology
Department of Large Animal Medicine and Surgery
Texas A&M University, College Station, Texas

Steven P. Brinsko
DVM, MS, PhD, Dipl ACT
Assistant Professor of Theriogenology
Department of Large Animal Medicine and Surgery
Texas A&M University, College Station, Texas

James Schumacher
DVM, MS, Dipl ACVS
Professor
Department of Surgery
Faculty of Veterinary Medicine
Ballsbridge, Dublin, Ireland

Sherri L. Rigby
DVM, PhD, Dipl ACT
Bayer Animal Health
Virginia Beach, Virginia

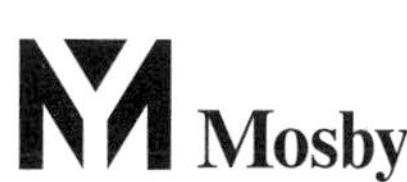

A Harcourt Health Sciences Company
St. Louis London Philadelphia Sydney Toronto

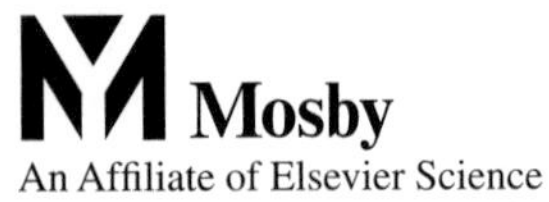

An Affiliate of Elsevier Science

11830 Westline Drive
St. Louis, MO 63146

MANUAL OF EQUINE REPRODUCTION
SECOND EDITION

ISBN 0-323-01713-4

NOTICE

Veterinary medicine is an ever-changing field. Standard safety precautions must be followed, but as new research and clinical experience broaden our knowledge, changes in treatment and drug therapy may become necessary or appropriate. Readers are advised to check the most current product information provided by the manufacturer of each drug to be administered to verify the recommended dose, the method and duration of administration, and contraindications. It is the responsibility of the treating veterinarian, relying on experience and knowledge of the patient, to determine dosages and the best treatment for each individual patient. Neither the Publisher nor the editor assume any liability for any injury and/or damage to persons or property arising from this publication.

The Publisher

First edition 1998

International Standard Book Number: 0-323-01713-4

Senior Editor: Elizabeth M. Fathman
Managing Editor: Teri Merchant
Project Manager: Peggy Fagen
Designer: Julia Dummitt

RT/MVY

Printed in the United States of America.

Last digit is print number: 9 8 7 6 5 4 3 2 1

DEDICATION

This textbook is dedicated to Dr. Robert M. Kenney, Professor Emeritus of Reproduction in the Section of Reproductive Studies, New Bolton Center, University of Pennsylvania School of Veterinary Medicine, and Dr. O.J. Ginther, Professor of Veterinary Science in the Department of Veterinary Science, University of Wisconsin-Madison. These two individuals have devoted their entire professional lives to advancements in equine reproduction and have served as invaluable resources and mentors for countless veterinary students, graduate students, clinical residents, university faculty, and practicing veterinarians. They can be considered true fathers of the modern-day discipline of equine reproduction.

Preface

We originally wrote this manual to serve as a textbook for veterinary students studying clinical reproduction in horses. We quickly found that the manual had become a popular resource for veterinarians practicing equine reproduction. In this thoroughly updated second edition, we have tried to maintain its easy readability and overwhelmingly clinical emphasis. Many new illustrations have been added to the expanded chapters, particularly those covering reproductive disorders of the mare and stallion. To evaluate fertility problems of stallions, a new chapter has been included on the use of breeding indices obtained from farm records.

Manual of Equine Reproduction is a practical field guide designed for both students and practitioners. It succinctly covers reproductive management of horses, including management of stallions, broodmares, and neonatal foals. The manual will also benefit animal scientists teaching reproductive physiology and artificial insemination. Horse owners will find useful information regarding reproductive management, breeding with transported cooled or frozen semen, and management of the pregnant/foaling mare and newborn foal.

Each chapter begins with a listing of important learning objectives, along with questions to guide self-study. More than 100 new illustrations, including many diagnostic ultrasound images, enhance understanding of diagnostic and treatment procedures, including broodmare hormonal therapy, diagnosis and treatment of abnormalities of the mare and stallion reproductive tracts, performance of routine reproductive surgeries, processing semen for cooling or freezing, and principles of embryo transfer.

Terry L. Blanchard
Dickson D. Varner
James Schumacher
Charles C. Love
Steven P. Brinsko
Sherri L. Rigby

Contents

1

Reproductive Anatomy of the Mare

OBJECTIVES

While studying the information covered in this chapter, the student should attempt to:

1. Acquire a working understanding of the anatomy of the reproductive organs of the mare.
2. Acquire a working understanding of how defects in anatomic development or changes in anatomy that occur with injury or age of the reproductive tract of the mare might adversely affect fertility.
3. Acquire a working understanding of procedures to be used for safely examining the reproductive tract of the mare per rectum.

STUDY QUESTIONS

1. Describe the normal nonpregnant equine reproductive tract, including location and shape of the ovaries, ovulation fossa, oviducts, uterus, cervix, vagina, vestibule, and vulva.
2. Describe normal equine ovarian structures, the process of ovulation and oocyte entry into the oviduct, the process of sperm entry into the oviduct, and the site of fertilization.
3. List structures that are physically isolated from the reproductive tract but play a central role in regulation of reproductive events in the mare.
4. List three major physical barriers to contamination of the mare's uterus.
5. Describe important guidelines to follow when performing an examination of the mare reproductive tract per rectum, including restraint, protective wear, lubrication, manure removal, guards against rectal perforation, and anatomic orientation.
6. Discuss congenital and acquired defects of the mare reproductive tract that could affect reproductive performance.

The reproductive system is made up of two groups of organs: (1) those structures that are intrinsic to the reproductive tract (ovaries and tubular genitalia) and (2) those structures that are physically isolated from the reproductive tract but play a role in the regulation of reproductive events (e.g., pineal gland, retina, hypothalamus, and pituitary gland).

The reproductive tract (Figures 1-1 through 1-4) consists of two ovaries and a tubular tract, including the paired oviducts and uterine horns, and a single uterine body, cervix, vagina, vestibule, and vulva. The lumen of the female reproductive tract is the only channel in the body that communicates between the abdominal cavity and external environment. Well over half of the reproductive tract lies within the abdominal cavity, and the remainder lies within the pelvic cavity. When

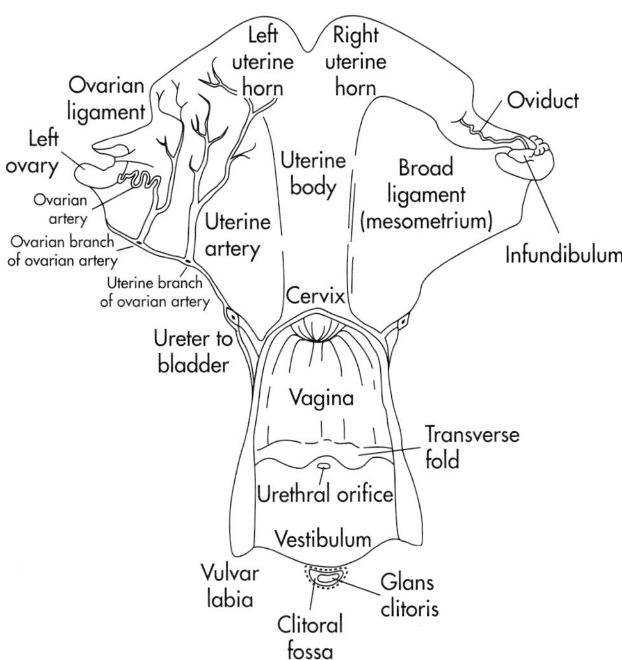

FIGURE 1-1. Dorsal view of the mare reproductive tract. Broad ligament attachments have been cut away from the abdominal and pelvic walls, and the dorsal vaginal wall has been cut open to reveal the mucosal surface of the external cervical os, vagina, and vestibule. (Modified from Sisson S, Grossman JD: *The anatomy of domestic animals*, ed 4, Philadelphia, 1953, WB Saunders.)

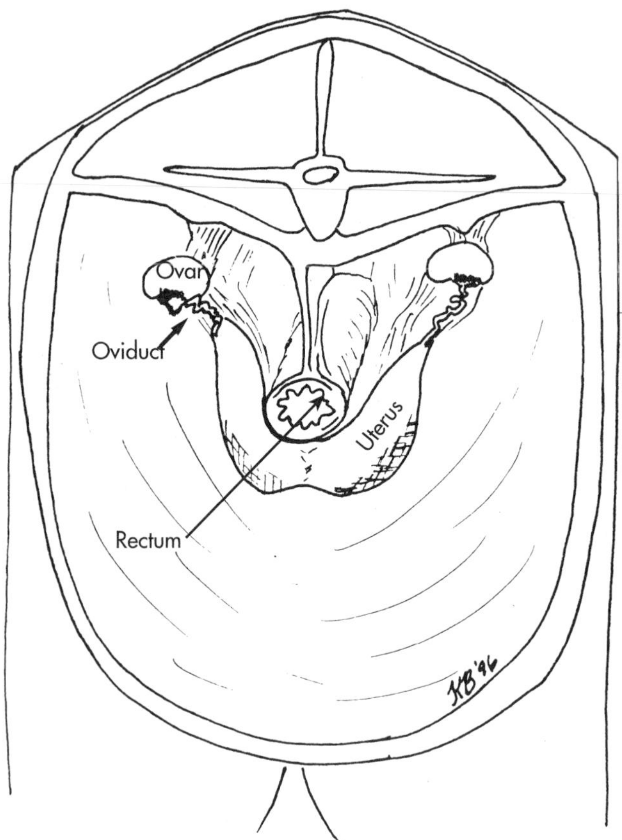

FIGURE 1-2. Frontal aspect of the suspended ovaries and uterine horns. The uterus is noncoiled and dorsally suspended by the broad ligaments. (Modified from Sisson S, Grossman JD: *The anatomy of domestic animals*, ed 4, Philadelphia, 1953, WB Saunders.)

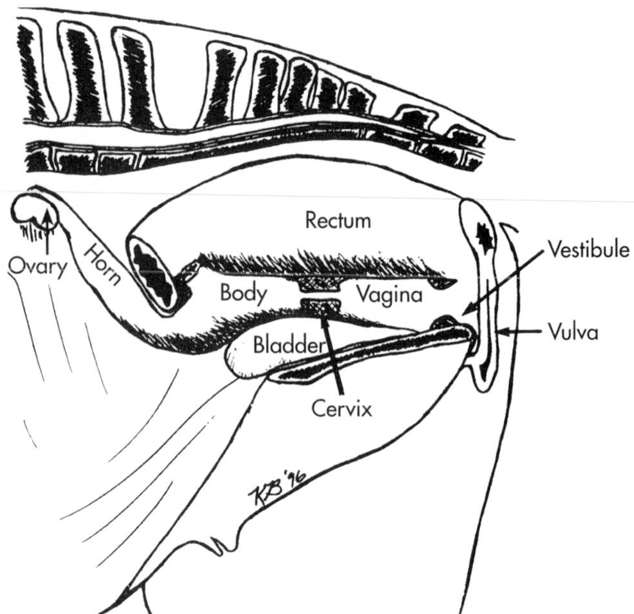

FIGURE 1-3. Lateral view of suspended ovary, oviduct, and uterine horn. One ovary and uterine horn has been removed, depicting a cross-sectional view of the collapsed uterine lumen. The ovaries of the mare are in the cranial-most transverse plane. (Modified from Sisson S, Grossman JD: *The anatomy of domestic animals*, ed 4, Philadelphia, 1953, WB Saunders.)

the *ovum* is discharged from the follicle at ovulation, it is received at the level of the *ovarian bursa*, which is thought to assist the passage of the ovum into the **oviduct**. The oviduct is responsible for movement of sperm and ova to a common site (the *ampulla*) for fertilization. The fertilized ovum (*embryo*) then travels down the oviduct and gains entrance into the uterus for gestational support. The **uterus** provides the proper environment for the embryo to develop.

The **cervix** accommodates the expanded glans penis of the stallion at estrus to allow intrauterine deposition of sperm and closes tightly during pregnancy to prevent ascending bacterial/fungal infection from the posterior tract. It also expands considerably at the time of parturition to accommodate passage of the foal. The caudal portion of the cervix projects into the lumen of the vagina (Figure 1-5). Longitudinal folds comprise the lining of the cervix and are continuous with the endometrial folds lining the uterine body. The cervix secretes two types of mucus: a thin mucus to lubricate the posterior genital tract in preparation for coitus and a more viscid mucus to help seal the cervical lumen during pregnancy.

The vagina is a potential space that expands to permit penile and foal passage. A transverse fold overlies the external urethral orifice and is the anatomical division between the

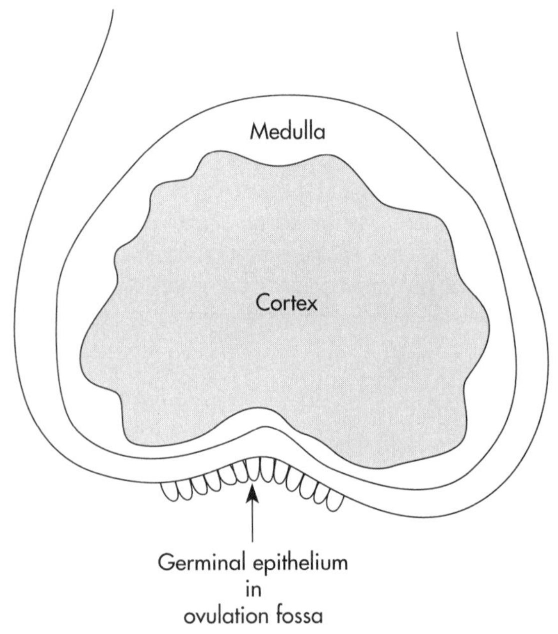

FIGURE 1-4. Schematic drawing of cortical and medullary areas of equine ovary. The germinal epithelium lines the surface of the ovulation fossa, where all ovulations take place. The oviductal fimbria (not pictured) pick up the ovulated oocyte and move it to the site where fertilization will take place. (Modified from Sisson S, Grossman JD: *The anatomy of domestic animals*, ed 4, Philadelphia, 1953, WB Saunders.)

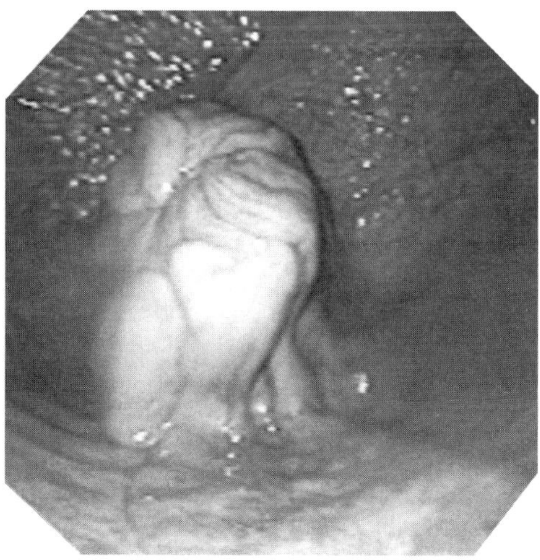

FIGURE 1-5. Per vagina view of external cervical os protruding into vaginal lumen.

vagina, which is anterior, and the **vestibule**, which is posterior. The juncture between the vestibule and vagina is referred to as the **vestibulovaginal ring**. When closed, this ring restricts entry of air and debris into the upper tubular tract. The **vulva** is limited to the external opening of the tubular tract.

OVARIES

The ovaries of the mare are usually the most anterior part of the reproductive tract in the nonpregnant mare (see Figure 1-3). The noncoiled and dorsally suspended uterus of the mare (compared with the coiled tract and more ventral and posterior [flank] broad ligament attachment in other farm animal species) accounts for the more cranial location of the ovaries. Thus in the mare, the ovaries are in the cranial-most transverse plane, whereas in other farm animal species a portion of the uterus is cranial to the ovaries. The ovaries, as well as follicles, are larger in the mare than in other farm species. Equine ovaries are bean-shaped and vary in size according to ovarian activity, being largest during the breeding season (spring and summer) and smallest during the nonbreeding season (winter anestrus). The average size of the ovaries is 6 to 8 cm in length and 3 to 4 cm in height and average weight is 70 to 80 g.

The ovaries are located in the sublumbar area (ventral to the fourth or fifth lumbar vertebra), suspended by long sheetlike **broad ligaments**, and are usually located several centimeters behind the corresponding kidney. The right ovary is typically more cranial (2 to 3 cm) than the left. Because the ovaries may be lifted by the intestines, their actual location in the body is quite variable. Therefore to facilitate locating the ovaries during palpation per rectum the authors recommend tracing the tip of each uterine horn to the associated ovary (because the ovary may be in contact with the ipsilateral uterine horn to within 5 cm of the tip). Each ovary consists of two surfaces (medial and lateral), two borders (attached [dorsal] and free [ventral]), and two poles (cranial [tubal] and caudal [uterine]). The caudal border is connected to the uterine horn by the ovarian ligament. Each ovary is kidney bean–shaped, with a very prominent depression on the free or ventral border. The convex dorsal border is sometimes called the greater curvature.

The ovarian surface is largely covered by peritoneum except at the attached border where nerves and vessels enter. The relationship between ovarian cortical and medullary areas is unusual in the mare (see Figure 1-4). The ovary of the mare is "inside-out" compared with ovaries of other farm animal species. In other words, the medullary or vascular zone is superficial and the cortical zone (which contains the follicles) is in the interior of the gland. The cortical tissue reaches the surface only at the depression of the ventral or free border. This is therefore the only area from which normal ovulation occurs and is appropriately termed the **ovulation fossa**. The ovulation fossa is covered by a layer of short polygonal cells, which are a remnant of the primitive germinal epithelium. The ovulation papilla of the corpus luteum does not project from the convex surface of the ovary as it does in other species, but rather from the ovulation fossa.

The ovary has both exocrine and endocrine functions. The **exocrine function** is development of gametes, and the **endocrine function** is production of hormones.

OVIDUCTS

The oviducts (Fallopian tubes and uterine tubes) are long tortuous ducts that measure 20 to 30 cm in length in horse mares when fully extended. Cilia are present on the epithelium of the oviduct and produce a current directed toward the uterus. The oviduct is divided into three parts: the **infundibulum** (funnel-shaped portion nearest the ovary), **ampulla** (expanded middle portion), and **isthmus** (narrowed portion connecting the ampulla to the uterine horn). The cranial edge of the infundibulum attaches to the lateral surface of the mare's ovary. At ovulation, this fan-shaped structure envelops the ovulation fossa to facilitate ovum entry into the oviduct. The ampulla is the middle part of the oviduct where fertilization and early cleavage of the fertilized ovum occur. The highly muscular isthmus transports the fertilized ovum (embryo) from the site of fertilization into the uterine lumen. The oviduct enters the uterus just caudal to the blunt end of the uterine horn through a distinct papilla (**oviductal papilla**) that is easily visualized from the uterine lumen (see Figure 4-31). Normal oviducts are not usually palpable per rectum.

Sperm gain access to the oviduct through the *uterotubal junction (UTJ)*, which is located in the center of the *oviductal papilla* that projects into the uterine lumen near the blunt end of the uterine horn. Deep, edematous longitudinal folds are present in the UTJ during estrus, and numerous sperm can be found "bound" to epithelial cells or "trapped" in these folds within 4 hours of breeding. The UTJ may play a role in the selection of morphologically normal sperm and may also act as a storage site for sperm awaiting transport into the oviduct. The muscular isthmus is believed to contract rhythmically after breeding in a fashion that propels sperm to the fertilization site in the ampulla. Adhesion of sperm to epithelial cells in the isthmus (and perhaps the UTJ) is thought to prevent premature capacitation and increase the lifespan of the sperm, resulting in a sperm reservoir awaiting the opportunity for release to fertilize the ovum.

UTERUS

The uterus consists of two horns and a singular body. The uterus has been described as T-shaped in the mare, but Y-shaped (see Figure 1-2) is probably a more accurate description of the organ when viewed dorsally in its natural position in the mare. The uterus is suspended within the pelvic cavity and abdomen by the broad ligament. The portion of the broad ligament that attaches to the uterus is called the **mesometrium**. In the mare, the mesometrium attaches to the dorsal surface of the uterine horns, whereas in the cow the attachment is on the ventrolateral surface. Therefore in mares the free (unattached) surface of the uterus is ventral to the broad ligament, whereas in cattle the free surface is dorsal to the broad ligament. This arrangement prevents digital evaluation of the uterine body and likewise prevents retraction of the uterus into the pelvic cavity during palpation of the mare per rectum. In contrast, in the cow these procedures are easily accomplished. The uterine horns of the mare are entirely in the abdominal cavity and "float" on or are intermingled with intestinal viscera.

The serosal layer of the uterus and the vascular layer plus longitudinal muscular layer are continuous with that of the broad ligament. The **myometrium** is composed of an inner circular layer and an outer longitudinal layer. Finally, the innermost layer of the uterus consists of the **endometrium**, which is glandular and secretory.

The uterine lumen in the normal nonpregnant state is nearly obliterated by the collapsed wall and prominent **endometrial folds**. The endometrial folds are arranged longitudinally in the uterus and are usually palpable per rectum when the uterus is "strummed" between the thumb and forefingers. The myometrium is quite thick and is responsible for variation in uterine tone of the mare during estrus versus during diestrus or early pregnancy. In contrast to that of the cow, the uterus of the mare is not coiled, the intercornual ligament is not prominent, the internal bifurcation is marked by a short uterine septum, and the body is longer.

The vasculature of the uterus is supplied on each side by three arteries and veins weaving their way through the broad ligament: the uterine branch of the **vaginal artery** and corresponding vein; the **uterine artery** (sometimes called **middle uterine artery**) and corresponding vein; and the uterine branch of the ovarian artery and corresponding vein. Rupture of these arteries sometimes occurs during parturition in aged mares, leading either to hematoma formation within the broad ligament or fatal hemorrhage into the abdomen. The **ovarian artery** is located in the cranial portion of the broad ligament and follows the course of the ovarian vein and the uterine branch of the ovarian vein; however, in contrast to ruminant species, the ovarian artery is not closely attached or applied to the ovarian vein. This has important functional considerations, namely, for countercurrent transport of prostaglandin-$F_{2\alpha}$ ($PGF_{2\alpha}$) from the veins draining the uterus into the ovarian artery. Because this countercurrent exchange is not efficient in the mare, *regression of the corpus luteum is induced by* $PGF_{2\alpha}$ *that reaches the ovary via the systemic circulation*, as opposed to ruminants, in which $PGF_{2\alpha}$ reaches the ovary in higher concentrations via the ovarian artery because of countercurrent exchange from the closely entwined uterine venous drainage.

CERVIX

The cervix is a versatile organ. It is lined internally by epithelium containing secretory cells that produce a thin mucus to serve as a lubricant during estrus and a thick mucus to occlude the cervical lumen during diestrus and pregnancy so that it is less permeable to bacteria and foreign objects. The longitudinal folds of the cervix are continuous with the endometrial folds present in the body of the uterus. The cervix expands to accommodate the stallion's penis during estrus and the foal during parturition, and it closes tightly during diestrus and even more so during pregnancy.

The thick-walled cervix is usually identifiable by palpation per rectum, particularly during diestrus or pregnancy, typically being 5 to 7.5 cm in length and 2 to 4 cm in diameter. During estrus, the cervix is quite flaccid and thus more difficult to feel by palpation per rectum.

The cervix of the mare differs from that of the cow in two ways: (1) the cervical lumen greatly expands and contracts during the estrous cycle because of a thick layer of circular muscle rich in elastic fibers, and (2) the cervix has only longitudinal folds with no obstructing transverse cervical rings. Therefore the uterus is more easily accessed through the cervix of the mare than through the cervix of the cow. The **external os of the cervix** protrudes into the vaginal lumen (see Figure 1-5) and is surrounded by the **vaginal fornix** (i.e., the area of reflection of vaginal mucous membrane onto the cervix).

VAGINA

The vagina is a tubular organ that extends horizontally for 15 to 20 cm through the pelvic cavity from the external os of the cervix to the **transverse fold** overlying the **external urethral orifice**. In maiden mares, this transverse fold is often continued on either side of the vagina, forming the hymen. Occasionally, the hymen completely encircles the vestibulovaginal junction and is imperforate (**persistent hymen**) (Figure 1-6), precluding breeding until it is removed. The vagina continues caudally as the vestibule.

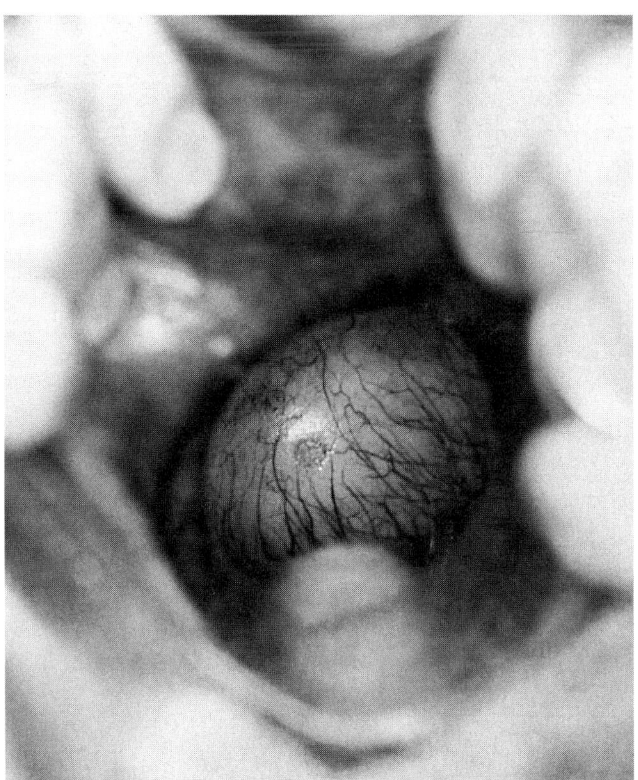

FIGURE 1-6. Persistent hymen in a maiden mare.

The lumen of the vagina is normally collapsed except during breeding and passage of the foal at parturition. The vagina, including its mucosa, is highly elastic and expands considerably to accommodate the passage of the foal. It becomes distended with air when the abnormal condition of **pneumovagina** exists. The lumen of the vagina is covered with stratified squamous epithelium. The cranial vagina is covered with serosa and lies within the peritoneal cavity. The posterior vagina is in a retroperitoneal position and therefore is not covered with serosa. Because *most of the vagina is retroperitoneal*, vaginal injuries (such as tearing during breeding) usually do not perforate into the peritoneal space, although this sometimes occurs. Unlike the uterus, cervix, and vestibule, the vagina contains no glandular structures.

VESTIBULE

The vestibule extends 10 to 12 cm from the transverse fold overlying the external urethral orifice to the vulva. A vestibulovaginal ring exists at the junction of the vestibule and vagina and, owing to the vulvar and vaginal constrictor muscles that encircle this area, forms a seal, thereby minimizing entry of foreign material into the upper tubular tract. This ring oftentimes is incompetent (weak or incapable of closing) when pneumovagina exists, allowing entry of air into the vaginal space. The vestibule contains vestibular glands ventrally that secrete mucus to provide lubrication of the posterior tubular tract.

VULVA

The vulva (Figure 1-7) refers to the external opening of the female reproductive tract and the structures surrounding it. The vertical vulvar opening normally begins 5 to 7 cm directly under the anus and is 12 to 15 cm in length. The dorsal commissure of the vulva normally is less than 5 cm above the ischium (floor of the pelvis). The mare is prone to aspiration of air into the vagina (**pneumovagina**) if the dorsal commissure is greater than 5 cm above the ischium, particularly if the anus is recessed (sunken) and the vulvar lips are tipped horizontally so the vulva is no longer vertical (Figure 1-8). The labia of the vulva contain underlying musculature that functions to close the vulvar opening, providing a further barrier to the entrance of foreign material into the tubular tract. The vulva contains much elastic tissue and expands greatly during passage of the fetus at parturition. The **clitoris**, a homolog of the penis, is located in a cavity just cranial to the ventral commissure of the vulvar opening (Figure 1-9). The **glans clitoris** is more prominent in the mare than in other farm animal species. Three **clitoral sinuses** are located on the dorsal aspect of the clitoris, and a large singular **clitoral fossa** is located ventral to the glans clitoris. The clitoral sinuses and fossa must be swabbed for bacteriologic culture to document freedom from infection with *Taylorella equigenitalis*, the organism causing contagious equine metritis.

EXAMINATION OF THE REPRODUCTIVE TRACT OF THE MARE PER RECTUM

Mare Restraint

It is essential that the mare be adequately restrained before one examines the reproductive tract. Such precautions protect both the mare and examiner from severe injury. Minimal, but effective, restraint is the key to a safe examination and will vary from mare to mare. The disposition of the mare should be determined before the examination is begun. Mares accustomed to periodic examinations per rectum tend to require little restraint, whereas mares not accustomed to such practices often become very anxious and sometimes explosive during the examination. In any case, never be careless. Always use caution. A strategically placed kick can quickly terminate your career! If stocks are available, all mares should be placed in them (Figure 1-10) before the examination. Ideally, the stocks should be equipped with a solid, padded rear door to help prevent leg extension if the mare does decide to kick and afford some protection against injury to the lower legs of the mare. The height of the door should not be greater than the mid-upper gaskin region of the mare's hindquarters. Higher doors could damage the examiner's arm if the mare abruptly squats while the arm is in the rectum. If stocks are not available, the mare should be examined by placing her in a doorway with the hindquarters remaining 2 feet beyond the doorway. The examiner is thus protected by the doorframe. If a mare must

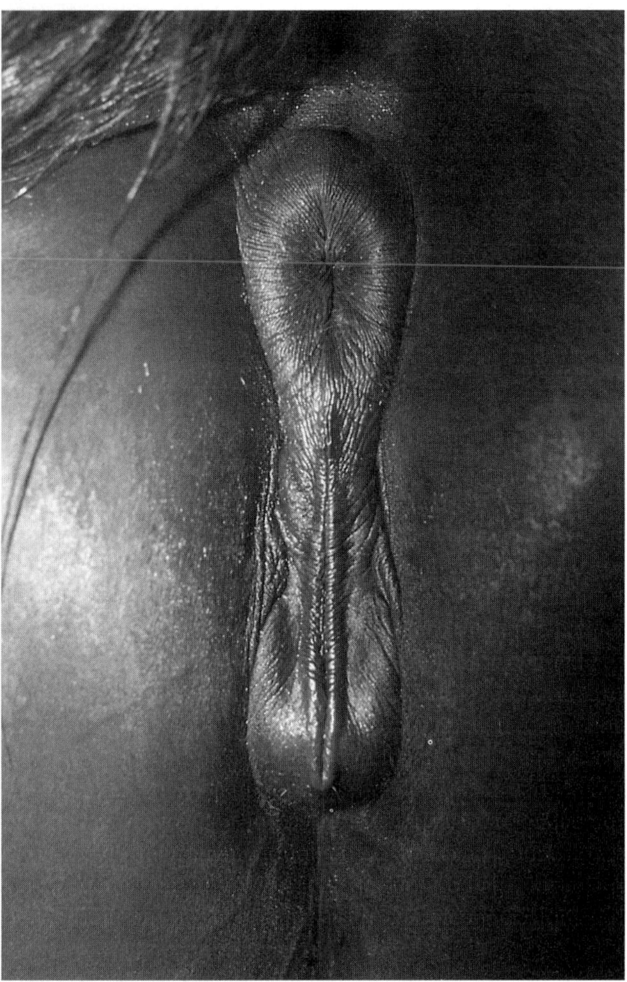

FIGURE 1-7. Normal vulva and anus of a mare.

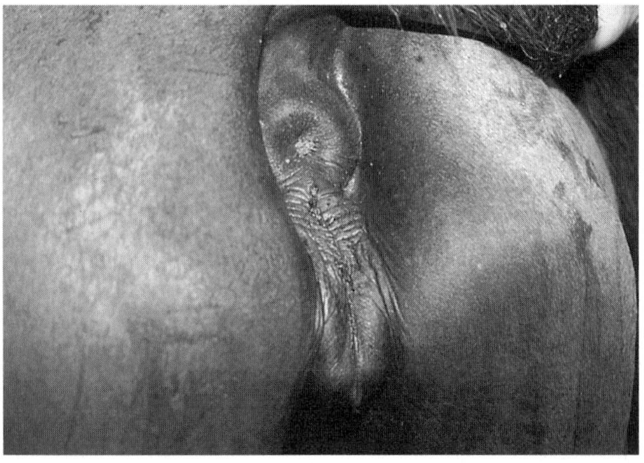

FIGURE 1-8. Sunken anus and tipped vulva in an aged mare.

be examined in an open area, breeding hobbles can be properly secured to the mare's hindlegs to reduce the range of limb motion, should she decide to kick. A leg strap can also be applied to a flexed front leg. Lifting the tail directly over the

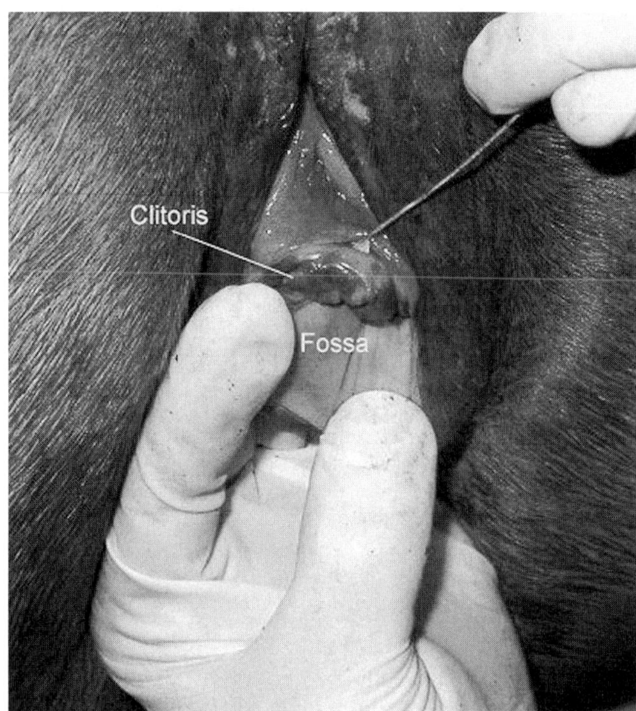

FIGURE 1-9. The clitoris (*arrow*) is located in a cavity just cranial to the ventral commissure of the vulva. A wire is placed within one of the clitoral sinuses located on the dorsal surface of the clitoris. Smegma can be seen being expressed from this clitoral sinus. The clitoral fossa that surrounds the clitoris ventrally has been partially everted to allow viewing of the clitoris.

back of the mare also helps distract her from the examiner's activities. If necessary a twitch can also be placed on the mare's muzzle as an additional means of physical restraint. Tranquilization may be required to adequately restrain an anxious mare. Remember, overrestraint can be as dangerous to the mare and examiner as underrestraint.

Never develop a false sense of security through the use of the above protective devices. Always take special precautions when walking around the hindquarters of a mare. Approach the mare from the front and work your way back to the hindquarters while quietly talking to her so she will be aware of your location. Never surprise her. Minimize the time spent directly behind the mare. Rather, stand to one side when possible. Stand close to the mare to reduce concussion, should you be in the line of fire if she decides to kick.

Technique

The first question that comes to mind is which arm to use to perform the examination. Ambidexterity may provide some advantage, but both hands will probably be equally clumsy when learning to palpate at the onset of your career. Therefore a general recommendation is to teach the off hand to palpate per rectum. The more commonly used hand can then perform other duties during the examination.

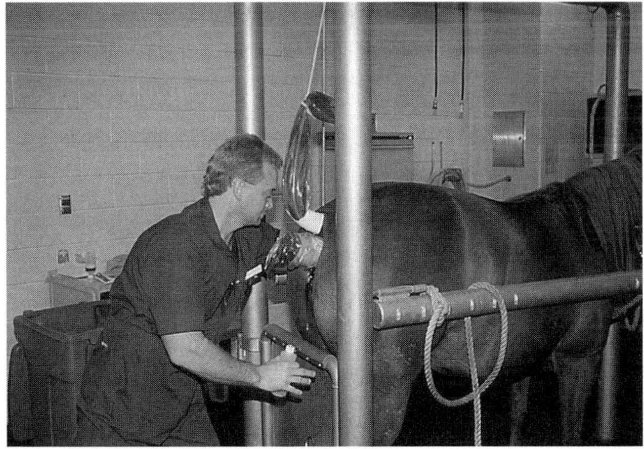

FIGURE 1-10. Mare being palpated in a stock with a padded kickboard.

Shoulder-length rubber obstetrical sleeves or disposable plastic sleeves can be used to protect the arm during the examination. Soft, pliable sleeves (approximately 3 mils thick) will increase sensitivity. Alternatively, the fingers can be removed from the plastic sleeve and replaced with a rubber surgical glove. To minimize horizontal disease transmission, sleeves should be changed between mares.

The protected hand should be well lubricated before use. A water-based lubricant such as methylcellulose can be used. The lubricated hand should then be shaped into a cone and gently inserted into the rectum through the tight anal sphincter. Slow rotation of the arm in conjunction with gentle forward pressure enhances advancement into the rectum. **DO NOT RUSH.** Rectal perforation is a common cause of malpractice claims against equine practitioners. Use extreme caution. Never perform forceful manipulations in the rectum against peristaltic waves or a tense rectal wall.

Manure in the rectum and distal colon should be removed before evaluation of abdominal and pelvic structures. This task is accomplished by passing the coned hand past a small amount of feces, then cupping the hand to facilitate removal of manure when the arm is withdrawn.

Two established principles for examination of the female reproductive tract per rectum are the following: (1) determine normal anatomical orientation, and (2) follow a thorough methodical approach. Adherence to these principles will reduce the chance of error.

Before placing emphasis on detection of the reproductive tract, the examiner should first become properly oriented by identifying topographical landmarks that are in a constant position such as the outlines of the pelvic cavity (the pelvic floor, sacrum, wings of the ilia, and pelvic brim). Once the examiner feels confident of his or her location in the pelvic and abdominal cavities, he or she may proceed to specific examination of reproductive structures.

Three initial landmarks have been described for locating the reproductive tract in the mare by various authorities on

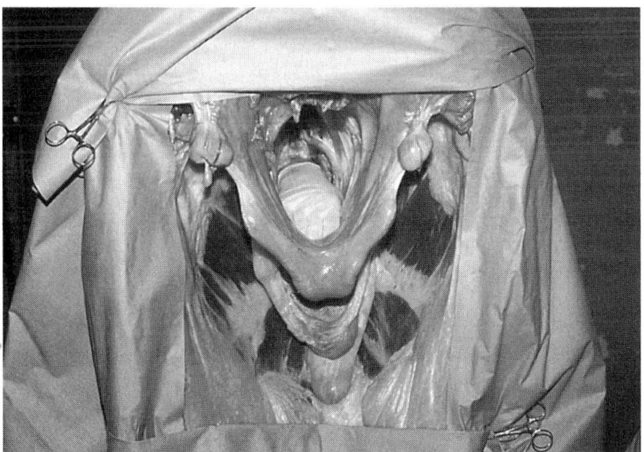

FIGURE 1-11. Procedure used to locate the cervix during palpation per rectum. A side-to-side motion is made with the extended hand in the pelvic cavity, using downward pressure with the fingers held together and the palm facing downward. The rectum and abdominal viscera have been removed to facilitate visualization.

the subject: the cervix, the leading edge of the uterus, and the ovary. The positions of all of these structures are relatively inconstant. The cervix of the nonpregnant mare is located in the pelvic cavity, whereas the leading edge of the uterus and the ovaries are always in the abdominal cavity. To locate the cervix of a nonpregnant mare, one should produce a side-to-side motion with the extended hand in the pelvic cavity, using downward pressure with the fingers held together and the palm facing downward (Figure 1-11). The cervix can be palpated in almost all instances but may relax during estrus to the point of becoming barely perceptible. It is also difficult to palpate the dilated cervix per rectum in the early postpartum period. Uterine contents (e.g., fetus or pyometra) may pull the cervix into an abdominal position.

The leading edge of the uterus can be detected by first inserting the arm deeply into the rectum, cupping the hand

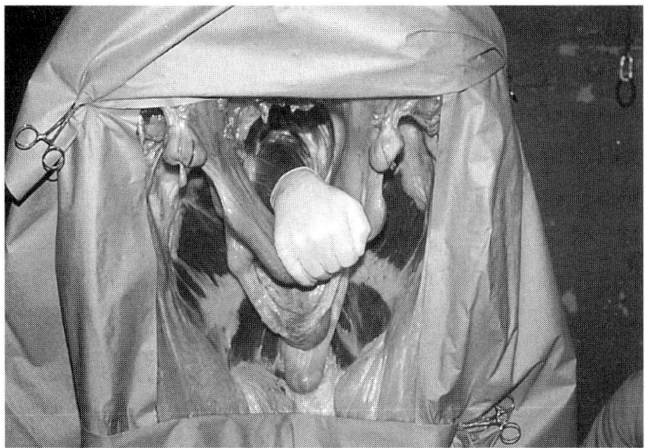

FIGURE 1-12. Palpation of uterine horns per rectum. The cupped hand is used to grasp the leading edge of the uterine horn. The rectum and abdominal viscera have been removed to facilitate visualization.

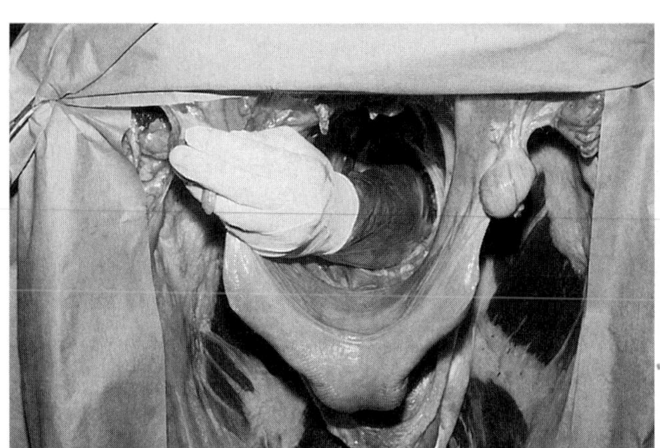

FIGURE 1-13. Palpation of an ovary per rectum. The ovary is gently grasped with the fingertips, enabling the examiner to identify raised and/or softened follicles. The rectum and abdominal viscera have been removed to facilitate visualization.

downward, then slowly retracting the arm (Figure 1-12). The cupped hand will "hook" the uterus if the technique is properly applied and if the uterus is a normal, nonpregnant size and in the usual location. Enlarged uteri that have begun descent into the lower abdomen are difficult to identify using this method.

The ovaries are located in the sublumbar area, caudoventral to the corresponding kidney. By placing the arm in the rectum and directing the hand to the estimated location of the ovary, the ovary can usually be located with the fingertips. Providing the rectal wall is relaxed, gentle grasping motions with the fingers together can be used to pick up the ovary (Figure 1-13). The ovaries will be pulled downward and toward the midline when the uterus becomes greatly enlarged (i.e., in the early postpartum period, in advanced pregnancy, or in some instances of pyometra).

After any of these landmarks is located, one should proceed with a methodical examination of the accessible reproductive tract. The examination should include both ovaries, the uterus, and the cervix. Structures caudal to the cervix do not lend themselves to palpation per rectum but, rather, are evaluated via the vulvar opening.

BIBLIOGRAPHY

Ginther OJ: *Reproductive biology of the mare: basic and applied aspects*, ed 2, pp 1-40. Cross Plains, WI, 1992, Equiservices.

Greenhoff GR, Kenney RM: Evaluation of reproductive status of nonpregnant mares. *J Am Vet Med Assoc* 167:449-458, 1975.

Sisson S, Grossman JD: *The anatomy of domestic animals*, ed 4, pp 606-614. Philadelphia, 1953, WB Saunders.

2

Reproductive Physiology of the Nonpregnant Mare

OBJECTIVES

While studying the information covered in this chapter, the student should attempt to:

1. Acquire a working understanding of the physiology of the estrous cycle of the mare.
2. Acquire a working knowledge of the criteria used for staging the estrous cycle of the mare.
3. Acquire a working understanding of seasonal control of reproductive function of the mare.

STUDY QUESTIONS

1. List the length of the estrous cycle, estrus, and diestrus in the mare.
2. Explain the endocrine events that occur during estrus, ovulation, formation of the corpus luteum, and luteolysis in the mare.
3. Explain why determination of the presence of a large follicle on an ovary is a poor predictor of estrus in the mare.
4. List the criteria that are useful in staging the estrous cycle by palpation per rectum in the mare.
5. Describe the effects of long and short photoperiods on control of reproductive function of the mare.
6. Describe seasonal effects on the incidence of ovulation in mare populations in the Northern Hemisphere.
7. Discuss effects of season on duration of estrus, including the first postpartum estrus (foal heat) in the mare.

THE ESTROUS CYCLE

The mare is a **seasonal polyestrous** animal; during the breeding season, the nonpregnant mare will have recurring estrous cycles. The estrous cycle is defined as the period from one ovulation to a subsequent ovulation, with each ovulation being accompanied by signs of estrus and plasma progesterone concentrations less than 1 ng/ml. The estrous cycle is divided into the ovulation process and an interovulatory period. The estrous cycle may also be considered to consist of a **follicular phase** (**estrus**—in which the mare is sexually receptive to the stallion and the genital tract is prepared to accept and transport sperm to the oviducts for fertilization) that involves the ovulation process, and a **luteal phase** (**diestrus**—in which the mare is not receptive to the stallion and the genital tract is prepared to accept and nurture the conceptus). The diestrus period ends with regression of the corpus luteum and initiation of the next follicular phase. The average length of the estrous cycle in the mare population during the physiologic breeding season is 21 to 22 days (ranging from approximately 18 to 24 days) with estrus comprising 4 to 7 of these days (Figure 2-1). The length of diestrus remains relatively constant at 14 to 15 days and is less affected by season than is the length of estrus. The length of estrus is more variable (ranging from 2 to 12 days or more), typically being of longer duration early in the breeding season, perhaps because of a less prominent luteinizing hormone surge during this period. The diameter of the largest follicle at the time of luteolysis affects the interval from onset of estrus to ovulation: larger follicles present at corpus luteum regression typically ovulate sooner, thus shortening the associated estrus period.

The regular pattern of the estrous cycle relies on the delicate balance among hormones produced by the pineal gland, hypothalamus, pituitary gland, ovaries, and endometrium (Figures 2-2 and 2-3). The neurosecretory cells in the hypothalamus produce **gonadotropin-releasing hormone (GnRH)**. Axons of these cells project into the perivascular space in the median eminence at the origin of the pituitary stalk and episodically release GnRH into the hypothalamic-hypophyseal (hypothalamic-pituitary) portal system, which transports the hormone to the anterior pituitary. GnRH stimulates the synthesis and release of the gonadotropins **follicle-stimulating hormone (FSH)** and **luteinizing hormone (LH)** from the anterior pituitary gland. These hormones enter the systemic circulation and, at the level of the ovaries, FSH is responsible for follicular recruitment, whereas LH is responsible for follicular maturation and production of estrogen, ovulation, and luteinization of the corpus luteum. The estrogen produced by maturing follicles has a positive feedback effect

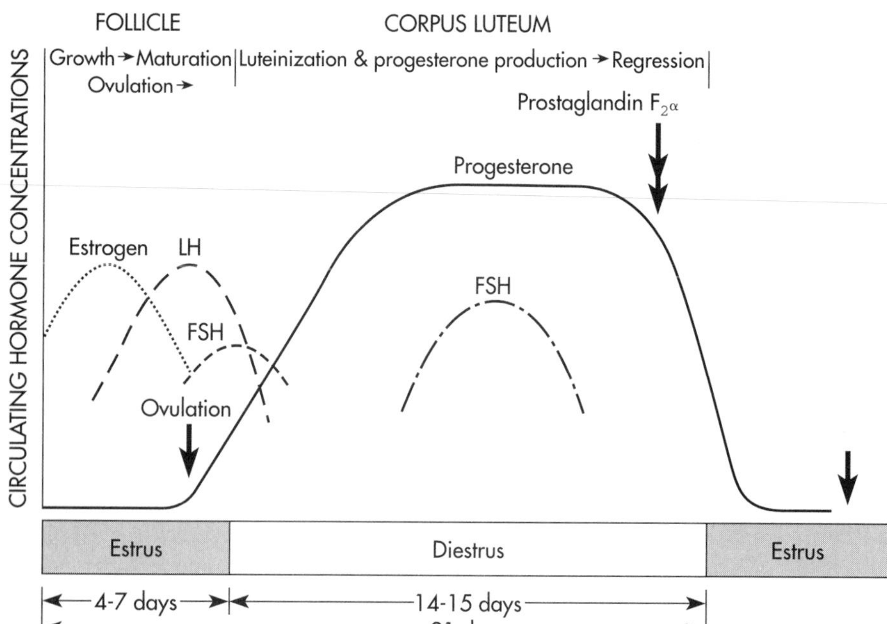

FIGURE 2-1. The estrous cycle of the mare averages 21 to 22 days with 4 to 7 days of estrus (sexual receptivity) and 14 to 15 days of diestrus (in which the mare is not sexually receptive to the stallion). Ovulation generally occurs 1 to 2 days before the end of estrus. (Modified from Irvine CHG: Endocrinology of the estrous cycle of the mare: applications to embryo transfer, *Theriogenology* 15:85, 1981; and Neely DP, Liu IKM, Hillman RB: *Equine reproduction*, Nutley, NJ, 1983, Veterinary Learning Systems.)

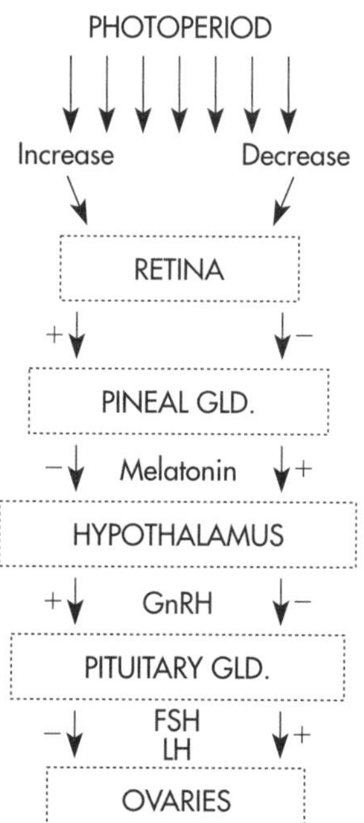

FIGURE 2-2. A simplified version of hormonal regulation of the estrous cycle of the mare. The regular pattern of the estrous cycle of the mare is controlled by the interplay between the pineal gland, hypothalamus, pituitary gland, ovaries, and endometrium. The role of the endometrium is depicted in Figure 2-3.

on LH release (i.e., it promotes further LH release) in the presence of a low concentration of circulating progesterone. **Inhibin** and estrogen produced by growing follicles have a negative feedback effect on release of FSH (i.e., they inhibit FSH release). Progesterone produced by the corpus luteum has a negative feedback effect on release of LH.

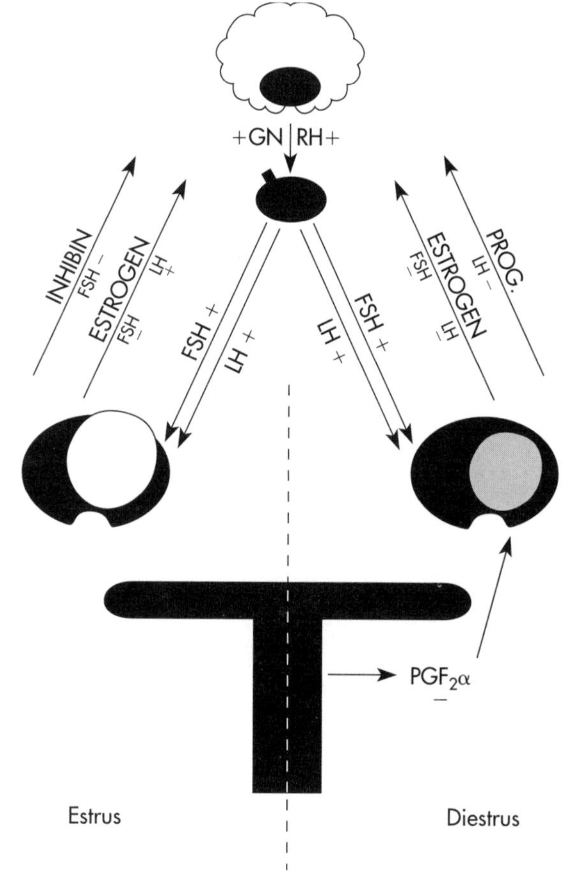

FIGURE 2-3. Schematic depiction of hormonal control of ovarian activity in the mare.

The follicular phase of the estrous cycle is characterized by follicular growth with **estrogen** production, resulting in behavioral estrus (Figure 2-4). Many follicles start the maturation process, but usually only one follicle becomes dominant and ovulates. Follicular development typically occurs in one or two major waves during the estrous cycle. The term *follicular wave* has been used to describe the initially synchronous growth of a group of follicles until one, or perhaps two, follicles begin preferential growth (i.e., become *dominant*) to the remaining follicles. The selected follicle(s) continues to grow (>30 mm diameter) until it either ovulates or regresses. For mares with one follicular wave during the estrous cycle, the wave emerges at mid-cycle (approximately day 10 postovulation). This *primary follicular* wave results in an ultrasonographically identifiable dominant follicle approximately 7 days before ovulation. For mares with two follicular waves during the estrous cycle, the dominant follicle selected during the first follicular wave (i.e., termed a *secondary follicular wave*) that begins during late estrus or early diestrus will sometimes ovulate (*diestrus ovulation*). Secondary follicular waves and diestrus ovulations are currently thought to occur more often in Thoroughbreds than in Quarter Horses and ponies and may contribute (when ovulation occurs) to prolonged diestrus intervals.

At the onset of luteolysis, the largest follicle is typically the one to enlarge and ovulate. Ovulation is a rapid process; the majority of the follicular fluid is released within 2 minutes and complete evacuation typically requires 2 to 7 minutes. The remainder of the follicles, which have already become atretic, eventually regress. Follicular diameter at ovulation normally ranges from 30 to 70 mm (seldom <35 mm) and usually is approximately 40 to 45 mm, although smaller or larger follicles sometimes ovulate. Ovulatory follicles are often larger early in the breeding season (March to May) compared with those that ovulate in the peak of the season (June and July). The majority of mares ovulate within 48 hours of the end of estrus; occasionally mares ovulate after the end of estrus (usually on the day when the intensity of estrus signs is decreasing). The average incidence of double ovulations is 16%, with Thoroughbred, Warmblood, and draft mares having the highest incidence of double ovulations, and Quarter Horse, Appaloosa, and pony mares having the lowest incidence.

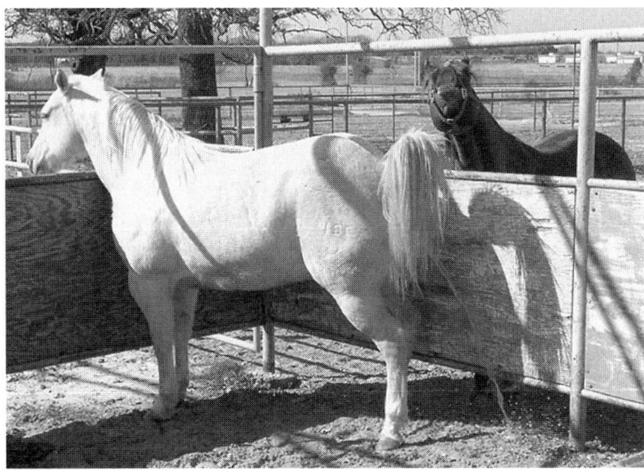

FIGURE 2-4. Mare showing typical signs of estrus: squatting with tail raised, urinating, and everting clitoris.

The luteal phase is initiated at ovulation by the formation of a **progesterone**-secreting corpus luteum, causing the mare to cease showing signs of behavioral estrus (Figure 2-5). Maximum circulating progesterone concentrations are reached by 6 days postovulation. A mare will rarely show behavioral signs of estrus when plasma progesterone concentrations exceed 1 to 2 ng/ml, even when large follicles are present on the ovaries. The life span of the corpus luteum depends on the endogenous release of **prostaglandin $F_{2\alpha}$ ($PGF_{2\alpha}$)** from the endometrium in bursts between days 13 and 16 postovulation. The $PGF_{2\alpha}$ is absorbed into the uterine venous drainage, enters the circulation, and reaches the ovaries by a systemic route. Rapid luteolysis is caused by the $PGF_{2\alpha}$, resulting in a decline in circulating progesterone concentration (a detectable decline occurs within 4 hours, with concentrations less than 1 ng/ml occurring within 40 hours of the initial $PGF_{2\alpha}$ release), which, in turn, releases the block to LH secretion. Follicular maturation and behavioral signs characteristic of the follicular phase of the estrous cycle then ensue. Deviations (of several days) in the length of the luteal phase are usually due to uterine disorders. Secretion of $PGF_{2\alpha}$ due to acute endometritis shortens diestrus. Persistent luteal function (prolonged diestrus) is caused by failure of the luteolytic mechanism, perhaps resulting from failure of the endometrium to release sufficient amounts of $PGF_{2\alpha}$ in late diestrus.

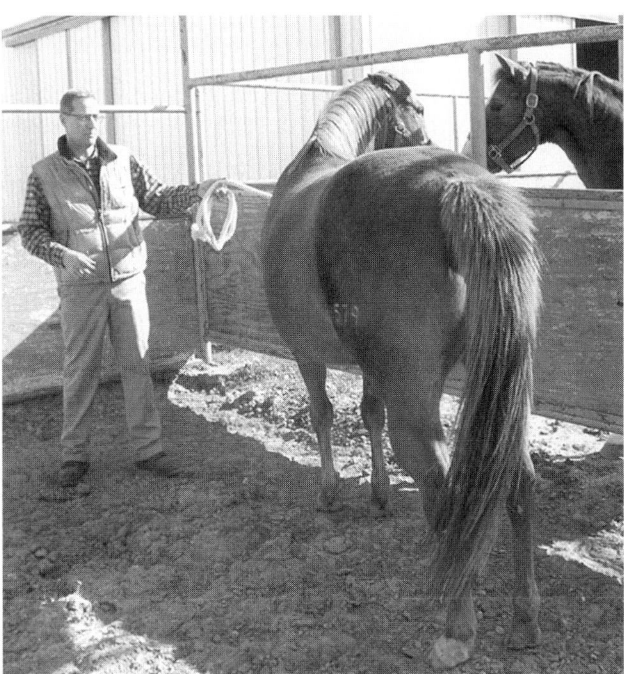

FIGURE 2-5. Mare showing typical signs of nonestrus: ears laid back, "switching" tail, and attempting to avoid the stallion.

STAGING THE ESTROUS CYCLE BY EXAMINATION

Determination of the stage of the estrous cycle can be made by examination of the reproductive tract. Criteria for determining the stage of the cycle include the size and softness of ovarian follicle(s) and relaxation of the uterus and cervix determined by palpation per rectum. With the exception of determining whether ovulation has occurred recently (i.e., typically within 0 to 2 days), palpation for the presence of a corpus luteum is not possible in the mare (e.g., the follicle ovulates into the ovulation fossa, and the corpus luteum does not protrude from the surface of the ovary). Transrectal ultrasonography is also used for staging the estrous cycle, because the size and character of the follicles can be determined, corpora lutea can be visualized, and the degree of edema present in the uterus can be measured. The state of the cervix—closed and dry or relaxed, edematous, and moist with cervical mucus—can be determined by palpation per rectum or per vagina and visualization per vagina. Finally, accurate teasing information, including the dates on which signs of estrus or nonestrus were determined when the mare was presented to the stallion, is very helpful in staging the cycle (Figures 2-4 through 2-8).

Large follicles can be present during any stage of the estrous cycle; thus *determination of follicular size, by itself, is not a reliable indicator of estrus or diestrus*. When a mare shows signs of estrus during teasing with a stallion, one or more large follicles are present on an ovary, and the uterus and cervix are soft and relaxed (edematous endometrial folds may also be seen on ultrasound examination), a determination of estrus can be made. The same criteria are used to predict time of ovulation for breeding of a mare in estrus. If the mare does not show positive behavioral signs of estrus when teased by a stallion, a corpus luteum is visualized on an ovary by ultrasound examination, the uterus is firm ("toned up") on palpation and exhibits uniform echodensity without edema being visualized in endometrial folds on ultrasound examination, and the cervix is narrow and tightly closed, diestrus can be identified. A summary of criteria used to stage the estrous cycle in the mare is shown in Table 2-1.

SEASONALITY

Seasonal variation in the duration of daylight has a profound influence on mare reproductive performance. The horse is a seasonal breeder, and this pattern is regulated by daylight or **photoperiod**. The reproductive system of the horse responds positively (by improved reproductive efficiency) to increasing amounts of daylight and negatively (by reduced reproductive efficiency) to decreasing amounts of daylight. Length of the photoperiod modulates reproductive activity through regulation of GnRH secretion. Although the efficacy of modulation of pineal activity on seasonality in the mare remains speculative, the **pineal gland** is thought to signal the hypothalamus through secretion of **melatonin**. Kentucky workers have shown that in most, but not all, mares melatonin secretion is increased during nighttime hours. When day length is short, melatonin released by the pineal gland is thought to suppress GnRH synthesis and release. When day length is long, melatonin secretion is reduced and the inhibitory influence on GnRH synthesis and secretion is removed (see Figure 2-2). These concepts are supported by studies from Florida on pinealectomy of equids. Additionally, French workers have shown that melatonin administration during the winter months can

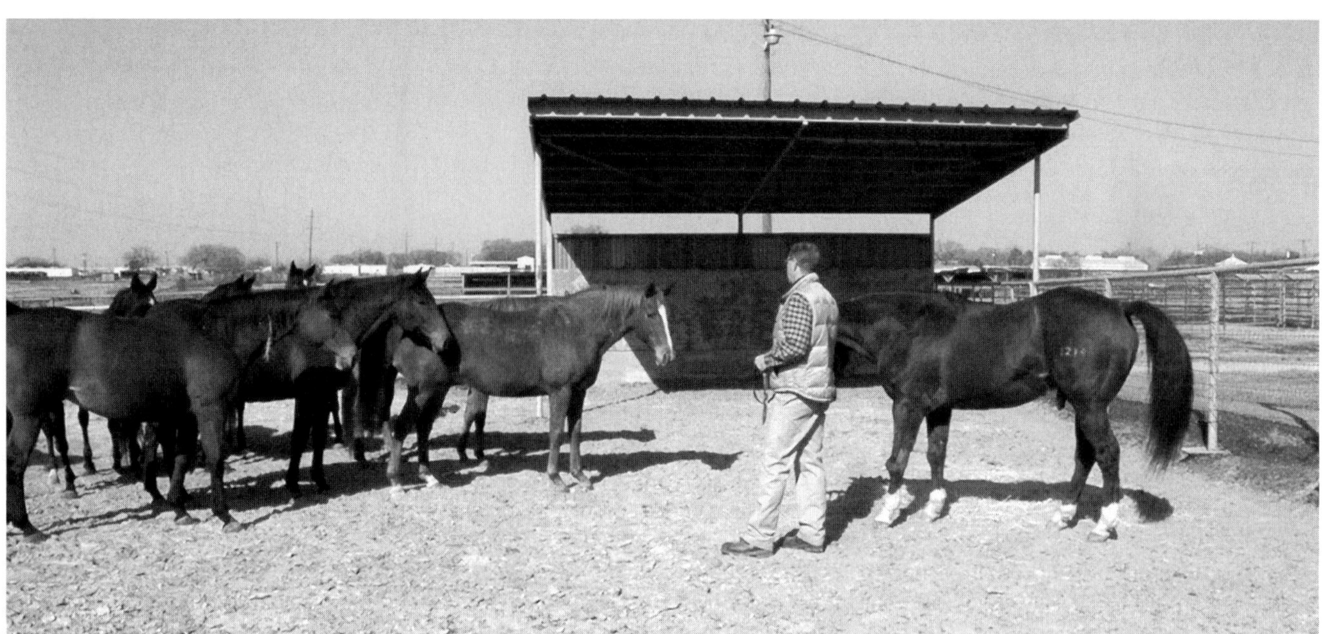

FIGURE 2-6. Method for teasing mares in a paddock with the stallion restrained on a lead.

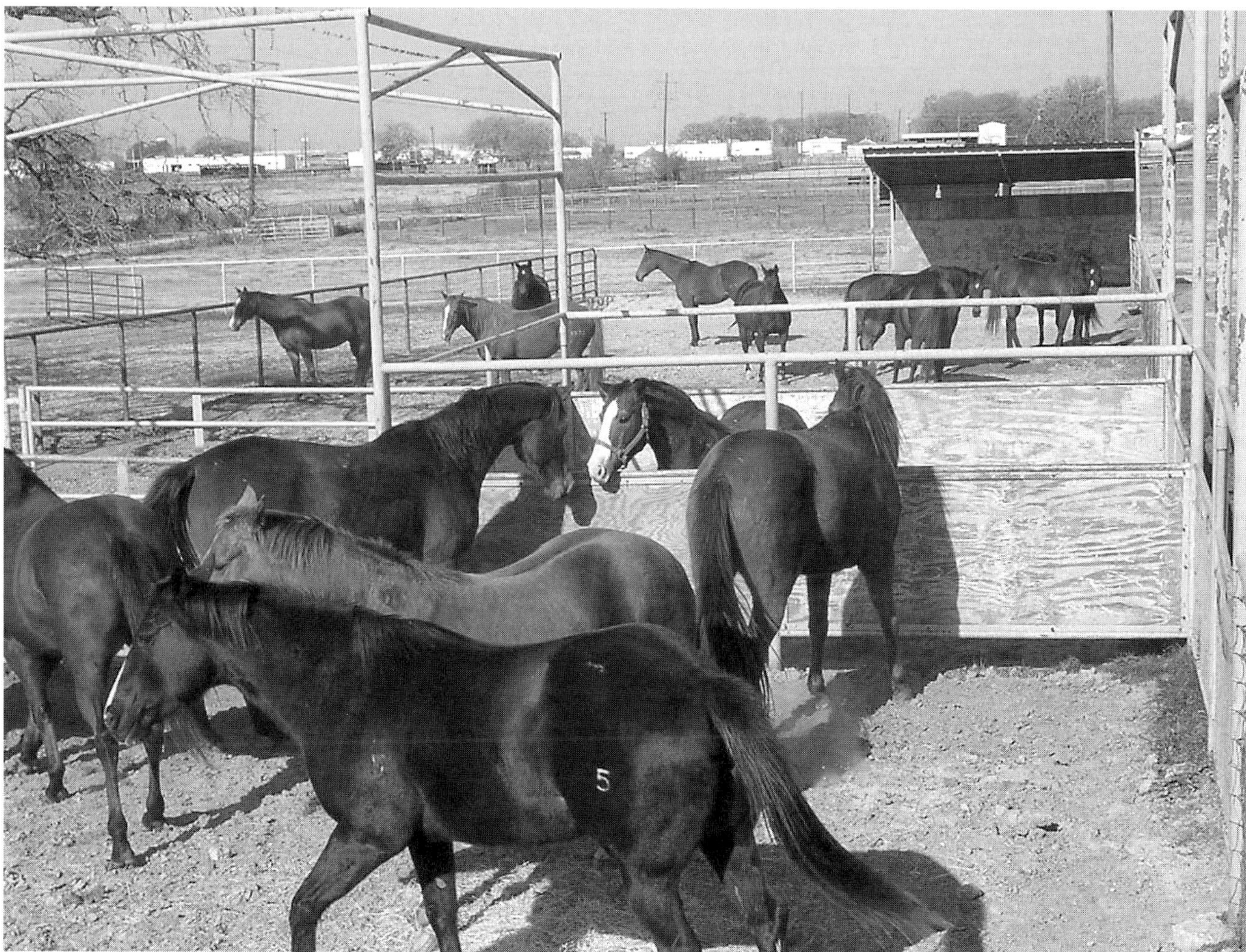

FIGURE 2-7. Method for teasing mares with the stallion in a box, allowing unrestrained mares in adjoining paddocks to approach the stallion at will.

block the stimulatory effect of artificially increased photoperiod and thus delay the onset of the breeding season. However, Kentucky workers found that the presence or absence of nighttime increases in melatonin concentrations did not predict whether mares would continue to have regular estrous cycles in winter and suggested that melatonin secretion during this time plays a limited role in controlling the onset of winter anestrus.

Opioids may participate in regulation of seasonal reproduction by modulating LH secretion during winter anestrus. Endogenous opioids are known to suppress gonadotropin secretion in farm animals, presumably by dampening the **GnRH pulse generator** (synchronous activation of GnRH neurons). New Zealand workers demonstrated that "opioid tone" was higher in mares during deep winter anestrus than during the breeding season, but the use of opioid antagonists in mares has failed to alter seasonality. Research on the role of endogenous opioids in reproductive seasonality in mares is continuing.

Whereas transition between seasons is a gradual, progressive process, the reproductive year for the mare population can be divided for descriptive purposes into four seasons that correspond with changes in day length. Pennsylvania workers have summarized these seasons as follows. The period of peak fertility (i.e., the physiologic breeding season or period of **ovulatory receptivity**) surrounds the longest day of the year or summer solstice (June 21). The mare then moves into a transitional period of **anovulatory receptivity** that coincides with the autumnal equinox (September 21) when day and night are of equal length. During this period, the mare exhibits erratic estrus behavior without corresponding ovulation. If ovulation does occur, corpus luteum function is not maintained. Mares then enter a state of **anestrus** or sexual quiescence that centers around and after the shortest day of the year or winter solstice (December 21). After this period, the mare enters another transitional period of **anovulatory receptivity** that corresponds with the vernal equinox (March 21). This period is characterized by a long and erratic heat period that

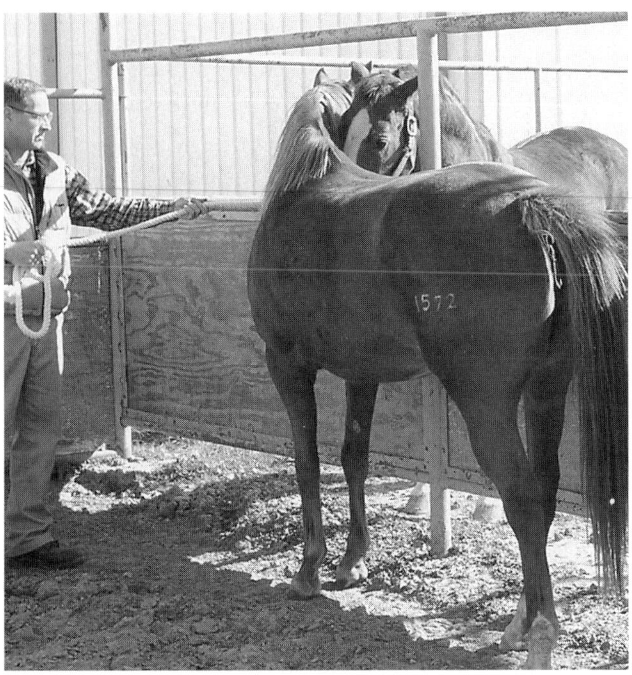

FIGURE 2-8. Method for teasing mares with the stallion unrestrained in a box and the mare on a lead taken to the stallion.

finally culminates in an ovulation, thus initiating the period of ovulatory receptivity. This cyclic pattern is a trend, and all mares are not included because a small percentage (approximately 15% to 20%) will have cycles regularly throughout the year. Even mare populations near the equator tend to show a seasonal pattern of reproductive cyclicity. Interestingly, Kentucky workers have recently demonstrated that, within a mare, the seasonal pattern of reproductive activity can vary considerably from year to year.

Reproductive seasonality effectively results in foals being delivered in the spring, when environmental conditions are favorable for foal survival. The role of seasonality on several aspects of reproductive performance helps exemplify this point. For instance, the initiation of estrus is under the direct influence of day length. As day length increases, the length of estrus decreases and the incidence of ovulation increases, both of which result in more conceptions for less work. The shortest heat periods and highest ovulation rates occur in June, thereby producing May foals. Furthermore, there are poorly understood factors that encourage a pregnant mare to foal during the physiologic breeding season. Mares with foals born near the first of the year tend to have a longer gestation length than mares with foals born late in the season. Another factor that favors May and June breeding occurs in mares that undergo **"foal heat" (first postpartum estrus)** near the first of the year because they tend to ovulate at a longer interval from parturition than those mares that enter foal heat later in the year. All these phenomena suggest that an inherent mechanism is present that pushes breeding and foaling toward the physiologic breeding season (May through July).

OPERATIONAL BREEDING SEASON

Horses have been described as inefficient breeders compared with other domestic species. This, however, is a fallacy and stems from humans' attempts to redesign the breeding season of the horse to meet their own needs. The operational breeding

TABLE 2-1

Criteria Used to Stage the Estrous Cycle of the Mare

Criteria	Estrus	Diestrus
Teasing with stallion	1. Tail raise 2. Squat, tip pelvis 3. Urinate 4. Evert clitoris	1. Switch tail 2. Kick, squeal 3. Attempt to bite stallion 4. Move away from stallion
Examination of ovaries	1. Large follicle(s) that may be soft 2. Follicle may be triangular with scalloped edges on ultrasound examination if mare is nearing ovulation 3. No corpus luteum on ultrasound examination	1. Presence of corpus luteum on ultrasound examination 2. Follicles of varying sizes, may be large
Examination of uterus	1. Relaxed with soft texture 2. Edematous endometrial folds visible on ultrasound examination	1. Firm texture ("good tone") 2. Uniform echogenicity on ultrasound examination
Examination of cervix	1. Shortening, widening 2. Relaxed with soft texture 3. Pink and drooping on vaginal floor when visualized through speculum 4. Lumen open 1-3+ fingers on digital examination per vagina	1. Long and narrow with firm texture 2. Pale, dry, and centrally located in cranial vagina when visualized through speculum 3. Closed lumen on digital examination per vagina

season for horses with a universal birthday of January 1 is often precariously assigned as the period from February 15 to the first week of July. This modified breeding season overlaps into the period of anovulatory receptivity, which is characterized by prolonged heats and delayed ovulation, thus indicating that the mares have not yet obtained their optimum reproductive potential. Breeding inefficiency in horses develops when they are bred out of the physiologic breeding season. Otherwise, intrinsic fertility is quite acceptable in the horse.

BIBLIOGRAPHY

Daels PF, Hughes JP: The normal estrous cycle. In McKinnon AO, Voss JL, editors: *Equine reproduction*, pp 121-132. Philadelphia, 1993, Lea and Febiger.

Daels PF, Fatone S, Hansen BS, et al: Dopamine antagonist-induced reproductive function in anoestrous mares: gonadotropin secretion and effect of environmental cues. In Proceedings of the 7th International Symposium on Equine Reproduction, University of Pretoria, South Africa, 1998, pp 45-46.

Fitzgerald BP, Schmidt MJ: Absence of an association between melatonin and reproductive activity in mares during the nonbreeding season, *Biol Reprod Monogr* 1:425-434, 1995.

Ginther OJ: *Reproductive biology of the mare. Basic and applied aspects*, ed 2, pp 41-74, 105-290. Cross Plains, WI, 1992, Equiservices.

Greenhoff GR, Kenney RM: Evaluation of reproductive status of nonpregnant mares. *J Am Vet Med Assoc* 167:449-458, 1975.

Grubaugh W, Sharp DC, Berglund LA, et al: Effects of pinealectomy in pony mares. *J Reprod Fertil* 32(Suppl):293-295, 1982.

Guillaume D, Arnaud G, Camillo F, et al: Effect of melatonin implants on reproductive status of mares. *Biol Reprod Monogr* 1:435-442, 1995.

Nishikawa Y, Hafez ESE: Horses. In Hafez ESE, editor, *Reproduction in farm animals*, pp 288-300. Philadelphia, 1975, Lea and Febiger.

Turner JE, Irvine CHG, Alexander S: Regulation of seasonal breeding by endogenous opioids in mares. *Biol Reprod Monogr* 1:443-448, 1995.

3

Manipulation of Estrus in the Mare

OBJECTIVES

While studying the information covered in this chapter, the student should attempt to:

1. Understand potential advantages of manipulating estrus in broodmares.
2. Acquire a working understanding of the principles by which manipulation of the photoperiod advances the onset of the breeding season in mares.
3. Acquire a working knowledge of the rationale for and efficacy of hormone administration for hastening the onset of the breeding season in mares.
4. Acquire a working knowledge of the use of various hormones for manipulating estrus, including the first postpartum estrus, in the cycling mare.

STUDY QUESTIONS

1. Describe the physiologic changes that occur during transition from seasonal anestrus through onset of the breeding season in mares in the Northern Hemisphere.
2. Define the following terms:
   a. seasonal (winter) anestrus
   b. transitional estrus
   c. ovulatory estrus
   d. artificial photoperiod
3. List guidelines to be followed when designing an artificial lighting program for broodmares in the Northern Hemisphere.
4. Discuss the rationale for using progestogens/progesterone to hasten the onset of ovulatory estrus in mares.
5. Outline a program (and include expected responses) for treating mares with altrenogest to:
   a. hasten the onset of ovulatory estrus early in the breeding season.
   b. synchronize estrus in cycling mares.
6. Outline a program (and include expected responses) for treating mares with progesterone and estradiol-17β plus prostaglandin $F_{2\alpha}$ to synchronize estrus and ovulation in cycling mares.
7. Outline a program (and include expected responses) for use of human chorionic gonadotropin or deslorelin (Ovuplant) to induce ovulation in mares:
   a. in late transitional estrus.
   b. having regular estrous cycles but that are to be bred at a precise time.
8. Outline a program (and include expected responses) for use of prostaglandin $F_{2\alpha}$ to:
   a. induce estrus in a mare with a functional corpus luteum.
   b. synchronize estrus in a group of cycling mares.
   c. induce earlier estrus in mares after their foal-heat ovulation.
9. Explain the rationale for the use of hormones to improve fertility in the early postpartum period.

INTRODUCTION

Registry-derived time constraints, in conjunction with a seasonal breeding pattern, result in the use of a narrowly confined breeding season for production of the majority of equine offspring. Early in the operational breeding season (February 15 through the first week in July), the veterinarian is often called on to assist in breeding mares to facilitate birth of foals as soon after January 1 as possible. Additionally, to maximally use genetically superior, popular stallions, veterinary management schemes have been developed to limit the number of services per estrus to the minimum necessary to establish pregnancy. The ascribed goal is one pregnancy per service per mare. To accomplish these ends, artificial lighting programs and hormone administration are used to (1) hasten the onset of the breeding season, (2) induce ovulation in cycling mares being bred, (3) synchronize estrus and ovulation in individual mares or groups of mares, and (4) increase the opportunity for establishment of pregnancy in foaling mares bred early in the postpartum period. The student is encouraged to refer to Table 3-1 for a summary of hormones commonly used in broodmare practice while studying the information in this chapter. This table also lists hormones used for purposes other than manipulation of estrus (e.g., induced abortion and induced parturition), which are discussed in later chapters.

TABLE 3-1

Hormones Commonly used in Broodmare Practice in the United States

Compound	Actions	Indications	Product	Source	Dosage	Comments
GnRH (gonadotropin-releasing hormone)	Release of FSH and LH from anterior pituitary gland	Stimulation of follicular growth Ovulation induction (?)	Cystorelin (synthesized native GnRH) Native GnRH	Ceva Veterinary pharmaceutical compounding companies	Suggested dosages of 500 μg twice daily or 250 μg 4 times daily; IM or SC	Not licensed for use in the horse. Long-term exogenous GnRH stimulates follicular growth in seasonally anestrous mares but may not be cost effective. Mares treated late in the transition period (larger follicles) are more likely to respond with follicular growth, ovulation, and formation of a normal corpus luteum and in less time than mares with static ovaries (winter anestrus) or in early transitional estrus (smaller follicules).
Deslorelin (GnRH analog)	Same, longer action, more potent	Ovulation induction	Deslorelin implant (Ovuplant)	Fort Dodge	Sustained release SC implant containing 2.1 mg of deslorelin acetate	Administer 1 implant once mare in estrus has a follicle ≥ 30 mm in diameter; >80% of mares ovulate within 48 hr. Extended interovulatory intervals occur in some mares that fail to become pregnant due to gonadotroph down-regulation. Removal of implant on day of ovulation will prevent this problem.
Oxytocin	Myometrial contractions	Parturition induction	Oxytocin	Several sources	40-100 IU IM (bolus injection or slow IV drip) or 15 IU IV or IM q 15 min until second stage of parturition	Can cause premature placental separation. Do not use in dystocia until fetal position is correct.
		Uterine evacuation (can be done in conjunction with uterine lavage)			20 IU IV or 20-40 IU IM	Ensure that cervix is patent before use.
		Expulsion of retained placenta			20 IU IV or IM, can repeat at 4- to 6-hr intervals as needed	May cause abdominal cramps or, rarely, uterine prolapse.
		Acceleration of uterine involution after dystocia			20 IU IM at 4- to 6-hr intervals	May cause abdominal cramps or, rarely, uterine prolapse. Will not accelerate uterine involution in normal foaling mares.
	Contraction of myoepithelial cells in mammary gland	Milk let-down			20 IU IV or IM	Generally unsuccessful in mares that are extremely nervous or have agalactia.

TABLE 3-1

(continued)

Compound	Actions	Indications	Product	Source	Dosage	Comments
Estrogens	Expression of estrus Maturation of reproductive tract and mammary glands Increased uterine circulation Uterine contraction	Expression of estrus in "jump" mare (for semen collection)	Estradiol cypionate (ECP)	Upjohn	1 mg IM	Only effective in the absence of progesterone. Investigational use during estrous cycle at breeding is lacking. Not approved for use in the horse.
	Cervical relaxation Resistance to uterine infection	Treatment of infectious endometritis (?)	Estradiol-17β	Chemical compounding companies *(no commercial preparations currently approved for use)*	10 mg/day IM for 1-3 days	Usefulness is questionable.
	Suppression of follicular growth to improve synchrony of ovarian response	Synchronization of ovulation	Estradiol-17β	Chemical compounding companies	10 mg/day IM for 10 days	Use in conjunction with progesterone in oil (150 mg/day for 10 days) and prostaglandin (on day 10 only).
		Postponement of "foal heat"	Estradiol-17β	Chemical compounding companies	10 mg/day IM for 1-5 days	Use in conjunction with progesterone in oil (150 mg/day).
Progestogens	Inhibition of LH release Suppression of estrus Reduce myometrial excitability Increase uterine tone	Shorten duration of transitional season	Progesterone in oil	Pharma-ceutical compounding companies	150 mg/day IM for 10-15 days	Can use in conjunction with estradiol-17β (10 mg/day IM for 10-15 days) and prostaglandin (on last day of treatment). Effective only in mares during late transitional phase; new research suggests this may not be effective.
			Altrenogest (Regu-Mate)	Hoechst	0.044 mg/kg/day orally for 10-15 days	Effective only in mares during late transitional phase; new research suggests this may not be effective.

TABLE 3-1

(continued)

Compound	Actions	Indications	Product	Source	Dosage	Comments
Progestogens *(continued)*	Endometrial gland growth	Suppression of estrus	Progesterone in oil		150 mg/day IM	May take 2-3 days for mare to go out of behavioral estrus.
	Cervical closure		Altrenogest (Regu-Mate)		0.044 mg/kg/ day orally	Does not appear to affect subsequent fertility when given for 30-60 consecutive days.
	Mammary gland development	Synchronization of ovulation	Progesterone in oil		150 mg/day IM for 10 days	Use in conjunction with estradiol-17β (10 mg/day) and prostaglandins (on day 10 only) for best results.
			Altrenogest (Regu-Mate)		0.044 mg/kg/ day orally for 10-15 days	
		Maintenance of pregnancy in ovariectomized recipient mare for embryo transfer	Progesterone in oil		300 mg/day IM	Begin injections 5 days before embryo transfer and continue for first 100-120 days of pregnancy.
		Pregnancy maintenance in habitually aborting intact mares; use questionable	Progesterone in oil Altrenogest (Regu-Mate)		150-300 mg/ day IM 0.044 mg/day orally	Efficacy is controversial. Should be given until at least day 100-120 of pregnancy, regardless of whether giving altrenogest or progesterone in oil; may be some risk of fetal mummification if fetus dies and is not expelled. For habitually late aborting mares or mares suspected to have impending abortion, should be given until just before expected parturition.
hCG (human chorionic gonadotropin)	Support of corpus luteum of pregnancy in women; has LH activity in the horse	Ovulation induction	hCG	Several sources	1500-3500 IU given IM or IV	Administer hCG once a ≥ 35-mm follicle is detected on the ovary during estrus. Ovulation usually occurs within 36-48 hr after hCG injection.
		Hasten ovulation in transitional mare	hCG	Several sources	1500-3500 IU given IM or IV	Administer hCG after a 40-mm follicle is detected. Not approved for IV use in the horse, but IV use may result in less antibody formation than IM use.
Prostaglandins ($PGF_{2\alpha}$)	Regression of corpus luteum Myometrial contractility	Shorten interovulatory period ("short-cycle" or induce estrus in cycling mares)	Dinoprost tromethamine (Lutalyse)	Upjohn	10 mg IM/ 1000 lb	Usually not effective if given before 5-6 days after ovulation is detected.
	Influence on numerous body functions		Cloprostenol (Estrumate)	Miles	250 µg IM/ 1000 lb	Not approved for use in the horses in the United States.
		Synchronization of estrus	Same as above	Same as above	Same as above	Give two injections, 14 days apart.

TABLE 3-1

(continued)

Compound	Actions	Indications	Product	Source	Dosage	Comments
Prostaglandins ($PGF_{2\alpha}$) *(continued)*						Effective only in mares with normal estrous cycles.
		Treatment of persistent luteal function	Same as above	Same as above	Same as above	Synthetics and "natural" prostaglandin (dinoprost) are equally effective in causing CL regression, but synthetic agents have the advantage of fewer side effects, such as sweating and abnormal cramping, although these are sometimes seen with cloprostenol.
		Shorten interval to second postpartum estrus	Same as above	Same as above	Same as above	Give prostaglandin 6-7 days after "foal heat" ovulation.
		Induction of abortion	Same as above	Same as above	Same as above	*Single injection* of prostaglandin is sufficient if given *by day 35 of pregnancy.* *Multiple injections* of prosta-glandin are required after supplementary corpora lutea are formed (*beyond days 36-40 of pregnancy*). Prostaglandins may be ineffective beyond 4 months of gestation.
		Acceleration of uterine involution	Sames as above	Same as above	1 dose twice daily for first 5-10 days after foaling	Usefulness is questionable in normal foaling mares.
		Induction of parturition	Cloprostenol (Estrumate)	Same as above	250 μg IM twice at 2-hr interval	Studies (limited) suggest that various prostaglandin analogs (not dinoprost) can be safely used to induce parturition; however, oxytocin remains the drug of choice.
Ergonovine	Smooth muscle contractions; also aids contraction of smooth muscle in vascular walls to control hemorrhage	Control of postpartum hemorrhage	Ergonovine maleate or methyler-gonovine maleate	Several sources	1-3 mg IM/ 1000 lb	Produces strong uterine contractions within 10-20 min after injection. Contractions may continue for up to 2-4 hr. Contractions are continuous rather than rhythmic, oxytocin-like contractions. Also aids in controlling certain types of uterine hemorrhage (i.e., uterine rupture; endometrial lacerations); ecbolics should not be used if uterine artery rupture is suspected.
		Hasten uterine involution	Same as above	Same as above	Same as above	Usefulness is unproven.

TABLE 3-1

(continued)

Compound	Actions	Indications	Product	Source	Dosage	Comments
Bromocryptine	Inhibits prolactin secretion	Spurious lactation in nongravid mares	Bromocryptine mesylate	Several sources	30-60 mg orally/1000 lb once daily for 3-7 days	Human product; not licensed for use in the horse.
Domperidone	Dopamine D-2 receptor antagonist Increases prolactin secretion	Agalactia	Domperiodone paste (Equidone)	Equitox, Center for Applied Technology	1.1 mg/kg orally once daily	Maintains elevated prolactin concentration for 7-9 hr. Increases prolactin to supraphysiologic levels within 7 days. Should be given daily to postpartum agalactic/hypogalactic mares until mare comes to full milk production. Foal may need additional nutritional supplementation. Can be started 10-15 days before expected foaling in mares grazing endophyte-infested fescue pastures to decrease parturient problems and agalactia.
		Anestrus	As above	As above	As above	Has been proposed as a treatment for anestrus to stimulate ovarian follicular activity and advance the first ovulation of the year. Dopamine is thought to inhibit gonadotrophin production; therefore, use of a dopamine antagonist is the rationale for its use. Because 2-4 weeks may be required to increase LH levels, begin treatment in late December or early January. Contradictory results were obtained in various studies.
Sulpiride	Dopamine D-2 receptor antagonist	Anestrus	No commercial preparation	Veterinary pharmacentical compounding companies	100-200 mg/454 kg body wt, once daily	Rationale is as proposed for domperidone, but sulpiride has been studied less.

PHYSIOLOGIC CHANGES DURING TRANSITION FROM SEASONAL ANESTRUS THROUGH ONSET OF THE BREEDING SEASON

The majority of mares in the Northern Hemisphere (approximately 85%) enter a period of reproductive quiescence ("winter or seasonal anestrus") during the late fall and winter (the period of shortened day length). During the period of seasonal anestrus, the hypothalamic-pituitary-ovarian axis is relatively inactive, with gonadotropin-releasing hormone (GnRH) content of the hypothalamus, luteinizing hormone (LH) content of the pituitary, and circulating concentrations of gonadotropins (LH and follicle-stimulating hormone [FSH]) and ovarian steroids (progesterone and estrogen) being decreased. In response to increasing day length, this axis becomes progressively more active, and pituitary stores of gonadotropins gradually increase. GnRH is released more often from the hypothalamus, as evidenced by an increase in LH pulse frequency. In mid to late transition, FSH concentrations are elevated while LH concentrations remain comparatively low, resulting in the growth of several follicles 20 to 35 mm in diameter that do not ovulate. Finally, as ovulation approaches, mean concentrations of LH increase while mean concentrations of FSH decrease. Apparently, once a dominant follicle develops (≥35 mm in diameter and becomes capable of producing significant amounts of estrogen) in concert with an increased pituitary store of LH, LH release is enhanced, causing ovulation to occur.

In general, once a mare ovulates and forms a corpus luteum, regular estrous cycles ensue (e.g., 14- to 16-day periods of diestrus; followed by a variable period of estrus, which may exceed 10 days early in the spring but eventually averages 4 to 7 days in late spring or summer). The physiologic breeding season, when the preponderance of mares are ovulating in concurrence with regular estrous cycles (**ovulatory estrus**), typically occurs during the late spring and summer months in the Northern Hemisphere (reviewed in Ginther, 1992).

As follicular growth and regression begin during the spring transitional period, mares typically show erratic signs of estrous behavior toward the stallion. This "**transitional estrus**" is variable in length and intensity, but frequently is of prolonged duration (i.e., sometimes a month or more in length). Because numerous follicles are growing and regressing during this period, it is difficult to predict when the mare will ovulate and thus determine the precise time the mare should be bred to maximize the opportunity to establish pregnancy. Interestingly, although the timing of this first ovulation is unpredictable, it is fertile. Colorado workers achieved normal pregnancy rates by breeding mares in transitional estrus every other day until their first ovulation of the year, even though some mares were bred more than 10 times during this estrus. Because it is not efficient to use stallions to breed mares during this long transitional estrus, efforts can be focused on (1) hastening the onset of regular estrous cycles by providing an **artificial photoperiod**, (2) shortening the duration of the late transition period by administering progestogen compounds, (3) hastening or ensuring ovulation of a dominant follicle within 48 hours after breeding by the stallion, or (4) waiting to breed the mare until regular estrous cycles occur naturally.

ARTIFICIAL LIGHTING

The physiologic breeding season can be successfully manipulated to fit into the operational breeding season by *artificially increasing the photoperiod.* The minimum length of light exposure required has not been established, but field experience indicates that provision of 14 to 16 hours of light stimulus (artificial plus natural) per day is adequate. A recent French study provided evidence that high light intensities may not require as many days of lighting to induce cyclicity in anestrous mares, and low light intensities may not be as efficacious in stimulating desired responses. Nevertheless, because lighting programs have traditionally been thought to require a minimum of 8 to 10 weeks for response, mares in the Northern Hemisphere are exposed to the lighting system by December 1 to establish normal cyclic activity by February 15. Various methods of light administration have been used successfully, the most common of which are (1) using a light source that is held steady at 14 to 16 hours/day throughout the entire stimulation period, or alternatively, (2) increasing light by small increments (similar to that which occurs naturally), usually by adding 30 minutes of daily light stimulation at weekly intervals until 14 to 16 hours of light exposure are achieved (e.g., 10 hours December 1, 10.5 hours December 8, and so on). After summarizing the results of various lighting programs, Sharp et al. (1993) suggested that the best results would be obtained when the supplemental light is either added to the end of the natural daylight period or split and added to both the beginning and end of the natural daylight period, instead of adding the supplemental light only at the beginning of the natural daylight period. Palmer and coworkers have described a technique for providing a 1-hour pulse of light 18.5 hours after the onset of daylight. This dark-phase light pulse has reportedly resulted in resumption of reproductive cyclicity similar to that produced by the more traditional lighting techniques. The efficacy of this lighting technique should be studied further before being applied to commercial operations.

For individual stall-lighting systems, Kenney et al. (1975) recommended that the mare should be within 7 to 8 feet of a 200-watt incandescent light bulb to provide adequate light exposure, and the stall should have sufficient window space to permit the same exposure during daylight. Minimal light intensities have not been adequately determined. Sharp et al. (1993) recommended a minimum intensity of 10 footcandles at mare eye level. The presence of shadows can prevent achievement of desired results, so care should be taken to eliminate them. Paddock lighting systems are also successful if light exposure is sufficient in all areas of the paddock. Guidelines for ensuring adequate light exposure in paddock lighting programs have been reviewed by Ginther (1992). A practical method for measuring light intensity has been described by Sharp et al. (1993) wherein the ASA reading of a 35-mm single-lens reflex camera is set to 400 and the shutter speed to $\frac{1}{4}$ second. The bottom of a Styrofoam cup is cut off and the cup is fitted over the lens to gather diffused light. If the aperture reading is ≥*f*4, light intensity is ≥10 footcandles.

If artificial lighting systems are used, it is widely believed that pregnant mares should also be exposed to lights. This is because early-foaling mares that are not exposed to lights are thought to be at risk for entering seasonal anestrus. Kentucky workers recently demonstrated that there is no consistency regarding when mares enter anestrus (e.g., an individual mare may enter seasonal anestrus in November of one year and in December or January of the next year, and an individual mare that cycled throughout one year may enter seasonal anestrus the next year), so it may be critical to provide artificial lighting to all mares to be bred on the farm if consistent responses to lighting are to be expected.

SHORTENING THE DURATION OF THE LATE TRANSITION PERIOD BY ADMINISTERING PROGESTOGENS

The rationale for the use of progestogen/progesterone treatment for hastening the onset of ovulatory estrus is the fact that mares in transitional estrus have insufficient storage/release of LH from the pituitary gland to promote maturation and ovulation of a dominant follicle. Progestogen treatment, which generally suppresses LH release during administration, has been hypothesized to provide for storage and subsequent release of sufficient LH to induce follicular maturation and ovulation once progestogen supplementation ceases. Administration of progesterone in oil (150 mg each day intramuscularly [IM]) or altrenogest (0.044 mg/kg each day by mouth) for 10 to 15 days may initiate slightly earlier and more predictable onset of ovulation and regular estrous cycles if it is given to mares in late transitional estrus. Initial experiments with altrenogest (a synthetic progestogen; Regu-Mate) tested the efficacy of treatment of mares in early transitional estrus (<20 mm diameter follicles) compared with treatment of mares in late transitional estrus (>20 mm diameter follicles) and revealed that altrenogest treatment did not induce an ovulatory response in mares in the early transition period. For the best results with altrenogest treatment, current recommendations are that the mare's ovaries be examined by palpation or ultrasound per rectum to ensure that multiple large (≥25 mm diameter) follicles are present before therapy is begun. Mares in early transitional estrus (i.e., smaller follicles only are present) are unlikely to respond. Although progestogen administration is expensive and time consuming, the best results may be achieved by longer (e.g., 2 weeks) durations of treatment, perhaps because of greater storage and subsequent release of LH. The interval to estrus is somewhat variable after cessation of progestogen administration, but averages 4 to 7 days, with ovulation usually occurring 7 to 12 days later.

Estradiol, in combination with progesterone, has also been used to slightly shorten the late transition period. The rationale and guidelines for its use are similar to those stated above for progestogens/progesterone alone. The addition of estradiol to progesterone results in greater suppression of follicular development than that seen with progestogen alone, so follicular size is smaller after cessation of steroid treatment. Therefore the mean interval to onset of estrus and thus ovulation is typically longer than those for progesterone treatment alone. Theoretically, the more uniform inhibition of follicular development associated with combined steroid treatment results in less diversity, and thus less variation, in the dynamics of follicular maturation and ovulation after cessation of treatment, thereby providing greater synchrony in mares ovulating on a given day. The dosage for estradiol/progesterone is 150 mg of progesterone and 10 mg of estradiol-17β IM once daily for 10 days. When an ovulation-inducing drug (human chorionic gonadotropin or deslorelin) is administered to mares after a dominant follicle (≥35 mm diameter) is achieved with this regimen, mares typically ovulate 18 to 23 days after the progesterone/estradiol treatment is begun. As with altrenogest treatment, mares should be in mid to late transition for treatment to be successful in initiating regular estrous cycles. The following results emphasize this point. Twenty 2-year-old anestrus mares in Southwest Texas were treated in early February for 10 days with progesterone plus estradiol but were not exposed to artificial lighting. Initiation of regular estrous cycles was not seen in any mares in this trial. None of the mares had follicles ≥15 mm diameter at the onset of treatment.

Progestogen/progesterone treatment, with or without estradiol, has also been used at the end of artificial lighting programs (about 60 days after initiation of artificial lighting) and appears to have an additive effect on induction of estrous cycles. It is possible that a combination of progesterone and estrogen may promote the onset of seasonal cyclicity more efficiently than progestogen/progesterone alone. No commercial preparation containing both progesterone and estradiol is currently licensed and available for use in mares, but practitioners can obtain the formulation from veterinary pharmaceutical compounding companies.

The reader should be aware that recent research at Colorado State University suggests progestogen/progesterone treatment does not promote pituitary storage of LH; in addition, the research revealed that beneficial effects are simply due to delaying the onset of the first ovulation of the year so that estrus can be synchronized.

HASTENING OVULATION DURING THE LATE TRANSITION PERIOD

Few studies have been performed on the use of **human chorionic gonadotropin (hCG)** to hasten the first ovulation of the breeding season in mares in the late transition period. Multiple injections of hCG (200 U) given late in the transition period resulted in fertile ovulations unaccompanied by LH surges, but mares tended to relapse into seasonal anestrus once ovulation had been induced. In mares with prolonged estrus early in the breeding season, hCG (1500 to 3500 U intravenously [IV] or IM) is routinely given when a preovulatory-sized follicle is present to increase the chance that ovulation will occur at a predictable time (approximately 48 hours after injection). Injection of hCG to mares in the late transition period can also be done any time a large follicle is present; however, administration of hCG in this manner does not ensure that ovulation will occur at a precise time. Many practitioners believe it is important for prominent edematous endometrial folds to be visible on transrectal ultrasonographic examination and for the cervix to be relaxed, in order for hCG administration to result in ovulation at a predictable time in mares in late transitional estrus. Perhaps this indirect evidence of estrogenic influence will prove to be clinically useful for predicting that a competent follicle capable of responding to hCG administration is present.

The integral role of hypothalamic GnRH in controlling recrudescence of ovarian cyclicity in the mare has led to numerous investigations of exogenous administration of native GnRH or its more potent agonists to stimulate follicular development and ovulation. In a review of the use of GnRH regimens used to induce ovulation during the anovulatory season, Ginther (1992) concluded that (1) pulsatile delivery systems may be most effective, (2) the percentage of mares ovulating as a result of treatment will increase as day length increases and diameter of the largest follicle increases, (3) not all mares with small follicles will respond to treatment, (4) some mares that ovulate as a result of treatment will revert to anestrus if they do not become pregnant, and (5) some mares treated when they have only small follicles present may be prone to higher than normal rates of embryonic loss, perhaps because of lower progesterone production from corpora lutea resulting from low LH secretion. In a recent retrospective study in central Kentucky, a 79% ovulation rate with a 53% pregnancy rate per cycle was achieved with ovulation occurring in 13.7 ± 7.4 days after twice daily intramuscular injections of 500 mg of native GnRH were begun in mares in anestrus or transitional estrus. Follicular size in that study was an important determinant of the interval from onset of native GnRH therapy to ovulation (Figure 3-1). The use of additional ovulation-inducing drugs (hCG or deslorelin implants) did not improve ovulatory response.

Attempts to use the GnRH analog deslorelin (Ovuplant) to hasten onset of regular estrous cycles in mares in either deep winter anestrus or early spring transitional estrus have mostly been unsuccessful. Australian researchers demonstrated that when ovarian follicles ≥35 mm diameter are achieved in mares late in the transition period, treatment with deslorelin implants every other day until ovulation results in approximately 80% of mares ovulating within 3 days of the beginning of treatment (requiring two implants). Further study of the use of GnRH analogs is warranted to refine the methodology of treatment during the transition period.

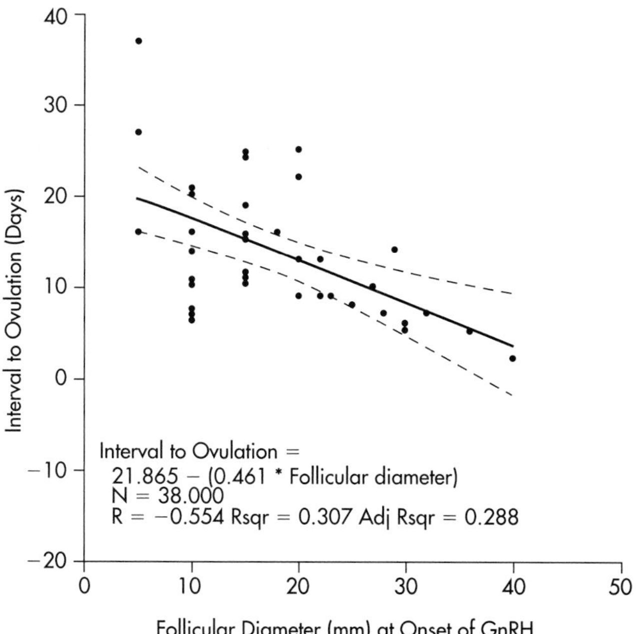

FIGURE 3-1. Relationship between follicular diameter (in millimeters) at the time of onset of native GnRH therapy and interval to ovulation in 38 Thoroughbred or Standardbred mares in central Kentucky. (From Morehead JP, Colon JL, Blanchard TL: Clinical experience with native GnRH therapy to hasten follicular development and first ovulation of the breeding season, *J Equine Vet Sci* 21:54, 81-88, 2001.)

WAITING TO BREED MARES UNTIL REGULAR ESTROUS CYCLES OCCUR

If teasing management practices are good, waiting to breed mares until they have established regular estrous cycles is a viable alternative to using more expensive, management-intensive practices to improve prediction of the onset of ovulatory estrus. This alternative is particularly viable when hormonal therapy is used to shorten the late transition period, which sometimes does not result in a significant savings in days to conception. The likelihood of achieving a time savings must be weighed against the time involved in hormonal treatment plus the waiting period after cessation of hormone treatment until ovulation occurs. Another practical approach is to administer prostaglandin $F_{2\alpha}$ ($PGF_{2\alpha}$) 1 week after the mare ceases behavioral estrus, or preferably 1 week after ovulation is confirmed by palpation or ultrasound examination per rectum, when the newly formed corpus luteum should be susceptible to its luteolytic effect. The mare should return to estrus and ovulate within 2 to 10 days.

INDUCTION OF OVULATION IN CYCLING MARES

To optimize fertility, it is commonly believed that ovulation should occur within 24 to 48 hours after the mare is bred to a fertile stallion. When cryopreserved semen or certain subfertile stallions are used for breeding, the fertilizable lifespan of spermatozoa may be reduced, requiring breeding closer to ovulation. At the present time in the United States, administration of either hCG or deslorelin remains the only reliable, practical method for inducing ovulation of a large, preovulatory follicle in cycling mares.

Injection of hCG (1000 to 3500 U IV or IM) is sufficient to induce ovulation of preovulatory follicles ≥35 mm in diameter in mares having regular estrous cycles. We have achieved similar success rates with intravenous administration of 1000, 1500, and 2500 U of hCG, although we most commonly administer 2500 U. When hCG is injected on the first day an estral mare develops a follicle ≥35 mm in diameter, the majority will ovulate within 48 hours (approximately 65% to 70% ovulation rates between 36 and 48 hours) (Figure 3-2). If the day of estrus is unknown and the follicle is larger than 35 mm in diameter, the interval to ovulation may be less predictable, sometimes occurring earlier after hCG administration. The drug is of most value when it is used in the early months of the breeding season when criteria used to predict ovulation in cycling mares (e.g., size and shape of follicle, thickness of follicular wall, softness of follicle, cervical relaxation, day of estrus, and degree of uterine edema) are less predictive of the interval to ovulation.

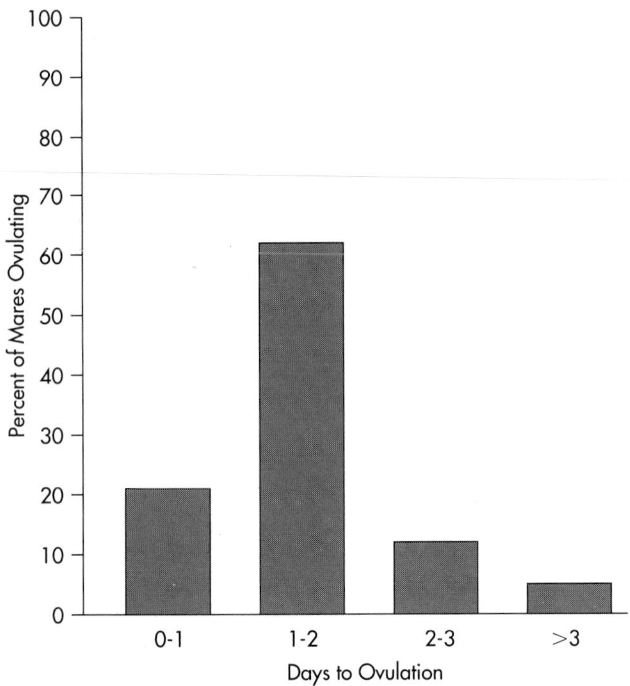

FIGURE 3-2. Intervals to ovulation in 214 estrous cycles of light-breed mares in southwest Texas after intravenous administration of 1000 to 2500 U of hCG during March through July 1999. Mares were in estrus with ≥35 mm diameter follicle(s) present at the time of treatment.

Antibodies to hCG are found in the serum of mares given repeated injections of the drug. Whether antibodies to hCG interfere with subsequent spontaneous ovulation in treated mares remains a controversial subject. Workers at Ohio State University claim that intravenous injection of hCG is less likely to induce an antibody response that delays ovulation than intramuscular injection of the drug. Despite evidence for antibody formation, we have achieved similar response rates at each injection of hCG in mares treated for up to four different estrous cycles within the same breeding season or up to seven different estrous cycles in two consecutive breeding seasons (i.e., mares were just as likely to ovulate within 2 days of hCG administration with their third or later injections as they were with their first or second injection). In contrast, Colorado workers have reported delayed intervals to ovulation after hCG injection in mares that have received the drug on more than two previous estrous periods, particularly when mares were treated on consecutive cycles.

hCG can be given in combination with other hormones used to synchronize estrus or shorten the duration of the late transition period. When hCG is used on the first day a ≥35 mm diameter follicle is present in cycling mares synchronized with a 10-day regimen of progesterone and estradiol, with $PGF_{2\alpha}$ given on the tenth day, approximately 80% to 85% of mares ovulate on days 19 to 22 after steroid treatment is begun (Figure 3-3).

The efficacy of GnRH to induce ovulation in other species and the ability of GnRH administered in a pulsatile fashion or by constant infusion for prolonged (28-day) periods to stimulate follicular development and ovulation in anestrous mares (reviewed by Ginther, 1992) have stimulated interest in its use to induce ovulation in cycling mares. Success in inducing ovulation in cyclic mares by administering single injections of native GnRH has generally been poor. Nevertheless, new analogs of GnRH that are more potent and have a longer half-life have been proven to be highly effective for inducing ovulation in cycling mares. Currently the only GnRH analog approved for use in horses in the United States is a 2.1-mg deslorelin implant (Ovuplant; Fort Dodge Laboratories). Administration (Figures 3-4 and 3-5) of implants containing deslorelin on the first day of estrus that a follicle ≥30 mm in diameter is detected results in a shortened time to ovulation and normal pregnancy rates in treated mares (reviewed by Jochle and Trigg, 1994).

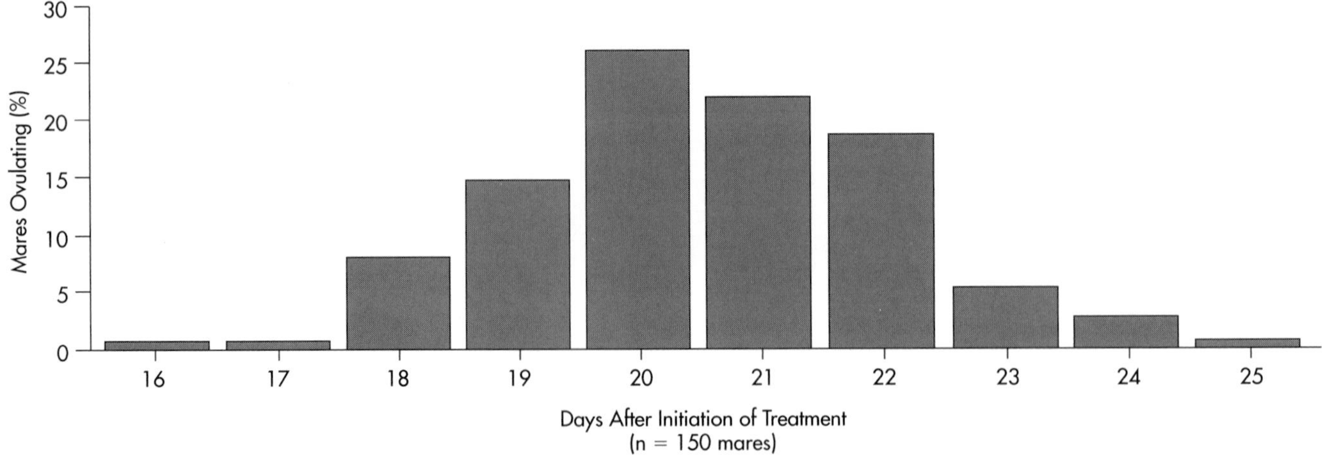

FIGURE 3-3. Intervals to ovulation in 150 estrous cycles of light-breed mares in southeast Texas after daily intramuscular injection for 10 days with 150 mg of progesterone and 10 mg of estradiol-17β, intramuscular injection of 10 mg of $PGF_{2\alpha}$ on day 10, and intravenous injection of 1500 to 2500 U of hCG on the first day a follicle ≥35 mm diameter was achieved.

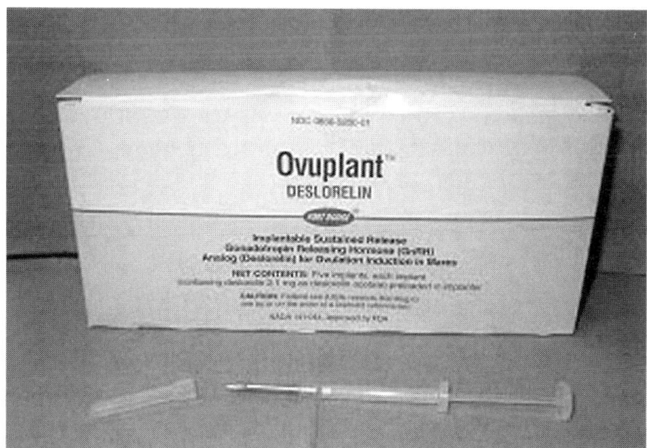

FIGURE 3-4. Deslorelin (Ovuplant) administration system. Implant containing deslorelin is contained within the large-bore needle to be inserted subcutaneously.

Few studies have directly compared the efficacy of deslorelin implants with that of hCG injections, but preliminary evidence suggests that use of either compound results in similar intervals to ovulation (Table 3-2) and fertility rates. One proposed advantage of using deslorelin is that antibodies against the compound that might diminish its effectiveness with repeated use are not formed.

A disadvantage of using deslorelin is the finding of extended interovulatory intervals in mares that fail to become pregnant, thereby delaying rebreeding. Follicular growth is suppressed early in diestrus, resulting in an average delay of 4 to 6 days before the next ovulation. A recent Kentucky study revealed that 10% of interovulatory intervals in deslorelin-treated mares were greater than 30 days, which can be problematic for the practitioner charged with ensuring that mares become pregnant as early as possible in the breeding season. Louisiana researchers recently confirmed that this prolonged interovulatory interval was due to suppressed follicular activity attributable to hyposecretion of gonadotropins from the

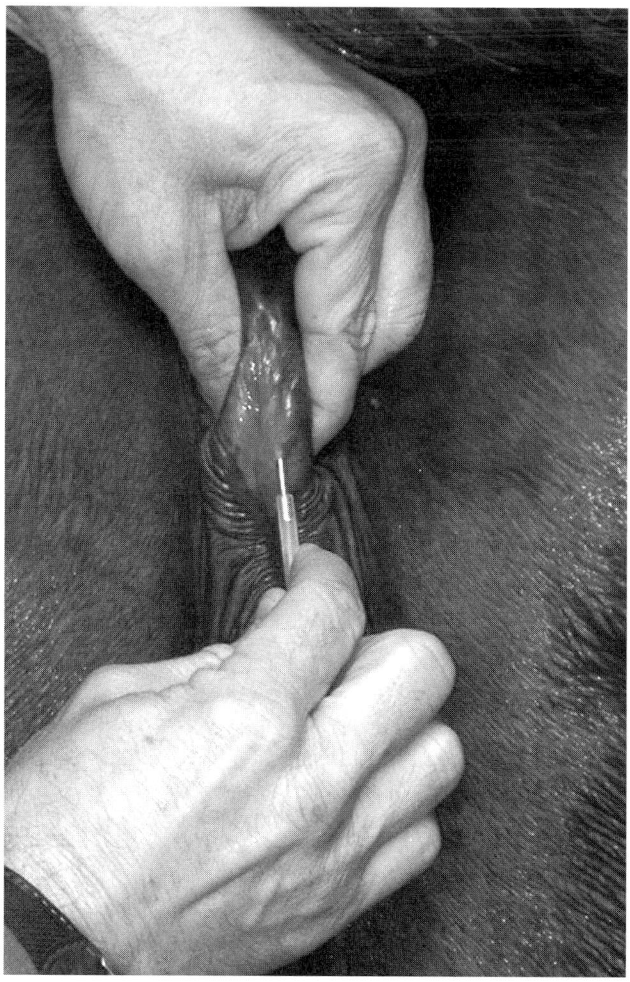

FIGURE 3-5. Administration of deslorelin (Ovuplant) beneath the mucosa of the dorsal vulvar labia. Before implant insertion, 1 cc of local anesthetic can be injected at the implant site. The needle should be inserted beneath the skin-mucosal junction, the plunger depressed to expel the implant, and the tissue pinched around the needle as the injection device is withdrawn. The implant should be palpable. Removal of the implant on the day of ovulation is recommended.

TABLE 3-2

Intervals to Ovulation and Interovulatory Intervals in 155 Thoroughbred Mares Receiving Either No Treatment, Deslorelin (Ovuplant) Implants, or Intravenous Injections of 2500 U of hCG during the 1999 Breeding Season in Central Kentucky

	No Treatment		hCG		Ovuplant	
	n	Mean ± SD	*n*	Mean ± SD	*n*	Mean ± SD
Follicular size at treatment (mm)	—	—	30	41.0 ± 5.2	204	42.0 ± 5.5
Interval to ovulation (days)	—	—	30	2.4 ± 1.0	204	2.1 ± 1.0
Interovulatory interval (days)	21	20.8 ± 1.7*	13	20.7 ± 2.0*	70	24.3 ± 6.2†

*, †Within row, means with different superscripts are significantly different ($P < 0.01$).

Modified from Morehead JP, Blanchard TL: Clinical experience with deslorelin (Ovuplant) in a Kentucky Thoroughbred broodmare practice, *J Equine Vet Sci*:358, 2000.)

pituitary gland. Presumably this finding was due to pituitary gonadotroph receptor down-regulation. Supporting this concept, Colorado researchers recently demonstrated that the gonadotropin response to native GnRH challenge 10 days postovulation in deslorelin-treated mares is attenuated.

Texas workers recently demonstrated that placement of the deslorelin implant beneath the dorsal vulvar mucosa (see Figure 3-5), with removal of the implant 2 days later, avoids the follicular suppression and delayed return to estrus that sometimes occurs with this drug.

SYNCHRONIZATION OF ESTRUS IN THE CYCLING MARE

The extended estrus period of the mare, with ovulation occurring variably from 1 to 10 days after the beginning of estrus, necessitates time-consuming, expensive reproductive management. Reproductive management of horses would be greatly benefited by development of an accurate, economical method for the precise control of estrus and ovulation in the mare.

Most synchronization methods used to control ovulation in domestic animals modify the **luteal phase** of the estrous cycle. $PGF_{2\alpha}$ has been administered to broodmares to shorten the lifespan of the corpus luteum and thus induce estrus. Treatment with $PGF_{2\alpha}$ is most often used for individual mares when the presence of a mature corpus luteum is suspected or known (e.g., when a breeding was missed or did not result in pregnancy or mismating has occurred). On average, $PGF_{2\alpha}$ treatment of mares with a mature corpus luteum results in estrus in 2 to 4 days and ovulation in 7 to 12 days (Table 3-3). The onset of estrus is more synchronized than the day of ovulation. Because of the greater role of the follicular phase in controlling the total length of the estrous cycle in mares, the time of ovulation after $PGF_{2\alpha}$-induced estrus in broodmares remains variable (2 to 12 days posttreatment). Mares in diestrus with large follicles present (≥35 mm diameter) will return to estrus and ovulate sooner than mares with smaller follicles present. In many such cases, behavioral estrus may not occur, may be partial, or may be abbreviated to 1 or 2 days. The average incidence of "silent estrus" (ovulation without accompanying signs of estrus) after prostaglandin injection is approximately 15% (Table 3-3). Therefore both estrus and ovulation can easily be missed if daily teasing and regular monitoring of follicular status are not initiated when $PGF_{2\alpha}$ is given.

Precise synchronization of estrus and ovulation in groups of mares is more difficult because of the incomplete sensitivity of the equine corpus luteum to $PGF_{2\alpha}$ administration before 6 days postovulation, and injection more than 9 days postovulation will not significantly shorten the interovulatory interval. These phenomena prevent *precise* synchronization of ovulation in groups of mares by single or multiple injections of $PGF_{2\alpha}$. However, because of cost, availability, and ease of administration, synchronization schemes using $PGF_{2\alpha}$, either alone or in combination with other hormones, are commonplace. A routine protocol used for synchronizing estrus in a group of mares is to administer two intramuscular injections of $PGF_{2\alpha}$ 14 days apart. The rationale for the two-injection scheme is that more mares will have corpora lutea that will regress after the second injection, permitting a greater percentage of mares to return to estrus in a synchronous manner. In a randomly cycling group of mares, approximately 50% will have a corpus luteum 5 to 15 days old that is capable of responding to a single injection of $PGF_{2\alpha}$, but most of the group of randomly cycling mares should have a corpus luteum capable of responding to the second injection of $PGF_{2\alpha}$ two weeks later. Typical responses to a two-injection scheme of $PGF_{2\alpha}$ are illustrated in Table 3-3.

TABLE 3-3

Efficacy of Two Intramuscular Injections of 10 mg of Prostaglandin $F_{2\alpha}$ Given 14 Days Apart to Synchronize Estrus in 33 Nonlactating Quarter Horse Mares

Estrus after 1st $PGF_{2\alpha}$	17/33 (52%)
Estrus after 2nd $PGF_{2\alpha}$	26/33 (79%)
Interval to estrus after 2nd $PGF_{2\alpha}$ (mean ± SD)	4.4 ± 1.7 days
Duration of estrus after 2nd $PGF_{2\alpha}$ (mean ± SD)	3.6 ±1.8 days
Ovulations after 2nd $PGF_{2\alpha}$	31/33 (94%)
Interval to ovulation after 2nd $PGF_{2\alpha}$ (mean ± SD)	7.2 ± 2.6 days (range 2-10 days)
Incidence of silent ovulations	5/31 (16%)
Incidence of treatment failures	2/33 (6%)

*Ovulation was induced with 1500 U of hCG injected intravenously after a 35-mm diameter follicle was detected.

Administration of progestogen, in the form of progesterone in oil (150 mg/day IM) or altrenogest (0.044 mg/kg/ day by mouth), to artificially prolong the luteal phase of the estrous cycle has been used to synchronize the ensuing estrus in mares. The rationale for the efficacy of progestogen therapy in synchronizing estrus is based on the fact that progestogens inhibit LH release and thereby block ovulation. When progestogens are administered long enough to cycling mares, corpora lutea regress and subsequent ovulation is blocked by inhibition of LH release by the exogenous progestogens. When progestogen administration ceases, mares return to estrus and ovulate. Administration of progestogens for 14 to 15 days should be more effective than administration for shorter periods because it allows sufficient time for spontaneous luteal regression to occur in mares with fresh ovulations at the onset of treatment. The interval to estrus is somewhat variable after cessation of progestogen administration, but it averages 4 to 7 days. Ovulation usually occurs, on average, 7 to 12 days after cessation of progestogen treatment. Because *follicular development is not uniformly inhibited*, even by relatively high doses of progestogens, a wide range of developmental stages of follicles exists after termination of treatment, resulting in highly variable intervals to ovulation among mares.

Control of follicular growth during the treatment period is required to achieve more precise control of ovulation in the mare. Several findings have led to development of more precise ovulation control in the mare. Daily administration of 10 mg of estradiol-17β was found to suppress follicular growth. Subsequently, it was hypothesized that daily administration of progesterone (to artificially prolong the luteal phase) in combination with daily administration of estradiol (to suppress follicular growth) might provide for a more predictable interval to ovulation after cessation of steroid treatment. This hypothesis was confirmed in cycling mares, postpartum mares, and maiden and barren mares that had been maintained under an artificially increased photoperiod for at least 60 days.

An additional problem contributing to variability in interval to ovulation has been the tendency for corpora lutea to persist (**persistent luteal function**) beyond cessation of progestogen treatment. This persistence occurs because (1) a number of mares ovulate after steroid treatment is initiated and the resulting corpora lutea continue to produce progesterone after cessation of exogenous progestogen treatment, and (2) the corpora lutea of some mares occasionally persist spontaneously longer than the usual diestrus period, thereby remaining functional after progestogen treatment is discontinued. Therefore administration of $PGF_{2\alpha}$ after cessation of progestogen treatment has been recommended to ensure that remaining corpora lutea regress and treated mares return to estrus in a timely manner. Loy's recommended protocol is 150 mg of progesterone plus 10 mg of estradiol-17β in oil injected daily for 10 consecutive days, combined with a single injection of $PGF_{2\alpha}$ on the last day of steroid treatment with the addition of 2500 U of hCG injected intravenously when a follicle ≥35 mm in diameter was first detected. With this protocol, approximately 80% to 85% of mares will ovulate 19 to 22 days after the first steroid injection on day 1 (ovulations typically range from 18 to 25 days after the last steroid injection) (Figure 3-3). Unfortunately, time-consuming daily injections of 150 mg of progesterone and 10 mg of estradiol-17β in oil are required, and *no commercial preparation containing estradiol-17β is approved* for veterinary use in the United States at this time. Thus progesterone and estradiol combinations must be obtained from veterinary pharmaceutical compounding companies.

Pharmaceutical companies are pursuing the development of implant technology that could provide sustained release of various compounds, including hormones, for prescribed periods of time. Such formulations have the advantage of having to be administered only once. Investigations have been performed with biodegradable microspheres containing progesterone and estradiol-17β. The microsphere preparations were formulated to release desired amounts of the hormones over a period of 12 to 14 days in mares. Field trials with these preparations were encouraging in that estrus and ovulation have been more precisely controlled, and fertility in treated mares has been normal.

HORMONAL THERAPY TO IMPROVE FERTILITY OF MARES EARLY IN THE POSTPARTUM PERIOD

The **first postpartum estrus**, commonly referred to as "**foal heat**," is characterized by normal follicular development and ovulation within 20 days postpartum. The onset of the foal heat occurs within 5 to 12 days after parturition in >90% of mares. In a study involving 470 Thoroughbred mares in central Kentucky, 43% had ovulated by day 9, 93% by day 15, and 97% by day 20 after parturition. The average interval to first ovulation was 10.2 ± 2.4 days. In a recent study of 93 Quarter Horse mares in southeast Texas, the day of the first postpartum ovulation was 12.3 ± 2.9 days and was significantly influenced by month of foaling, with ovulations in June-foaling mares occurring 3 days earlier than ovulations in March-foaling mares. This study revealed that the day of ovulation was not influenced by age or parity of the mare.

Pregnancy rates achieved by breeding during foal heat are generally reported to be 10% to 20% lower than those obtained by first breeding at subsequent estrous periods. The decreased pregnancy rate associated with foal heat breedings has been suggested to be due to failure of the uterus, particularly the endometrium, to be completely restored and therefore ready to support a developing embryo. In support of this hypothesis, the pregnancy rate from foal heat breedings is higher in mares that ovulate after 10 days postpartum compared with those that ovulate before this time. Because a 5-day interval after ovulation is required before the embryo enters the uterus, ovulation after day 10 postpartum ensures that the histologic appearance of the endometrium has returned to normal, and fluid normally present within the uterine lumen during the first week or two postpartum has been fully expelled before embryo entry. It is also of interest that, in the previously cited Kentucky study, foal heat pregnancy rates were farm dependent (i.e., on some farms pregnancy rates achieved were decidedly lower when mares were bred on the first postpartum estrus compared with mares bred on the second postpartum estrus, although no significant differences in pregnancy rates were found between these breedings at other farms). This emphasizes the need for the practitioner to use common sense in evaluating the practice of breeding on first versus second postpartum estrus, taking farm (management) practices and previous success rates on a given farm into consideration.

Attempts to improve pregnancy rates from breeding in the early postpartum period have been focused on either attempting to enhance the rate of uterine involution or delaying breeding until involution is more complete. To enhance fertility achieved on foal heat breeding, several methods have been used in an attempt to speed uterine involution in normal foaling mares. Some of the methods tested include repeated uterine lavage during the first week postpartum, repeated administration of uterine ecbolics (e.g., prostaglandins, oxytocin, and methylergonovine) to promote uterine contraction and evacuation during the first 10 days postpartum, and administration of steroid hormones (progestogens, progesterone, estradiol, and progesterone plus estradiol) during the first few days to 2 weeks postpartum. None of the methods tested has enhanced uterine involution rate (measured by gross uterine involution, histologic repair of the endometrium, or evacuation of uterine fluid) in normal foaling mares. Therefore we feel that at this time the best method to enhance fertility of mares in the early postpartum period is to delay breeding until histologic involution and expulsion of intrauterine fluid is complete.

There are two methods used at this time to postpone breeding in the postpartum period until normal pregnancy rates can be achieved: (1) to delay the onset of the foal heat or (2) to shorten the interval to the second postpartum estrus. Pregnancy rates achieved by breeding on foal heat appear to be higher in mares in which estrus is delayed by progestogen therapy. Altrenogest has been given daily for 8 or 15 days after foaling. Prostaglandin should be administered on the last day of treatment because progestogen therapy alone may not prevent ovulation from occurring even though estrus is suppressed. Daily treatment with a combination of progesterone and estradiol-17β for as few as 5 days has also been used to delay onset of the first postpartum estrus and ovulation. Treatment should commence as soon as practical on the day of foaling before gonadotropin surges responsible for follicular recruitment occur.

The major objection to the use of progestogen therapy for several consecutive days, beginning at the time of foaling, is that the treatment delays the onset of the first postpartum estrus sufficiently so that foaling intervals are not significantly reduced. If treatment of postparturient mares for 2 or 3 days after foaling would only delay ovulation until just after day 10 postpartum, progestogen treatment might offer the best method for increasing the pregnancy rate without significantly extending the parturition-to-breeding interval in early postparturient mares. Preliminary trials using 150 mg of progesterone and 10 mg of estradiol-17β daily for the first 2 days postpartum, or at twice this dose only on the first day postpartum, have been encouraging in this respect, ensuring that no treated mares ovulated before day 10 postpartum.

Administration of $PGF_{2\alpha}$ at 5 to 7 days after the first postpartum ovulation will hasten onset of the second postpartum estrus, which would normally not occur until approximately 30 days postpartum. Although this management technique is expected to increase the pregnancy rate at the first breeding postpartum, this is not always the case. Additionally, when compared with breeding during the foal heat, the parturition-to-breeding interval will be delayed approximately 2 weeks (i.e., approximately 1 week is saved compared with waiting and breeding on the second postpartum estrus). The authors believe the best method for using this technique is to monitor postparturient mares closely, by transrectal palpation and ultrasonographic evaluation, for ovulation and uterine fluid accumulation. Mares are bred on foal heat if they do not ovulate before day 10 postpartum and little or no fluid remains in the uterus. If ovulation occurs before day 10 postpartum or if significant fluid accumulation is present in the uterus, instead of breeding during the foal heat the mare can be injected with $PGF_{2\alpha}$ 5 to 6 days after ovulation and bred on the subsequent induced estrus.

BIBLIOGRAPHY

Alexander SL, Irvine CHG: Control of the onset of the breeding season in the mare, its artificial regulation by progesterone treatment. *J Reprod Fertil* 44(Suppl):307-318, 1991.

Burns SJ, Irvine CHG, Amoss MS: Fertility of prostaglandin-induced oestrus compared to normal postpartum oestrus. *J Reprod Fertil* 27(Suppl): 245-250, 1979.

Fitzgerald BP, Schmidt MJ: Absence of an association between melatonin and reproductive activity in mares during the non-breeding season. *Biol Reprod Monogr* 1:425-434, 1995.

Ginther OJ: *Reproductive biology of the mare. Basic and applied aspects*, ed 2, pp. 158-161. Cross Plains, WI, 1992, Equiservices.

Jochle W, Trigg TE: Control of ovulation in the mare with Ovuplan®. A short-term release implant (STI) containing the GnRH analogue deslorelin acetate: studies from 1990–1994. *J Equine Vet Sci* 14:632-644, 1994.

Kenney RM, Ganjam VK, Bergman RV: Noninfectious breeding problems in mares. *Vet Scope* 19:16-24, 1975.

Loy RG: Characteristics of postpartum reproduction in mares. *Vet Clin North Am Large Anim Pract* 2:345-358, 1980.

McCue PM, Nickerson KC, Squires EL et al: Effect of altrenogest on luteinizing hormone concentrations in mares during the transition period. *Proc Am Assoc Equine Practnr* 47:249-251, 2001.

Morehead JP, Blanchard TL: Clinical experience with deslorelin (Ovuplant®) in a Kentucky Thoroughbred broodmare practice. *J Equine Vet Sci* 20: 358-402, 2000.

Morehead JP, Colon JL, Blanchard TL: Clinical experience with native GnRH therapy to hasten follicular development and first ovulation of the breeding season. *J Equine Vet Sci* 21:54, 81-88, 2001.

Sharp DL, Cleaver BD, Davis SD: Photoperiod. In McKinnon AO, Voss JL, editors: *Equine reproduction*, Philadelphia, 1993, Lea and Febiger.

Squires EL, Heesemann CP, Webel SK et al: Relationship of altrenogest to ovarian activity, hormone concentrations and fertility of mares. *J Anim Sci* 56:901-910, 1983.

Taylor TB, Pemstein R, Loy RG: Control of ovulation in mares in the early breeding season with ovarian steroids and prostaglandin. *J Reprod Fertil* 32(Suppl):219-224, 1982.

Wendt K, Stich K, Blanchard T: Effects of deslorelin administration in vulvar mucosa, with removal in 2 days, in foal-heat mares, *Proc Am Assoc Equine Practnr* 2002 (in press).

4

Breeding Soundness Examination of the Mare

OBJECTIVES

While studying the information covered in this chapter, the student should attempt to:

1. Acquire a working understanding of the procedures used for performing a breeding soundness examination of the mare.
2. Acquire a working understanding of how abnormalities of the genital tract may adversely affect fertility of the mare.

STUDY QUESTIONS

1. List information (history) that should be obtained to assess prior reproductive performance and to identify potential problems to be looked for in a breeding soundness examination of a mare.
2. Describe procedures that are integral parts of the breeding soundness examination of the mare (e.g., assessment of vulvar conformation, vaginal speculum examination, procurement of specimens for uterine cytology, and culture and biopsy).
3. List benefits of a properly taken and interpreted uterine cytologic specimen.
4. List abnormalities that can be detected only by uterine biopsy.
5. List abnormalities that can be detected by intrauterine endoscopy.
6. Summarize the purposes for performing a breeding soundness examination of a mare.

HISTORY

A breeding soundness examination should begin with a gathering of all pertinent reproductive history about the mare. The examiner may uncover information about a mare that may not otherwise be obtained. For instance, the following queries should be answered: How old is the mare? Has the mare been bred previously? If so, has she become pregnant and delivered any foals? How many foals? How long has it been since she last foaled? Has she been bred each year? Has she been bred to fertile stallions using good breeding management procedures? Has she been bred to different stallions each year? Has she experienced any difficulties associated with foaling? Were any diagnoses of early pregnancy loss confirmed? Has she experienced any abortions or stillbirths? If so, at what gestational ages were pregnancies lost? Has the mare had any genital discharges? Has the mare previously been treated for genital infection? If so, what treatments were administered and when?

One should also collect information regarding the mare's estrous cycle. Mares are seasonal breeders with the peak of fertility corresponding to the longest days of the year. Mares typically have normal estrous cycles during the physiologic breeding season (spring and summer), and then enter a state of reproductive dormancy in the late fall, as day length decreases. Mares that are reproductively normal generally enter into estrus (heat) every 18 to 24 days (approximately every 3 weeks) during the breeding season, with heats typically lasting for a period of 4 to 7 days (see Chapter 2). Because of seasonal variations in the duration of estrus, a better indicator that the mare has regular estrous cycles is that the period between heats is 14 to 16 days. This interval remains relatively constant regardless of season. One should note whether or not the mare has normal estrous cycles and exhibits strong outward signs of heat (i.e., is sexually receptive) when exposed to a stallion during estrus. Additionally, the method of teasing should be obtained because most mares fail to show strong signs of estrus unless teased by a stallion. Many owners of mares believe otherwise; however, we have teased mares with a stallion when the owners thought the mares were showing heat to a gelding or another mare and have often found that the mares were not in estrus. In contrast, we have also teased mares thought by owners to be out of heat when we suspected they actually were in heat (based on palpation findings) and usually found that the mares would express behavioral estrus when presented to a stallion.

Shortened estrous cycles (e.g., less than 18 days) suggest the possibility of an underlying uterine infection (i.e., acute endometritis causing premature luteolysis). Lengthened estrous cycles in nonbred mares suggest the possibility of prolonged luteal function, whereas in mares that have been bred the possibility for early embryonic or fetal death exists. A less likely cause of irregular estrous cycles is endocrine dysfunction. If a

Mare Information:
Name:
Case #:
Age:
Breed:
Color:
Lip Tattoo #:
Registration #:
Markings / Brands:
Present Breeding Status:

Owner/Agent:
Address:

Telephone:
Facsimile:

Referring Veterinarian:
Address:

Telephone:
Facsimile:

History:

General Body Condition:

Genital Examination:
Method(s) Used: ☐ Palpation ☐ Ultrasound
- Anus/Perineum:
- Vulva:
- Clitoris:
- Vestibule:
- Vagina:
  - ☐ Speculum examination:
  - ☐ Digital examination:
- Cervix:
  - ☐ Palpation per rectum:
  - ☐ Speculum examination:
  - ☐ Digital examination:
- Uterus:
  - Right horn:
  - Left horn:
  - Body:
- Ovaries:
  - Right:
  - Left:
- Mammae:
- Other Findings:

Laboratory Tests:
☐ Endometrial culture:
☐ Endometrial biopsy:
  Category:
  Diagnosis:
☐ Endometrial cytology:
☐ Other tests performed:

Prognosis for supporting foal to term:

Diagnosis/Recommendations:

Signature: Date:

FIGURE 4-1. Example of a breeding soundness examination form for the mare.

mare has regular estrous cycles, the likelihood of endocrine dysfunction is low.

If possible, the examiner should collect previous breeding and medical records for the mare of interest and determine specifically whether the mare has developed any reproductive or general medical problems that have required treatment. A variety of ailments exist that may reduce or abolish a mare's reproductive potential. An illustration of a breeding soundness examination form for recording of history, examination findings, diagnosis and treatment recommendations is provided in Figure 4-1.

GENERAL PHYSICAL EXAMINATION

Just because a mare is being examined for reproductive potential does not mean that one should ignore her general body condition. Good general health extends the longevity of broodmares and aids the ability of a mare to support a pregnancy to term and provide sufficient high-quality colostrum/milk for adequate foal development. All body systems (e.g., digestive, respiratory, urinary, cardiovascular and nervous systems, and special senses) should receive at least a cursory examination to prevent overlooking conspicuous problems. Common laboratory tests (Coggins' test, urinalysis, blood analysis, and fecal egg counts) can be used in conjunction with a physical examination to assess the general health of a mare. It may also be prudent to evaluate conformation for defective traits that are potentially heritable.

REPRODUCTIVE EXAMINATION

Restraint

When a mare's reproductive tract is examined, it is important to ensure that she is properly restrained. Such precautions will prevent or reduce undue injury to the mare or veterinarian during the examination process. Methods of restraint are the same as those discussed for palpation per rectum (Chapter 1).

Examination of the External Genitalia

The first part of the reproductive examination involves a thorough inspection of the external genitalia. Conformation of the vulva, perineum, and anus are closely evaluated. To prepare the area for examination, the tail can be wrapped in a plastic sleeve, which is itself secured at the base of the tail with tape. The tail is then elevated by lifting it directly over the mare's rump to improve visualization of the external genitalia (Figure 4-2). Another useful method is to wrap the tail in a gauze bandage, pull the tail up to the side, and tie the gauze around the mare's neck. The disadvantage of this method is that exposure of the perineal area is reduced; however, it is useful for keeping the tail out of the way when a stock is not available.

The long axis of the vulva should be vertical, with the vulvar labia well apposed to produce an intact vulvar seal against contamination (see Figure 1-7). Any conformational abnormalities

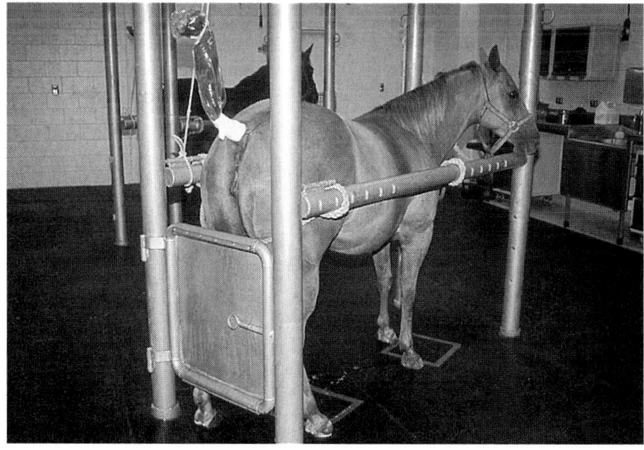

FIGURE 4-2. Mare placed in a stock with tail wrapped in a plastic sleeve and tied overhead in preparation for a breeding soundness examination.

or vulvar discharge is noted. The perineum should be intact, and the anus should not be recessed (sunken) (see Figure 1-8), because this conformation would predispose the mare to excessive vulvar contamination at the time of defecation. The labia of the vulva can be parted gently to document that the mare has an intact vestibulovaginal seal. If the vestibulovaginal seal is incompetent, parting the vulvar lips will result in aspiration of air, which is heard as a "sucking" noise. This seal is also important to deter ascending uterine infection.

Palpation per Rectum

Using the arm protected with a plastic sleeve, a veterinarian can palpate the internal genital organs of the mare. It is important that the mare be adequately restrained before this procedure is conducted, to avoid injury to the mare or veterinarian. With a systematic approach, the ovaries, uterus, and cervix are evaluated for normalcy (see Figures 1-10 through 1-13). The uterus should be examined for evidence of pregnancy before one proceeds with more thorough palpation. If the mare is determined to be nonpregnant, the examination is continued.

The ovaries of the mare are generally "bean-shaped" and range in size from that of a golf ball to a tennis ball (see Chapter 1). Mares can develop ovarian tumors that result in a substantial increase in ovarian size (Figure 4-3). Ovarian size can also be markedly increased with hematoma formation (Figure 4-4), which occurs when excessive bleeding follows ovulation and formation of the corpus hemorrhagicum. The ovaries are examined for follicles (Figure 4-5) or corpora lutea (Figure 4-6), activity that suggests that the mare is having normal estrous cycles. Occasionally, incidental parovarian cysts are detectable, but these seldom interfere with fertility. Cysts formed in the fossa region are thought to be peritoneal fragments that become embedded in the serosal surface of the ovary after ovulation. Other parovarian cysts are likely to be distended remnants of the embryonic mesonephric system or paramesonephric tubules or ducts and are located on the

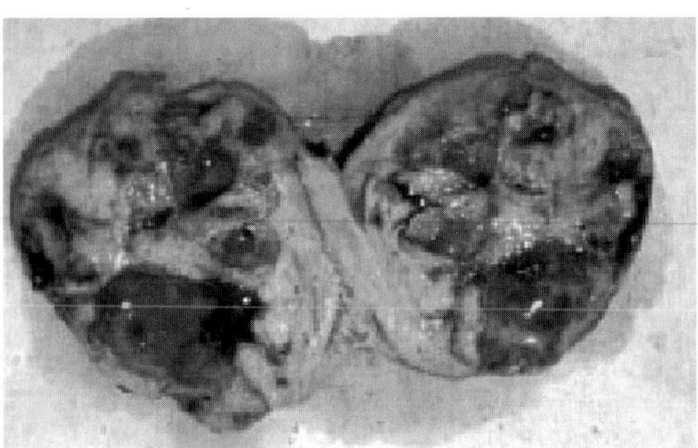

FIGURE 4-3. Surgically removed granulosa cell tumor of an ovary of a mare. The affected ovary was enlarged and firm, whereas the contralateral ovary was atrophied (small and inactive). The mare was behaviorally anestrus with elevated circulating concentrations of inhibin and testosterone.

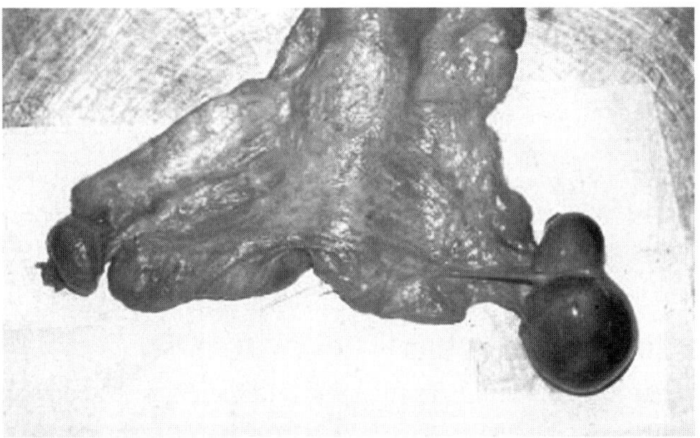

FIGURE 4-4. Ovarian hematoma of a mare. Mares with ovarian hematomas usually continue to have regular estrous cycles and do not have contralaterally atrophied ovaries. The enlarged ovary shrinks over time. Hormone assays reveal no abnormalities in hormone concentrations.

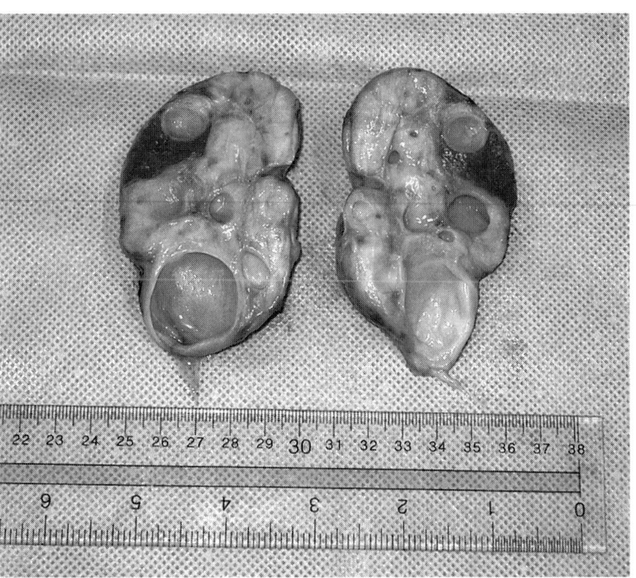

FIGURE 4-5. Cross-sectional view of a mare ovary with follicles of various sizes present.

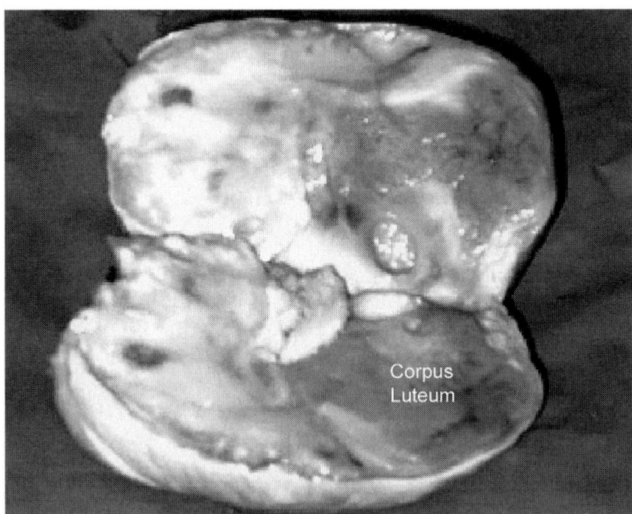

FIGURE 4-6. Cross-sectional view of a mare ovary with functional corpus luteum present.

mesovarium near the ovary (Figure 4-7) or on the ovary (epoophoron). Very small (1 to 2 cm in diameter) hypoplastic ovaries are sometimes found, in which case gonadal dysgenesis as a result of sex chromosome abnormalities should be suspected. Sometimes, one or both ovaries may be absent. If only one ovary is missing, it was probably removed previously because of an ovarian tumor. Some owners have both ovaries surgically removed from performance mares which become difficult to handle while in estrus. If an ovariectomized mare is sold, the new owner may be unaware that the ovaries have been removed.

The uterus of the nonpregnant mare is T (or Y)-shaped, consisting of two uterine horns and singular uterine body (see Chapter 1). It is palpated in its entirety for size, symmetry between uterine horns, and evidence of luminal contents. Many uterine abnormalities can be detected by palpation per rectum, including atrophy of endometrial folds (Figure 4-8), localized atrophy of uterine musculature, lymphatic cysts (Figure 4-9), uterine tumors (Figure 4-10), and the presence of large quantities of purulent material or other abnormal fluid within the lumen of the uterus (Figure 4-11).

The cervix, a tubular structure that connects the uterus with the vagina, can be easily palpated per rectum. It is primarily evaluated to aid in estimating the stage of the estrous cycle, being closed when a mare is in diestrus (i.e., out of heat) and dilated when a mare is in estrus (heat). Most abnormalities of the cervix affect its lumen and cannot be readily identified by palpation per rectum. For this reason, the cervix is also evaluated by visual inspection and digital palpation per vaginam. For digital palpation, the index finger is inserted into the

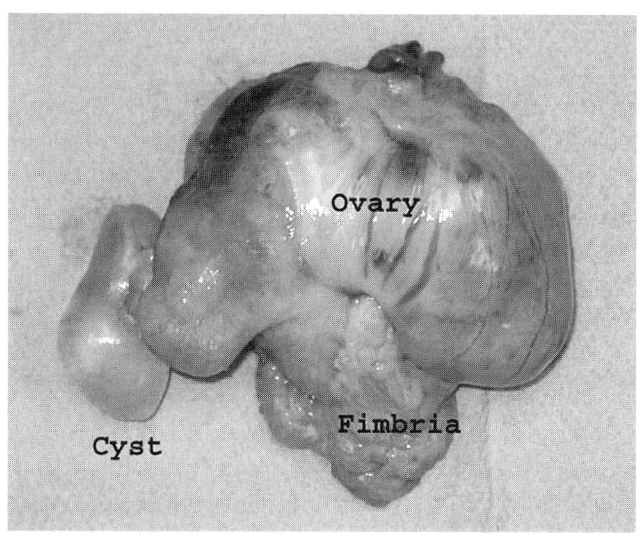

FIGURE 4-7. Parovarian cyst next to an ovary from a mare. Such cysts are not uncommon, and are not believed to interfere with fertility.

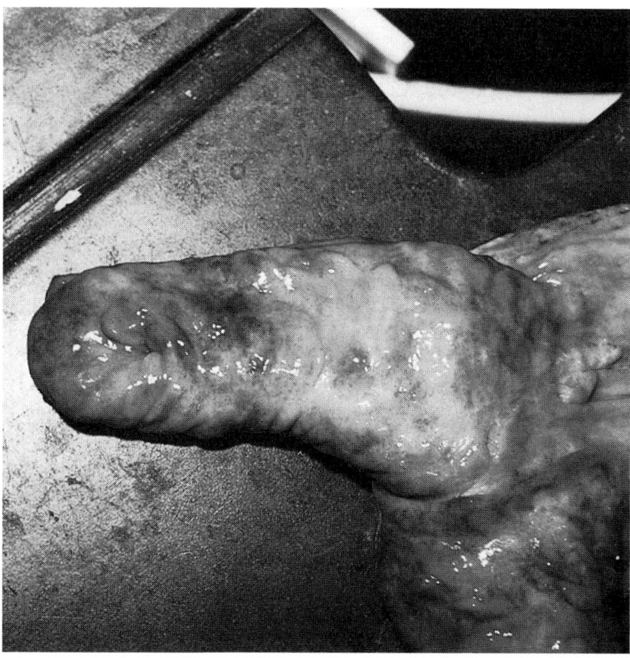

FIGURE 4-8. Uterus of a mare with atrophied endometrial folds. The uterus has been turned inside out so the endometrial surface is outermost.

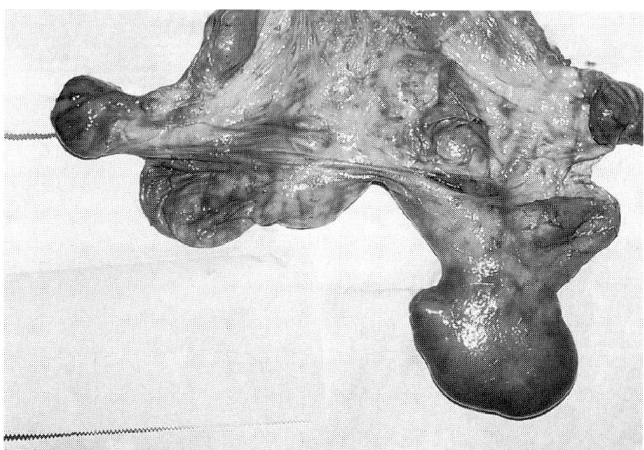

FIGURE 4-9. Large endometrial lymphatic cyst evident at the base of the uterine horn. The uterine wall was thin (atrophied) and a prominent sacculation was present at the base of one uterine horn during palpation per rectum.

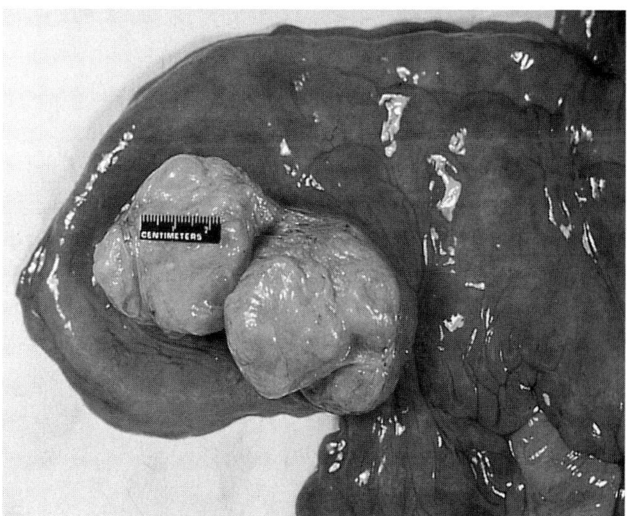

FIGURE 4-10. Uterine tumor (leiomyoma) near the end of the right horn of a mare uterus. The cut surface is shown with the endometrium outermost. On palpation per rectum, the tumor was firm and easily mistaken for the ovary, except that the tumor was contained within the uterus and the ovary was palpable just beyond the tip of the uterine horn.

cervical lumen, the thumb is apposed on the outside of the protruding cervix, and the entire circumference of the cervix is palpated between the thumb and forefinger to determine if muscle separations or lacerations are evident (Figure 4-12). Luminal adhesions can also be detected by advancing the index finger along the entire length of the cervical lumen.

One part of the internal reproductive tract that cannot be examined readily by palpation per rectum is the oviduct. The mare has two oviducts. These tiny tubes connect the uterine horns with their corresponding ovaries, serve as a sperm reservoir after breeding, are the site of fertilization, and transport fertilized oocytes to the uterus for continued development. Oviductal problems that interfere with fertility in mares are considered to be rare. However, this opinion may change as improved technology allows better assessment of oviductal function.

VAGINAL SPECULUM EXAMINATION

After the vulva and surrounding areas are critically cleansed to avoid contamination of the reproductive tract with bacteria,

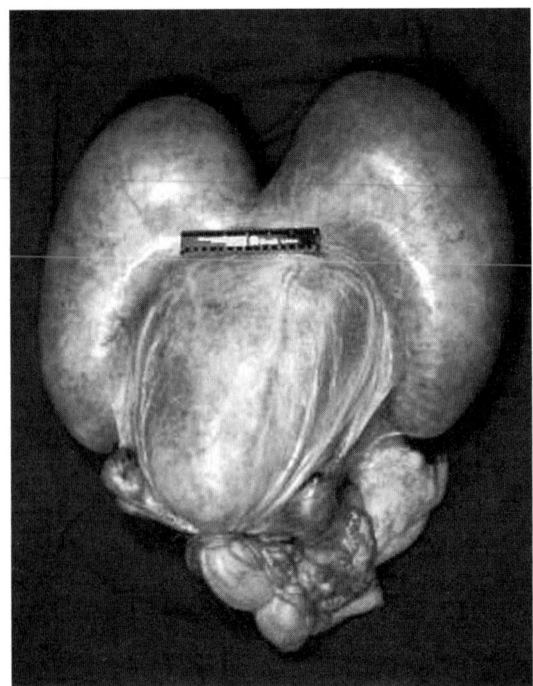

FIGURE 4-11. Uterine distension with purulent material from a mare with chronic pyometra.

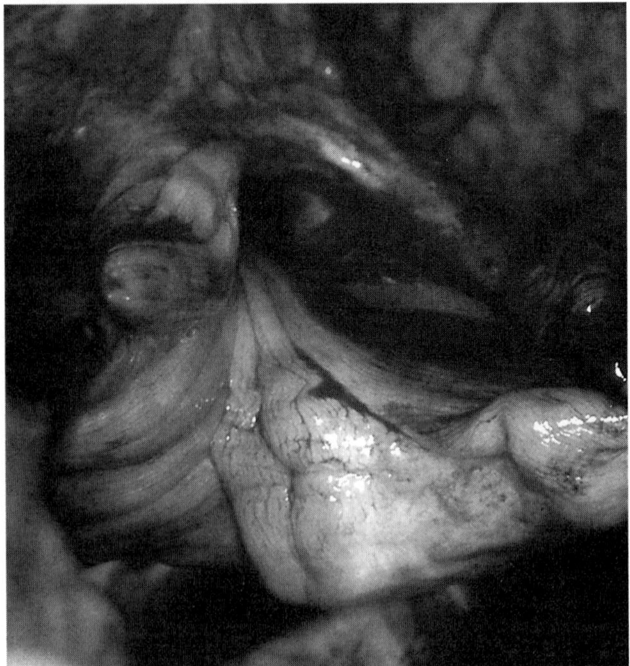

FIGURE 4-12. Pie-shaped cervical laceration evident during speculum examination of a mare cervix.

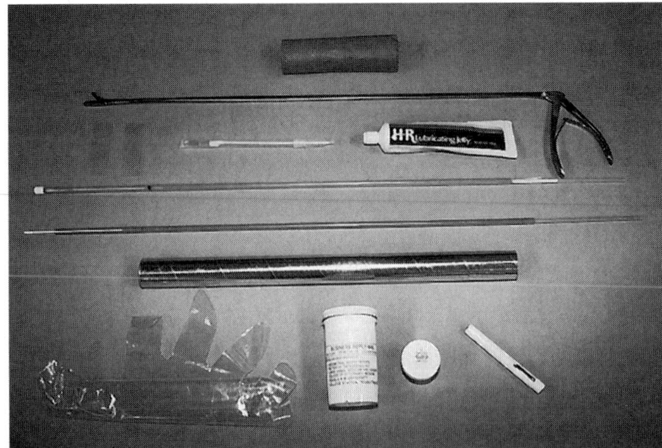

FIGURE 4-13. Equipment used for performing a breeding soundness examination in the mare. From *top to bottom*: gauze tail wrap; alligator-type uterine biopsy forceps for procuring an endometrial biopsy specimen; microscope slides for making of endometrial cytologic preparations for staining; transport medium to contain the uterine swab during shipment to the bacteriology laboratory; sterile, nonbactericidal/nonbacteriostatic lubricant; guarded and unguarded (i.e., no distal occlusion) culture instruments for taking of samples for uterine culture or cytologic analysis; disposable vaginal speculum; rectal sleeve; fixative vial and shipping container for transport of endometrial biopsy sample to reference laboratory; and light for illumination of vagina during viewing through a speculum.

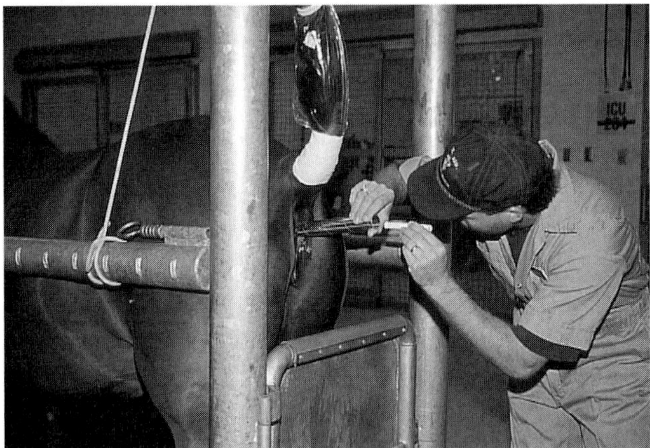

FIGURE 4-14. Procedure for viewing of the vagina and external os of the cervix through a tubular vaginal speculum.

fungus, or debris, a tubular vaginal speculum can be inserted into the vaginal cavity to allow examination of this area (Figures 4-13 and 4-14). A small amount of sterile lubricant is placed on the speculum before insertion into the vagina, and a light is used to illuminate the vagina through the speculum. The entire vagina and external cervical os can be viewed by this approach (Figure 4-14). Abnormalities that may be detected by a vaginal speculum examination include persistent hymen (see Figure 1-6), vaginitis/cervicitis, vaginal varicosities (Figure 4-15), adhesions (scarring of the cervical opening or vaginal vault), lacerations or tears of the posterior cervix (see Figure 4-12) or vaginal walls, and accumulation of purulent material or urine in the vaginal cavity (Figure 4-16).

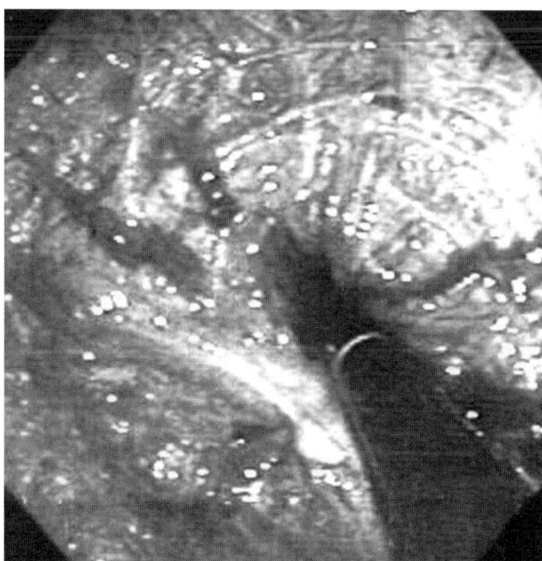

FIGURE 4-15. Vaginal varicosities on the cranial aspect of the vestibular fold and caudal vagina. The flexible endoscope was passed into the cranial aspect of the vagina and turned to permit viewing of the front side of the vestibular fold. The mare had a history of recurrent episodes of hemorrhage from the vulva.

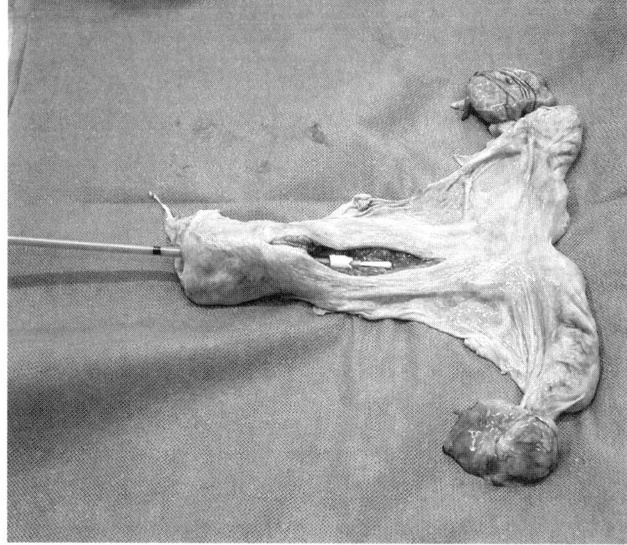

FIGURE 4-17. Method used for transcervical procurement of uterine swabbing for bacteriologic culture or cytologic analysis. The body of the uterus has been cut open to facilitate viewing of the extended swab.

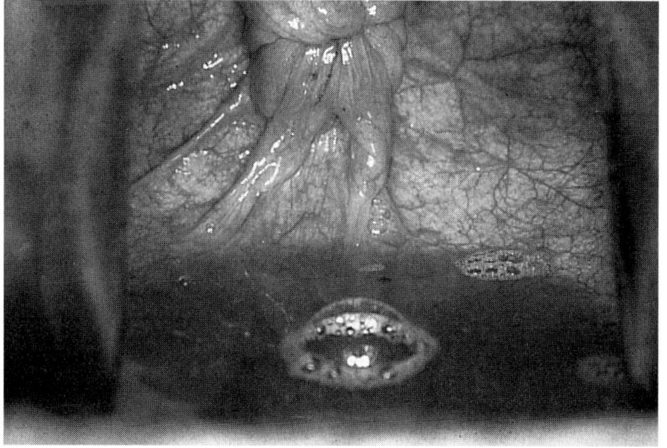

FIGURE 4-16. Urine and debris pooled in the anterior vaginal vault of a mare with urovagina.

UTERINE (ENDOMETRIAL) CULTURE

A uterine culture can yield valuable information about a mare's reproductive potential, provided it is properly obtained and interpreted. The objective of a uterine culture is precisely to determine if any microorganisms (i.e., bacteria or fungi) are present within the cavity of the uterus. Unfortunately, it is extremely easy to contaminate a uterine swab with microorganisms originating from the outside environment or vagina. Such contamination could lead to the false impression that a mare has a uterine infection. Hence, it is imperative to aseptically prepare the mare's hindquarters and use a guarded swab and sterile equipment when swabbing the endometrium for bacteriologic culture (see Figure 4-13). To procure a swabbing for culture, one of two methods can be used. The first method involves carrying the guarded swab into the vagina with a sterile gloved hand. The index finger is placed in the cervical lumen, and the guarded swab is guided into the uterine lumen where the swab is then exposed (Figure 4-17). The swab should be retracted back into the guard before removing it from the uterus. In the other method, a sterile vaginal speculum is passed into the cranial vagina to the cervical os. A light is used for illumination, and the sterile guarded swab is passed through the speculum and cervix into the uterine lumen where the swab is then exposed. Again, the swab should be retracted back into the guard before removing it from the uterus.

To further increase the chance that culture of the endometrial swabbing accurately reflects the status of the uterus, the culture must be handled correctly upon transit to the laboratory for testing. We recommend use of a transport medium, such as Amie's charcoal or Stuart's medium, that maintains organism viability without encouraging overgrowth of bacteria if much time will elapse between obtaining of the sample and inoculation of the swab on the culture media. Additionally, we recommend that culture results be obtained from direct inoculation on media rather than from broth cultures that encourage overgrowth of contaminant bacteria. Finally, growth should be quantified in some fashion, because heavy growth at 24 or 48 hours of incubation is more likely to be significant than recovery of only a few colonies. If the practitioner prefers to perform his or her own cultures, 5% blood agar plates and MacConkey's agar can be inoculated with the uterine swabbing. Incubating these media under aerobic conditions is adequate for recovery of the vast majority of potential pathogens found in the mare reproductive tract (the exception being the need for microaerophilic or anaerobic conditions for the mare with septic postparturient metritis). Antimicrobial sensitivity testing is also desirable to aid in selection of the proper drug for treatment of uterine infections.

To minimize misinterpretation of culture results, the findings should be compared with those of uterine cytologic analysis or endometrial biopsy. These latter procedures allow one to detect endometrial inflammation, a process that would accompany the presence of microorganisms if a mare truly has infectious endometritis.

UTERINE CYTOLOGIC ANALYSIS

By using a swab (the same method as that described for obtaining a swabbing for culture) or other device, cells can be retrieved from the uterine cavity to check for the presence of an active inflammatory process that would accompany infectious endometritis. If a swab is used to collect material for cytologic analysis, it should immediately be gently rolled across the surface of a microscope slide, allowed to air dry, labeled, and stained with a suitable stain such as Diff-Quik. If a loop or small scoop is used to collect a specimen for cytologic analysis, the fluid from the collection device should be gently tapped onto a microscope slide, allowed to air dry, and stained as before. Stained cytologic preparations are examined under a microscope for the presence of white blood cells (usually neutrophils), microorganisms, and healthy or unhealthy luminal epithelial cells. Normal endometrial cytologic preparations contain sheets and individual columnar epithelial cells with a healthy appearance, few or no white blood cells, and no bacteria, fungi, or yeast organisms (Figure 4-18). Cytologic preparations from mares with acute or subacute endometritis contain increased numbers of white blood cells and may also have degenerate, vacuolated epithelial cells.

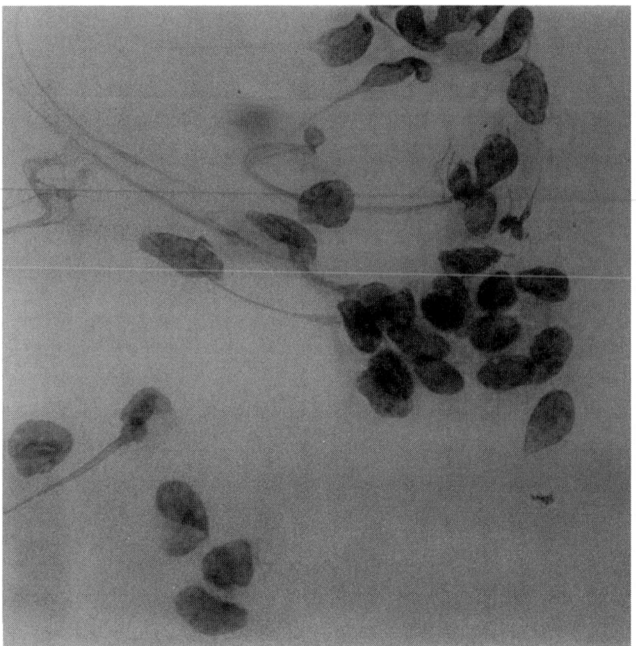

FIGURE 4-18. Cytologic preparation (Diff-Quik stain) showing normal endometrial cytology. Normal endometrial cytology will include simple columnar epithelial cells, often in clumps, that appear healthy and few or no neutrophils.

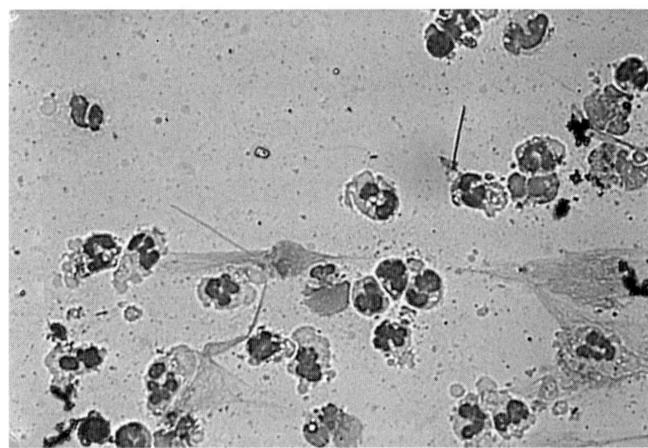

FIGURE 4-19. Cytologic preparation (hematoxylin-eosin stain) of acute endometritis associated with *Streptococcus* infection. Cytologic preparations from mares with acute or subacute endometritis yield numerous neutrophils that are often degenerate and may contain phagocytosed bacteria along with many singular, degenerate epithelial cells.

The value of uterine cytologic analysis is usually limited to documentation of an active (i.e., acute or subacute) inflammatory response because neutrophils are a prominent luminal component of endometritis (Figure 4-19). Additionally, staining of uterine cytologic preparations remains the best way to demonstrate infection with yeast or fungi (Figure 4-20), because these organisms tend to proliferate in the uterine lumen and on the endometrial surface (luminal epithelial cells). However, more subtle inflammatory changes of the endometrium, such as chronic endometritis, are usually not detectable by this approach. Nevertheless, uterine cytologic analysis can provide a gauge of the representativeness of uterine culture results, particularly when time is of the essence. For example, when a mare is presented for examination early during estrus, if the uterine cytologic analysis and culture results suggest that inflammation is not a problem, the mare can be bred during the same estrus. Likewise, if evidence of only a mild infection exists, treating the uterus before and after breeding is sometimes an option (see Chapter 6). If the practitioner has to wait for biopsy results, breeding on that estrus would most likely have to be skipped (e.g., ovulation would occur before biopsy results were available).

Uterine (Endometrial) Biopsy

Providing that results of the examination of the gross physical condition of the mare and reproductive tract are within normal limits, evaluation of an endometrial biopsy is probably the single most important means of assessing the mare's potential

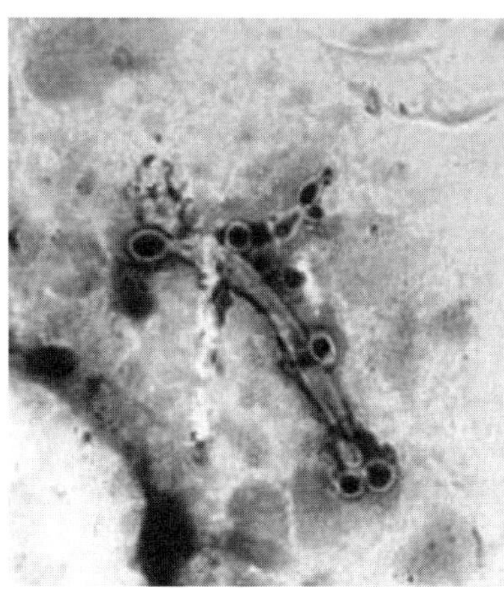

FIGURE 4-20. Cytologic preparation (Diff-Quik stain) from a mare with fungal endometritis.

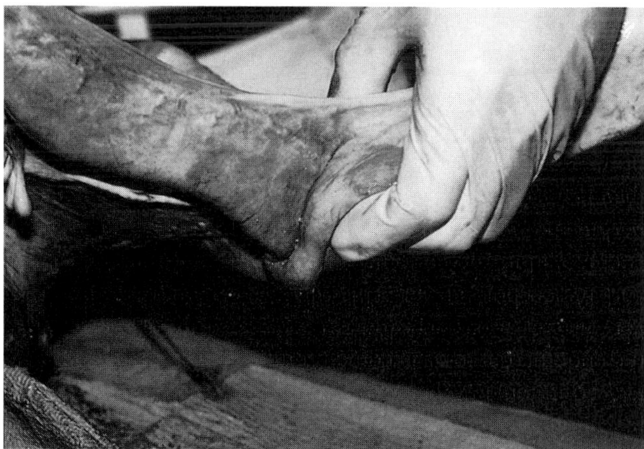

FIGURE 4-21. Procurement of endometrial biopsy specimen from the ventral surface of the uterus. The uterine wall is gently lifted with the finger(s) into the jaws of the biopsy punch and held in this position until the jaws are closed, thereby clipping off a portion of the endometrium.

as a broodmare. In other words, biopsy results can be categorized according to the prognosis for the mare to become pregnant and carry a foal to term:

Category I—better than 80% chance
Category IIA—50% to 80% chance
Category IIB—10% to 50% chance
Category III—less than 10% chance

A sample for biopsy can easily be taken from the endometrium by passing an appropriately designed instrument through the cervix and into the uterus. The aseptic procedure is the same as that for procuring an endometrial swabbing for culture, except that it is important to pass the closed biopsy punch as far as is safely possible into the uterus to ensure that a representative specimen of endometrium is obtained. Endometrial specimens obtained too near the cervix have reduced glandular density and shallow gland penetration into the lamina propria, which prevent accurate assessment of glandular normalcy or pathologic changes. After the biopsy punch is inserted into the uterus, one hand is inserted into the rectum while the other hand holds the biopsy grip. By using the hand in the rectum, the biopsy punch can be further guided to the base of one of the uterine horns. The jaws of the biopsy punch are opened, and the uterine wall is lifted (if sample is to be procured from the ventral surface of the uterine horn) (Figure 4-21) or pressed (if the sample is to be procured from the dorsal surface of the uterine horn or body) (Figure 4-22) into the jaws and they are closed, thereby clipping off a portion of the endometrium. The biopsy punch is removed from the mare's reproductive tract, and the endometrial specimen is placed in a suitable fixative, such as Bouin's solution, and transported to a reference laboratory for interpretation.

Many abnormalities that can adversely affect a mare's fertility can be detected *only* by microscopic evaluation of an endometrial biopsy specimen. Examples include periglandular fibrosis, cystic glandular distention, lymphatic distension, and chronic inflammatory changes within the endometrium (Figures 4-23 through 4-28). Biopsy evaluation is also an excellent way to

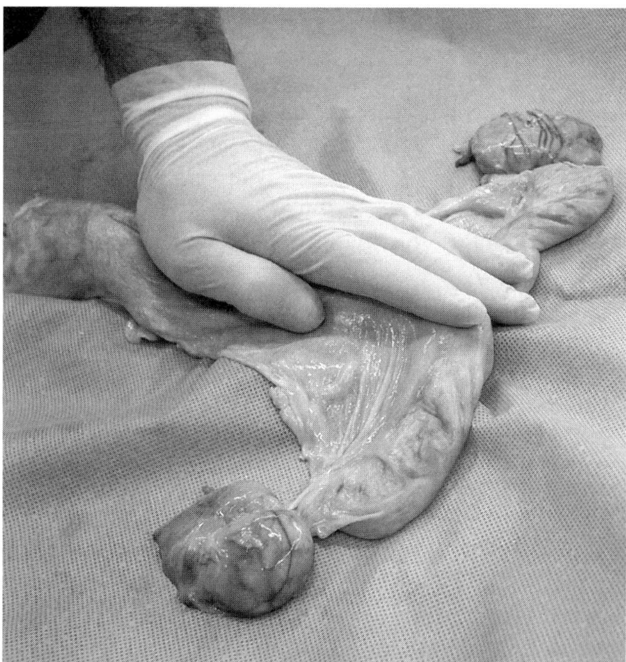

FIGURE 4-22. Procurement of endometrial biopsy from the dorsal surface of the uterus. The uterine wall is gently pressed into the underlying jaws of the biopsy punch and held in this position until the jaws are closed, thereby clipping off a portion of the endometrium.

monitor patient response to therapy when uterine infections or other endometrial abnormalities are diagnosed and treated. Workers in the United Kingdom have shown that biopsy scores after treatment (i.e., whether pathologic changes detected in a previous endometrial biopsy have improved or not) are more closely related to subsequent fertility of mares than prognosis based on results of a single pretreatment biopsy.

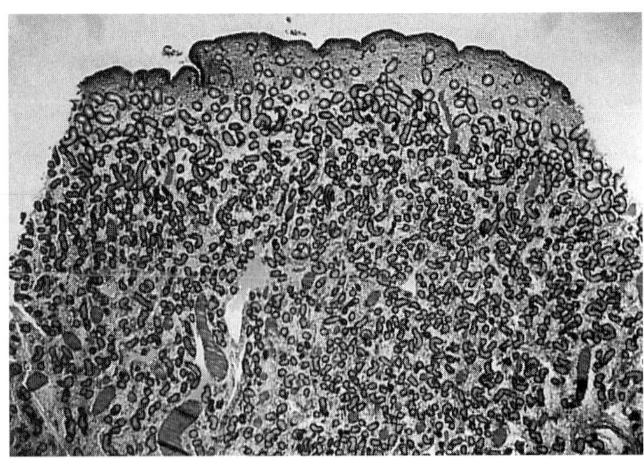

FIGURE 4-23. Normal, active endometrium (category I: 80% or better chance of foaling). Glands are numerous, randomly dispersed, and active. Inflammatory cells are absent or occur infrequently.

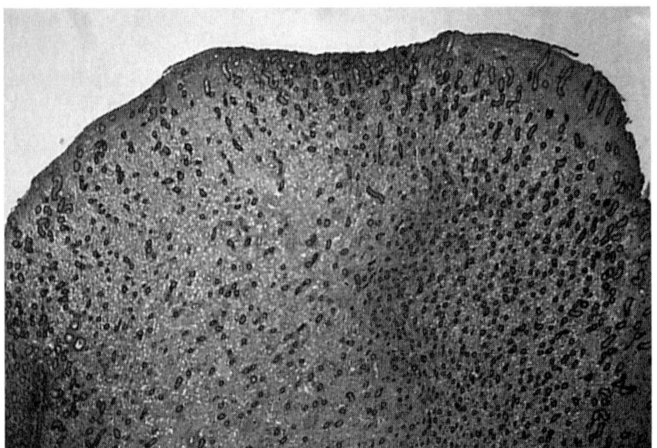

FIGURE 4-24. Seasonal endometrial atrophy. Atrophy of glands (shrunken, straight, and nontortuous) and luminal epithelium (flattened and cuboidal) is evident during seasonal atrophy. Fertility is likely to be reduced until seasonal atrophy is corrected.

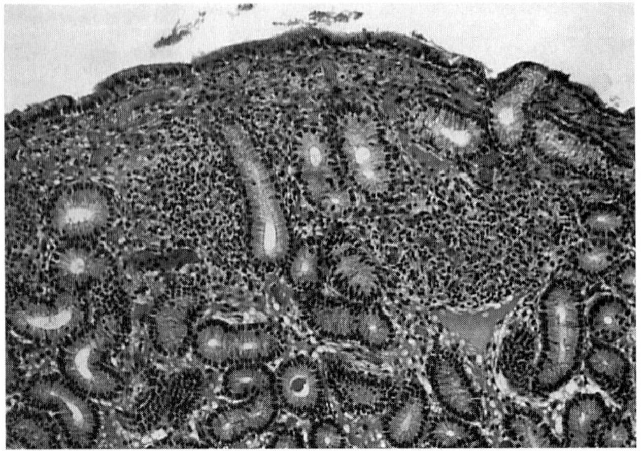

FIGURE 4-25. Chronic endometritis with lymphocyte infiltration into lamina propria (category IIA: 50% to 80% chance of foaling). This type of inflammation may not be detected with uterine cytologic analysis.

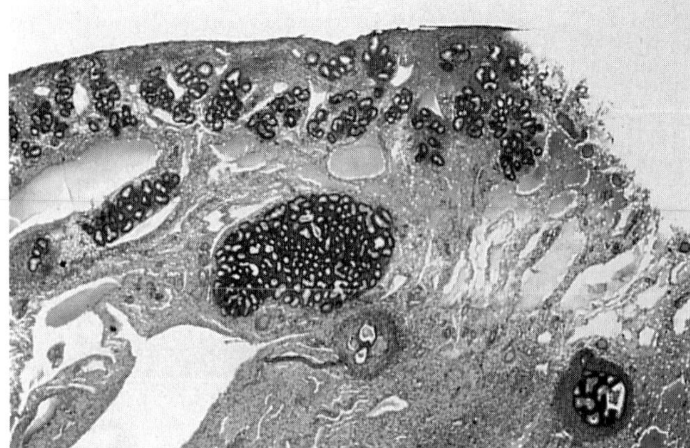

FIGURE 4-26. Widespread, moderately frequent periglandular fibrosis (category IIB: 10% to 50% chance of foaling). Clumped (nested) glands are distended and are surrounded by a few layers of connective tissue.

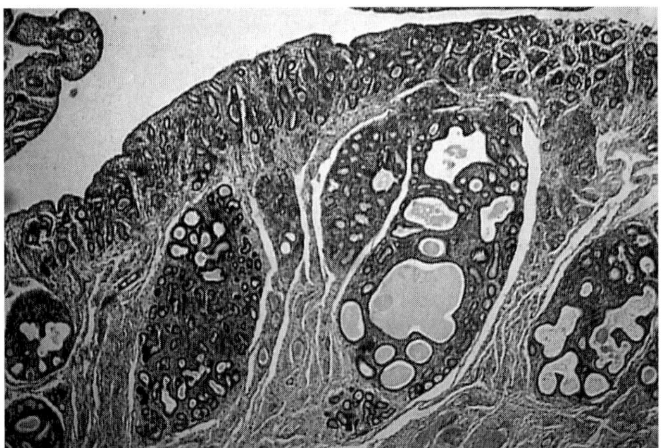

FIGURE 4-27. Widespread, frequent periglandular fibrosis (category III: less than 10% chance of foaling). Gland nesting (clumping) due to fibrosis is so frequent as to affect almost all glands within the stratum spongiosum (deeper lamina propria).

OTHER DIAGNOSTIC AIDS

Additional diagnostic tests can be incorporated into a breeding soundness examination if it becomes necessary to ascertain more information about a mare to judge her breeding potential. Two of the more commonly used procedures are transrectal ultrasonographic examination of the reproductive tract and transcervical endoscopic examination of the uterine cavity. Ultrasonographic examinations use high-frequency sound waves to visualize reproductive structures (e.g., the ovaries and uterus, that are otherwise "hidden" from view) using a relatively noninvasive approach. They permit easier diagnosis of several reproductive abnormalities, including ovarian tumors or hematomas; uterine tumors, cysts, or abscesses; and pathologic fluid accumulations within the uterine cavity.

Endoscopic examinations allow direct visualization of the uterine cavity. A specialized viewing instrument (disinfected

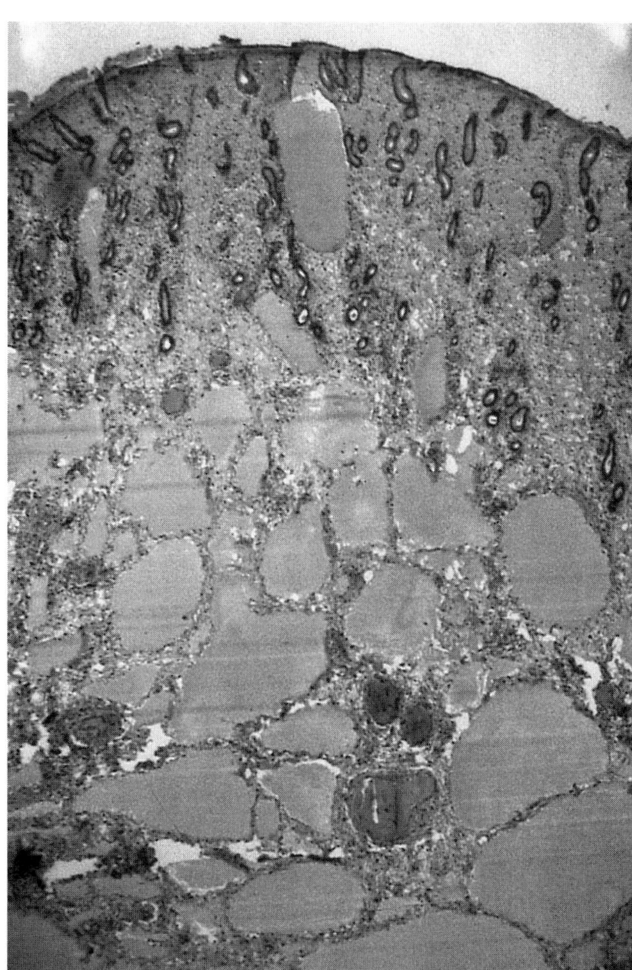

FIGURE 4-28. Widespread, frequent lymphatic lacunae (category IIB: 10% to 50% chance of foaling). Lymphatic vessels, particularly in the core areas of the lamina propria, are distended with homogeneous, eosinophilic fluid.

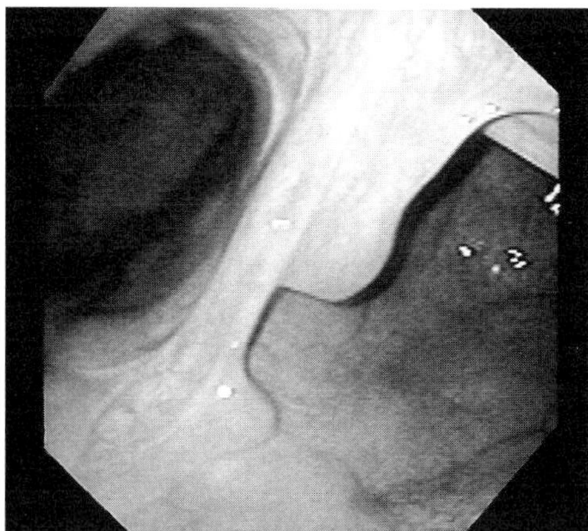

FIGURE 4-29. Endoscopic view of bifurcation of uterine horns. The uterus must be partially distended with air or fluid to visualize the interior of the uterus.

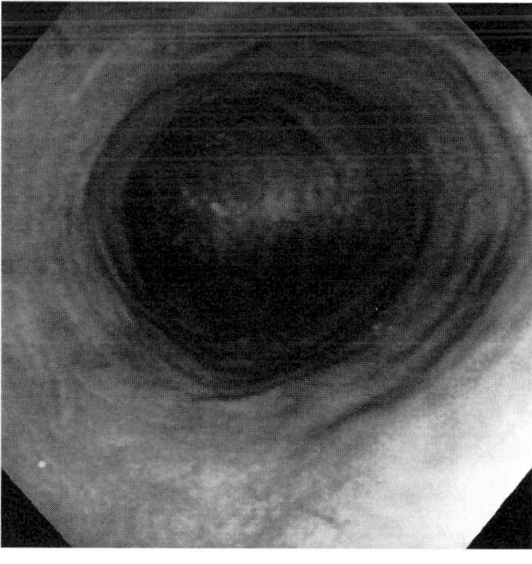

FIGURE 4-30. Endoscopic view of the lumen of a uterine horn. Endometrial folds are not apparent because of distention of the uterine horn with air to facilitate visualization.

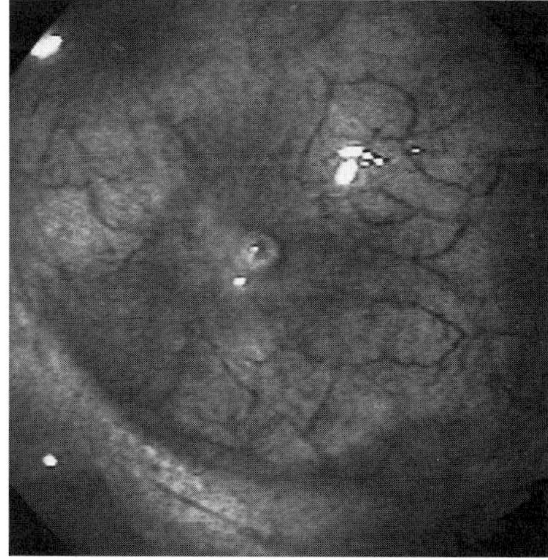

FIGURE 4-31. Endoscopic view of the oviductal papilla, the location at which the oviduct empties into the uterus.

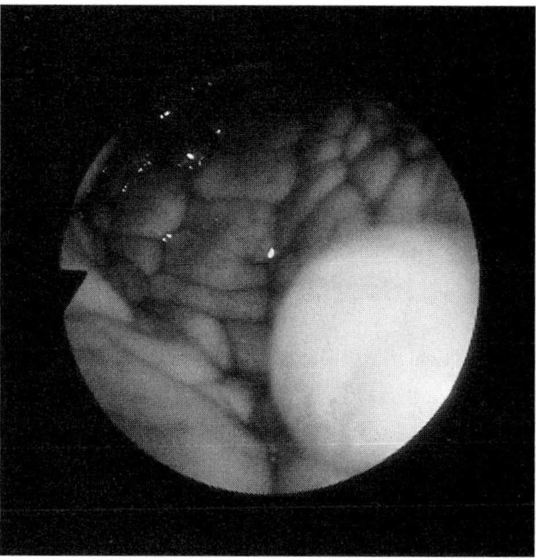

FIGURE 4-32. Endoscopic view of an endometrial cyst.

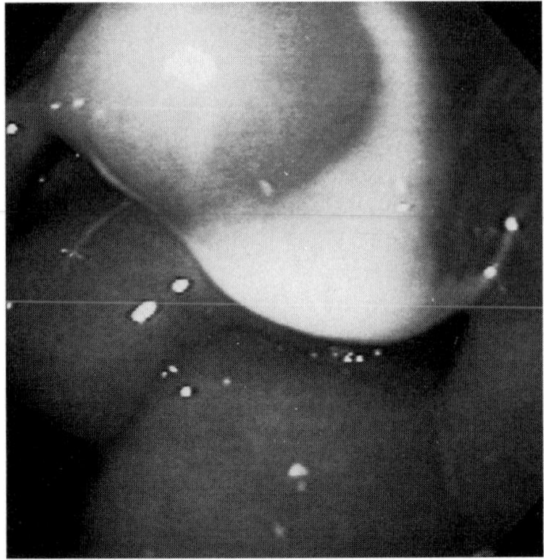

FIGURE 4-33. Endoscopic view of the uterine lumen, with purulent material on the luminal epithelium.

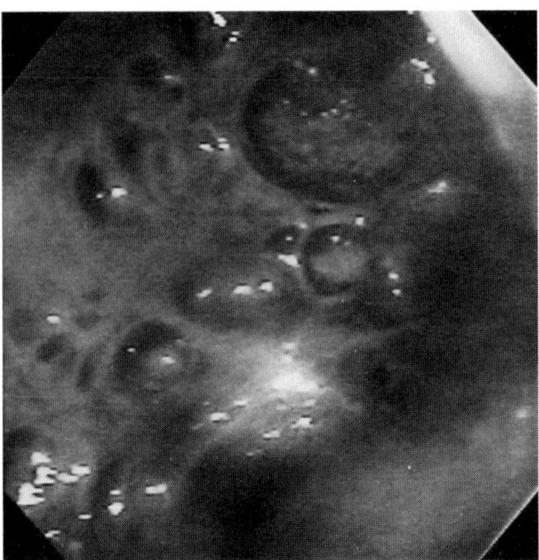

FIGURE 4-34. Endoscopic view of extensive transluminal adhesions occluding the uterine lumen.

endoscope or videoscope of sufficient length to fully visualize the entire uterus) is passed directly into the uterine cavity via the cervix. The uterus is insufflated with sufficient air to dilate the uterine cavity, and the endoscope is advanced to the internal bifurcation (Figure 4-29) and then to the end of a uterine horn (Figures 4-30 and 4-31). After one uterine horn is viewed in its entirety, the endoscope is retracted and passed to the end of the other uterine horn in the same manner. The entire inner surface of the uterus can thus be viewed, permitting definitive diagnosis of abnormalities such as endometrial cysts (Figure 4-32), foreign bodies (e.g., cotton swabs that had been broken off in the uterine cavity during a previous attempt at obtaining a uterine culture), purulent luminal contents (Figure 4-33), transluminal adhesions (Figure 4-34), or other space-occupying lesions (Figure 4-35).

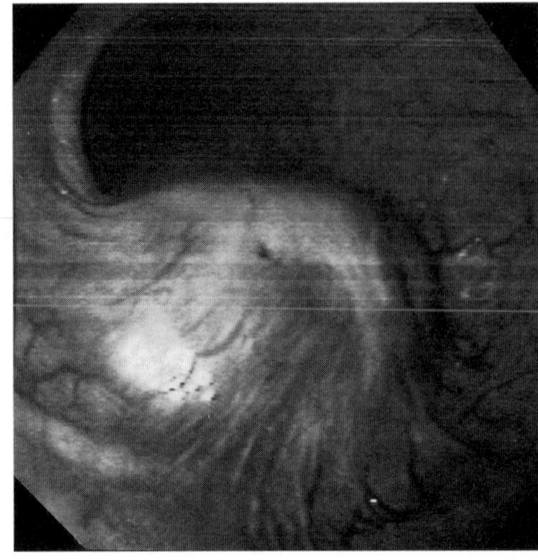

FIGURE 4-35. Endoscopic view of a leiomyoma (uterine smooth muscle tumor) impinging on the uterine lumen as a space-occupying mass.

WRITTEN SUMMARY FOR CLIENT/OWNER

As with any type of soundness examination, a written report should be given to the client/owner that summarizes findings, including any definitive diagnosis, recommended treatment, and prognosis for future fertility. This document is also useful for review in determining response to treatments and in assessing breeding outcome.

BIBLIOGRAPHY

Baker B, Kenney RM: Systematic approach to diagnosis of the infertile or subfertile mare. In Morrow DA, editor, *Current therapy in theriogenology*, pp 721-736. Philadelphia, 1980, WB Saunders.

Brook D: Uterine cytology. In McKinnon AO, Voss JL, editors, *Equine reproduction*, pp 246-254. Philadelphia, 1993, Lea and Febiger.

Kenney RM: Cyclic and pathologic changes of the mare endometrium as detected by biopsy, with a note on early embryonic death. *J Am Vet Med Assoc* 172:241-262, 1978.

Kenney RM, Doig PA: Equine endometrial biopsy. In Morrow DA, editor, *Current therapy in theriogenology*, pp 723-729. Philadelphia, 1980, WB Saunders.

Kenney RM, Ganjam VK, Bergman RV: Non-infectious breeding problems in mares. *Vet Scope* 19:16-24, 1975.

5

Transrectal Ultrasonography in Broodmare Practice

OBJECTIVES

While studying the information covered in this chapter, the student should attempt to:

1. Acquire a working understanding of the principles and equipment used for performing ultrasonographic examination on the mare reproductive tract.
2. Acquire a working knowledge of the ultrasonographic appearance of the normal reproductive organs of the mare.
3. Acquire a working understanding of the ultrasonographic appearance of the mare reproductive tract and conceptus during the estrous cycle and early pregnancy.
4. Acquire a working understanding of how abnormalities of the mare reproductive tract appear ultrasonographically.

STUDY QUESTIONS

1. List the components and characteristics of an ultrasound machine suitable for use in examining the mare reproductive tract.
2. Describe the technique for safely performing a transrectal ultrasonographic examination of the mare reproductive tract. Emphasize the importance of using a systematic approach to ensure thorough scanning of the uterus of a mare for early pregnancy diagnosis.
3. Describe the ultrasonographic appearance of:
   a. The anestrous ovaries.
   b. A preovulatory follicle.
   c. A recently ovulated follicle (within 24 hours after ovulation).
   d. The developing corpus luteum.
   e. The mature corpus luteum.
   f. The estrous uterus.
   g. The diestrous uterus.
   h. An anovulatory follicle.
   i. An ovarian hematoma.
   j. A granulosa cell tumor.
   k. Uterine lymphatic cyst(s).
   l. Intrauterine fluid accumulation associated with endometritis.
4. Summarize the characteristic location and transrectal ultrasonographic appearance of the equine conceptus at the following days of pregnancy:
   a. 12 to 14 days.
   b. 17 to 18 days.
   c. 20 to 21 days.
   d. 28 to 30 days.
   e. 34 to 36 days.
   f. 38 to 40 days.
   g. 45 to 50 days.
   h. 60 to 65 days.

In 1980, real-time ultrasonography was first reported as a potentially valuable diagnostic modality in the discipline of equine reproduction. Since this original report, applications of diagnostic ultrasonography in equine reproduction have expanded to the point that the instrument has become a fundamental, almost indispensable, tool for both veterinary clinicians and research scientists.

The two-dimensional gray-scale image produced by *B-mode* (brightness-modality) *real-time ultrasonography* provides a detailed cinematographic view of the structure(s) being studied. For the first time the observer can actually visualize "hidden" reproductive organs and follow various reproductive events in a noninvasive manner, with no apparent adverse biologic effects being incurred by the patient. Although the technology behind real-time ultrasonography is quite complex, operation of the unit is relatively simple for the trained theriogenologist, requiring only good palpation skills and a basic knowledge of ultrasound principles and the ultrasonic anatomy of the reproductive tract.

INSTRUMENTATION

A B-mode real-time ultrasound system consists of a *transducer,* which is connected by a long cord to a base unit containing a *display monitor* and *control panel* (Figure 5-1). The transducer transmits and receives *high-frequency sound waves* to produce images of soft tissues and organs on the display monitor. The echogenicity of tissues varies (i.e., their ability to

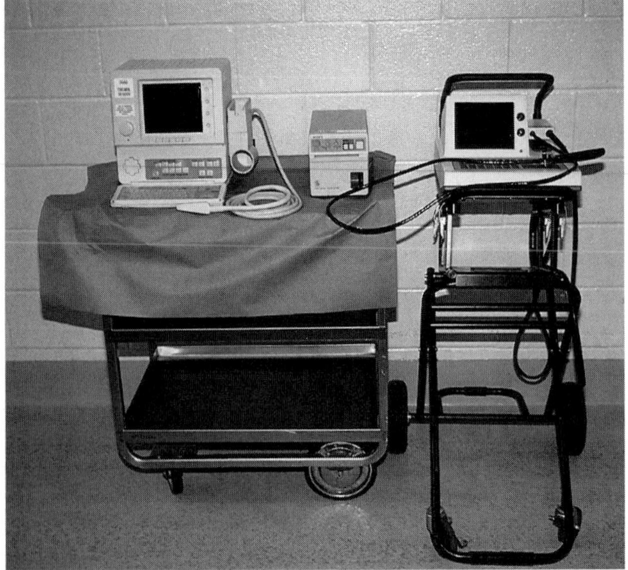

FIGURE 5-1. Two ultrasound systems for use in transrectal ultrasonographic examination of the mare. Shown on the *left* is a portable unit with a display monitor and fold-down control panel, 5-MHz transducer, and attached cord. A thermal image printer is shown in the *middle* of the photograph. Printers are attached to the video-out jacks on most ultrasound monitors, and print images that have been "frozen" on the monitor. Mavipad recorders are also available for storage of images in a digital format on diskettes. The stored images can be accessed for viewing, enhancement, sending as a viewable image over the Internet, and printing. The portable ultrasound system shown on the *right* is mounted on a rolling, foldable transport stand. It also has a 5-MHz transducer and attached cord. The control panel does not fold down on this model. Most portable ultrasound systems can be purchased with a number of different probes for varied uses.

propagate or reflect sound waves); therefore the proportion of reflected sound waves depends on the innate characteristics of the tissues or fluids being examined. For instance, fluids readily propagate sound waves, whereas air and dense tissues reflect most or all sound waves. Reflected sound waves received by the transducer are then converted to electronic impulses and subsequently displayed on the monitor. The monitor consists of a two-dimensional array of closely aligned dots. The brightness of the dots is directly proportional to the amplitude of the echoes (or reflected sound waves). Hence, highly *echogenic* tissues (e.g., bone or connective tissue) appear *white* on the ultrasound monitor, whereas nonechogenic *(anechoic)* fluids are *black*. A continuum of gray shades between white and black allows one to distinguish tissues of intermediate echogenicity. The control panel of the ultrasound unit allows the operator to adjust the quality of the image and label or measure structures of interest.

Linear-array 5- to 6-MHz transducers are adequate for most needs encountered in equine reproduction. The higher resolving power of 7.5- to 8-MHz transducers allows a more detailed study of structures, but the tissue-penetrating capacity of these transducers is more limited. Transducers with lower sound-wave frequencies (e.g., 3 MHz) permit greater tissue penetration, so they may be more useful for evaluation of the uterus and its contents during advanced pregnancy; however, image resolution is reduced accordingly. Sector or curvilinear probes available for transcutaneous abdominal imaging can be useful for monitoring fetal viability (e.g., heartbeat and activity), character, and amount of amnionic or allantoic fluid, uteroplacental thickness, and separation of the placenta.

PROCEDURAL CONSIDERATIONS

Ultrasonic evaluation of the mare's reproductive tract is generally performed by a transrectal approach. Usefulness of transcutaneous ultrasonography is limited to evaluation of the uterus and fetus during advanced (3 to 4 months to term) pregnancy.

Precautions regarding mare restraint and reproductive examination per rectum are similar to those stated for palpation per rectum. Minimal but effective restraint of the mare to be examined will greatly reduce the likelihood of equipment damage or injury to the mare or operator during the examination process. When the mare's reproductive tract is examined by transrectal ultrasonography, the following steps should be taken:

1. All manure is removed from the rectum using a well-lubricated arm. Care is taken to avoid entry of air into the rectum during the manure-evacuation process, because air will effectively prevent transmittance of ultrasound waves into surrounding structures.
2. The internal genital organs are palpated in their entirety and in a systematic manner.
3. Palpation per rectum is followed by an ultrasonographic examination, with the transducer well shielded by the examiner's hand to avoid undue trauma to the wall of the rectum. A methodical approach should be used during the examination.
4. The transducer should be well lubricated and should have good contact with the rectal wall. Manure or air should not be interposed between the transducer and the tissue of interest.
5. If the mare resists excessively, the examination should be discontinued or the mare should be sedated or, in rare cases, epidural anesthesia can be performed before continuing. If the mare is sedated or if an epidural anesthetic is administered, the reproductive tract should be examined as soon as deemed prudent to prevent pneumorectum, which occurs with anal sphincter relaxation. The presence of pneumorectum increases the risk of injury to the rectum during the examination and often interferes with transducer contact with the rectum, thereby reducing image clarity.

For ultrasound examination of the mare reproductive tract per rectum, we prefer to advance the transducer over the cervix and body of the uterus until the bifurcation of the uterus is visualized (Figures 5-2 through 5-5). The transducer

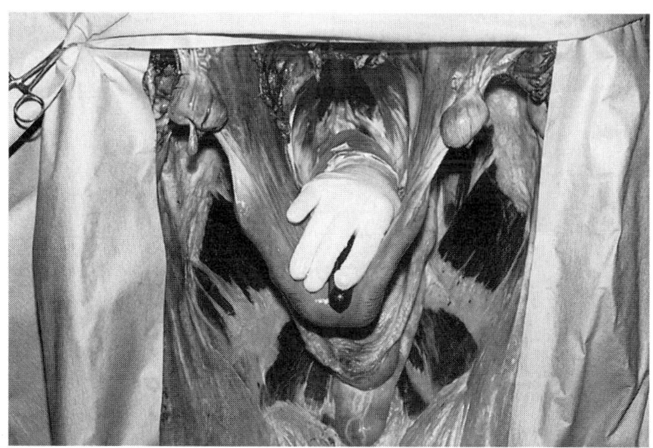

FIGURE 5-2. Examiner advancing the ultrasound transducer to the bifurcation of the uterus.

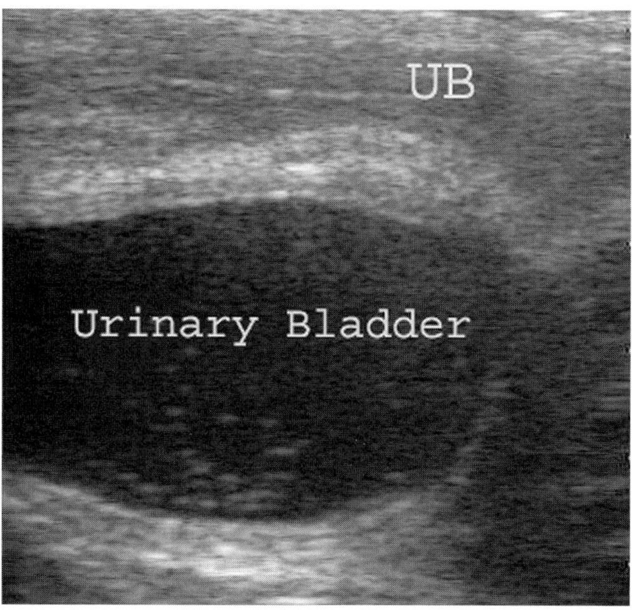

FIGURE 5-3. Transrectal ultrasound image of a longitudinal section through the cervix and uterine body (UB) of a mare in diestrus. The white spectral reflection delineating the mucosal surface of the uterine lining is often visualized at this time.

is slowly moved toward the tip of one uterine horn, taking care to ensure that the image of the uterine horn in cross-section remains in the center of the monitor screen. As the transducer moves beyond the tip of the uterine horn, the ovary is scanned (Figure 5-6) in its entirety. The transducer is then moved slowly back down the uterine horn to the bifurcation, and the remaining uterine horn and ovary are scanned in a similar manner. After the opposite ovary is scanned, the transducer is moved slowly back to the bifurcation and is rotated slightly in a back-and-forth motion across the uterine body and cervix as it is withdrawn from the rectum. This

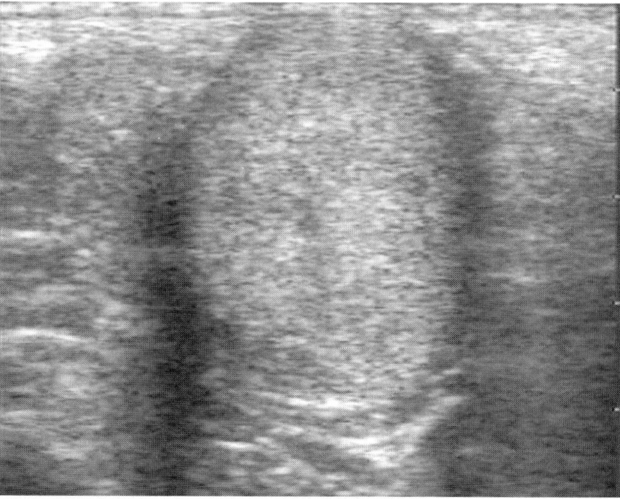

FIGURE 5-4. Transrectal ultrasound image of a cross-section through the base of a uterine horn.

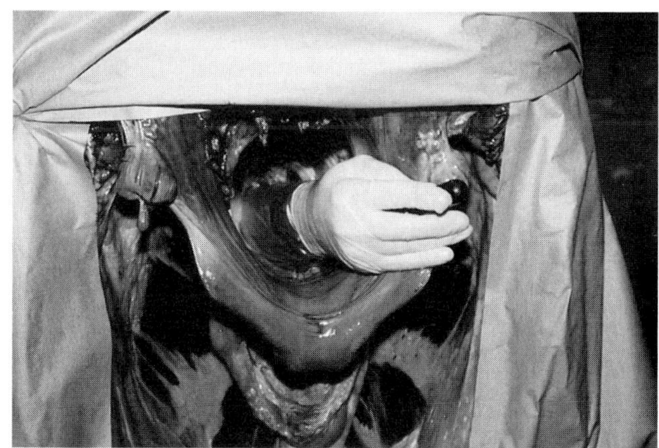

FIGURE 5-5. Examiner moving the ultrasound transducer to the tip of the uterine horn and ovary.

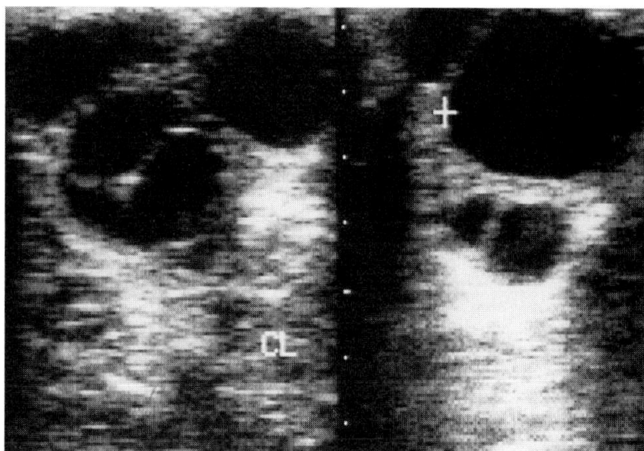

FIGURE 5-6. Ultrasonographic image of mare ovaries containing anechoic (black) follicles.

systematic scanning procedure ensures that the entire reproductive tract is examined twice, permitting accurate identification of the location of singleton or multiple pregnancies and uterine pathologic conditions, and provides assurance that any conceptus(es) was (were) not overlooked during the examination process.

Transabdominal ultrasonography allows maximum visualization of the fetus and placenta, sometimes beginning as early as 60 to 80 days of gestation. Linear, curvilinear, and sector transducers can be used. Sector transducers may be more useful during early pregnancy when accessibility of the uterus in the inguinal area is important. At later gestation times, it is usually helpful to use low-frequency transducers (2.5 to 3.5 MHz), because maximum penetration into the ventral abdomen is necessary. Clipping the skin closely from the xiphoid portion of the sternum to the udder and to the level of the lower flanks on either side of the midline will improve contact and thus image clarity. Application of ultrasound gel or alcohol is also helpful. The transducer is placed between the sternum and mare's udder for locating more advanced pregnancies and is then moved slowly from side to side and forward and backward until the fetus is located. Often, fetal membranes are visualized within intrauterine fluid that can be helpful in orientation. Fetal heart rate, movement, amount of fluid (amnionic/allantoic), uteroplacental thickness, and evidence of separation between the uterus and placenta are typically assessed to determine normalcy. Examination for two fetuses may be important to eliminate the possibility of twin pregnancy.

Diagnostic ultrasonography is used in the broodmare for (1) evaluation of ovarian activity, (2) detection and evaluation of pregnancy, and (3) diagnosis of pathologic changes in the reproductive tract. Transrectal ultrasonography is emphasized in this chapter; transabdominal ultrasonographic images are contained in Chapters 7 and 8.

EXAMINATION OF THE OVARIES

The ovaries of the mare are easily visualized by transrectal ultrasonography. The connective tissue stroma is uniformly echogenic (white). Follicles are fluid-filled and, hence, represented as circular or irregularly shaped anechoic (black) images on the ultrasound monitor (see Figure 5-6). The ultrasonic appearance of corpora lutea is variable and ranges from a uniformly hyperechoic image (Figure 5-7) to a heterogeneous or mottled image, where only a portion of the gland contains echogenic material. Because of their distinct border, many corpora lutea can be distinguished from the surrounding stroma throughout their life span.

Estimating the Stage of the Estrous Cycle by Ovarian Characteristics

Owing to the ease with which follicles and corpora lutea can be detected by transrectal ultrasonography, this technique can be used to approximate the stage of the estrous cycle in mares. One can also distinguish mares that exhibit reproductive cyclicity from those that are seasonally anestrous or in transitional estrus.

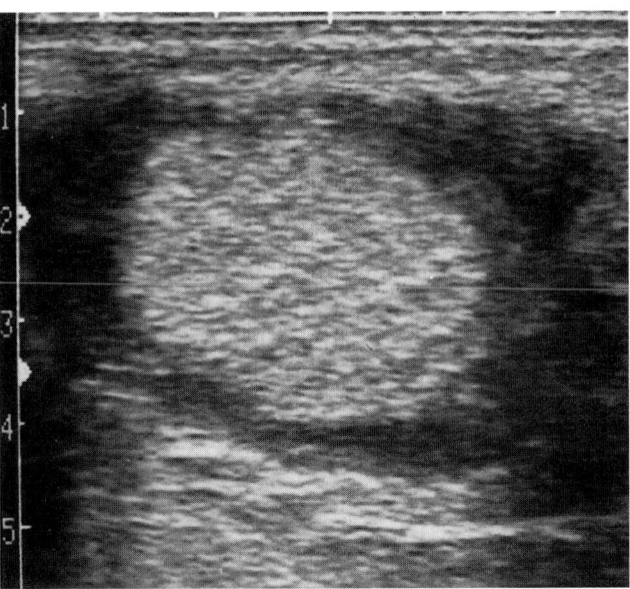

FIGURE 5-7. Ultrasonographic image of a mare ovary containing a hyperechoic (white) corpus luteum.

The advent of high-quality real-time ultrasound imaging has permitted detailed study of follicular dynamics in mares throughout the estrous cycle. Mares tend to have either one or two follicular waves during the estrous cycle, with one follicular wave being the most common pattern. In either case, the ovulatory follicle becomes ultrasonically identifiable approximately 10 to 12 days before ovulation (see Chapter 2). Diestrous follicles (i.e., large follicles detected while a functional corpus luteum is present) sometimes become quite large (e.g., >35 mm diameter), although the preovulatory follicle of estrus is generally the largest follicle of the estrous cycle.

Follicles destined to ovulate tend to grow rapidly (approximately 3 mm/day increase in mean diameter) beginning approximately 7 days before ovulation, with corresponding atresia of other follicles within the same follicular wave. If a 5-MHz transducer is used for the examination, corpora lutea tend to be identifiable throughout their functional life span (generally about 13 to 14 days). Occasionally, the gland remains ultrasonically visible through the following ovulation. Unless a clear border is visible around the corpus luteum, it may be difficult to differentiate between a corpus luteum and the ovarian stroma, both of which are echogenic. "Mare-side" progesterone assays can be of help in such cases. If the progesterone concentration in the blood is high, a functional corpus luteum must be present; if the progesterone concentration is low, the echogenic tissue in the ovary is more likely stroma or a regressed corpus luteum. When all of the ultrasonographic features of the ovarian structures are used in conjunction with the echotexture of the uterus and relaxation of the cervix, the stage of the estrous cycle can be predicted much more accurately than by palpation per rectum alone.

Ovarian inactivity (i.e., small ovaries with minimal or no follicular activity and no luteal structures) is typical of mares in seasonal **anestrus. Transitional estrus** is characterized by protracted and pronounced follicular activity (i.e., multiple follicles of varying size) in the absence of detectable corpora lutea, and the lack of a pronounced edematous appearance characteristic of the uterus and cervix seen during an ovulatory estrus.

Prediction or Detection of Ovulation

Using transrectal ultrasonography, the cross-sectional size and shape of follicles and the echogenicity of the follicular fluid can be used to aid in prediction of ovulation. The diameter of preovulatory follicles generally ranges from 40 to 50 mm. However, the size may be smaller, especially for double unilateral preovulatory follicles. Within 24 hours before ovulation, the shape of most, but not all, follicles tends to change from spherical to a conical or "pear" shape, and the follicular wall may become "scalloped" or thickened in appearance (Figure 5-8). The apex of the conical follicle will be located at the ovulation fossa. Occasionally, the echogenicity of the follicular fluid will increase slightly just before ovulation, but this is not a reliable indicator of impending ovulation.

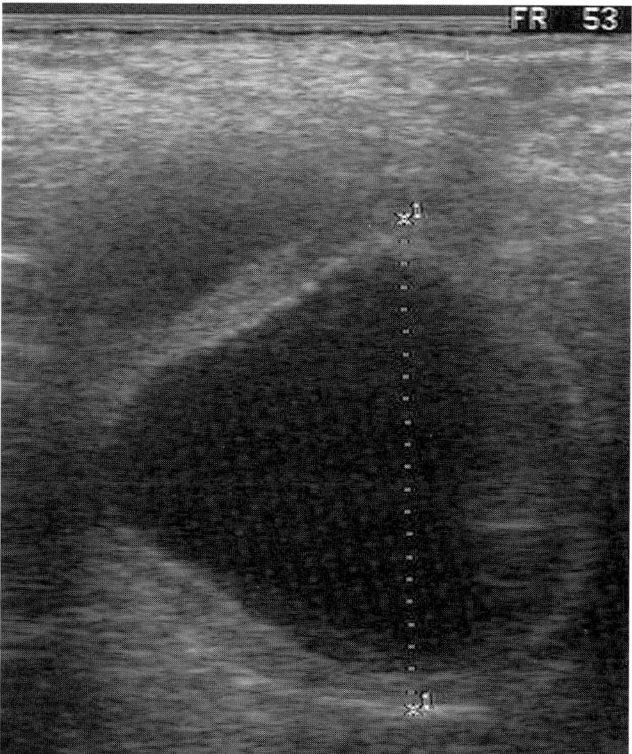

FIGURE 5-8. Ultrasonographic image of a typical preovulatory follicle (within 1 day before ovulation). In contrast to the follicles seen in Figure 5-6, note the thickened borders of the follicular wall, loss of round shape, and conical appearance near the center of the ovary (i.e., near the ovulation fossa).

At the time of ovulation, follicular fluid may be discharged either abruptly or gradually (i.e., within a 1- to 7-minute period). The echogenicity of the follicle changes from a predominantly anechoic appearance to a heterogeneous echotexture as the fluid is released and luteal development begins. The developing corpus luteum usually contains a small anechoic center resulting from retained follicular fluid or blood or, alternatively, may retain variable echolucent areas within or surrounding it for several days. Rarely, regressing follicles may collapse without subsequently forming a corpus luteum.

Ultrasonic examination of a mare's ovaries during the periovulatory period ensures precise determination of the number, location, size, and shape of ovarian follicles. In contrast with palpation per rectum, the ultrasonographic method can accurately detect multiple ovulations of adjacent follicles on a single ovary.

Diagnosis of Pathologic Conditions

Ultrasonography has been useful for diagnosis of various ovarian abnormalities.

Anovulation. This is a common and normal phenomenon during transitional estrus in the spring or fall; however, it occurs less commonly during the ovulatory season and is considered abnormal during that time. The cause of anovulation during the ovulatory season is not known. Although some anovulatory follicles simply seem to regress, they more commonly are considered to be hemorrhagic preovulatory follicles and are usually characterized ultrasonographically as large (6- to 10-cm) follicular (hypoechoic) structures that gradually begin to show echogenic specks within the follicular antrum. They may have a highly echogenic rim, possibly associated with some luteinization of the follicular wall (Figure 5-9). Maximum size is usually reached during this apparent "consolidation" process. After the structure ceases to grow, organization becomes apparent with "fibrinous" strands appearing within the cavity (Figure 5-10), and the hemorrhagic follicle slowly decreases in size over a 3- to 6-week period until it is nonapparent.

Whether hemorrhagic follicles are more common in mares with normally appearing follicles that are treated with human chorionic gonadotropin (hCG) is not known at present. In a discussion of these structures, Ginther (1992) suggested that they may be associated with deficient estrogen production because uterine echotexture during the estrus in which they develop is often reduced or absent. He also stated that, in some instances, hemorrhagic follicles that occur during the breeding season are associated with prolonged interovulatory intervals and may be associated with low levels of progesterone production. Clinical experience suggests that once hemorrhagic follicles have formed they do not predictably respond to treatment with either hCG or deslorelin by either ovulating or organizing into an luteal structure as seen

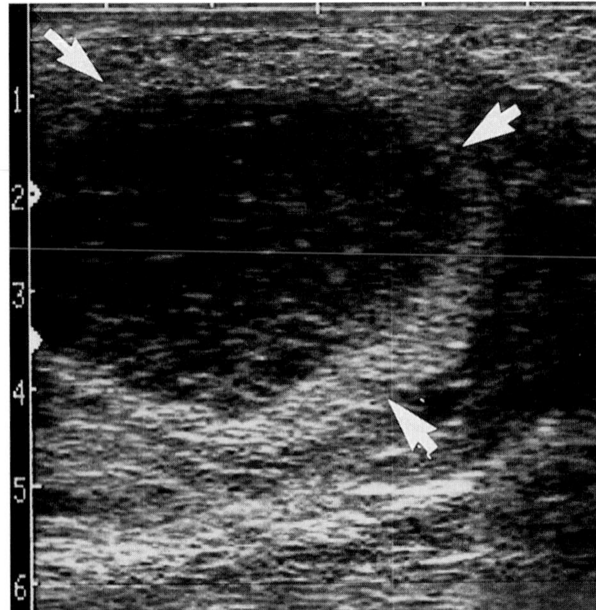

FIGURE 5-9. Ultrasonographic image of a hemorrhagic anovulatory follicle. Fluid in the follicle is slightly echogenic *(white speckling)* and the follicular wall *(arrows)* is greatly thickened.

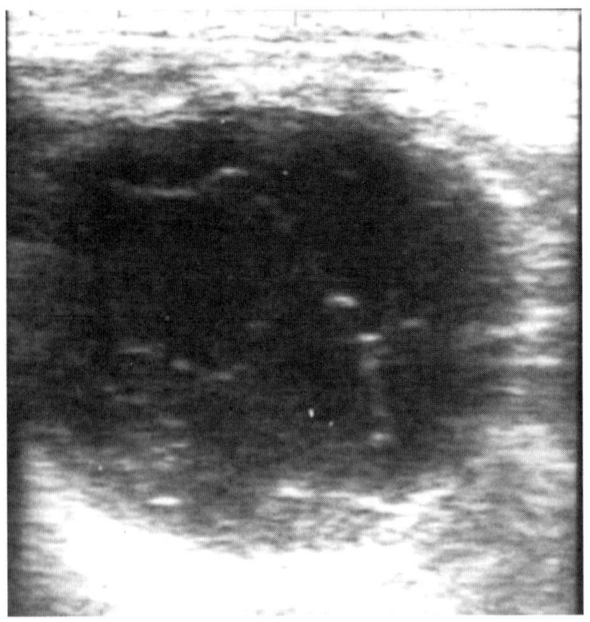

FIGURE 5-10. Ultrasonographic image of a hemorrhagic follicle that has become more "fibrinous" in appearance.

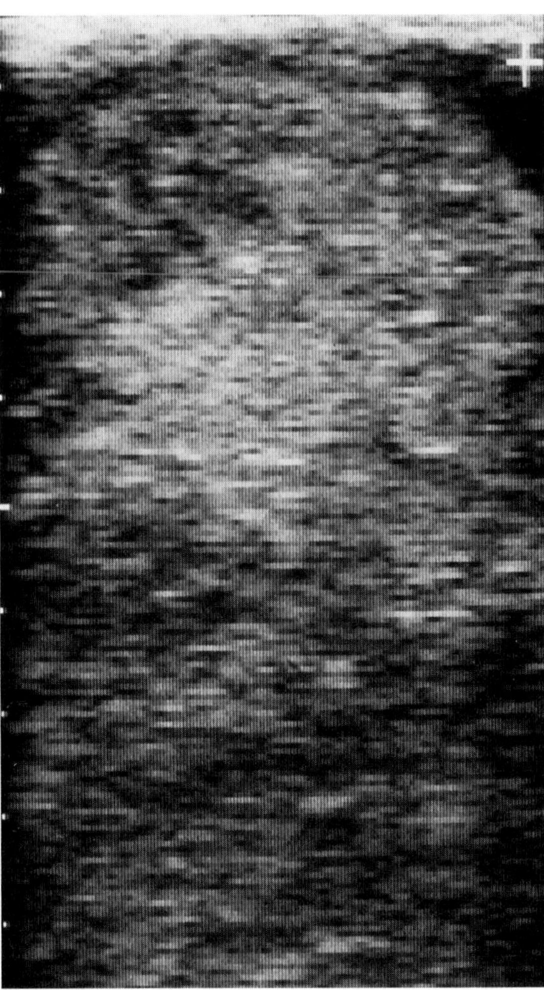

FIGURE 5-11. Ultrasonographic image of a large ovarian hematoma. Hematomas typically appear with a mottled or "spiderweb" pattern. Corpora hemorrhagica and corpora lutea sometimes also have this ultrasonographic appearance, but they are not as large as ovarian hematomas and they become echogenic as a result of organization much sooner than ovarian hematomas.

ultrasonographically. We have also noted that in some mares in which hemorrhagic follicles develop during the breeding season, the level of progesterone production is low, and predicting a response to prostaglandin $F_{2\alpha}$ administration is unreliable. Most descriptions of their occurrence and subsequent extension of the interovulatory interval are anecdotal. Further investigation of their cause and occurrence is indicated before effective methods of treatment can be devised.

Ovarian Hematoma. Ovulation tends to be a hemorrhagic event in the mare; hence hematomas sometimes develop on the ovary, presumably at the time of ovulation (see Figure 4-4). Affected ovaries sometimes are quite large (e.g., 10 to 30 cm in diameter), although smaller hematomas are probably more common. When the ovary rapidly fills with blood and ovarian tissue becomes dwarfed in comparison, its ultrasonographic appearance is initially hypoechoic. As the blood clots, the echotexture first becomes "fibrinous" or "honeycombed" and eventually becomes mottled to be heterogeneous in pattern (Figure 5-11). Regression of large ovarian hematomas is slower than that of anovulatory hemorrhagic follicles, and sometimes it takes months for the ovary to return to its normal size and ultrasonographic appearance. Mares usually continue to have

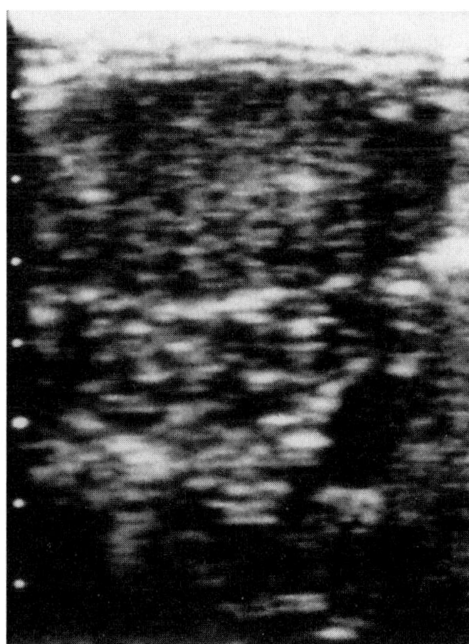

FIGURE 5-12. Ultrasonographic image of an anestrous ovary, devoid of developing follicles or corpora lutea.

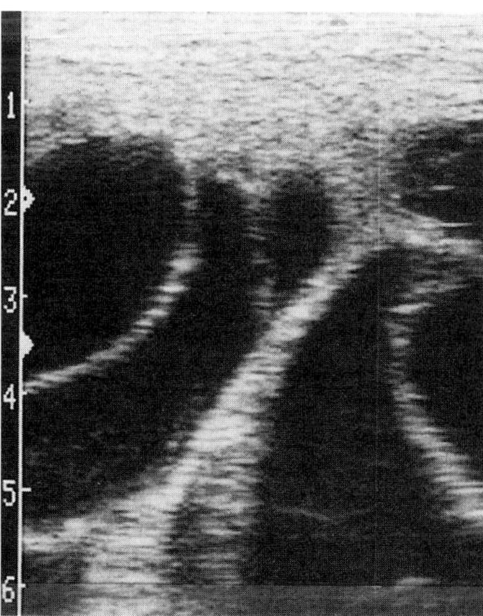

FIGURE 5-13. Ultrasonographic image of a multicystic granulosa cell tumor of mare ovary illustrating "honeycomb" appearance. The tumor was too large to permit complete visualization with a 5-MHz probe.

regular estrous cycles even though ovarian hematomas are present.

The effects of ovarian hematomas on fertility are not well documented. Large ovarian hematomas tend to pull the uterus into a pendant position, which might interfere with uterine motility and thus maternal recognition of pregnancy, thereby causing embryonic death. Large ovarian hematomas might also interfere with oocyte pick up by the associated fimbria, which would result in failure of the mare to become pregnant. We have observed smaller ovarian hematomas (8 to 12 cm in diameter) in mares that became pregnant and maintained pregnancy to term. No treatment is generally necessary for ovarian hematomas. They must be differentiated from ovarian tumors, which usually do interfere with fertility.

Inactive Ovaries. Ovarian activity normally subsides as mares enter seasonal anestrus. Inactive ovaries are also observed in prepubertal fillies and sexually senescent mares. Ovarian inactivity of a pathologic nature primarily results from malnutrition or abnormalities involving the sex chromosomes. Malnutrition or lactational anestrus leads to ovarian atrophy, whereas chromosomal abnormalities usually result in profound ovarian hypoplasia. Ovarian inactivity is characterized by small (4 × 3 × 3 cm or less) echodense stroma with few (very small) or no follicles visible by ultrasonographic imaging (Figure 5-12). Profound ovarian hypoplasia (≤1 to 2 cm in diameter) caused by sex chromosome abnormalities can be confirmed by karyotyping studies. The most commonly identified sex chromosome abnormality associated with this condition is Turner's syndrome (63 X,O).

Ovarian Neoplasia. Ovarian neoplasia is rather common in mares, with granulosa-thecal cell tumors (see Figure 4-3) and teratomas being detected most often. The ultrasonographic appearance of granulosa-thecal cell tumors varies, depending on their structure and composition. They may be uniformly echogenic (if the tumor is solid), heterogeneous with a honeycomb appearance (if the tumor is multicystic) (Figure 5-13), or largely hypoechoic or anechoic (if the tumor consists primarily of a single fluid-filled cyst). Hypoechoic or anechoic granulosa cell tumors are usually quite large with a thick (up to 1 to 2 cm), echodense wall and are sometimes stippled with echogenic material (probably clotted blood, because the tumors are highly vascularized). The ultrasonographic characteristics of granulosa-thecal cell tumors are too inconsistent to enable definitive identification, but they may aid in narrowing the differential diagnoses when used in conjunction with other diagnostic measures (e.g., historical findings and evaluation of the contralateral ovary, which is typically atrophied and inactive, and hormonal assay). The ultrasonographic characteristics of teratomas may mimic those of granulosa-thecal cell tumors, unless the tumor contains highly echogenic components such as cartilage, teeth, or bone (Figure 5-14). Demonstration of high testosterone and/or inhibin concentrations in hormonal assays from a mare with an enlarged, firm ovary and atrophy of the contralateral ovary will confirm the diagnosis of granulosa-thecal cell tumor.

Treatment for an ovarian tumor is surgical removal of the affected ovary. After removal of a secretory granulosa-cell tumor, most, but not all, mares will begin having regular estrous cycles during the next breeding season.

EVALUATION OF THE TUBULAR TRACT

Although the oviducts cannot be easily detected using a 5-MHz transrectal transducer, the remainder of the tubular

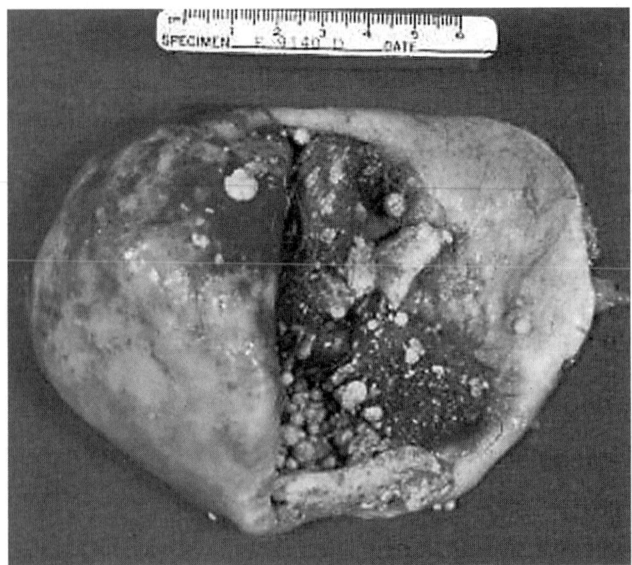

FIGURE 5-14. Ovarian teratoma of a mare ovary. The mare could produce a foal when ovulating from the other ovary. Ultrasonographic appearance of the teratoma was multicystic with "bright" hyperechoic areas present within the parenchyma. Hair, cartilage, and bone were found within the ovarian stroma.

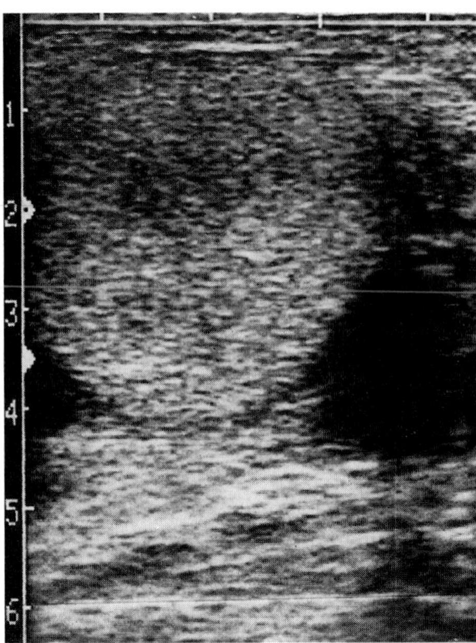

FIGURE 5-15. Ultrasonographic image of a cross section of a uterine horn of a mare in diestrus. The echotexture is homogeneous and nonedematous.

tract can usually be imaged in its entirety. The exception is a uterus that is greatly enlarged as a result of (1) incomplete involution during the early postpartum period, (2) advanced pregnancy, or (3) pathologic conditions (e.g., pyometra, mucometra, or large endometrial-lymphatic cysts or leiomyomas). In these instances, only a portion of the uterus can be viewed because of incomplete penetration of sound waves emanating from the transducer. With a linear-array transducer, the uterine horns are typically scanned in a transverse (cross-sectional) plane, and the uterine body and cervix are scanned in a longitudinal plane.

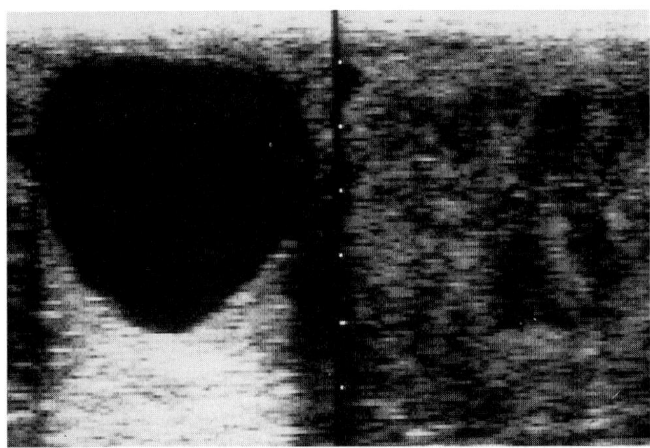

FIGURE 5-16. Ultrasonographic appearance of a cross section of a uterine horn and an ovary containing a 45-mm-diameter follicle of a mare in estrus. Note the edematous (hypoechoic), "starfish-like" appearance of the uterine horn cross-sectional image, which is caused by accumulation of fluid within the edematous endometrial folds.

Estimating the Stage of the Estrous Cycle by Uterine Characteristics

Uterine echotexture can be used to differentiate diestrus (i.e., the luteal or progesterone-dominated phase of the estrous cycle) and estrus (i.e., the follicular or estrogen-dominated phase of the estrous cycle). The diestrus uterus is characterized by a relatively *homogeneous echotexture* (Figure 5-15). The uterine lumen and endometrial folds are not discernible during diestrus (approximately days 2 to 3 through days 14 to 16 postovulation during the breeding season). A bright reflection (white line) often identifies the lumen of the uterus viewed in longitudinal section during diestrus. During estrus, the endometrial folds become prominent and the uterus has a very *heterogeneous appearance* (i.e., a mixture of hyperechoic and hypoechoic areas). This ultrasonic pattern results from edema within the endometrium and, occasionally, free fluid within the uterine lumen. A characteristic "starfish" pattern may be evident in cross-sectional images of the uterine horns of mares in estrus (Figure 5-16). The degree of uterine heterogenicity (i.e., endometrial edema) tends to peak approximately 1 to 3 days before ovulation and begins to decrease within a day preceding ovulation, and a homogeneous uterine echotexture typical of diestrus is restored within 1 to 3 days after ovulation. Changes from homogeneous to heterogeneous patterns (and vice versa) are more gradual during the fall months in mares that are still having regular estrous cycles.

The cervix of mares in diestrus is well demarcated, hyperechoic, and contracted. During estrus it becomes less distinct and relaxed, and loses some of its echogenicity. The cervical lumen is more likely to be visualized ultrasonographically during estrus than during diestrus.

DIAGNOSIS AND EVALUATION OF PREGNANCY BY TRANSRECTAL ULTRASONOGRAPHIC EXAMINATION

One of the first uses of diagnostic ultrasound in mares was early pregnancy detection. With a high-quality ultrasound unit equipped with a 5- to 8-MHz transrectal transducer, embryonic vesicles can be detected within the uterine lumen as early as 9 to 10 days postovulation. The embryo proper is visible by days 20 to 21 postovulation, and the heartbeat of the embryo is discernible ultrasonically by days 24 to 26 postovulation. The sex of the fetus can also sometimes be determined; the optimal time for sex determination is days 60 to 70 postovulation. At this stage of gestation, the location of the *genital tubercle* can be used to aid in differentiating the sex of the fetus. The genital tubercle is under the tail of the female fetus and just behind the umbilical cord of the male fetus. Estimation of conceptus age during early pregnancy (i.e., days 10 to 50 postovulation) can be made using the above information in addition to the following:

- Size and shape of the embryonic vesicle (Figures 5-17 through 5-19).
- Location and fixation of the embryonic vesicle within the uterine lumen. The embryonic vesicle typically becomes fixed at the base of one uterine horn approximately 16 days postovulation (see Figure 5-18).
- Percentage of the embryonic vesicle occupied by yolk versus allantoic fluid (e.g., the allantois occupies 25% of the vesicle at 25 to 26 days; 50% of the vesicle at 28 to 30 days; 75% of the vesicle at 34 to 36 days; and nearly 100% of the vesicle at 38 to 40 days) (Figures 5-20 through 5-23).
- Location of the embryo (or fetus) within the vesicle (e.g., the embryo is located ventral in the vesicle at 21 days

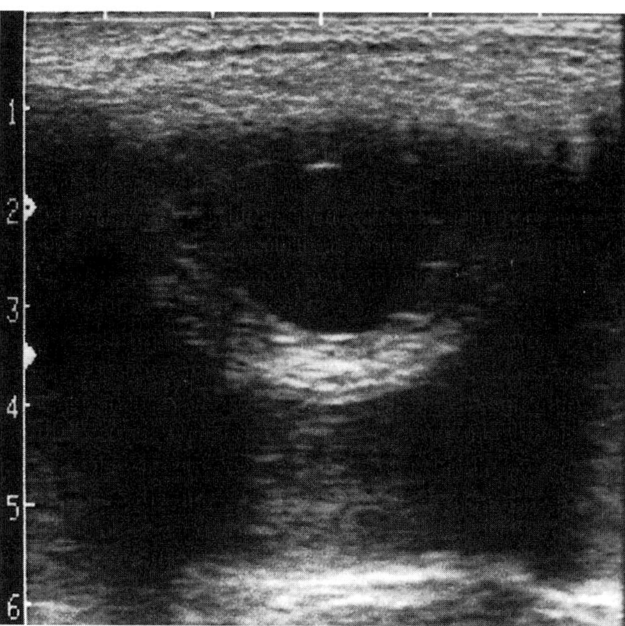

FIGURE 5-17. Transrectal ultrasonographic image of an equine pregnancy 12 days after ovulation. The pregnancy is located in a uterine horn in this mare but can be located anywhere throughout the uterus during the prefixation stage, often being found in the body of the uterus.

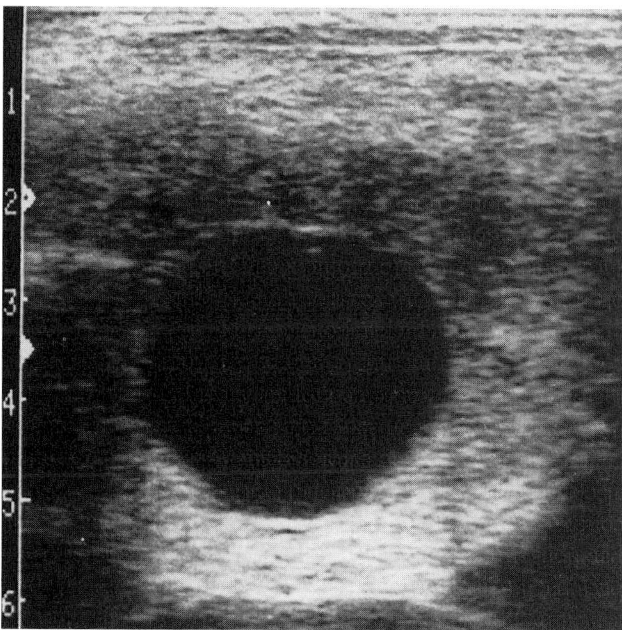

FIGURE 5-18. Transrectal ultrasonographic image of an equine pregnancy 16 days after ovulation. The pregnancy is located at the base of the uterine horn and is round.

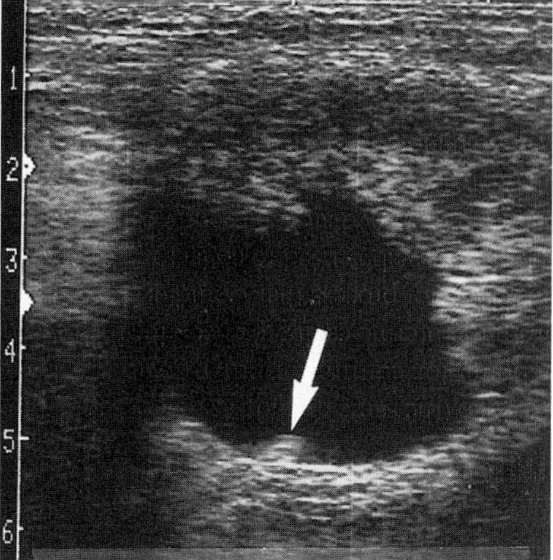

FIGURE 5-19. Transrectal ultrasonographic image of an equine pregnancy 21 days after ovulation. The pregnancy is located at the base of the uterine horn and is no longer round, gaining a triangular or "guitar pick" shape caused by hypertrophy of the dorsal uterine wall. The embryo proper *(arrow)* can be visualized at the base of this vesicle.

and rises to a dorsal position by 38 days; the fetus then descends to a ventral position by 45 to 50 days) (Figures 5-20 through 5-25).

Our understanding of events during early pregnancy in the mare (e.g., the role of conceptus mobility in maternal recognition of pregnancy, the incidence of twin pregnancy [both unicornuate and bicornuate], embryonic development, and natural mechanisms involved in twin elimination) is markedly improved as a result of transrectal ultrasonography. This new knowledge has led to advancements in breeding management and to improved methods for manual reduction of twin pregnancies to singleton pregnancies. Better ways for assessing conceptus viability may now also be used.

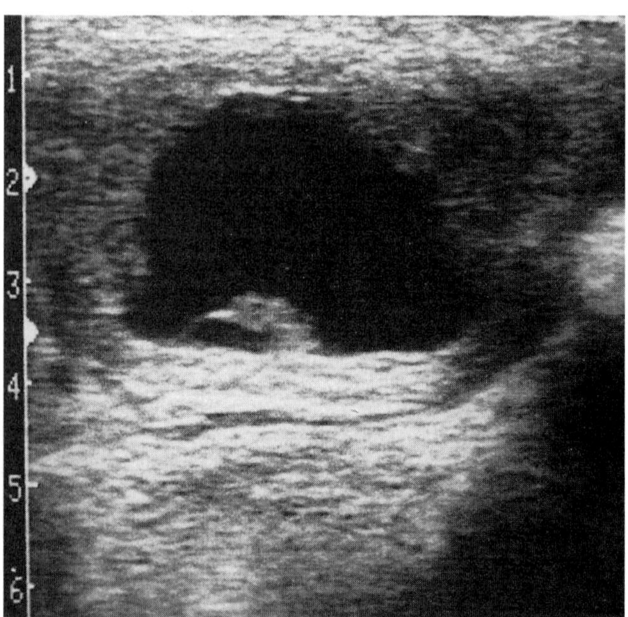

FIGURE 5-20. Transrectal ultrasonographic image of an equine pregnancy 22 days after ovulation. The embryo can be visualized at the bottom of the embryonic vesicle, and the allantois is beginning development.

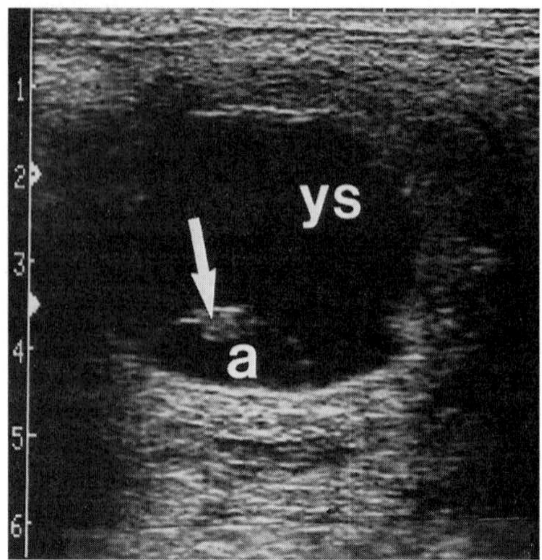

FIGURE 5-21. Transrectal ultrasonographic image of an equine pregnancy 26 days after ovulation. The embryo *(arrow)* and allantois *(a)* occupies the bottom portion of the vesicle, whereas the yolk sac *(ys)* occupies the top portion.

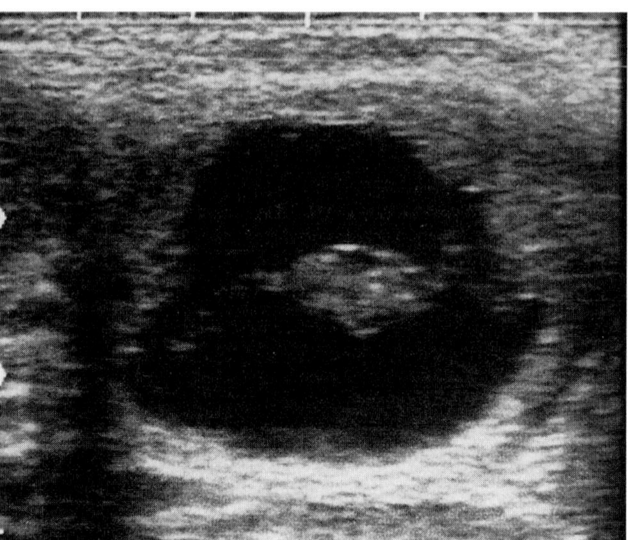

FIGURE 5-22. Transrectal ultrasonographic image of an equine pregnancy 28 days after ovulation. The embryo is positioned at the center of the vesicle, with the regressing yolk sac located above and the developing allantois located below.

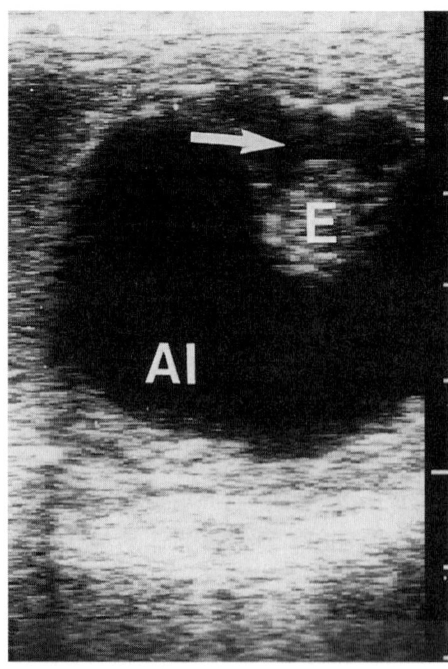

FIGURE 5-23. Transrectal ultrasonographic image of an equine pregnancy 36 days after ovulation. The embryo *(E)* is positioned near the top of the vesicle, and the yolk sac *(arrow)* is mostly resorbed. The allantois *(Al)* occupies the greatest portion of the vesicle at this time.

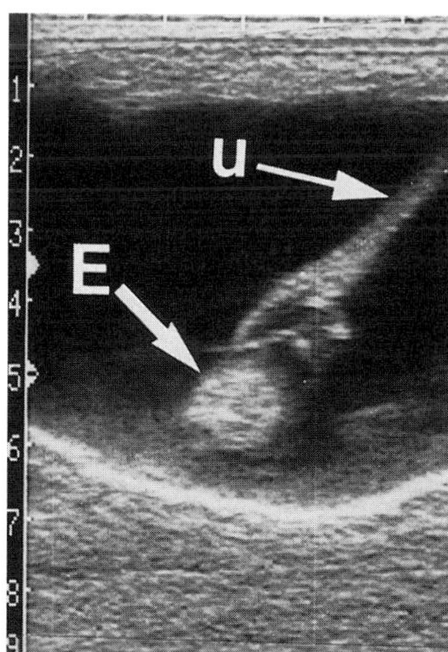

FIGURE 5-24. Transrectal ultrasonographic image of an equine pregnancy 47 days after ovulation. The embryo *(E)* is positioned near the bottom of the vesicle, and the umbilicus *(U)* is prominent.

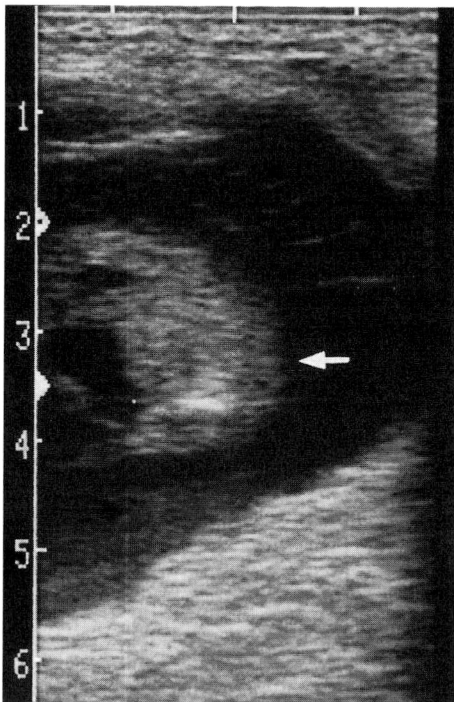

FIGURE 5-25. Transrectal ultrasonographic image of an equine pregnancy at 52 days after ovulation. A sagittal view of the fetus *(arrow)* can be visualized within the amnion. The head, neck, trunk, one forelimb, and two hindlimbs are shown.

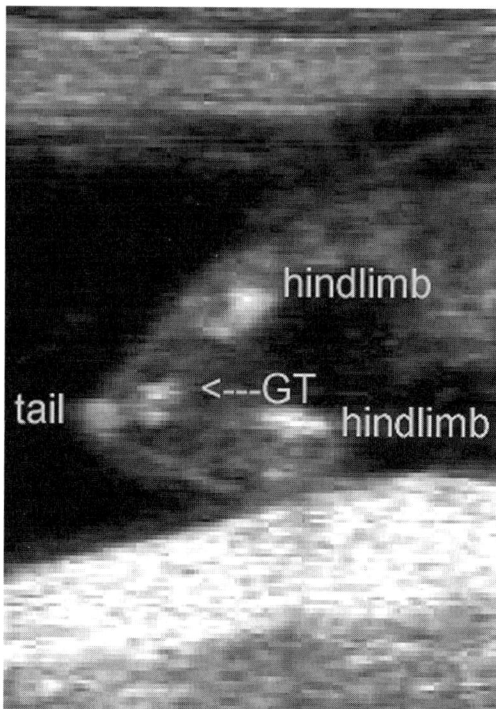

FIGURE 5-26. Transrectal ultrasonographic image of a 65-day-old filly fetus. The genital tubercle *(GT)* represents the clitoris and is located within the triangle formed by the coccygeal vertebrae of the tail and the long bones of the two hindlimbs.

DETERMINATION OF FETAL GENDER BY TRANSRECTAL ULTRASONOGRAPHY

In the past 10 years, transrectal ultrasonography has been increasingly used to determine the gender of the fetus ("fetal sexing"). Considerable study and practice are required to become proficient in this technique. The ability to determine fetal gender with this method is based on assessing the location of the **genital tubercle,** which is the embryonic process that differentiates into either the **penis** (male) or **clitoris** (female). As differentiation progresses, associated structures (i.e., the **prepuce** in the male, which is identifiable by gross inspection by day 77 and pendulous by day 115 of gestation; **vulvar lips** in the female, which begin extending dorsally from the clitoris by 55 days of gestation) develop sufficiently to lend additional echogenic patterns that aid in determining location of the genital tubercle. The undifferentiated genital tubercle is located between the hindlimbs midway between the anus and umbilicus. As fetal growth occurs, the genital tubercle becomes relatively closer to the umbilicus in males or to the anus in females. The ideal time for determining fetal gender by transrectal ultrasonography is between 60 and 70 days of gestation, when the genital tubercle location is sufficiently obvious to reduce the incidence of mistaken diagnoses (Figures 5-26 and 5-27). Determination of fetal gender is possible by transrectal ultrasonography beyond 70 days of gestation (Figure 5-28), but because of the size and location of the enlarging pregnancy, proper imaging of the desired area of the fetus becomes increasingly difficult. However, other organs develop sufficiently to aid in gender determination beyond 80 to 115 days of gestation (e.g., mammary buds, prepuce, and scrotum).

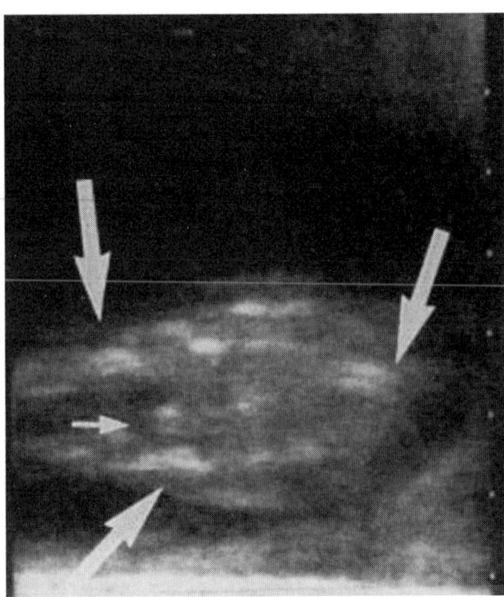

FIGURE 5-27. Transrectal ultrasonographic image of a male fetus 65 days after breeding. The genital tubercle *(small arrow)* represents the prepuce/penis and is located between the hocks of the two hindlimbs and the tailhead *(large arrows)*.

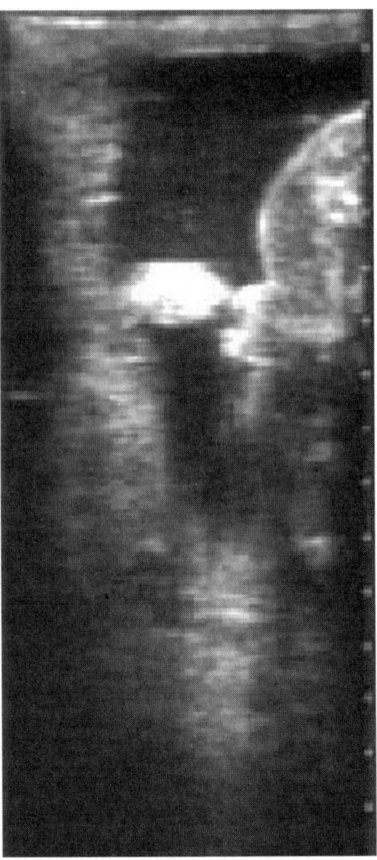

FIGURE 5-28. Transrectal ultrasonographic image of a female fetus 193 days postovulation. The fetus lies on its side, with the tail, labia, and buttocks visible (from *left to right*) in this image.

DIAGNOSIS OF PATHOLOGIC UTERINE CONDITIONS BY TRANSRECTAL ULTRASONOGRAPHY

Ultrasongraphy has been quite useful in the diagnosis of uterine cysts and pathologic fluid accumulations within the uterine lumen. Other pathologic conditions (e.g., leiomyomas, abscesses, and periuterine masses) may also be examined ultrasonically, but their incidence is low.

Uterine Cysts

Uterine cysts that can be identified ultrasonically are generally of lymphatic origin and are more commonly located in the endometrium than in other uterine layers. Lymphatic cysts range in size from microscopic to several centimeters in diameter, and cysts as small 2 to 5 mm can oftentimes be detected with a 5- to 8-MHz transducer. They can be unilocular or multilocular (Figures 5-29 and 5-30), with the larger cysts obviously protruding into the uterine lumen. The cysts are anechoic, but they can have hyperechoic trabeculae if they are compartmentalized. The incidence of endometrial cysts in mares is fairly high (possibly 10% to 15% and up to 27%), being more common in mares older than 10 years. Although cysts may be located anywhere within the uterus, they may be predisposed to develop in the ventral surfaces of the corpus cornual junctions.

The presence of endometrial cysts is important because (1) they can be mistaken for an embryonic vesicle during early pregnancy examinations and (2) they may increase pregnancy wastage, especially if sufficiently numerous or large enough to

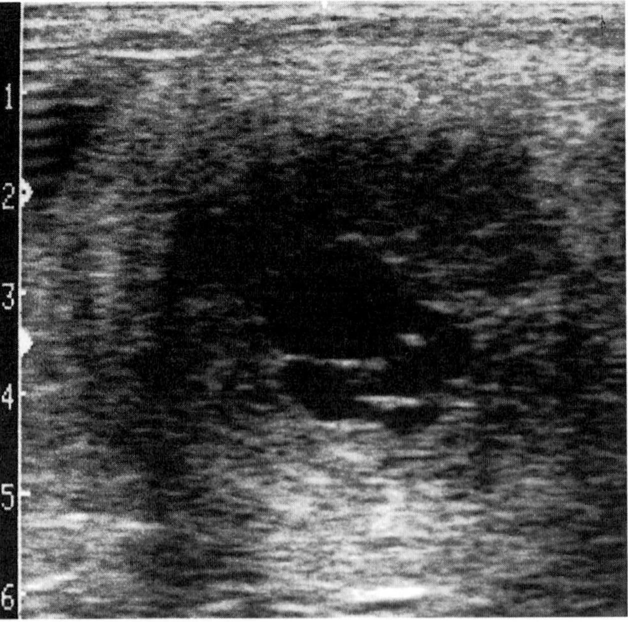

FIGURE 5-29. Ultrasonographic image of a multilocular uterine lymphatic cyst in the uterus of a mare.

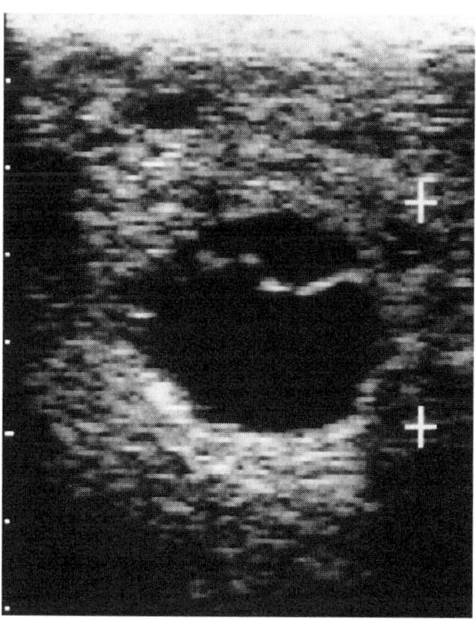

FIGURE 5-30. Ultrasonographic image of a two-chambered lymphatic cyst in the uterine horn of a mare. The structure mimics an equine pregnancy except that an embryo proper is not present.

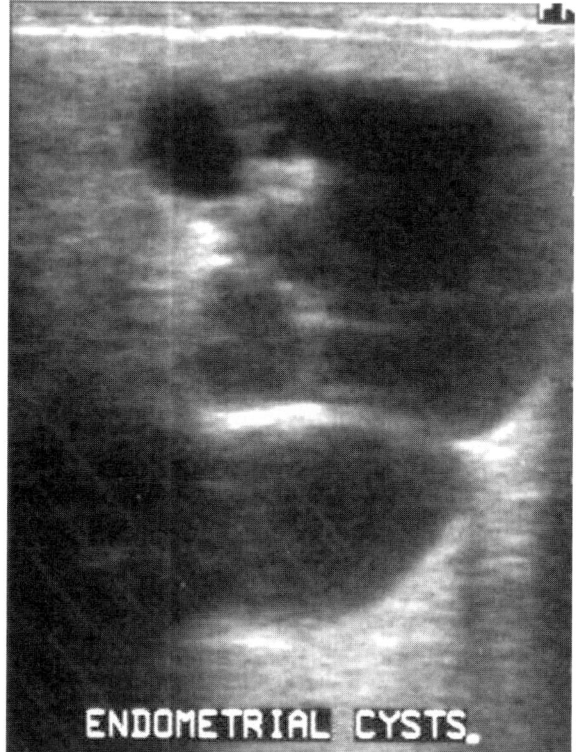

FIGURE 5-31. Ultrasonographic image of a large (5 cm) compartmentalized uterine cyst, adjacent to smaller cysts, located at the base of a uterine horn in a mare. Such a large cyst may interfere with embryo mobility and result in failure to maintain pregnancy, may interfere with ability of the inseminate to reach the oviductal papillae, thereby preventing fertilization, or may prevent uterine flushing to effectively remove an embryo-for-embryo transfer.

interfere with conceptus mobility (Figure 5-31) or placental-endometrial interaction.

Whether endometrial cysts depress fertility in the absence of other uterine pathologic conditions remains controversial. Ginther (1986) suggested that single cysts and groups of small cysts do not adversely affect fertility. A subsequent Wisconsin study found a tendency for mares with more than five cysts or cyst(s) larger than 1 cm in diameter to have lower 40-day pregnancy rates than mares with smaller or fewer cysts. Louisiana workers recently reported that in 215 Thoroughbred mares, the number and size of cysts were unrelated to the ability of mares to become pregnant or to maintain their pregnancy to term. We have certainly noted that some mares presented for examination because of failure either to become detectably pregnant or maintain pregnancy have numerous endometrial cysts of varying size without accompanying severe changes in endometrial biopsy specimens.

Until further research better characterizes the potential adverse effects of endometrial cysts on fertility, we make the following recommendations concerning treatment: (1) treatment of endometrial cysts is seldom necessary if cysts are small (≤2 to 3 cm in diameter) and few (fewer than five located throughout the uterus), and if they are not grouped together at the corporocornual junction; and (2) other potential causes of fertility problems have been eliminated. Although the relationship between lymphatic lacunae and endometrial cysts remains conjectural, if extensive pooling of lymphatic fluid in the endometrium (we recommend examining biopsies from each uterine horn, which show many widespread, medium to large lymphatic lacunae) is present, we believe the mare is a poor candidate for treatment (i.e., because cysts seem to be more likely to recur).

If cyst removal is elected, it can be done through an endoscope. A pedunculated cyst can be removed by use of a snare passed through the biopsy channel and looped around

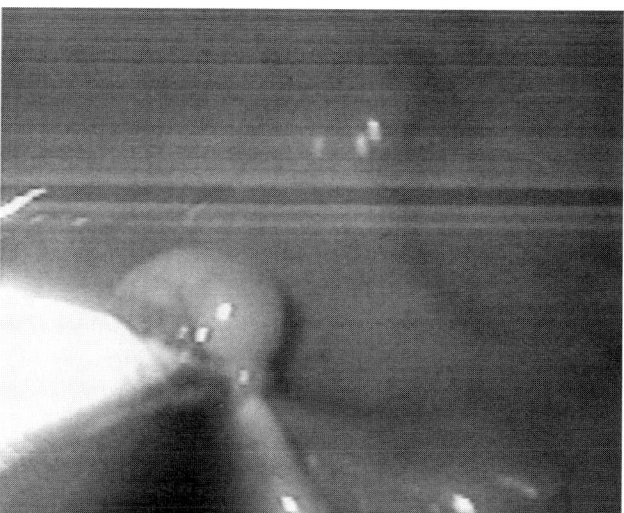

FIGURE 5-32. Endoscopic view of an endometrial cyst being removed by YAG laser surgery.

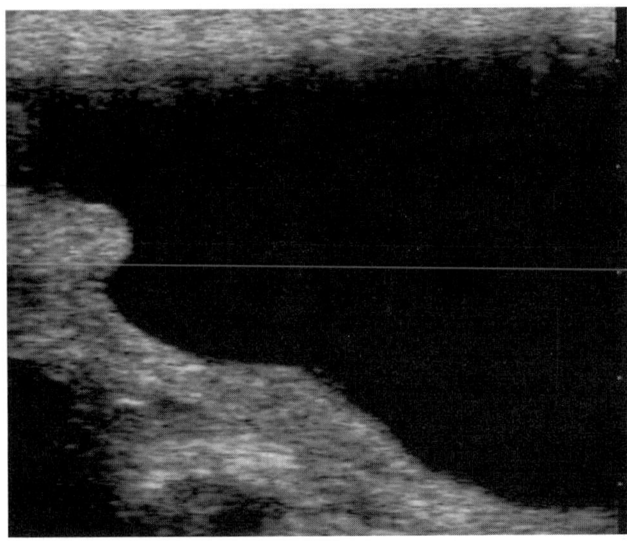

FIGURE 5-33. Ultrasonographic image of anechoic fluid present within the uterine lumen.

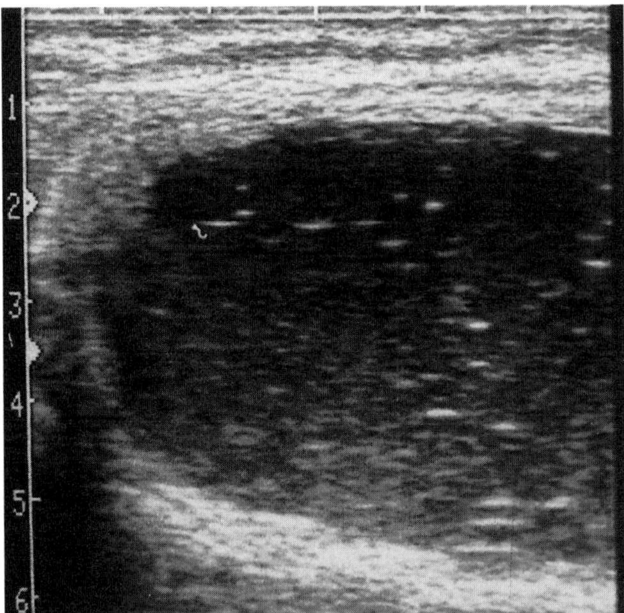

FIGURE 5-34. Ultrasonographic image of intrauterine fluid accumulation in a mare. Note the intermediate echogenicity of the fluid, suggesting the presence of inflammatory products and debris.

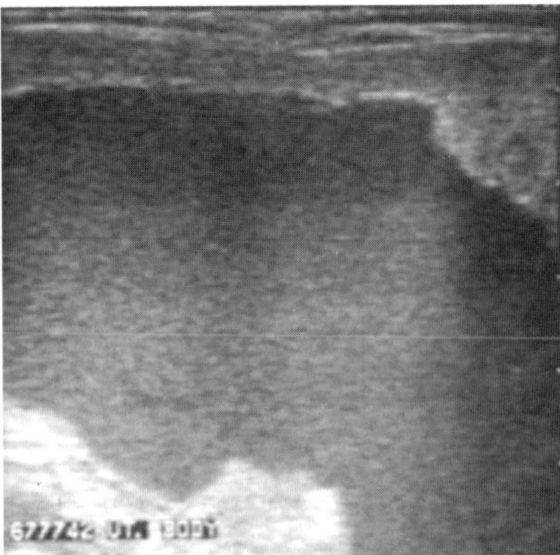

FIGURE 5-35. Ultrasonographic image of pyometra in a mare. Note the hyperechoic nature of the fluid. No fetus or fetal membranes were detected.

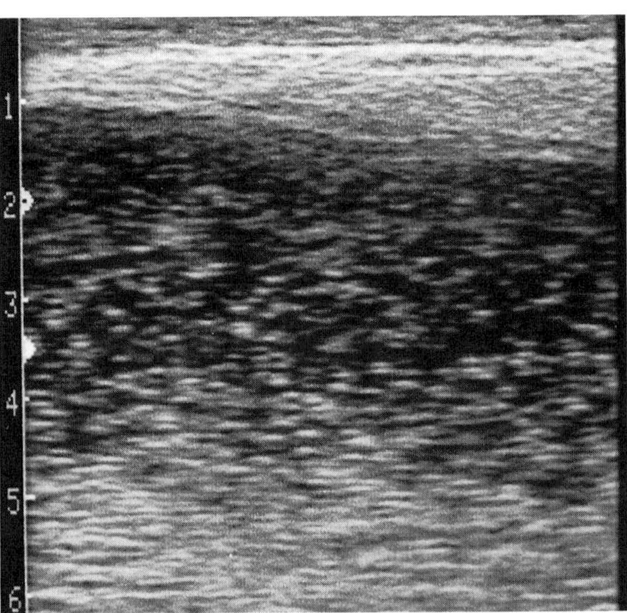

FIGURE 5-36. Contents of the urinary bladder can sometimes be confused with uterine contents during an ultrasonographic examination.

the base. If a cyst is located just cranial to the cervix, blind transcervical removal of the cyst may be performed with either a snare or biopsy punch guided by a finger through the cervix. When nonpedunculated cysts are present, which is commonly the case, yttrium-aluminum-garnet (YAG) laser surgical removal via endoscopy is recommended. The cysts are lysed and sufficient tissue in the wall of the cysts is burned (taking care not to damage the rest of the endometrium) until necrosis and sloughing of the cyst is ensured (Figure 5-32). Postsurgical uterine lavage and infusion of broad-spectrum antimicrobial agents are recommended at intervals for up to 1 week to minimize the chance of development of intraluminal adhesions, to remove sloughed necrotic cyst tissue, and to prevent infection. Because underlying uterine problems may be contributing to further cyst formation, treated mares should be bred as soon as possible after endometrial healing.

Uterine Intraluminal Fluid Accumulations

A small amount of anechoic free fluid is sometimes detected within the uterine lumen of reproductively normal mares during estrus. It has generally been thought that if the volume of fluid is large (i.e., 1 to 3 cm or greater height of luminal distension) or echogenic (Figures 5-33 and 5-34; see also

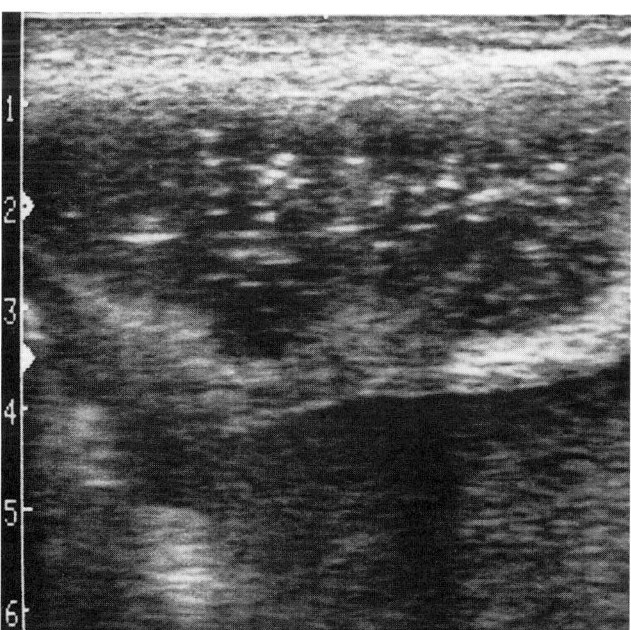

FIGURE 5-37. Numerous hyperechoic "flecks" in the uterine body can be indicative of pneumouterus (air within the uterus) and should be differentiated from pyometra.

Figure 6-4), it is considered abnormal. However, it is possible that even lesser accumulations of anechoic fluid during diestrus or particularly during the immediate postovulation period could adversely affect fertility. Wisconsin workers have demonstrated that any free fluid within the uterine lumen during diestrus should be considered abnormal and is associated with reduced pregnancy rates and increased embryonic losses. Such fluid accumulations are indicative of **endometritis** (perhaps identifying mares inefficient at mechanically evacuating the uterus; see Chapter 6) and should be treated accordingly. The degree of fluid echogenicity is related to its concentration of inflammatory cells and debris. Pyometra or mucometra can also be easily distinguished from advanced pregnancy with ultrasonography because of their lack of hypoechoic or anechoic appearance and the failure to detect an embryo/fetus, umbilicus, or fetal membranes (Figure 5-35). The contents of the urinary bladder can sometimes be confused with uterine contents with transrectal ultrasonography, so it is imperative to distinguish between the two organs when the examination is performed (Figure 5-36).

Pneumouterus

Hyperechoic areas in the uterus may be an indication of pneumouterus (air in the uterus) (Figure 5-37). If the condition is not associated with examination or treatment procedures that resulted in entry of air into the uterus, pneumovagina and/or cervical incompetency should be suspected. Treatment measures for pneumouterus caused by pneumovagina or cervical incompetency are surgical.

BIBLIOGRAPHY

Adams GP, et al: Effect of uterine inflammation and ultrasonically detected uterine pathology on fertility in the mare. *J Reprod Fertil* 35(Suppl): 445-454, 1987.

Curran S, Ginther OJ: Ultrasonic diagnosis of equine fetal sex by location of the genital tubercle. *J Equine Vet Sci* 9:77-83, 1989.

Curran S: Fetal gender determination. In Rantanen NW, McKinnon AO, editors, *Equine diagnostic ultrasonography*, Baltimore, 1998, Williams & Wilkins.

Eilts BE, et al: Prevalence of endometrial cysts and their effect on fertility. *Biol Reprod Monogr* 1:527-532, 1995.

Ginther OJ: *Ultrasonic imaging and reproductive events in the mare,* Cross Plains, WI, 1986, Equiservices.

Ginther OJ: *Reproductive biology of the mare: basic and applied aspects,* ed 2, pp. 173-230, 305-311, 392-396. Cross Plains, WI, 1992, Equiservices.

McGladdory A: Fetal ultrasonography. In McKinnon AO, Voss JL, editors, *Equine reproduction,* Philadelphia, 1993, Lea and Febiger.

McKinnon AO, Carnevale EM: Ultrasonography. In McKinnon AO, Voss JL, editors, *Equine reproduction,* Philadelphia, 1993, Lea and Febiger.

6

Endometritis

OBJECTIVES

While studying the information covered in this chapter, the student should attempt to:

1. Acquire a working understanding of the mechanisms by which normal, fertile mares are able to eliminate potentially pathogenic organisms from the genital tract.
2. Understand the anatomical and physiologic deficiencies that contribute to establishment of uterine infections in the mare.
3. Understand how persistent postmating endometritis differs from chronic infectious endometritis and be able to discuss methods used to reduce the incidence of embryonic loss associated with persistent postmating endometritis.
4. Acquire a working understanding of rationales for selecting methods for treatment of genital infections in the mare.

STUDY QUESTIONS

1. Review the barriers to uterine infection in the mare.
2. Discuss potential roles for the following factors in eliminating microorganisms from the uterus of the mare:
   a. immunoglobulins.
   b. neutrophil migration.
   c opsonins.
   d. physical clearance mechanisms.
      1) secretions.
      2) uterine tone and contractility.
      3) lymphatic drainage.
      4) transcervical drainage.
3. Regarding mares considered susceptible to postmating endometritis, discuss how you would recognize which mares might be affected and how you would optimize management during estrus to enhance resolution of the postmating endometritis.
4. Regarding treatment of uterine infections in the mare, discuss the rationale for and procedures used in:
   a. local antibiotic therapy.
   b. uterine lavage.
   c. administration of oxytocin or prostaglandins.
   d. infusion of immunity enhancers (colostrum, plasma, or bacterial filtrates).
   e. uterine curettage.
   f. hormonal therapy.
5. List the most common locations for genital infections in the mare.
6. List the most common organisms associated with genital infections in the mare.
7. Discuss signs of and techniques for diagnosing endometritis in the mare.
8. Discuss methods for preventing genital infections in the mare.

TERMINOLOGY FOR GENITAL INFECTIONS

The majority of uterine infections in the mare involve only the endometrium *(endometritis)*. Very few endometrial infections progress into deeper uterine tissues such as the myometrium *(metritis)*. If infection progresses this deeply into the uterine wall, it can result in perimetritis and peritonitis, as well as lead to septicemia and laminitis. The cervix can become involved *(cervicitis)*, as can the vagina *(vaginitis)*, usually as an extension of endometritis. Fortunately, infection of the oviducts *(salpingitis)* is rare because of the tight uterotubal junction in the mare. Even in the mare with a distended uterus due to pyometra, the exudate rarely penetrates through the oviduct papilla to enter the oviduct.

ENDOMETRITIS

Endometritis has long been recognized as a major cause of reduced fertility in mares. Sources of uterine contamination that lead to development of endometritis include parturition, reproductive examination (even under strictly hygienic conditions), artificial insemination or natural mating, and self-contamination owing to conformational characteristics. Reproductively normal mares respond to uterine contamination with a transient inflammatory response that includes the activation of humoral or antibody-mediated defense mechanisms, recruitment of polymorphonuclear cells for bacterial phagocytosis, the release of prostaglandins, and increased uterine contractility to mechanically rid the uterus of luminal contents. These normal defense mechanisms render the reproductively normal mare *resistant* to persistent endometritis.

Mares that are not reproductively normal experience a breakdown in this natural defense mechanism and are considered to be *susceptible* to persistent endometritis. Some of the mechanisms proposed for development of persistent endometritis include insufficient opsonization of bacteria by polymorphonuclear neutrophils within the uterine lumen and defective physical clearance of uterine contents. Defective physical clearance of uterine contents can result from dysfunctional uterine contractility, obstruction of physical clearance due to failure of cervical relaxation, and conformational changes (e.g., pendulous uterus) that make physical removal of intrauterine contents more difficult. Persistent endometritis can be divided into two categories: *persistent, postmating endometritis* and *chronic infectious endometritis*.

Persistent, Postmating Endometritis

After mating or insemination, reproductively normal mares experience a transient inflammatory reaction within the uterus (in response to the presence of bacteria and spermatozoa), which is quickly resolved (i.e., within 24 to 48 hours). This efficient clearance of the uterus after mating provides ample time for the intrauterine environment to return to normal, thus allowing for embryonic survival when the embryo enters the uterus 5 to 6 days after ovulation. In contrast, mares in which postmating endometritis fails to resolve within 48 to 72 hours are considered to have a persistent, postmating endometritis. In a field fertility study including more than 700 mare cycles, Zent et al. (1998) reported that 14% of Thoroughbred mares developed a persistent, postmating endometritis. They noted that mares that accumulated a large amount of fluid after breeding tended to have lower pregnancy rates.

Management of Mares Susceptible to Persistent, Postmating Endometritis. The key to enhancing fertility of mares susceptible to persistent, postmating endometritis is to identify them before breeding and then to manage them in a manner to aid physical clearance of uterine contaminants during and immediately after the estrus of breeding. In general, mares susceptible to persistent, postmating endometritis are multiparous and older in age. However, older maiden mares may also be predisposed to this problem because of a tight cervix that fails to adequately relax during estrus, leading to retention of semen, bacteria, and inflammatory by-products within the uterus. The result is a sustained inflammatory response that renders the environment incompatible with establishment of pregnancy.

Reproductively normal mares may accumulate a small volume of fluid within the uterus during estrus. Ultrasound examination of normal mares during estrus reveals evidence of edema within the endometrium with no or less than 1 to 3 cm of anechoic fluid within the lumen of the uterine horns or uterine body. One can often visualize the uterus contracting and moving fluid toward the cervix in such mares during transrectal ultrasonographic examination. In contrast, most mares that are susceptible to persistent, postmating endometritis tend to accumulate larger than normal volumes of fluid within the uterus during estrus (>3 cm in luminal distension), and fluid may become hyperechoic in nature. These mares have been hypothesized to have deficient lymphatic drainage of endometrial edema, resulting in dramatic endometrial edema patterns when viewed ultrasonographically. It is important to note that uterine fluid during estrus is probably sterile unless the uterus has been contaminated. The contamination that results from breeding leads to infectious endometritis in the mare whose uterus fails to clear the bacterial contaminants.

Prudent management of the mare susceptible to persistent, postmating endometritis includes routine ultrasound examination during the estrus before insemination and treatment as needed with uterine ecbolics (i.e., oxytocin or prostaglandin) to stimulate uterine contractility and expel uterine contents. Uterine lavage before breeding may be indicated in those mares in which systemic treatment with ecbolics is unsuccessful in controlling intrauterine fluid accumulation.

It is also important to minimize uterine contamination and inflammation. Problems encountered during breeding that contribute to increased contamination of the uterus include excessive trauma to the genital tract, improper hygiene during breeding, excessive breeding, and a large bacterial inoculant in the stallion ejaculate. Iatrogenic contamination during artificial insemination or during examination and treatment of the genital tract can also contribute to an overwhelming inoculum. A nonsterile, reusable vaginal speculum used for vaginal or cervical examination is a common culprit. Insemination should be performed under strict hygienic conditions, and semen should first be mixed with a suitable extender that contains broad-spectrum antibiotics to control bacterial growth. Ideally, breeding should only be done once within 24 to 48 hours before ovulation. Mares that must be bred by natural service may benefit from infusion of 30 to 50 ml of prewarmed antibiotic-containing semen extender into the uterus immediately before mating.

Postbreeding uterine lavage as early as 4 to 8 hours after insemination/mating will aid in removal of uterine contents, yet apparently will not interfere with spermatozoal colonization of the oviducts. Intrauterine infusion of antibiotics after lavage has improved pregnancy rates after breeding of Thoroughbred mares in some studies. However, infusion of an antibiotic-containing solution into the uterus of a mare might be counterproductive if the solution remains retained within the uterus. Therefore, uterine lavage and/or infusion should be accompanied by the use of ecbolics to promote clearance of the fluid from the uterus. Unfortunately, the ideal interval for ecbolic administration after the uterus is infused remains unstudied. The practitioner is faced with the knowledge that administration of an ecbolic too soon after infusion could result in expulsion of the antibiotic before it may exert its beneficial effects on resident bacteria. When endometrial concentrations of various antimicrobials infused into the uterine lumen of cows and mares were evaluated, results suggested relatively rapid penetration of the few drugs studied. Therefore, until further research is done, we offer the following recommendations:

1. If uterine lavage results in complete evacuation of uterine contents, antimicrobial infusion can immediately follow the lavage. If ecbolic administration is desired, the ecbolic can be administered 4 to 8 hours later. Hopefully this would allow sufficient time for beneficial effects of the antimicrobial drug to be exerted before being expelled from the uterus.
2. If uterine lavage is accompanied or followed immediately by ecbolic administration, sufficient time should be allowed for uterine contractility to diminish before the antimicrobial infusion. Because oxytocin administered intravenously commonly results in increased uterine contractility for 20 to 50 minutes, the antimicrobial infusion could be performed as soon as 1 hour after lavage and ecbolic administration. Because the prostaglandin analog cloprostenol has been reported to result in 2 to 4 hours of sustained uterine contractions, antimicrobial infusion would have to be delayed by at least this interval of time.
3. If oxytocin is administered intravenously immediately before uterine lavage and if uterine lavage requires 20 to 30 minutes to complete, the antimicrobial could be infused immediately after lavage when uterine contractility from oxytocin administration should be diminishing.

Mares susceptible to persistent endometritis should be reevaluated daily after breeding by transrectal ultrasound examination until ovulation is confirmed. Uterine lavage and systemic treatment with ecbolics may be indicated daily (or perhaps twice daily) to rid the uterus of fluid. Oxytocin administration for ecbolic effects has been shown to be safe for 2 or perhaps 3 days postovulation. However, research has shown that administration of prostaglandins during the early postovulatory period (0 to 3 days) will lower corpus luteum production of progesterone during the ensuing diestrus. Because of the fear that this process may contribute to early embryonic death, the use of prostaglandins for their ecbolic effect is not recommended after ovulation has occurred. The use of oxytocin and prostaglandins during estrus and postovulation is further discussed later in this chapter.

Chronic Endometritis

Infectious agents are capable of causing disease if the mare has a defective uterine clearance mechanism or the reproductive system is overwhelmed by a large and/or repeated inoculum. A common underlying problem associated with genital infection in the mare is **pneumovagina**, which can lead to **pneumouterus**. The presence of these conditions implies aspiration of air and debris into the genital tract. When these conditions exist, one or more of the three physical barriers to contamination of the uterus must be disrupted: the vulvar seal, the vestibulovaginal sphincter, and/or the cervix. Continuing insult, coupled with the inability to overcome infection, results in chronic endometritis. Longstanding, more severe disease shows significant infiltration of the endometrium with lymphocytes and plasma cells, confirming the chronicity of the infection. Plasmacytic infiltration implies the continuing presence of antigen, and therefore the prognosis is guarded.

Causes of Infectious Endometritis

Numerous causes of infectious endometritis in the mare have been identified. They include bacteria (both aerobic and anaerobic), fungi, and yeasts. The role of mycoplasmas, chlamydias, and viruses is thought to be relatively insignificant, but few studies have focused on identifying these organisms as causes of genital infections in the mare.

Diagnosis of Endometritis

Treatment of genital infections in the mare should always be preceded with a proper diagnosis. Mares are sometimes treated empirically without first pursuing a diagnosis to justify treatment. To substantiate a diagnosis of endometritis, *signs of inflammation* (e.g., the presence of hyperechoic fluid in the uterus or genital discharges, particularly from the uterus) should be present. The endometritis is easily confirmed with uterine cytologic analysis or biopsy. Recovery of the offending organism on *culture* and determination of its *in vitro sensitivity to antimicrobial agents* will allow selection of a suitable drug for treatment. The earlier the diagnosis is made, the less likely irreversible damage will occur. For this reason, mares found to be barren during fall pregnancy rechecks should be examined and treated as soon as possible.

Diagnostic aids/criteria for genital infections follow.

External Signs of Infection

- These are rarely seen with low-grade endometritis.
- Possible *matting of tail hairs* from chronic discharges is present.
- Occasional *exudate* is seen at the ventral commissure of the vulva.
- Obvious exudate is seen at the vulva with an open cervix pyometra or metritis.

Findings on Examination per Rectum (by Either Palpation or Ultrasound)

- *Fluid accumulation in the uterine lumen* is indicated by an enlarged uterus. An echogenic character to the fluid often indicates the presence of purulent material. Extensive fluid accumulation in diestrus, even when it is anechoic, has also been correlated with endometritis. However, the presence of small amounts of anechoic intrauterine fluid during estrus sometimes occurs without endometritis being present. A small volume of anechoic intrauterine fluid during estrus (<1 to 3 cm of intraluminal distension) is often seen in reproductively normal mares. Excessive

intrauterine fluid during estrus (>3 cm) suggests poor uterine clearance mechanisms.
- Massage of the uterus/vagina per rectum may *express contents* through a dilated cervix or vagina that become evident as vulvar discharge.
- A slight *thickening of the uterine wall* may be detected in some mares with acute endometritis, but "poor tone" of the uterus is not a reliable indicator of endometritis.

Findings on Vaginal Speculum Examination
- Presence of inflammation indicated by *reddening* or *increased vascularity.*
- Presence of *discharge through the cervix.*
- Presence of *urine pooled* in the anterior vagina.
- Presence of *debris* (such as manure) in the anterior vagina.

Endometrial (Uterine) Swabbing for Culture
- *Avoid contamination of swab.* Use a *guarded culture instrument* (i.e., a distal occlusion should be present on the swab container that prevents exposure of the swab until it is placed within the uterus), and properly clean the hindquarters of the mare. One can pass the culture instrument through a speculum to obtain a swabbing; however, with this technique it may be difficult to pass the instrument through the cervix of maiden mares or mares not in estrus.
- *Perform culture when appropriate.* Culture is best done in early estrus when the cervix is relaxed and the uterus is more resistant to infection, but the uterus can be cultured during any stage of the cycle. However, the cervix must be dilated manually to accomplish swabbing of the uterus during diestrus.
- *Avoid interpretive error.* Compare the results of the culture to the presence of signs of inflammation (particularly biopsy) to determine the significance of results. Isolation of bacteria alone is not evidence of endometritis. Even when guarded uterine culture swabs are used, disagreement between culture and biopsy sometimes occurs. This disagreement means that positive cultures can be obtained from mares without endometritis, and negative cultures can be obtained from mares with endometritis.

Bacterial endometritis. The following four organisms are responsible for the vast majority of confirmed cases of endometritis in the mare:
- *Streptococcus zooepidemicus*
- *Escherichia coli* (also *Enterobacter* spp.)
- *Pseudomonas aeruginosa*
- *Klebsiella pneumoniae*

α-Hemolytic streptococci, *Staphylococcus* spp., and other bacteria may be recovered, but should be regarded as contaminants unless accompanied by significant signs of inflammation.

Another organism less commonly linked to endometritis in the United States is *Taylorella equigenitalis*, a microaerophilic, Gram-negative coccobacillus believed to have originated in Thoroughbreds in France and Ireland. *T. equigenitalis* is the cause of *contagious equine metritis.* This organism is *venereally transmitted* to mares at breeding by stallions, which serve as lesionless carriers of the organism. Some mares develop a copious gray vaginal discharge within 2 to 10 days after breeding, whereas other mares may show no clinical signs except shortened diestrous periods. Some mares recover spontaneously, whereas others remain chronic carriers. Codes of practice have been developed to control spread of this disease, which must be reported to federal authorities if discovered.

Yeast and fungal endometritis. *Candida* spp., *Aspergillus* spp., and *Mucor* spp. are the most common organisms seen. These organisms are *more likely to be detected in cytologic specimens than in biopsy preparations.* Yeast and fungal infections are usually superficial, in which case they often readily respond to treatment; however, they may also result in chronic, deep endometritis that responds poorly to treatment.

Endometrial Cytologic Analysis. Endometrial cytologic analysis, although it does not provide as definitive a diagnosis of endometritis as biopsy, does provide an immediate indicator of acute endometrial inflammation. A suitable sample for cytologic analysis can be obtained from a uterine swabbing or various custom-made cell accumulation devices. It is important that guarded instruments be used for collection of samples to ensure that inflammatory cells collected are from the uterus (endometrium). A uterine flushing can also be centrifuged and cells harvested for the cytologic specimen.

Usually the prepared slide is air-dried, fixed, and stained. Diff-Quik is a commonly used stain for air-dried specimens. New methylene blue is a commonly used stain for cover-slipped wet mounts. The slide is observed under a microscope for the presence and condition of epithelial cells, bacteria, yeast or fungi, and inflammatory cells. The presence of a significant number of *neutrophils,* which may be degenerate and may contain phagocytized bacteria, indicates an acute inflammation.

Endometrial Biopsy. An endometrial biopsy is obtained using a stainless steel uterine biopsy punch. The biopsy can provide information on *various types of endometrial pathologic conditions,* including *acute* or *chronic endometritis.* The biopsy is considered to be the definitive test for endometritis. In some cases, special stains can be used to identify the types of pathologic organisms involved. Proper interpretation of the endometrial biopsy will enable the interpreter to suggest types of treatment that may be beneficial in an individual mare.

TREATMENT OF GENITAL INFECTIONS

For successful treatment of genital infections, any underlying problems that contribute to reinfection must be eliminated. Problems requiring surgical correction include **pneumovagina, urovagina, cervical lacerations, perineal lacerations,** and **rectovaginal fistulas. Retained placenta** or **delayed uterine involution** should be treated early in the postpartum period to overcome uterine contamination. Finally, poor management practices, such as *unhygienic breeding/ examination* or excessive breeding should be corrected to minimize contamination of the genital tract.

The organism that is causing the infection must be identified and eliminated. A number of techniques are commonly used by veterinarians to eliminate uterine infections, including the following.

Uterine Lavage

Uterine lavage is an important therapeutic tool for treatment of uterine infections. Reasons for uterine lavage include (1) removal of microbes, nonfunctional neutrophils, and other substances (e.g., proteolytic enzymes), which are likely to interfere with the function of potentially useful neutrophils or antibiotics; (2) stimulation of uterine contractility to aid in the physical clearance of uterine contents; and (3) recruitment of fresh neutrophils and possibly opsonins (through mechanical irritation of the endometrium) to combat infectious agents.

Typically, the uterus is lavaged by gravity-driven instillation and removal of 1 to 2 liters of warmed (42° to 45° C) solution through a large-bore (e.g., 8-mm inside diameter) catheter with a balloon cuff to facilitate retention in the uterus (the balloon is distended with air after passage beyond the cervix) (Figures 6-1 through 6-3). The procedure is oftentimes combined with uterine massage per rectum to further stimulate uterine contraction and more thoroughly distribute the solution within the uterine lumen. This process is generally repeated two to three times in sequence and may be performed for several consecutive days.

Isotonic saline or balanced salt solutions are generally preferred for uterine lavage, but dilute povidone-iodine solutions have also been used. Studies involving other species (e.g., human, rat, dog, and rabbit) indicate a dose-dependent inhibition of neutrophil migration in vitro at povidone-iodine

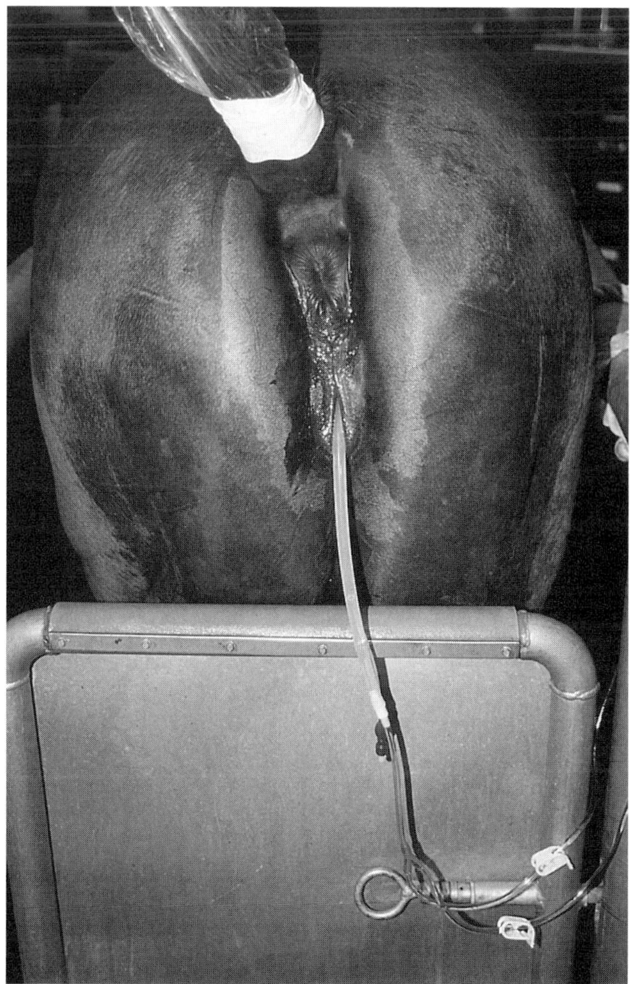

FIGURE 6-2. Performing uterine lavage in a mare. Fluid is instilled into the uterus by gravity flow; return effluent is caught for examination of character.

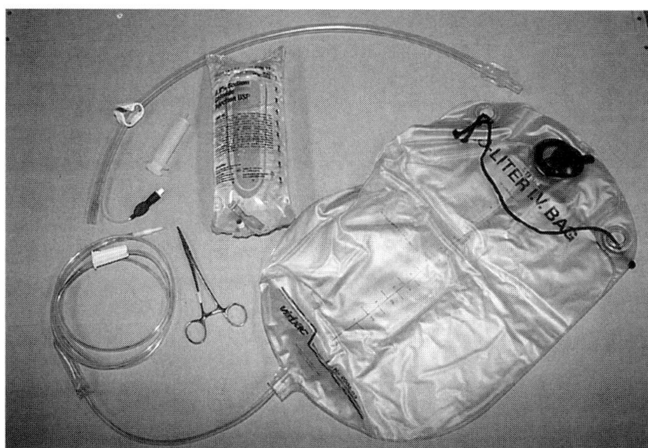

FIGURE 6-1. Equipment used to perform uterine lavage. A modified Foley catheter with balloon cuff, a syringe for filling the cuff with air, lavage fluid, a lavage bag to contain fluid with attached tubing and connector, and forceps for controlling the flow of fluid through the catheter are shown.

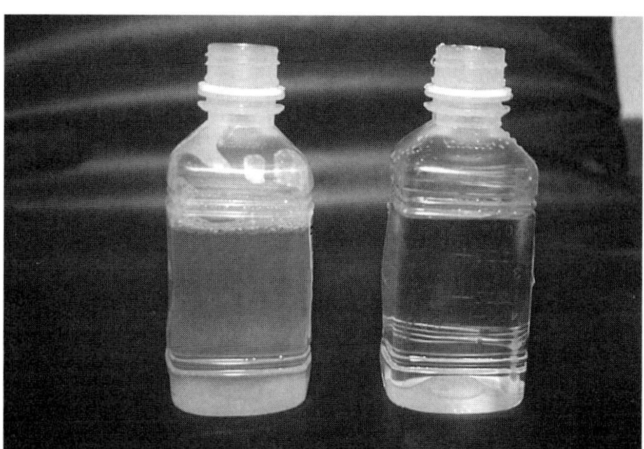

FIGURE 6-3. During uterine lavage, the uterus is successively filled with 250 ml to 1 liter of sterile saline solution and drained. Lavage is generally continued until resulting effluent is clear. The bottle on the *left* contains the initial cloudy effluent obtained from a mare with subacute endometritis. The bottle on the *right* contains clear effluent obtained at end of the lavage procedure.

concentrations >0.05%. Work specific to the horse revealed no depressive effect of povidone-iodine on directional or random migration of neutrophils in vitro at concentrations ≤0.02%, but a complete inhibition of neutrophil motility at povidone-iodine concentrations ≥0.2%. Differences noted in neutrophil sensitivity between the two investigations may have been due to greater resistance of horse neutrophils to damage or simply to differences in experimental designs (e.g., methods of in vitro motility analysis). It is interesting to note that normal cellular morphology of horse neutrophils was maintained at higher povidone-iodine concentrations than those observed in other species, suggesting enhanced resistance of horse neutrophils to the cytotoxic effects of povidone-iodine solution. Because the inhibition of neutrophil motility was associated with detectable cytotoxic effects (i.e., cellular pyknosis and lysis), it is probable that phagocytic activity would be rendered nonfunctional at similar povidone-iodine concentrations. A suitable lavage solution can be made by mixing 10 ml of Betadine Veterinary or 5 ml of Betadine in 1 liter of sterile saline or lactated Ringer's solution.

Administration of Ecbolics

Because some mares susceptible to endometritis have been found to be unable to physically expel uterine contents through the cervix and to have impaired lymphatic drainage from the uterus, injection of uterine ecbolics (stimulate myometrial contraction) such as oxytocin (with or without concurrent uterine lavage) has been proposed as an adjunctive treatment for endometritis (Figures 6-4 and 6-5). Oxytocin (20 units intravenously, or 20 to 40 units intramuscularly) is the most commonly used uterine ecbolic in equine practice, and it is often combined with uterine lavage to treat endometritis. Whether administration of oxytocin by the intramuscular route is superior to intravenous administration is not known, but intramuscular administration has been shown to prolong the duration of uterine contractions in other species. Some practitioners administer oxytocin several times on a given day. Information on the ability of the equine uterus to respond repeatedly to routinely administered doses of oxytocin or the importance of the dose of oxytocin used to the type of uterine contraction(s) generated (i.e., spasmodic versus peristaltic) is lacking. However, Florida workers have suggested that administration of more than 20 units of oxytocin intravenously or administration more often than once every 4 to 6 hours induces spasmodic uterine contraction(s) that are likely to be unproductive in eliminating uterine fluid. Treatment with oxytocin should be repeated for 1 to 2 days if uterine lavage effluent remains cloudy or intrauterine fluid accumulation remains evident on ultrasound examination. Texas workers demonstrated that once daily injection of oxytocin (20 units intravenously) during estrus had no detrimental effect on fertility, provided that treatment is postponed until 4 hours postbreeding on the same day that a mare is bred. Oxytocin treatment near the time of breeding is currently discouraged because it has been shown recently that it may decrease fertility, perhaps because semen is expelled from the uterus before adequate numbers of spermatozoa access the oviduct. Treatment more than 2 to 3 days post-ovulation is generally discouraged.

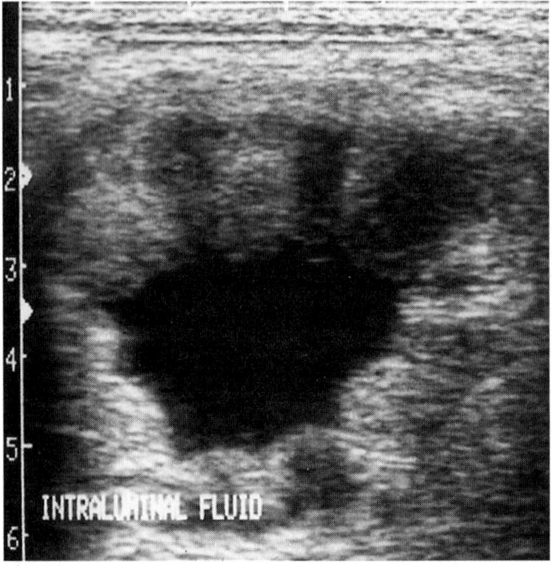

FIGURE 6-4. Ultrasonographic image of intrauterine fluid accumulation in a mare.

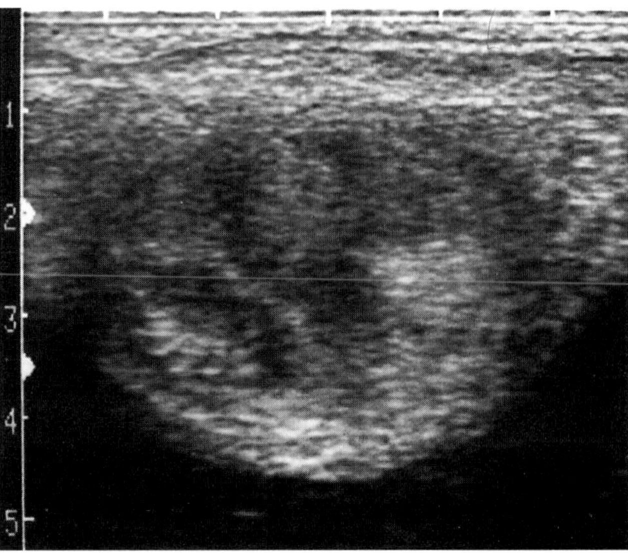

FIGURE 6-5. Ultrasonographic image of the uterine horn shown in Figure 6-4 30 minutes after intravenous administration of 20 units of oxytocin. Fluid retention was not ultrasonographically detectable anywhere within the uterus at this time, indicating that evacuation of fluid from the uterus had been achieved.

Intramuscular administration of 250 μg of cloprostenol (Estrumate, Bayer Corp.), a prostaglandin analog, has been advocated by Florida workers to aid in evacuation of uterine contents in mares being treated for endometritis. The analog results in a longer duration of induced uterine contractions

(2 to 4 hours) compared with oxytocin administration (30 minutes to 1 hour). Cloprostenol (or prostaglandin $F_{2\alpha}$) should not be administered to mares after ovulation has occurred. Colorado and Oregon workers demonstrated that administration of prostaglandins on the day of ovulation or 1 to 2 days postovulation lowered serum progesterone concentrations during the ensuing diestrus. If intrauterine uterine fluid continues to accumulate in the postovulatory period, uterine lavage and/or oxytocin administration would be preferred treatments. Cloprostenol is not approved for use in horses in the United States, but it is in some other countries. Side effects are reportedly minimal, although we have noted abdominal cramping (colic) in some mares after treatment with this compound and, rarely, have seen some mares sweat after its administration. Studies directly comparing the effects of oxytocin versus prostaglandins on pregnancy rates are lacking.

Antimicrobial Therapy

Some commonly used antimicrobial drugs and dosages for treatment of uterine infection in mares are provided in Table 6-1. The antibiotic chosen should be selected based on the susceptibility pattern obtained from culture. Distribution patterns of several antibiotics in reproductive tissues of the mare have been studied after intrauterine infusion. With standard infusion doses, endometrial and uterine lumen levels of most antibiotics (penicillin, ampicillin, chloramphenicol, gentamicin, amikacin, etc.) remain at or above bacteriostatic/bacteriocidal concentrations for at least 24 hours. In contrast, higher doses and administration more often (two to four times daily) is usually required to achieve the same levels in the endometrium and uterine lumen after systemic administration of these same antibiotics. Therefore most veterinary practitioners prefer to administer antibiotics by once-daily intrauterine infusion. In general, we recommend once daily infusion for 3 days for treatment of slight endometritis (as judged by endometrial biopsy), for 5 days for treatment of moderate endometritis, and for 7 days for treatment of severe endometritis. To enhance efficacy, particularly if aminoglycosides are used, uterine lavage to remove organic material and particulate matter should be done before infusion. This procedure is thought to help avoid inactivation of the antibiotic infused.

Some antibiotics have a very acidic or alkalotic pH, which can be quite irritating to the endometrium if they are not buffered to a more neutral pH before infusion. Gentamicin and amikacin have an acidic pH, but when buffered with sodium bicarbonate, they can be infused with minimal irritation to the endometrium. In contrast, enrofloxacin has a basic pH. Unfortunately, when buffered to a more neutral pH, enrofloxacin has been reported to be less effective for bacterial killing, and infusion of unbuffered enrofloxacin may be very irritating to the genital tract. If the susceptibility patterns of bacterial infection suggest the use of enrofloxacin, systemic treatment is recommended. Pennsylvania workers found oral administration of 5 mg/kg enrofloxacin twice daily resulted in endometrial levels of enrofloxacin that were above the minimum inhibitory concentration of many bacteria that can cause endometritis.

One consideration for antibiotic selection is the antibiotic-neutrophil interaction in microbial killing. Some antibiotics (e.g., polymyxin B and tetracycline) are readily capable of penetrating phagocytes and thus may cause enhanced intracellular killing of microbes. Other antibiotics (e.g., penicillins, streptomycin, and gentamicin) only pass into phagocytes with difficulty. Once intracellular access is attained, these antibiotics may augment bacterial killing. However, ingested bacteria can also be protected from the action of extracellular antibiotics, allowing some bacteria to actually continue multiplication within neutrophils.

Many studies have been conducted to evaluate the effect of various antibiotics on specific aspects of neutrophil function (e.g., chemotaxis, phagocytic activity, and oxidative metabolism). Several antibiotics have been incriminated as damaging to neutrophil chemotaxis (e.g., tetracyclines, gentamicin, or amikacin), phagocytosis (e.g., tetracyclines or polymyxin B) or oxidative metabolism (e.g., tetracyclines or polymyxin B) in other species. However, conflicting reports make data interpretation difficult. One investigation specific to the horse revealed that gentamicin or amikacin significantly reduced in vitro phagocytic activity of neutrophils, whereas phagocytosis was unchanged in the presence of penicillin or ticarcillin.

During the breeding season, many mares are treated concurrently during the same estrous cycle in which they are bred. Such treatments most commonly involve intrauterine infusion of antibiotic (with or without prior uterine lavage) either early in the estrous cycle before breeding or late in the estrous cycle after breeding, often after ovulation is confirmed. Infusion of antimicrobials on the day of breeding (i.e., before breeding) should probably not be done because many antimicrobials have spermicidal properties when present in high concentrations. In some instances, practitioners will lavage and infuse the uterus after a mare is bred. It is critical that any intrauterine treatment not be done less than 4 hours after breeding so that oviductal colonization with spermatozoa is not disturbed. Additionally, we do not recommend intrauterine treatment for more than 2 to 3 days after ovulation for fear of causing sufficient endogenous prostaglandin release to impair corpus luteum function.

Intrauterine Infusion of Disinfectant

Although intrauterine infusion of disinfectants is widely practiced, precautions should be taken when a disinfectant is chosen and used. Some disinfectants are quite irritating to tissues, including Lugol's iodine and chlorhexidine, particularly when they are not sufficiently diluted. Severe irritation from inadequate dilution has resulted, in some cases, in the formation of transluminal adhesions of the tubular tract. Intrauterine deposition of disinfectants has also been shown

TABLE 6-1

Guidelines for the Administration of Some Commonly Used Intrauterine Drugs

Drug	Dosage	Comments
Penicillin (Na^+ or K^+ salt)	5 million U	Very effective for streptococci; economical and commonly used.
Gentamicin sulfate	500-1000 mg	Highly effective; generally nonirritating when mixed with an equal volume of $NaHCO_3$ and diluted in saline.
Ampicillin	1-3 g	Use at high dilutions because it can be irritating; Na^+ salt leaves a precipitate on the endometrium that remains in the uterus for a prolonged period.
Carbenicillin	2-6 g	Use is reserved for persistent *Pseudomonas* (synergistic efficacy with aminoglycosides); usually given on alternate days with aminoglycosides; slightly irritating.
Ticarcillin	1-3 g	Use for *Pseudomonas*; do not use for *Klebsiella*.
Timentin	3-6 g	Broad-spectrum activity against many Gram-positive and -negative bacteria; contains ticarcillin and clavulanic acid to protect ticarcillin against degradation by β-lactamase enzyme-producing bacteria.
Amikacin sulfate	1-2 g	Use for *Pseudomonas, Klebsiella,* and persistent Gram-negative organisms; mixed with equal volume of $NaHCO_3$ and diluted in saline.
Ceftiofur sodium (Naxcel)	1 g	Third-generation cephalosporin; has been used empirically once daily either intramuscularly or by intrauterine infusion; broad-spectrum effectiveness against Gram-positive and -negative bacteria.
Cefazolin sodium	1 g	First-generation cephalosporin; has been used empirically once daily intramuscularly for 2-3 weeks; broad-spectrum effectiveness against Gram-positive and -negative bacteria.
Kanamycin sulfate	1 g	Do not use close to breeding, because it is toxic to spermatozoa.
Polymyxin B	1 million U	Use for Gram-negative bacteria, particularly *Pseudomonas*.
Neomycin sulfate	3-4 g	Use for sensitive *Escherichia coli;* can be irritating; routine postbreeding use of oral preparations containing neomycin mixed with other antimicrobials has lowered pregnancy rates in mares.
Chloramphenicol	2-3 g	Can be very irritating, especially in the oral form.
Nitrofurazones	50-60 ml	Effectiveness is highly questionable.
Povidone-iodine (5ml of stock solution of Betadine, diluted in 1 L)	1 liter (lavage solution)	If solutions are too concentrated, severe endometritis may result and/or impair neutrophil function. In vitro bactericidal activity is maintained at concentrations as low as 0.01%-0.005%; indicated for lavage of uteri with nonspecific inflammation or fungal/yeast infections; should not be left in uterus.
Nystatin	500,000 U	Used primarily for yeast (e.g., *Candida albicans*) in the growing phase; dilute in 100 to 250 ml sterile water; makes an insoluble suspension that must be vigorously mixed immediately before infusion.
Amphotericin B	200 mg	Used for infections with *Aspergillus, Candida, Histoplasma,* or *Mucor;* dilute in 100 to 250 ml sterile water; makes a relatively insoluble suspension.
Clotrimazole	700 mg	Used for yeast infections (*Candida* spp.); available as cream, tablets, or suppositories; preferable treatment is with tablets crushed and mixed with 40 ml sterile water; generally infused after uterine lavage.
Miconazole	200 mg	Is most efficacious for yeast infections (*Candida* spp.) but has been used by some practitioners for resistant fungal infections in mares by infusing once daily for up to 10 days; dilute in 40-60 ml sterile saline before infusion.
Fluconazole	100 mg	Synthetic triazole antifungal agent; proposed as infusion for treatment of fungal or *Candida* endometritis once daily for 5-10 days; adjust pH to 7 if necessary as pH varies from 4-8.
Vinegar	2% (v/v) 20 ml/L of saline	Used empirically as an adjunct for treating yeast endometritis; 1-liter uterine lavage; efficacy not tested.
Dimethyl sulfoxide (5% of stock solution)	50-100 ml	Used as penetrating agent to carry drugs; effectiveness and safety unknown.
Mannose	50 g/L of saline as a lavage solution	In vitro study demonstrated that mannose decreased adhesion of *E. coli, Pseudomonas aeruginosa,* and *Streptococcus zooepidemicus* to equine endometrial cells in culture; proposed as therapy in uterine lavage; bacteria bind to the sugar and are removed in lavage effluent; not critically tested in naturally infected mares.
EDTA-Tris (1.2 g NaEDTA + 6.05 g Tris/L of H_2O, titrated to pH 8.0 with glacial acetic acid)	250 ml, then infuse antibiotic 3 hr later	EDTA theoretically binds Ca^{2+} in bacterial cell walls, making cell wall permeable to antibiotic and thus more susceptible; use confined to persistent *Pseudomonas* infections.

to kill neutrophils, possibly interfering with an important cellular immune defense mechanism.

Povidone-iodine solution (0.2%, 500 ml) has been used successfully as a uterine treatment in mares with endometritis, when infused during the estrus before breeding. This povidone-iodine concentration induces a marked inflammatory response by the endometrium, which generally subsides within 7 days after treatment. Higher iodine concentrations are generally not recommended.

Because no controlled studies have demonstrated a superior efficacy of disinfectants over antibiotics or antifungal agents when instilled into the uterus, we tend to avoid their use except in certain instances. For example, when lavage of the postpartum uterus must be performed in a field setting where large volumes of sterile solution are not available, a tamed iodine solution (such as povidone-iodine) can be prepared by mixing 30 ml of Betadine Veterinary solution with 1 gallon of clean, warm tap water to which 34 g of NaCl is added. Similar dilutions of tamed iodine solutions (mixed in sterile saline) are also sometimes used to treat yeast or fungal infections of the uterus of the mare.

Intrauterine Infusion of Plasma

Intrauterine plasma infusion, combined with uterine lavage, is one approach for treatment of chronic infectious endometritis, owing to the neutrophil-enhancing properties of serum and the reported success of this treatment combination. Only heparin or citrate should be used as an anticoagulant during the plasma collection process because EDTA will inactivate complement, the principal opsonin in serum. *Autologous plasma* is often recommended for intrauterine infusions, because transmission of infectious agents or immunologic incompatibilities are possible when heterologous plasma is used. However, use of heterologous plasma is commonplace. The plasma is generally infused in 50- to 100-ml aliquots once daily for 4 to 5 days. Suitable plasma can be stored for later use for 100 days if frozen at −20 °C. Aminoglycosides are believed to interfere with plasma function, whereas penicillin and ticarcillin do not.

Two studies found no improvement in infectious endometritis after intrauterine plasma infusions, but the therapeutic protocol in each study was different from that originally proposed by Florida workers. By contrast, in an Australian study involving 1341 breeding cycles in 905 Thoroughbred mares, lactating and barren mares treated with intrauterine antibiotics and autologous plasma once 12 to 36 hours after breeding had better pregnancy rates than similar mares either not treated or only treated with antibiotics. More studies are needed to definitively verify or reject intrauterine plasma infusions, in conjunction with uterine lavage or other therapies, as an important therapeutic strategy.

Uterine Curettage

Benefits have been reported from mechanical curettage of uteri in mares with persistent endometritis. Improvement is thought to be gained by inducement of acute inflammation, with attendant movement of neutrophils and serum-derived opsonins into the uterine lumen. Infusion of strongly irritating solutions has been advocated as a method of uterine curettage (e.g., termed "chemical" curettage). Chemical curettage is accomplished by infusing irritating solutions (e.g., strong disinfectant solutions, diluted kerosene, or magnesium sulfate solution) that cause endometrial necrosis. Direct comparisons between mechanical and chemical methods of inducing uterine inflammation have not been made. Overzealous curettage, be it by mechanical or chemical means, can incite excessive tissue damage and permanent infertility. The practitioner is cautioned that more controlled experimentation with the technique of mechanical or chemical curettage is needed to justify its appropriateness as a treatment modality for any form of endometrial pathologic changes, including endometritis.

Colostrum Infusions

Equine colostrum, an abundant source of immunoglobulins, has been reported as a successful treatment for infectious endometritis in mares. Although not critically studied, its efficacy remains questionable because the uteri of mares susceptible to endometritis apparently do not have a quantitative deficiency of immunoglobulins. Continued studies will be required to more completely understand the effects of the uterine environment on biologic activity of immunoglobulins. As with plasma, heterologous colostrum is a potential means of disease transmission or cause of immunologic complications. Additionally, aseptic collection and storage of colostrum would be essential to avoid iatrogenic induction or propagation of infection.

Hormonal Therapy

Existing studies indicate that mares under estrogen influence are more capable of eliminating uterine infections than mares under progesterone influence. Improved microbial clearance in estrous mares may be due to enhancements in migrational capacity of neutrophils, neutrophil phagocytic and/or microbicidal ability, uterine physical clearance mechanisms, or a combination thereof. Given the potential advantages of an estrous over a diestrous state to eliminate uterine infections, a logical approach to treatment includes increasing the percentage of time that a mare is in physiologic estrus. This effect can be achieved in the cyclic mare by administering an exogenous prostaglandin 5 to 6 days after ovulation to reduce the length of diestrus.

Advantages of exogenous estrogen for treatment of endometritis in cyclic mares have not been demonstrated. It is possible that diestrus (i.e., progesterone influence) may mask any beneficial effects exerted by exogenous estrogen therapy. Many commercially available estrogens are esterified, resulting in heightened potency and prolonged (and unpredictable) duration of action; hence, complications may arise from their use. When estrogen therapy is contemplated by the practitioner, small doses (e.g., 0.5 to 1.0 mg of estradiol cypionate or

5 to 10 mg of estradiol-β) should be used. Estrogens are not currently approved for use in horses.

Locally Applied Prostaglandin E

Some mares that tend to repeatedly accumulate fluid within the uterus, often as a result of endometritis, seem to have insufficient relaxation of the cervix during estrus. Because cervical relaxation is required to allow expulsion of uterine contents, we have tried local application of either 2 mg of prostaglandin E_2 (Sigma Chemical Co.; mixed in 2 to 4 ml of lubricating jelly and deposited in the cervical canal and external cervical os) or 200 µg of misoprostol (prostaglandin E_1 analog) tablets (Cytotec, G. D. Searle and Co.; softened in a small volume of sterile saline or lubricating jelly and inserted into the external cervical os) once daily. Use of these compounds appears to result in cervical softening and dilation that facilitates uterine drainage in such mares. Further investigation on use of prostaglandin E in mares is warranted.

Use of "Immunonormalizers"

Some products have been used empirically in an attempt to stimulate immunity to overcome uterine infection. Such treatments remain unstudied and of questionable efficacy. Products that have been used include the following:

- **Levamisole** given once daily (1 mg/lb) for 3 days, then stopped for 4 days and then repeated for three to four series of treatments. Severe anaphylaxis and colic are potential side effects, so this treatment should be used with caution.
- **Mebendazole (Telmin)** given once daily (1 mg/lb) for 3 days, then stopped for 4 days and then repeated for three to four series of treatments. Apparently, side effects are unlikely with this treatment, although we have no personal experience with it.
- An immunostimulant made from the bacteria *Propionibacterium acnes* **(EqStim)** was reported to be efficacious when injected intravenously (4 ml/454 kg body weight) on days 1, 2, and 7 after diagnosis of endometritis. We are unaware of controlled studies performed to evaluate the success of this regimen.

PREVENTION OF GENITAL INFECTION

Prevention is of paramount importance for controlling genital infections of mares. Prevention techniques are varied, but involve common sense. Conditions such as pneumovagina or urovagina should be controlled by corrective surgery. Proper hygiene during parturition, breeding, and genital examination is critical. Artificial insemination using a suitable antibiotic-containing semen extender or infusion of 30 to 50 ml of antibiotic-containing extender into the uterus of the mare immediately before natural cover can be of benefit in preventing infection of the genital tract.

BIBLIOGRAPHY

Asbury AC: Bacterial endometritis. In Robinson NE, editor: *Current therapy in equine medicine,* Philadelphia, 1983, WB Saunders.

Brendemuehl JP: Influence of cloprostenol, $PGF_{2\alpha}$ and oxytocin administered in the immediate postovulatory period on corpora luteal formation and function in the mare. *Proc Equine Symp Soc Theriogenol* p. 267, 2000.

Evans MJ, Hamer JM, Gason, LM et al: Factors affecting uterine clearance of inoculated materials in mares. *J Reprod Fertil* 35(Suppl):327-334, 1987.

Giguere S, Sweeney RW, Belanger M: Pharmacokinetics of enrofloxacin in adult horses and concentration of the drug in serum, body fluids, and endometrial tissues after repeated intragastrically administered doses. *Am J Vet Res* 57:1025-1030, 1996.

Gunthle LM, McCue PM, Farquhar VJ et al: Effect of prostaglandin administration postovulation on corpus luteum formation in the mare. *Proc Equine Symp Society for Theriogenol* 139, 2000.

Hughes JP, Loy RG: Investigations on the effect of intrauterine inoculations of *Streptococcus zooepidemicus* in the mare. *Proc Am Assoc Equine Pract* 15:289-292, 1969.

LeBlanc MM: Recurrent endometritis: is oxytocin the answer? *Proc Am Assoc Equine Pract* 40:17-18, 1994.

Liu IKM: Uterine defense mechanisms in the mare. In Van Camp SD, editor: *The veterinary clinics of North America: equine practice,* vol 4, Philadelphia, 1988, WB Saunders.

Neely DP: Evaluation and therapy of genital disease in the mare. In Neely DP, Liu IMK, Hillman RB, editors, *Equine reproduction,* Nutley, NH, 1983, Veterinary Learning Systems.

Pascoe DR: Effect of adding autologous plasma to an intrauterine antibiotic therapy after breeding on pregnancy rates in mares. *Biol Reprod Monogr* 1:532-543, 1995.

Peterson FB, McFeely RA, David JSE: Studies on the pathogenesis of endometritis in the mare. *Proc Am Assoc Equine Pract* 15:279-287, 1969.

Scott MA, Liu IKM, Overstreet JW: Sperm transport to the oviducts: abnormalities and their clinical implications. *Proc Am Assoc Equine Pract* 41:1-2, 1995.

Troedsson MHT: Uterine clearance and resistance to persistent endometritis in the mare. *Theriogenology* 52:461-471, 1999.

Troedsson MHT, Liu IKM, Thurmond M: Function of uterine- and blood-derived polymorphonuclear neutrophils in mares susceptible and resistant to chronic uterine infection: phagocytosis and chemotaxis. *Biol Reprod* 49:507-514, 1993.

Watson ED: Uterine defence mechanisms in mares resistant and susceptible to persistent endometritis: a review. *Equine Vet J* 20:397-400, 1988.

Zent WA, Troedsson MHT, Xue J-L. Postbreeding uterine fluid accumulation in a normal population of Thoroughbred mares: a field study. *Proc Am Assoc Equine Pract* 44:64-65, 1998.

7

Pregnancy: Physiology and Diagnosis

OBJECTIVES

While studying the information covered in this chapter, the student should attempt to:

1. Acquire a working understanding of the physiologic events of pregnancy in the mare.
2. Acquire a working knowledge of the procedures used to diagnose pregnancy in the mare.

STUDY QUESTIONS

1. Discuss the following physiologic events of pregnancy in the mare:
   a. entrance of embryo into the uterus.
   b. conceptus mobility throughout the uterus.
   c. embryonic vesicle fixation.
   d. maternal recognition of pregnancy.
   e. endometrial cup formation.
   f. supplementary corpora lutea formation.
   g. placentation.
2. Describe the hormonal events of pregnancy in the mare, paying particular attention to source and timing of progesterone production (i.e., primary corpus luteum of pregnancy, supplementary corpora lutea of pregnancy, and placental progestogen production). Also include in your description the concentrations of estrogen and equine chorionic gonadotropin in the bloodstream of the mare.
3. Discuss methods of pregnancy detection at various stages of gestation in the mare. Include advantages and disadvantages of each method.
   a. behavioral assessment.
   b. progesterone assays.
   c. vaginal speculum examination.
   d. palpation per rectum.
   e. transrectal ultrasonographic examination.
   f. equine chorionic gonadotropin detection.
   g. serum estrone sulfate detection.
   h. urinary estrone sulfate detection.

EARLY EVENTS OF PREGNANCY

Hormonally, the first 14 days of pregnancy are quite similar to the same time period in the nonpregnant mare in diestrus. If the mare is not pregnant, the endometrium will release prostaglandin $F_{2\alpha}$ ($PGF_{2\alpha}$) on approximately days 14 to 15 after ovulation, which causes regression of the corpus luteum and permits the mare to return to estrus. The corpus luteum does not undergo lysis on days 14 to 15 if the mare is pregnant, but it persists and continues to secrete progesterone, which is responsible for pregnancy maintenance.

The embryo enters the uterine lumen approximately 6 days after ovulation. The **embryonic vesicle** is quite *mobile* after its descent into the uterus (at least after it is detectable by ultrasound examination beginning on day 9 to 10), migrating through both uterine horns and the uterine body. Mobility is maximal on day 11 or 12 and is maintained to approximately day 16. Movement of the embryonic vesicle is passive, being dependent on uterine contractions, which force it through the uterine lumen. Movement throughout the uterus is thought to be important for the conceptus to "signal" the dam that pregnancy has occurred, thereby preventing luteolysis (this process whereby luteolysis is prevented by the presence of the conceptus is referred to as *maternal recognition of pregnancy*). The corpus luteum, called the *primary corpus luteum (CL) of pregnancy*, can be visibly identified in the ovary for up to 180 to 220 days. The primary CL regresses at approximately the same stage of gestation as the supplementary corpora lutea.

The *critical time for maternal recognition of pregnancy, to prevent luteolysis of the primary CL and subsequent loss of the pregnancy, is thought to be 14 to 16 days after ovulation in the mare*. Conditions that prevent the conceptus from migrating throughout the uterus (e.g., blocked uterine horn) interfere with maternal recognition of pregnancy, resulting in failure to prevent endometrial production and release of $PGF_{2\alpha}$, and the mare will return to estrus despite conceiving.

The embryonic vesicle becomes stationary by approximately day 16 after ovulation. This process is referred to as *fixation* and is apparently caused by restriction of the enlarging conceptus at the base of one uterine horn. The process of embryonic vesicle fixation should not be confused with the process of fetal-maternal attachment. Soon after the time of fixation, the cross-sectional shape of the embryonic vesicle typically changes from circular to *triangular;* this change in shape is identified by transrectal ultrasonographic examination. The change in vesicle shape is caused by thickening *(hypertrophy)* of the dorsal uterine wall (see Figures 5-17 through 5-19).

When the reproductive tract is under progesterone influence from the primary CL of pregnancy and estrogen influence from the developing conceptus (estrogen is produced by day 12), the uterus begins to develop a characteristic shape with marked *tone* that becomes readily apparent on palpation per rectum by days 16 to 18 postovulation (Figure 7-1). Examination by palpation per rectum usually reveals suggestive, but not definitive, evidence of early pregnancy at this point, because the conceptus is not yet palpable. The advent of ultrasonography has allowed considerable progress in pregnancy diagnostics in the mare, because this technique enables detection of embryonic vesicles in the uterus as early as 10 to 12 days postovulation. The conceptus does not begin attaching to the endometrium until days 40 to 45 of gestation, so the increased tone of early pregnancy is thought to help keep the embryo and developing membranes in close apposition with the endometrium during this time period to maximize nutrient transfer. During uterine examination at 25 to 35 days of gestation the pregnancy can usually be confirmed by palpation per rectum.

The process of *fetal-maternal attachment* is gradual. The vascularized trophoblast is closely associated with the uterine epithelium by day 25. Beginning interdigitation of **trophoblastic microvilli** and uterine epithelium has been described by days 38 to 40. Fetal **macrovilli** (not the same as microvilli; macrovilli will become the **microcotyledons**) begin appearing by day 45 as rudimentary structures and gradually develop until full placental attachment occurs in the form of well-developed **microplacentomes** (microcotyledons with maternal microcaruncles) by day 150 (Figure 7-2).

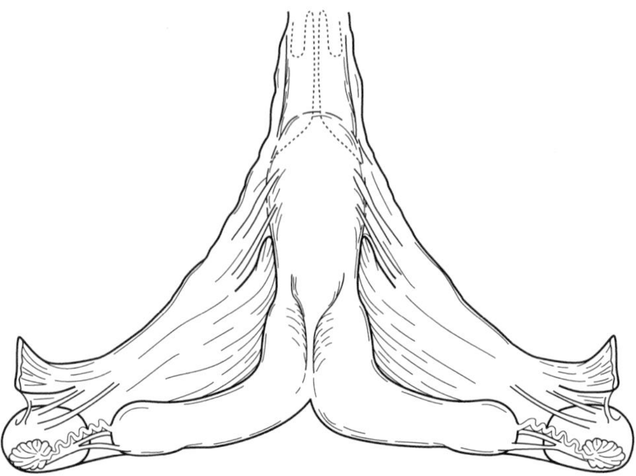

FIGURE 7-1. Drawing of the uterus during day 18 of pregnancy. The cervix is elongated and firmly closed. The uterine horns are palpably turgid, making the bifurcation between the two uterine horns prominent on palpation per rectum.

ENDOMETRIAL CUP FORMATION

A unique feature of the equine placenta is the development of endometrial cups early in gestation. On about day 25 of gestation, a specialized annular band of the **trophoblast** undergoes cellular changes to form the **chorionic girdle** at the junction of the developing allantois and regressing yolk sac. These trophoblastic cells of the chorionic girdle invade the adjacent uterine epithelium on approximately day 38 of gestation, migrating into the underlying lamina propria to develop into the prominent decidua-like cells of the **endometrial cups**. The endometrial cups are identified as a circular or "horseshoe" arrangement of pale, irregular outgrowths on the luminal surface of the gravid uterine horn (Figure 7-3). They attain maximum size at about day 70 of gestation and then begin to undergo degeneration and eventually are sloughed, which is complete by approximately day 130 of gestation. The endometrial cups secrete a hormone known as *equine chorionic gonadotropin (eCG),* previously termed *pregnant mare serum gonadotropin.* eCG is first detectable in maternal blood on days 35 to 42, its concentration rapidly increases to peak levels on days 55 to 65, and then concentrations decline slowly to low or nondetectable levels by days 100 to 150. This hormone is believed to assist in the formation of supplementary corpora lutea and apparently is also thought to be a necessary stimulus for maintenance of the primary CL during approximately days 35 to 120. Progesterone output from the primary CL actually increases during days 35 to 40, before aquisition of significant progesterone production by the supplementary corpora lutea. eCG is also thought to play an important immunoregulatory role during pregnancy.

Endometrial cup formation is an important consideration in the management of early embryonic loss. If pregnancy loss occurs before the formation of the endometrial cups (days 36 to 40), the mare will return to estrus within a short period of time (less than 1 month). Because only the primary CL is present, a single injection of $PGF_{2\alpha}$ will promote CL regression and a return to estrus. *If pregnancy loss occurs after endometrial cup formation, eCG production continues and the mare may not return to estrus for 3 months when the endometrial cups degenerate, thereby allowing supplementary corpora lutea to regress.* Additionally, a mare that loses a conceptus after days 36 to 40 of gestation will continue to show positive results for pregnancy according to eCG detection tests (e.g., Equi-Check, Endocrine Technologies, Inc.) for up to 3 months, because these tests assay for presence of circulating blood levels of eCG, not pregnancy itself. *Of additional importance, repeated $PGF_{2\alpha}$ injections may cause a mare that has aborted after 40 days of gestation to return to estrus by inducing regression of supplementary corpora lutea, but the estrus is seldom fertile as long as endometrial cups remain.* Another aggravating problem when

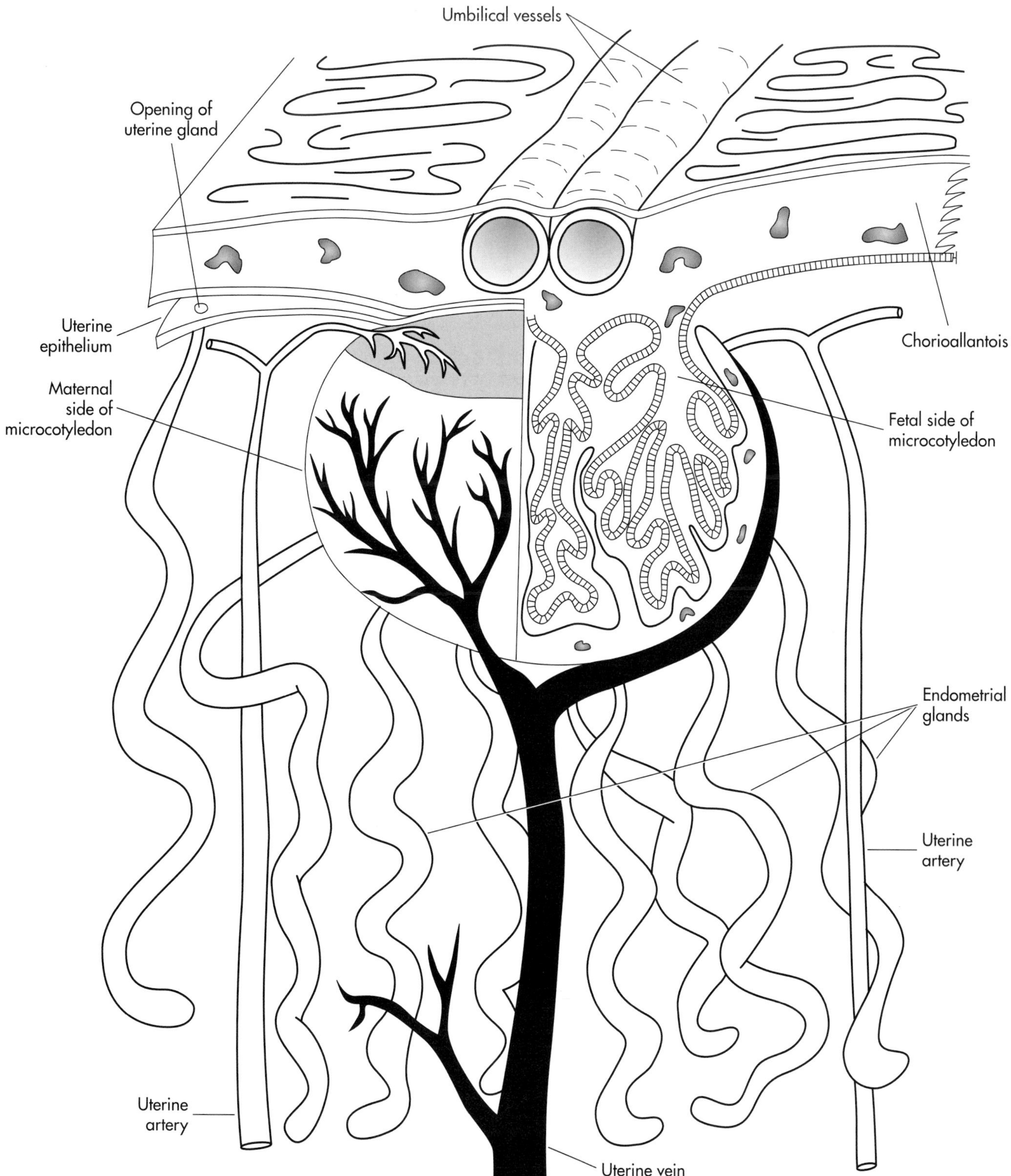

FIGURE 7-2. Drawing of mature microplacentomes composed of fetal microcotyledons and maternal microcaruncles. (Modified from Steven DH, Samuel CA: Anatomy of the placental barrier in the mare. *J Reprod Fertil* 23[Suppl]:579, 1975.)

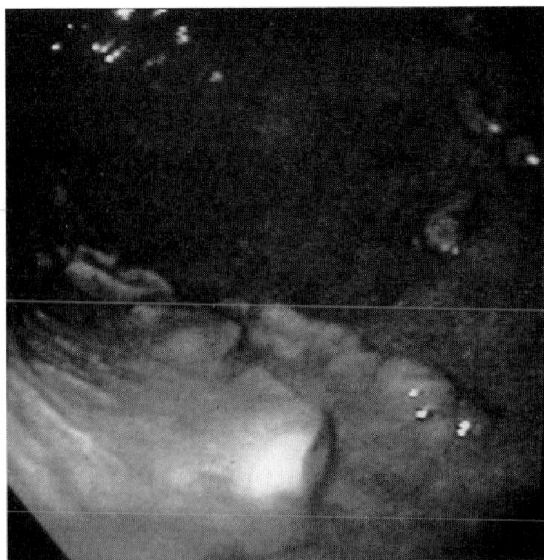

FIGURE 7-3. Endoscopic view of endometrial cups present in the uterus after pregnancy termination at day 70 of gestation.

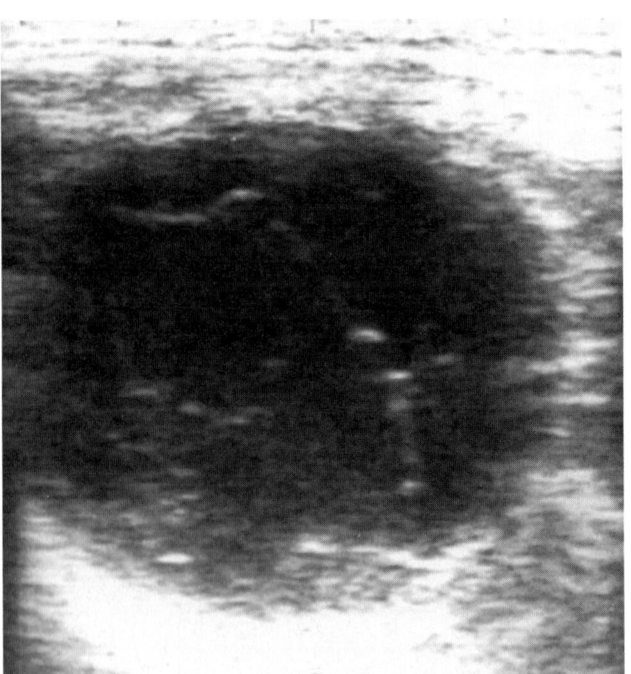

FIGURE 7-4. Anovulatory follicle in a mare that aborted between 70 and 75 days of gestation. Multiple $PGF_{2\alpha}$ injections were given to regress corpora lutea and bring the mare into estrus for rebreeding, but ovulation failed. (Photo courtesy Dr. James Morehead, Equine Medical Associates, PSC, Lexington, KY, 2001.)

one attempts to rebreed a mare that has endometrial cups remaining after abortion, even when the mare has been induced to return to estrus with repeated $PGF_{2\alpha}$ injections, is the tendency for follicles to fail to ovulate. Mares with this problem have also been noted to ovulate smaller-than-normal follicles, luteinize follicles that do not ovulate, or form structures similar in appearance to hemorrhagic anovulatory follicles (Figure 7-4).

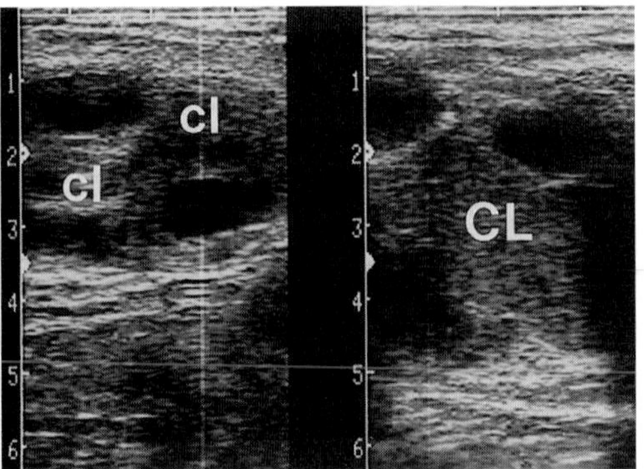

FIGURE 7-5. Ultrasonograph of the ovary of a pregnant mare (65 days of gestation) depicting the primary corpus luteum *(CL)* of pregnancy on the right ovary and supplementary corpora lutea *(cl)* on the left ovary.

DEVELOPMENT OF SUPPLEMENTARY CORPORA LUTEA

Through the control of the pituitary gland and endometrial cups, the ovaries begin to develop supplementary corpora lutea about day 40 of gestation. In response to increasing eCG levels, progesterone production increases from resulting **secondary corpora lutea** (which arise from ovulations over days 40 to 70) and **accessory corpora lutea** (which arise from luteinization of existing follicles over days 40 to 150). The secondary corpora lutea and accessory corpora lutea together are referred to as **supplementary corpora lutea** (Figure 7-5). The additional progesterone produced by supplementary corpora lutea contributes to that produced by the primary corpus luteum in supporting the pregnancy during the first 5 months of pregnancy. *All corpora lutea degenerate by days 150 to 200 of gestation, and the placenta assumes the sole role of progestin secretion (and thus pregnancy maintenance) until parturition.*

In rare instances, mares may not develop supplementary corpora lutea. This phenomenon has been described as one potential cause of abortion in mares at less than 100 to 150 days of gestation. During the transition from pregnancy dependence on ovarian progesterone to placental progestin, the mare may experience increased susceptibility to abortion from adverse environmental influences. Abortion may occur during this time span (days 70 to 150 of gestation) from stress-related causes such as unaccustomed exercise, trucking, inclement weather, or maternal illness.

PROGESTIN PRODUCTION BY THE FETOPLACENTAL UNIT

The fetoplacental unit synthesizes and secretes high levels of *progestins* (primarily 5α-pregnanes) into the maternal circulation during mid to late pregnancy. These progestins first appear in the maternal circulation between days 30 and 60

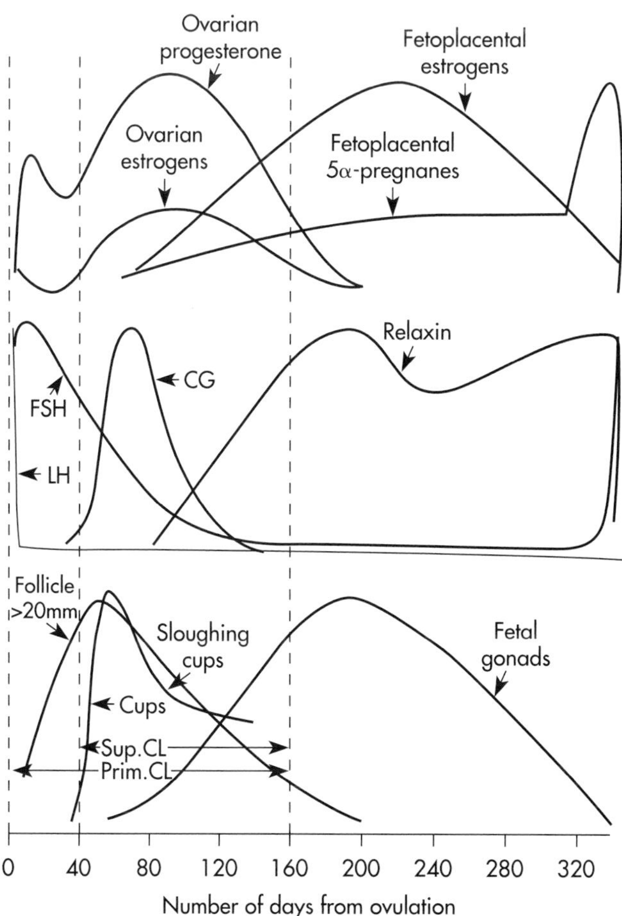

FIGURE 7-6. Graphic summary of the hormonal and reproductive changes that occur during equine pregnancy. (Modified from Ginther OJ: *Reproductive biology of the mare: basic and applied aspects,* ed 2, Cross Plains, WI, 1992, Equiservices.)

and increase gradually through day 300 of gestation. Fetoplacental progestin production is sufficient to maintain pregnancy in mares in mid to late gestation. Studies involving ovariectomy during different gestational stages have led to the conclusion that an ovarian source of progesterone is required to maintain pregnancy in some mares as late as day 70 but is not essential beyond days 100 to 140 of gestation. Indeed, many ovariectomized mares will maintain pregnancy in the absence of exogenously administered progesterone from day 100 of gestation to term. A summary of hormonal and reproductive changes that occur during pregnancy in the mare is provided in Figure 7-6.

☐ Summary of Methods of Pregnancy Diagnosis

Several methods of pregnancy detection are available to the veterinarian. The type of diagnostic aid used depends on equipment availability, clinician expertise, and stage of pregnancy. Some methods of pregnancy diagnosis currently used are outlined below.

Behavioral Assessment

Monitor sexual behavior of mare by daily teasing with a stallion. A mare that is not pregnant should demonstrate behavioral estrus approximately 16 to 20 days after ovulation. Failure of the mare to return to estrus suggests pregnancy.

False-positive and false-negative results are likely to occur. Some pregnant mares will exhibit behavioral estrus. Persistent luteal function and early embryonic death (after day 14 of gestation) may result in uninterrupted signs of diestrus in a nonpregnant mare.

This is a nonspecific indicator of pregnancy.

Serum/Milk Progesterone Assay

Progesterone assay is performed 18 to 20 days after ovulation. A high progesterone level implies the presence of a functional CL, thereby suggesting pregnancy.

False-positive results can result from a persistent luteal function (spontaneous or owing to early embryonic death after maternal recognition of pregnancy has occurred that prevents CL regression).

This is a nonspecific indicator of pregnancy.

Vaginal Speculum Examination

Vaginal speculum examination is performed 18 to 21 days after ovulation, usually in conjunction with examination of the reproductive tract per rectum. Speculum examination is not indicated unless results of per rectum examination are equivocal. The presence of a dry, pale, tightly closed cervix with the external os protruding into the center of the cranial vagina suggests pregnancy.

This is a nonspecific indicator of pregnancy, simply suggesting the presence of a functional CL that is secreting progesterone.

Palpation of the Reproductive Tract per Rectum

Palpation of the reproductive tract per rectum is the most common and rapid pregnancy detection method in current use. It can be used to detect pregnancy at almost any stage of gestation.

Detection of Early Pregnancy at 18 to 20 Days after Ovulation (Figure 7-1). During this time period, *increased tone and tubularity of the uterine horns* are noted. The increase tone makes the external bifurcation between the two uterine horns noticeable as a prominent "cleft" or indentation. *Ovarian follicular activity is usually quite pronounced, and the cervix is elongated, firm, and tightly closed.* The cervix is so prominent that it feels much like a pencil per rectum, being longer than is usual for a mare in diestrus. In maiden mares with a small uterus, a small swelling at the base of a uterine horn may occasionally be detected. False-positive and false-negative results may occur with early embryonic death or persistent luteal function. Transrectal ultrasound

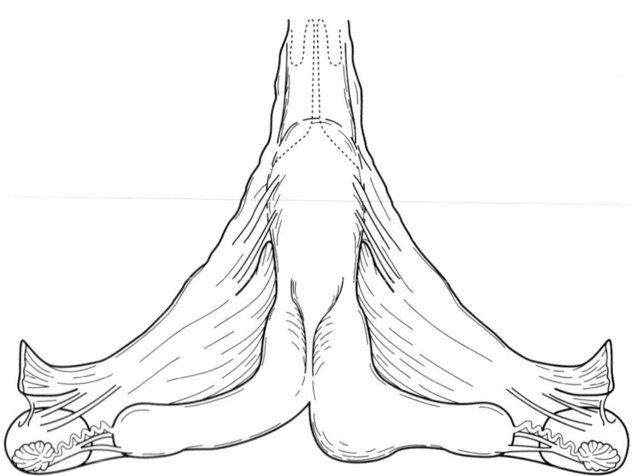

FIGURE 7-7. Drawing of the appearance of the uterus of a mare at 25 to 30 days of gestation. The pronounced uterine tone and tubularity typical of early pregnancy remain, along with the palpably elongated cervix. A resilient spherical or ovoid bulge approximately the size of a golf ball or hen's egg is often palpable at the base of one uterine horn.

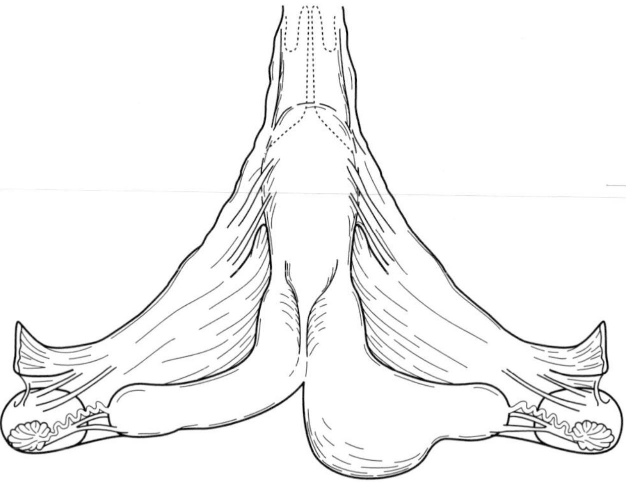

FIGURE 7-8. Drawing of the appearance of the uterus of a mare at 35 to 40 days of gestation. The pronounced uterine tone and tubularity typical of early pregnancy remain, along with the palpably elongated cervix. A resilient spherical or ovoid bulge approximately the size of a tennis ball or baseball is present at the base of one uterine horn.

examination is usually required to confirm pregnancy at this stage.

Detection of Pregnancy at 25 to 30 Days after Ovulation (Figure 7-7). The prominent uterine tone and tubularity, elongated cervix, and pronounced follicular activity noted at 18 to 21 days of gestation are still present. In addition, *a resilient spherical or ovoid bulge* (approximately the size of a golf ball or hen's egg) can often be noted on the anteroventral aspect of the uterine horn near the external bifurcation. It is critical that the ventral surface of the uterine horns be gently picked up in the fingers, because the bulge of early pregnancy is easy to miss if only the dorsal surface of the uterine horns is palpated. The uterine wall over the bulge is thin-walled with less tone than the adjacent uterine wall, feeling much like a balloon filled with water.

Detection of Pregnancy at 35 to 40 Days after Ovulation (Figure 7-8). Palpation per rectum of the mare that is 35 to 40 days pregnant reveals the above findings plus a *resilient spherical-to-ovoid bulge (approximately the size of a tennis ball or baseball)* at the base of one uterine horn.

Detection of Pregnancy at 45 to 50 Days after Ovulation (Figure 7-9). Palpation per rectum of the mare that is 45 to 50 days pregnant reveals the above findings plus a *resilient spherical-to-ovoid bulge (approximately the size of a softball)* that fills the palm and fingers of the hand. The ventral uterine wall typically feels thin-walled and more fluid-filled than earlier in the pregnancy.

Detection of Pregnancy at 60 to 65 Days after Ovulation (Figure 7-10). Although the cervix remains quite elongated and firm, the progressive filling of the uterus as pregnancy advances tends to feel less tonic than earlier in the pregnancy. Additionally, the pregnancy is *beginning to expand into the uterine body,* and the uterus begins to descend into the ventral abdomen as pregnancy progresses. The uterine bulge tends

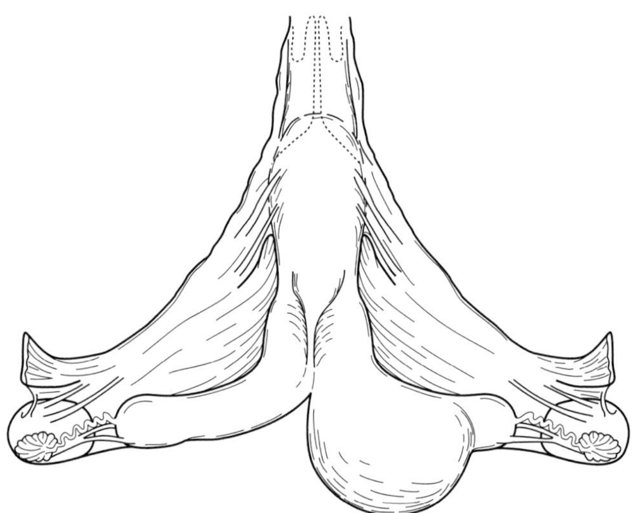

FIGURE 7-9. Drawing of the appearance of the uterus of a mare at 45 to 50 days of gestation. The elongated cervix and increased uterine tone remain. A resilient spherical or ovoid bulge approximately the size of a softball or grapefruit is present at the base of one uterine horn.

to lose some of its earlier resiliency. The uterine bulge is *approximately the size of a cantaloupe or small football.*

Detection of Pregnancy at 100 to 120 Days after Ovulation (Figure 7-11). The pregnancy continues its expansion into the uterine body, being easier to detect here than in the uterine horn. The pregnancy is easily felt more dorsally than before, with the bulge being *the size of a volleyball or basketball.* The fetus may sometimes be ballotted within the uterus, although ballottement is more difficult at this stage of pregnancy than in the cow. *It is quite easy to mistake a full urinary bladder for pregnancy at this stage, so the examiner must take care to ensure*

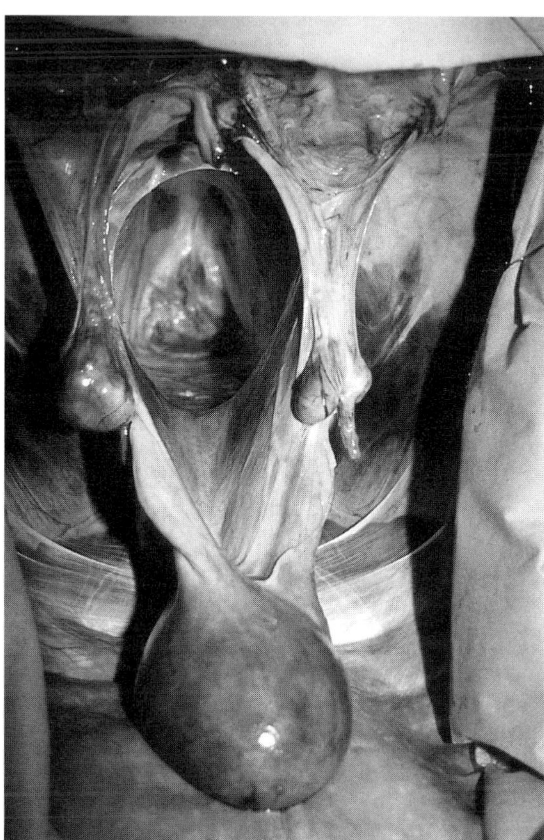

FIGURE 7-10. Appearance of the uterus of a mare at 60 to 65 days of gestation. The rectum and abdominal viscera have been removed. The elongated cervix remains readily palpable per rectum, and the bulge at the base of one uterine horn is moving into the body of the uterus and is the size of a cantaloupe or small football.

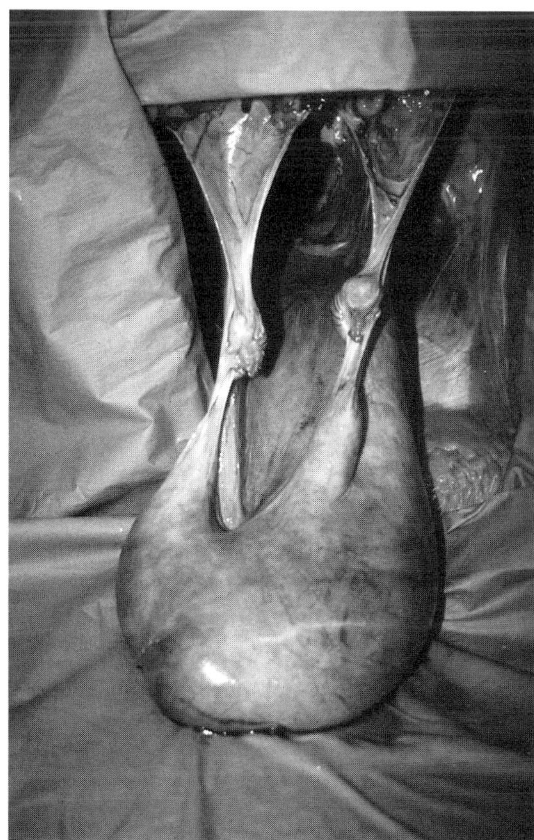

FIGURE 7-11. Appearance of the uterus of a mare at 100 to 120 days of gestation. The rectum and abdominal viscera have been removed. The elongated cervix remains readily palpable per rectum, and the bulge in the uterus typically is the size of a volleyball or basketball.

that the fluid being felt is within the uterus. Tracing the fluid-filled organ back to the cervix will confirm that it is the uterus and not the urinary bladder. If the cervix is not located, the examination must be repeated, taking even more care to search for anatomical markers of the reproductive tract, including the ovaries.

Detection of Pregnancy at 150 to 210 Days after Ovulation. As pregnancy progresses and the uterus enlarges, the heavy uterine contents pull the suspending broad ligaments and ovaries into a more medioventral position. Uterine descent into the ventral abdomen is complete at 150 to 210 days of gestation, and the pregnant uterus is too large to be encompassed with the outreached arm. The fetus is located in the ventral abdomen but may usually be detected by ballottement.

Detection of Pregnancy at 240 Days of Gestation to Term. The enlarging uterus begins to expand upward, with the majority of fetal growth occurring during this period. As the fetus enlarges markedly, there is proportionately less fluid present in the uterus, making the hard fetus easy to feel. Although the position and approximate size of the fetus can usually be detected, a precise estimation of the gestational age of the fetus is quite difficult.

DETECTION OF PREGNANCY BY ULTRASOUND EXAMINATION

Major advantages of transrectal ultrasonography for pregnancy detection in the mare are the following:

- Allows the earliest positive detection of pregnancy, with the embryonic vesicle being visible as early as days 10 to 12 of gestation. The accuracy of vesicle detection approaches 99% by 15 days of gestation.
- Provides embryonic vesicle and embryo growth charts (sometimes programmed into the ultrasound computer) that permit more accurate determination of embryo/fetal age.
- Permits early detection of twin pregnancy, allowing superior methods of intervention to be pursued.
- Permits assessment of early embryonic loss by comparing expected development based on ovulation or breeding dates against actual values.
- Permits assessment of embryonic and fetal viability (i.e., heartbeat, movement, and expected development for age).
- Allows fetal sexing at approximately days 60 to 70 of gestation.

Transrectal ultrasonography does have its limitations. It cannot replace palpation per rectum; indeed, to effectively use ultrasonography the veterinarian must first be an accomplished palpator. The equipment is expensive, so some clients will find the charges for ultrasound pregnancy diagnosis to be prohibitive. Interpretive errors are also possible. Finally, the fetus is often difficult to visualize by transrectal ultrasonography between 3 to 5 or 6 months of gestation because progressive enlargement of the gravid uterus causes it to be beyond the reach of the examiner. Transabdominal ultrasonography using a 2.5- to 3.5-MHz curvilinear or sector probe is often helpful in assessing fetal viability during this period of mid-term gestation as well as during late-term gestation.

Refer to Chapter 5 for a discussion of characteristics of early pregnancy that are detectable by transrectal ultrasonographic examination.

EQUINE CHORIONIC GONADOTROPIN DETECTION

Recall that eCG is produced by endometrial cups in the pregnant mare uterus, beginning on days 36 to 40 of gestation. The period of detection of eCG in mare serum is limited to days 40 to 120 of gestation.

To test for the presence of eCG, serum can be submitted to a reference laboratory for testing, or serum can be analyzed using a commercially available "mare-side" kit. Using a mare-side kit, the test can be completed in approximately 30 minutes.

False-positive reactions are possible. If a pregnancy is lost after days 36 to 40 of gestation, when endometrial cups are already developed in the endometrium, a false-positive result will occur (i.e., eCG is present despite pregnancy loss).

False-negative reactions occur if serum is evaluated before days 36 to 40 of gestation, when concentrations of eCG in the mare's serum may be too low to detect, or after day 120 of gestation, when concentrations have declined after endometrial cup regression. Additionally, false-negative results are very common (81%) in mares carrying mule fetuses.

ESTROGEN DETECTION IN BLOOD OR URINE

The developing conceptus has a remarkable estrogen-producing capability as early as day 12 of pregnancy. Concentrations of estrogens in the blood and urine parallel each other. By days 60 to 100 of pregnancy, estrogen concentrations in blood or urine exceed those noted during estrus. Because the estrogens are secreted primarily by the fetoplacental unit, the assay for estrogens has been advocated as a noninvasive means for assessing fetal viability during pregnancy. The concentration of estrogens in feces has even been reported for pregnancy diagnosis in feral horses. Blood serum or plasma can be submitted to a reference laboratory for measurement of estrogen concentration. The circulating estrogen concentration peaks at day 180 to 240 of gestation, then slowly declines until parturition. The test has been advocated for diagnosing pregnancy and fetal viability or stress from 60 to 80 days of gestation through term. We have noted some pregnant mares with equivocal or negative test results (estrone sulfate concentrations below that expected for pregnant mares) at 60 to 70 days of gestation that became positive (estrone sulfate concentrations consistent with viable pregnancy) at 80 days of gestation.

BIBLIOGRAPHY

Bergfeldt DR, Adams GP, Pierson RA: Pregnancy. In Rantanen NW, McKinnon AO, editors, *Equine diagnostic ultrasonography,* Baltimore, 1998, Williams & Wilkins.

Ginther OJ: *Reproductive biology of the mare—basic and applied aspects,* ed 2, Cross Plains, WI, 1992, Equiservices.

McKinnon AO: Diagnosis of pregnancy. In McKinnon AO, Voss JL, editors, *Equine reproduction,* Philadelphia, 1993, Lea and Febiger.

Neely DP: Equine gestation. In Neely DP, Liu IMK, Hillman RB, editors, *Equine reproduction,* Nutley, NY, 1983, Veterinary Learning Systems Co.

8

Pregnancy Loss

OBJECTIVES

While studying the information covered in this chapter, the student should attempt to:

1. Acquire an understanding of the factors that contribute to pregnancy losses in the equine embryonic, fetal, natal, and neonatal periods.
2. Acquire a working knowledge of the signs of placental and fetal infection.
3. Acquire a working knowledge of procedures to be followed to maximize the chance of diagnosing the cause of an abortion.
4. Acquire a working knowledge of the more common gestational abnormalities in the mare, including management of each condition.

STUDY QUESTIONS

1. Give the length of the embryonic, fetal, and neonatal periods of the horse.
2. List signs of embryonic loss in the mare, and discuss methods that can be used to confirm it.
3. Discuss management options for embryonic death in the mare.
4. List the causes of placental dysfunction in the mare.
5. List the more common infectious and noninfectious causes of abortion in the mare.
6. Explain why most aborted fetuses submitted for examination are 6 to 11 months of gestational age.
7. Explain how placentitis results in abortion.
8. Give the routes of placental and fetal invasion by microorganisms.
9. Design a thorough diagnostic approach to an abortion problem on a broodmare farm.
10. Describe the more common gestational abnormalities in the mare, and discuss methods of diagnosis, treatment, and probable outcomes for each.

Equine pregnancy loss occurs more often early in pregnancy than later. Bain reported that, of pregnancies that were lost, 55% occurred by day 39 of gestation and 75% by day 49. The rate of pregnancy loss apparently diminishes after days 60 to 75 of gestation. Among individual mares that suffer early loss of pregnancy, the rate of subsequent pregnancy loss is reportedly not different from that of the rest of the mare population (i.e., pregnancy loss is no more likely to recur than in mares not previously having a pregnancy loss). Despite this report, some mares seem to be predisposed to recurring pregnancy losses. Additionally, pregnancy loss rates tend to gradually increase when broodmares exceed 12 to 15 years of age.

Many genetic, maternal, and environmental factors can contribute to pregnancy loss during critical periods of development. These include the **embryonic period** (conception through organogenesis), **fetal period** (completion of organogenesis through end of gestation), **natal period** (birth), and **neonatal period** (first 28 days of life).

The susceptibility of the embryo to injurious agents varies with the stage of development. Cattle and sheep embryos less than 14 days of age (period of preattachment) are resistant to teratogens but susceptible to genetic mutations and chromosomal abnormalities. During the rest of the embryonic period, the embryo is highly susceptible to teratogens until this susceptibility begins to decrease as the various organ systems develop. The *embryonic period in the horse includes the period from conception to 40 days of gestation* (according to a review by Ginther in 1992).

Limitations in accurately determining that conception has occurred prevent accurate assessment of the incidence of **embryonic death** in most animals. For the horse, the rate of pregnancy loss between days 15 and 50 after ovulation has been reported to be 10% to 15%. These estimates are based on losses that occur after early pregnancy diagnosis by transrectal ultrasonography. Rates of earlier pregnancy loss (i.e., before ultrasonographic detection is possible at 10 to 14 days post-ovulation) are more difficult to assess but have been obtained from flushing uteri on different days (7 to 10 days post-ovulation) and comparing actual embryo recovery rates at those times with known fertilization rates obtained in other populations of mares (by determining whether ova are cleaved in the oviducts). The presence of nonrecovered oocytes or embryos, a problem with any recovery methodology, adds a measure of inaccuracy to such estimates.

Estimates for embryonic death rates in the horse vary from 5% to 24%; the average is approximately 20% from conception to day 40 of gestation in groups of fertile mares. Because fertilization rates are generally quite high in both fertile and subfertile mares (exceeding 80% to 90%), a significant cause of subfertility is early embryonic death. New York researchers reported the incidence of embryonic death before day 14 of gestation to be seven to eight times greater for aged, subfertile mares than for young, fertile mares. Other investigators found that older mares are more likely to produce defective oocytes; if these are fertilized, presumably, higher rates of embryonic death are seen.

The nonviable embryo is resorbed or expelled from the uterus and is therefore seldom observed. If embryonic death occurs before maternal recognition of pregnancy, affected mares will return to estrus at the usual time expected if they had failed to conceive. In such cases, early embryonic death would not be suspected.

CAUSES OF EMBRYONIC DEATH

Possible causes of embryonic mortality include infectious agents, chromosomal abnormalities, teratogenic agents, immunologic reactions, genetic abnormalities, local uterine disturbances, nutritional factors (particularly deficient dietary energy or protein intake), and temperature stress. Ball (1993) divides potential factors contributing to embryonic mortality into three general areas: (1) maternal, (2) external, and (3) embryonic.

Maternal Factors

- Endocrine—low progesterone production from *failure of maternal recognition of pregnancy, primary luteal deficiency,* or *uterine-induced luteolysis* caused by endometrial irritation.
- Oviductal environment—improper timing of oviductal transport; *salpingitis.*
- Uterine environment—commonly including *endometritis* and *periglandular fibrosis;* intraluminal fluid accumulation (often caused by endometritis) during early pregnancy; endometrial cysts when embryonic vesicle fixation occurs at cyst location.
- Age—increased embryonic death rates as mares age, attributed in part to age-related degeneration of the uterus and/or oocyte viability.
- Lactation—if nutritional demands result in *declining body condition, delayed uterine involution,* or *persistent endometritis.*

External Factors

- Stress—hypothesized to decrease progesterone production, which may result in pregnancy loss.
- Inadequate nutrition—particularly when mares lose body condition in late gestation and/or early lactation.

Embryonic Factors

- Small size; morphologic defects.
- Reduced viability of embryos from aged, subfertile mares when transferred to uteri of normal recipient mares.
- Chromosomal abnormalities originating from *gamete aging* or other causes.

DIAGNOSIS OF EMBRYONIC DEATH (AFTER ULTRASONOGRAPHIC DETERMINATION OF PREGNANCY)

In a thorough discussion of ultrasonographically detectable signs of impending embryonic loss, Newcombe (2000) suggests the following criteria for predicting its occurrence.

Small-for-Age Embryonic Vesicles

Embryonic vesicles are sometimes visible as early as days 10 to 11 postovulation, at a diameter of 3 to 4 mm. Vesicle size (diameter, top to bottom) typically increases 3 to 4 mm in diameter each day until day 16, plateaus at days 17 to 25, and resumes increasing in diameter by 1.8 mm/day by day 28 (Ginther, 1986). Whenever the diameter of the vesicle (through 30 days) is retarded in development by more than 1 to 2 days, particularly when it is undersized on more than one examination, embryonic viability should be questioned (Figure 8-1). Colorado workers recently found that the percentage of examinations during which the vesicle was undersized was significantly higher for abnormal conceptuses (44.4%) than for normal conceptuses (<1%). Some veterinary ultrasound machines are programmed with gestation tables that permit the practitioner to estimate gestational age based on ultrasonographic measurements, which is very useful for determining whether conceptuses are small for gestational age.

Anembryonic Vesicles

On occasion, vesicles fail to develop an embryo (Figure 8-2). Such vesicles often are first noted to be small for gestational

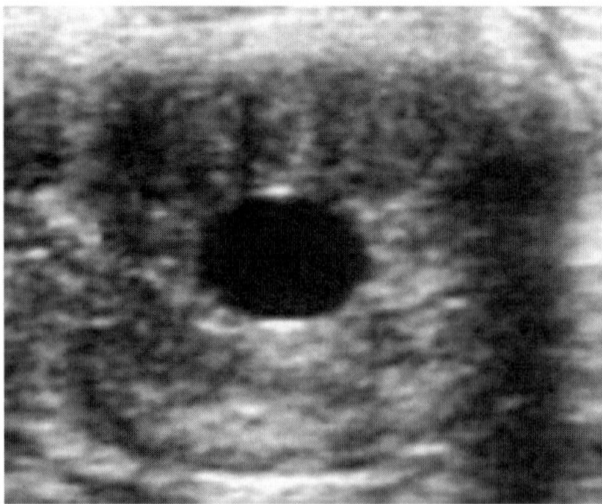

FIGURE 8-1. Transrectal ultrasonographic image of an embryonic vesicle 16 days postovulation. The vesicle was smaller than expected (being only approximately 1 cm in diameter) for gestational age, and the pregnancy was lost by day 21.

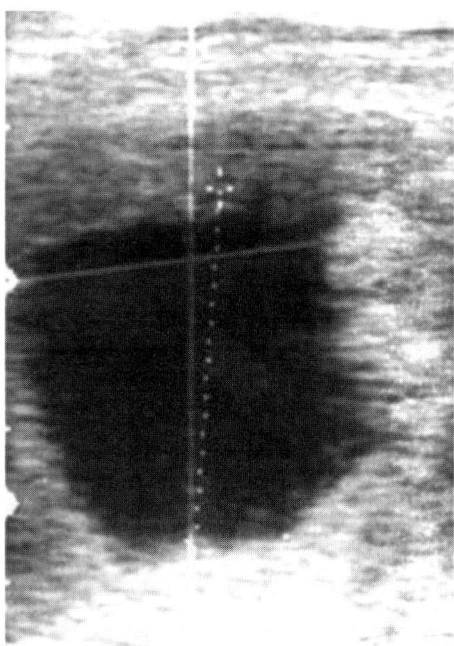

FIGURE 8-2. Transrectal ultrasonographic image of a small-for-gestational-age embryonic vesicle on day 32 postovulation. The vesicle had been normal sized on days 14 and 16 postovulation, but no embryo was visualized on days 27 or 32 postovulation. The conceptus was no longer detectable by day 36 postovulation.

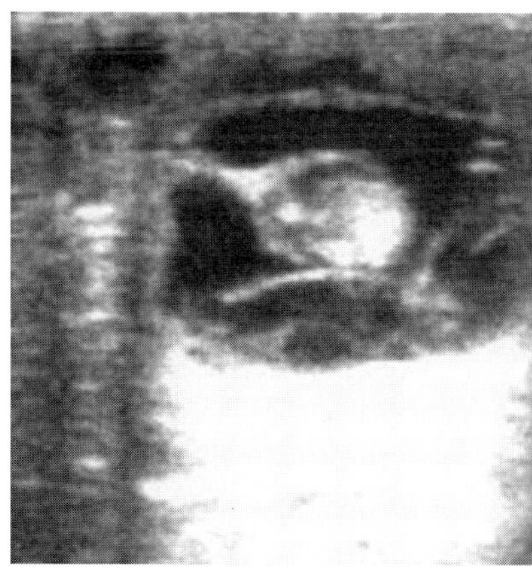

FIGURE 8-3. Abnormal pregnancy with impending loss is evident in this transrectal ultrasonographic image of a day 38 postovulation conceptus. An embryonic heartbeat was not present, and the chorioallantois had separated from the endometrium.

age when they are detected early in pregnancy before the embryo would be ultrasonographically visible (typically by days 20 to 21 of gestation). If an embryo is not visible by days 24 to 26, embryonic viability should be questioned. Colorado workers found the incidence of anembryonic vesicles to be 4.4%.

Retarded Development of the Embryo

Normal progression in embryo development, as outlined in Chapter 5, should be apparent during examination for pregnancy. Briefly, the embryo is typically apparent by 21 days, the embryonic heartbeat can be seen by 24 to 25 days, and the allantois should occupy approximately one-half of the vesicle by 28 to 30 days and most of the vesicle (with the embryo having migrated dorsally within the vesicle) by 33 to 36 days, and migrate to the ventrum of the allantois by 48 to 50 days. The embryo should also increase in size and development during this time. When development is retarded, heartbeat is lost, allantoic shrinkage occurs, or separation of membranes from the endometrium occurs (Figure 8-3), impending pregnancy loss should be suspected.

Abnormalities of Embryo Location and Orientation

The embryo normally appears in the 6 o'clock position within the vesicle, is lifted dorsally to the 12 o'clock position within the vesicle as the allantois develops, and then migrates ventrally as the umbilicus lengthens. Although altered orientation within the vesicle is noted with many singleton pregnancies, variations from the usual have not been proven to predict embryonic death. However, when the embryonic vesicle develops within the body of the uterus *(body pregnancy)* instead of at the base of one of the uterine horns, the pregnancy is thought to be prone to failure even though early development appears normal.

Development Adjacent to Endometrial Cyst(s)

The influence of endometrial cysts on fertility was discussed previously in Chapter 5. Whether endometrial cysts affect fertility independent of mare age (because of age-related changes in the endometrium that are often present in addition to cysts) is still an area of controversy. When the embryonic vesicle develops over a cyst, there may be an increased likelihood of pregnancy failure. Certainly many such pregnancies develop normally, and normal foals are delivered at term, so the size of the cyst(s) and orientation of the embryo in relation to the cyst may be important (Figure 8-4). Newcombe (2000) hypothesized that when the embryo begins development over the uterine wall, it is likely to develop normally, whereas if it begins development directly over the cyst, nutrient deprivation that will result in pregnancy loss is more likely to occur.

DEVELOPMENT OF UTERINE EDEMA DURING EARLY PREGNANCY

On occasion a mare in early pregnancy (15 to 17 days postovulation) will develop pronounced uterine edema, sometimes associated with behavioral estrus. Measurement of the progesterone concentration usually reveals low values consistent with estrus. Some of these pregnancies can be salvaged by immediate administration of progesterone or progestogen, which should be continued until either another ovulation occurs and a functional corpus luteum is formed, or progesterone supplementation is no longer deemed necessary to support

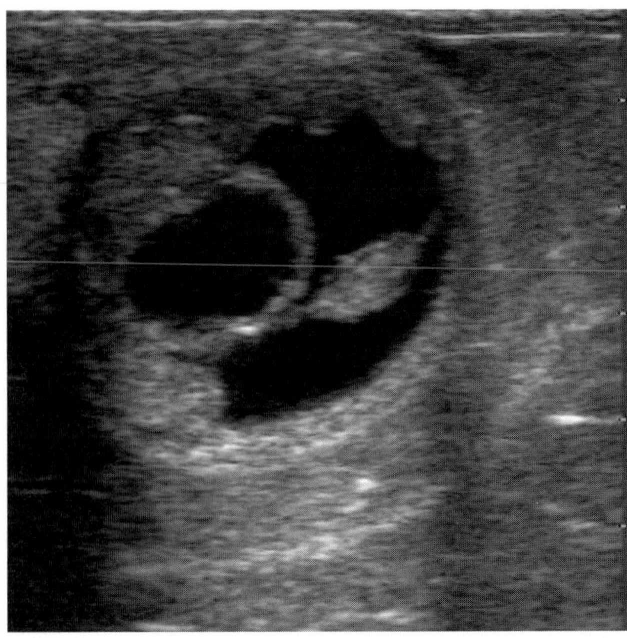

FIGURE 8-4. Transrectal ultrasonographic image of a day 28 post-ovulation embryonic vesicle developing adjacent to an endometrial cyst.

the pregnancy (usually 100 to 150 days of gestation). Newcombe (2000) suggested that conceptuses in such mares are more likely to be abnormal, particularly when embryonic vesicles are smaller than expected at 12 to 14 days post-ovulation; thus these pregnancies are more likely to fail even though progesterone supplementation is implemented. Close monitoring of embryonic development is warranted in mares given progesterone for these reasons.

MANAGEMENT OF MARES WITH SIGNS OF ABNORMAL EMBRYONIC DEVELOPMENT

With the exception of progesterone/progestogen supplementation of mares developing uterine edema during early pregnancy, the most prudent management of mares with signs of abnormal embryonic development is serial reexaminations at 1- to 3-day intervals. Colorado workers suggested that if an embryo and heartbeat cannot be identified ultrasonographically by day 25, monitoring through day 30 is indicated. If a viable embryo with an evident heartbeat does not become apparent by this time, prostaglandin $F_{2\alpha}$ should be administered to induce luteal regression and a return to estrus for rebreeding. Newcombe (2000) also suggested that manual crushing of the conceptus at the time of induced luteolysis, followed by uterine lavage to remove any remaining embryonic debris at the time of induced estrus, might improve the chances of conception when such mares are immediately rebred.

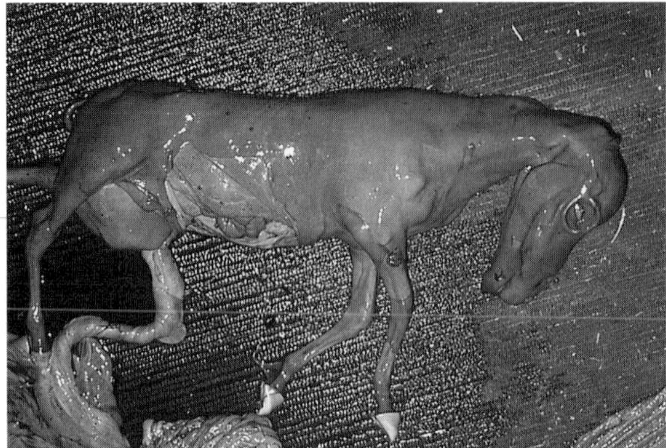

FIGURE 8-5. Intrauterine growth retardation (undersized for gestational age) is apparent in this aborted, autolytic equine fetus.

PREGNANCY LOSS BEYOND THE EMBRYONIC PERIOD

Fetal susceptibility to teratogens decreases with increasing age, except for those structures that differentiate later such as the cerebellum, palate, and urogenital system. The extent of fetal damage that occurs with infection depends on fetal age at the time of infection, degree of fetal immunocompetence, virulence of the infectious agent, and extent of placental lesions and degree of placental dysfunction.

Although the exact level of function necessary to support fetal life and development is difficult to define, a critical level of placental function is deemed necessary to support the developing embryo and fetus to term. Therefore **placental dysfunction** is a common cause of pregnancy loss. Possible causes of placental dysfunction include acute or chronic *placentitis, hypoxia* resulting from alterations in the perfusion ratios between uterine and placental blood flow (e.g., with uterine torsion), a *defective placenta* (e.g., in hydrallantois), *inadequate placental implantation* or *attachment, edema of the placenta,* local immunologic reactions in the placenta, and *maternal disease* or *malnutrition.* Placental dysfunction may result in a malformed fetus, fetal death, mummification, abortion, retarded fetal growth (Figure 8-5), prematurity, full-term stillbirth, and neonatal weakness and death.

Low birth weights of neonates are often attributed to placental dysfunction caused by infection with microorganisms. Signs in the neonate (such as neonatal weakness and septicemia) resulting from fetal infection in utero are usually encountered in the first week of life, particularly within the first 24 hours.

ABORTION

Abortion is the termination of pregnancy before the fetus is capable of extrauterine life. There are both *infectious* and *noninfectious* causes of abortion. The overall rate of abortion in the horse population reportedly varies from 5% to 15%. Observed abortions after 4 months of gestation usually account for a small fraction of equine pregnancy wastage; however, abortions before 4 months of gestation are rarely observed because fetal/placental tissues are small and often overlooked in bedding or on the pasture, and genital discharges are usually scant after abortion at this early stage. Therefore most aborted fetuses examined are 6 to 11 months of gestational age. The majority of equine abortions are caused by placental dysfunction.

Abortions may be *acute* or *chronic*. Acute abortions, such as those caused by equine herpesvirus (EHV-1), occur with no premonitory signs, whereas chronic abortions, such as those caused by twins and mycotic and most bacterial infections, follow premonitory signs. The fetus usually dies in utero, but some fetuses may be delivered alive but nonviable. When abortion occurs, the placenta, fetus, and fluids should be regarded as *potential sources of infection* to other pregnant mares until EHV-1 and *Salmonella abortus-equi* have been eliminated as causes. The percentage of equine abortions for which a cause can be determined is approximately 60%.

A summary of more common causes of equine abortion and recommendations for prevention is given in Table 8-1.

Placentitis is the lesion most commonly found in infectious abortion. In *acute placentitis,* hyperemia and hemorrhage occur, which lead to degeneration and necrosis that extends from the chorionic villi to the surrounding chorioallantois. Organisms and toxins then invade and kill the fetus. In *chronic placentitis,* infection extending through the placenta leads to edema and thickening of the chorioallantois, causing gradual separation of affected chorionic villi. As the edema progresses, the affected chorioallantois changes color from bright red to yellow and even to a leathery brown (Figures 8-6 and 8-7).

Placental invasion by microorganisms can occur hematogenously (e.g., leptospirosis), by extension from the uterus, or more commonly by ascent from the vagina (e.g., streptococci and fungi) (see Figure 8-6). Microorganisms invade the fetus *directly* (via the umbilical vein) or *indirectly* (via the amnionic fluid through fetal inhalation or ingestion or by invasion through the skin).

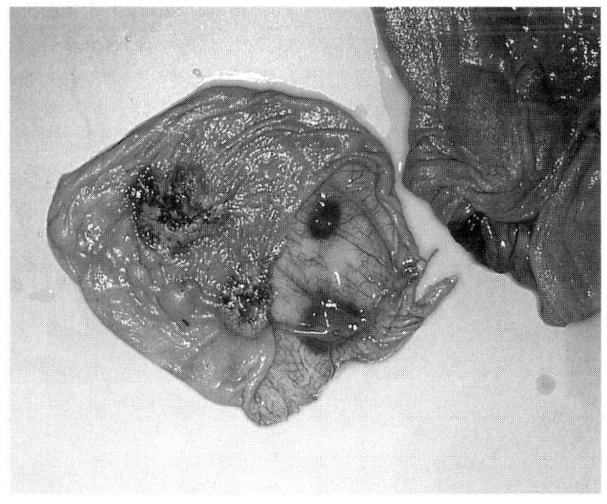

FIGURE 8-7. Section of placenta illustrating focal necrotic placentitis typical of fungal infection.

Dennis (1981) explained that aborted fetuses may be broadly divided into three groups: (1) those with no evidence of infection; (2) those with evidence of infection; and (3) those that are too autolytic to evaluate. Lesions detected in aborted fetuses are associated with the time of fetal death. Fetuses aborted at 4 to 6 months of gestation are usually autolytic and the cause is often bacterial septicemia. Fetuses aborted at 6 to 8 months of gestation are usually less autolytic, and placental lesions are more discernible. Fetuses aborted at 8 to 11 months of gestation are likely to be accompanied by apparent placental lesions (if the placenta was involved) as well as evident fetal lesions (because the fetus is becoming progressively more immunocompetent, permitting inflammatory reactions to occur). Full-term fetal deaths occur with *stillbirth* (i.e., a term, full-sized fetus that, although it was alive in utero, was born dead). Stillbirths occur commonly with

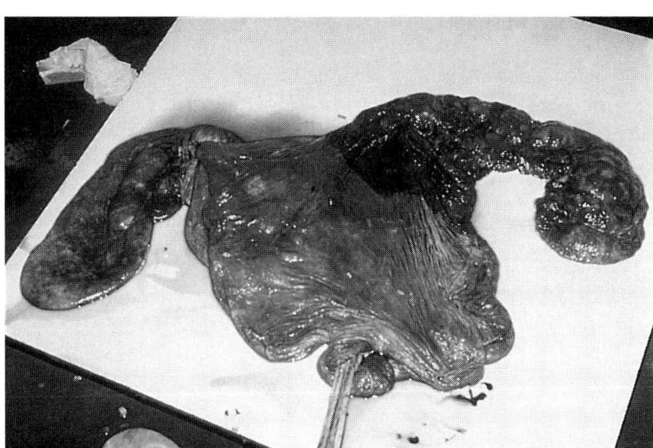

FIGURE 8-6. Thickened, yellow-brown areas of chronic placentitis. An ascending pattern of placentitis is apparent.

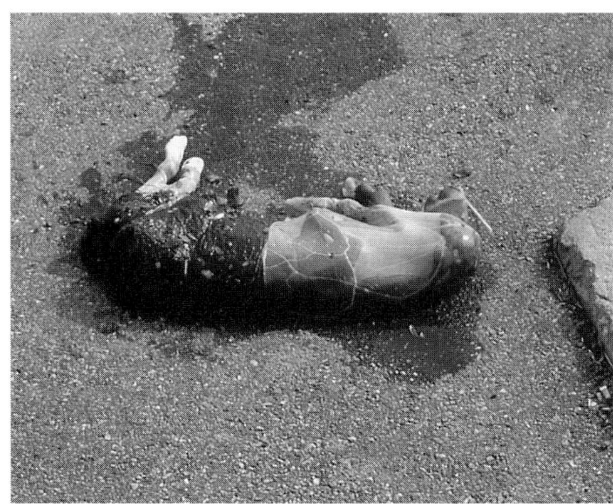

FIGURE 8-8. Fresh stillborn fetus delivered encased in the placenta. Viral isolation procedures yielded EHV-1.

TABLE 8-1

Diagnostic Summary of Some Common Abortion-Causing Diseases of Horses

Disease	Etiology	Clinical Signs	Placental Lesions	Fetal Lesions	Laboratory Diagnosis	Other
Equine rhinopneumonitis (EHV-1)	Equine herpes virus 1 Incubation up to 4 mo; abortions 1-4 mo after respiratory outbreak in weanlings	Primarily a respiratory disease, but also causes late abortions (>5 mo), stillbirths, or weak, infected foals (septicemia, viremia); can produce abortion storms (1%-90%) Respiratory disease and abortions rarely seen concurrently Occasionally seen with neurologic form of disease	None apart from some edema Chorioallantois usually separates from endometrium, thus fetus usually expelled fresh and often *within* the intact fetal membranes Usually no retained fetal membranes	*Fresh*—little or no autolysis; mild icterus, hydrothorax, hydroperitoneum; multifocal hepatic necrosis (1-2 mm diameter foci); pulmonary edema and/or congestion Histopathologic findings: necrotic foci in liver with eosinophilic *intranuclear inclusions* in surrounding hepatocytes Inclusions may also be in bronchiolar and alveolar epithelium, spleen and adrenal cortex	Histopathologic findings: *pathognomonic intranuclear inclusions* Fluorescence antibody test (FAT): fetal liver, lung, thymus Viral isolation Serology: not a definitive test (just indicates exposure to virus); rising complement fixation (CF) titer in paired sera may aid in diagnosis	Presumptive diagnosis with fresh fetus and gross lesions Vaccine does not guarantee protection against abortion, but should reduce the incidence of EHV-1 abortion in a herd Until more is known about vaccine protection, avoid switching types or brands of vaccine during pregnancy Management: isolation of weanlings and yearlings, aborting mares; separation of pregnant mares; closed herd
Equine streptococcal abortion	*Streptococcus zooepidemicus*	Sporadic abortion often <200 days, but can occur at any stage	*Chronic placentitis:* may show ascending pattern	Septic fetus, variable degrees of autolysis; congestion, yellow-red dirty discoloration of tissues Excessive fluid in pleural and peritoneal cavities, scattered petechiae	*Culture:* placenta, fetus, uterine discharge Organism readily isolated Direct smear of placental surface: Gram-positive cocci Histopathologic findings: Gram-positive cocci and low-grade inflammation	Most common *bacterial* cause of abortion No vaccine; prevent ascending infection
Nocardioform placentitis abortion	Unclassified Gram-positive filamentous branching bacteria	Sporadic abortions, usually occurring in late gestation (8-11 mo) with extensive placental involvement; usually accompanied with impending signs of abortion such as premature lactation	Focally extensive placentitis predominantly evident in the portions of the placenta occupying the base of the uterine horns or cranial uterine body	Fetus may be small for gestational age and emaciated; may be expelled alive	*Culture:* placenta, fetus, uterine discharge; demonstration of organism in placental lesions; bacteria grow slowly on blood agar	No effective treatment developed as yet because disease is incompletely understood Has become most commonly identified cause of placentitis in central Kentucky in recent years

TABLE 8-1

(continued)

Disease	Etiology	Clinical Signs	Placental Lesions	Fetal Lesions	Laboratory Diagnosis	Other
Other bacterial abortions	*Escherichia coli, Pseudomonas aeruginosa*	Sporadic abortions often >200 days, but can occur at any stage	*Chronic placentitis:* may show ascending pattern	No specific lesions; septic fetus, variable degrees of autolysis	*Culture:* placenta, fetus, uterine discharge; organism readily isolated Direct smear of placental surface; Gram-negative rods Histopathologic findings: Gram-negative rods and low-grade inflammation	*E. coli* second most common bacterial cause of abortion No vaccine; prevent ascending infection
Equine mycotic abortion	*Aspergillus fumigatus, Allescheria boydii, Mucor* spp.; primarily ascending infection	Sporadic abortions, usually occurring at 5-11 mo of gestation (majority around 10 mo)	*Chronic placentitis:* chorion is extensively involved; edematous and necrotic, with adherent viscous exudate, typical plaques are round with necrotic centers Amniotic lesions in only 10% of cases; necrotic plaques	Fetus small for gestational age and emaciated (as with any chronic placental dysfunction); may be expelled live; rare lesions—occasional 1-3 mm gray-white nodules in lungs (2% of cases); skin lesions quite rare	*Culture:* placenta, fetus (lung, liver); *hyphae* in chronic placental lesions and fetal stomach contents	May account for 5%-30% of all infectious abortions No vaccine; prevent ascending infection
Leptospirosis	*Leptospira interrogans;* serotypes: *pomona,* canicola, autumnalis*	Mild disease in horses except for periodic ophthalmia (moon blindness) Abortion is rare; occasionally follows mild illness by 1-3 wk Late abortions >6 mo	Not specific	Usually autolytic	*Culture:* leptospires in fetal fluid or blood; laboratory animal inoculation; dark-field or phase-contrast microscopy FAT Serology-paired sera	Diagnosis often unsuccessful Leptospirosis endemic in horses (i.e., in some studies, 50% of horses have titer of 1:400-1:800). No vaccine prepared for the equine; protection afforded by cattle vaccines questionable
Equine infecious anemia (EIA)	Retrovirus	Abortions usually last half of gestation; low incidence	Not specific	Not specific	Isolate virus Agar gel immuno-diffusion test: mare sera (100% of horses have titer by 45 days postinfection	No vaccine; no effective treatment
Protozoal abortion (piro-plasmosis	*Babesia caballi* or *equi*	Some severely stressed mares abort	Not specific	Excessive fluid in pleural and peritoneal cavities	FAT: fetal RBC of foal or dam CF test: mare sera	Primarily limited to Florida

TABLE 8-1

(continued)

Disease	Etiology	Clinical Signs	Placental Lesions	Fetal Lesions	Laboratory Diagnosis	Other
Protozoal abortion *(cont'd)*		Mares may have pronounced icterus or hemoglobinuria		Mild icterus sometimes		
Equine viral arteritis (EVA)	Togavirus	Rare outbreaks of severe systemic and respiratory disease with abortion as a complication; abort within 1-14 days of onset of clinical signs in these cases; however, abortions reported to occur with only mild or no visible illness of mares No retained fetal membranes	Autolytic	Autolytic No specific gross lesions Histologic findings: necrosis in media of small arteries	FAT: fetal tissues Viral isolation (culture of aborted fetus) Histologic findings: arteries Serology (virus neutralization test): antibodies develop 1-2 wk after infection and persist for years Clinical findings in aborting mares	Can be transmitted venereally by infected semen Infection is endemic in Standardbred horses Vaccine available, but generally requires approval of state and federal authorities (i.e., live virus vaccine); mares bred to known shedding stallions should be vaccinated before breeding
Twinning	Placental insufficiency 65%-70% of twins are aborted or stillbirths	Majority abort by 8-11 mo of gestation, but can occur at any stage Abortion often follows premature mammary development	Contacting surfaces of twin placentae are devoid of chorionic villi	Retarded growth Often have mummification of one of the twin fetuses	Placenta (lack of chorionic villi on portion of chorion that contacts placenta of twin) Twin fetuses, sometimes mummies	A common cause of equine abortion (20%-30% of all diagnosed abortions)
Uterine body pregnancy	Placental insufficiency	Majority abort by 8-11 mo of gestation, but can occur at any stage Abortion often follows premature mammary development	Placenta fails to extend fully into uterine horns (short placental horns noted during examination of expelled fetal membranes)	Retarded growth	"Short-horned" placenta	Uncommon occurrence

dystocia, asphyxia, or sometimes with EHV-1 infection (Figures 8-8 and 8-9). *Dysmature fetuses* (small and underdeveloped for gestational age) are also often delivered as stillbirths or as weak, emaciated neonates (Figure 8-10).

Signs of Intrauterine Infection

Gross signs suggesting intrauterine infection of the fetus include the following:

- Incomplete development of the fetus.
- Fetal edema.
- Fibrin stands or sheets in serous cavities of the abortus.
- Necrotic foci in the abortus liver and other organs.
- Variable degrees of fetal autolysis.

Microscopic lesions associated with intrauterine infection are found most commonly in the placenta and in fetal liver, lung, and intestine.

Diagnosis of Abortions

Each abortion should be regarded as a potential source of infection to other pregnant mares in contact with the mare that aborted until proven otherwise. When more than one pregnant mare is present on the premises, an abortion should

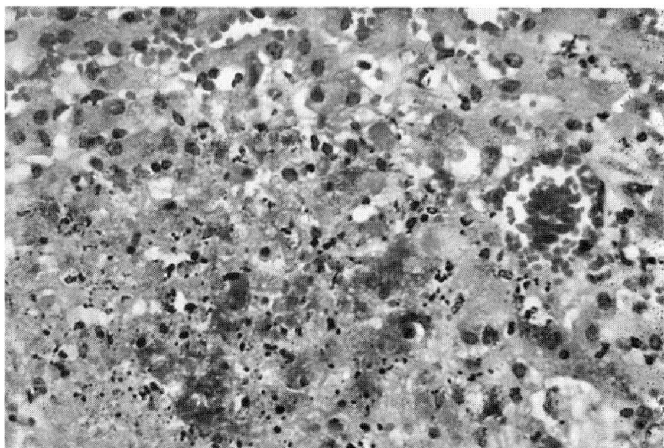

FIGURE 8-9. Focal hepatic necrosis in fetus aborted because of EHV-1 infection.

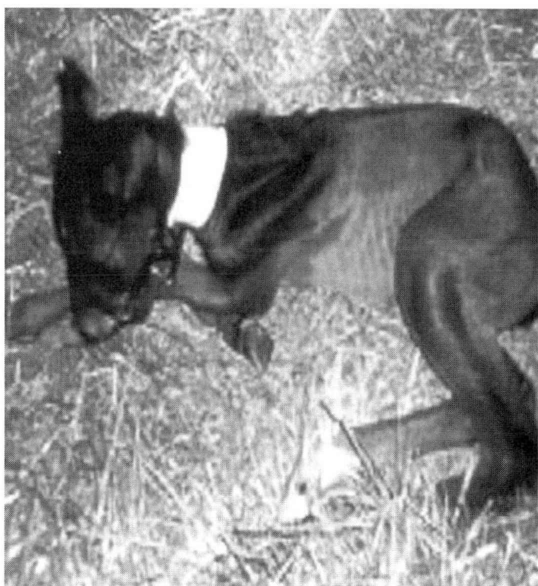

FIGURE 8-10. Weak, emaciated Thoroughbred foal delivered at 343 days of gestation. The foal was euthanized 7 days later because of toxemia and renal failure. The dam had begun premature udder development and lactation at 9 months of gestation, and placental separation was confirmed by transabdominal ultrasound examination. Treatment of the pregnant mare included administration of broad-spectrum antimicrobials for 3 weeks and an oral progestogen (Regu-Mate) daily through term. The fetal heart rate remained within normal limits through birth. At delivery, the chorion of the placenta was covered with a thick, tenacious brown exudate and had extensive villous atrophy and a chronic, necrotizing placentitis caused by a Gram-positive branching bacillus. (Photo courtesy Dr. D. Konkle, Equine Medical Associates, PSC, Lexington, KY.)

be treated as a potential herd problem. Because the gross placental and fetal findings resulting from most causes of infectious abortion are similar and nonspecific, practitioners require laboratory assistance for diagnosis. The quality of laboratory assistance depends primarily on the practitioner. Laboratory assistance typically involves serologic, microbiologic, and histopathologic procedures.

History

A complete history should be submitted with specimens sent to a diagnostic laboratory and should include the following:

- Reproductive history of the mare.
- Stage of pregnancy at which abortion occurred.
- Other pregnant animals involved (i.e., an abortion outbreak) or in contact with (exposed to) the mare aborting.
- Clinical signs observed before and after abortion.
- Herd or group history—vaccinations, diseases, closed or open herd, other animals transported to and from competition events or shows, etc.
- Housing and environment of the dam.
- Sources of feed and water.

Submitting Specimens

Specimens submitted to the diagnostic laboratory should be collected and sent as promptly as possible to avoid development of autolytic changes that interfere with making a diagnosis. The best specimen to submit is the *aborted fetus and placenta*. They should be placed in a leakproof plastic bag/container and should be transported *chilled* (not frozen). If it is not practical to submit the entire fetus and placenta, a field postmortem examination should be performed and the following samples should be submitted to the diagnostic laboratory in separate, labeled containers:

1. Intact *stomach and contents*. Tie off the esophagus and duodenum.
2. *Liver.*
3. *Lung.*
4. *Kidney.*
5. *Spleen.*
6. *Adrenal glands.*
7. *Placenta.* Submit as much of the placenta as possible. Although isolation of an infectious agent from the placenta does not establish pathogenicity, with histologic involvement diagnosis can sometimes be made directly from the placenta for mycotic abortions (see Figure 8-7), as well as for occasional bacterial abortions.
8. *Uterine fluid.*

Although the method is less desirable, instead of submitting the fetus or tissue samples for bacteriologic examination, swabs can be taken from abdominal and thoracic fluids, stomach contents, liver, lung, spleen, and cardiac blood. With a badly decomposed fetus, brain contents can be collected aseptically for bacteriologic examination. Uterine swabbings can also be taken from the aborting dam for culture. Items 2 to 7 should also be submitted in 10% buffered neutral formalin for histologic evaluation.

Fetal Serum

Fetal serum (if possible) and peritoneal fluid can be submitted for serologic examination. *Paired serum samples* should be submitted from the dam. Collect *acute* (i.e., at the time of abortion) and *convalescent* (i.e., approximately 2 to 3 weeks later) serum samples from the dam and submit as paired samples to the diagnostic laboratory. An increasing or decreasing serum titer for a given infectious agent after abortion provides circumstantial evidence for it as the causative agent. However, an increasing titer is often not seen if the abortion follows infection by a few weeks or more. Interpretation of serologic data is most reliable when microbiologic, histologic, and cytologic data are also taken into consideration.

Noninfectious Causes of Abortion

Noninfectious causes of abortion also exist for the mare. The most common noninfectious cause of abortion is twinning (see "Gestational Abnormalities"). Other noninfectious causes of abortion include fescue toxicosis, congenital anomalies, uterine body pregnancy, maternal stress and malnutrition, and possible hormonal abnormalities.

GESTATIONAL ABNORMALITIES

The more common gestational abnormalities in the mare include twinning, premature placental separation, uterine torsion, hydrallantois, and ruptured prepubic tendon. Pathologic prolonged gestation is a rare condition in the mare and is usually related to fescue toxicosis. Fetal mummification, with the exception of a mummified twin, is a rare occurrence.

Twinning

Twinning is an undesirable condition in the mare. If twins are not reduced to singletons at an early stage of gestation, the usual outcome is late-term abortion (Figures 8-11 and 8-12). Few twins are carried to term and survive. Complications that can arise with late-term abortion of twins or delivery of twins at term include dystocia, retained placenta, delayed uterine involution and metritis, and, of course, death of one or both twins. Virtually all twins arise from double ovulations, meaning the twins are dizygotic. As one

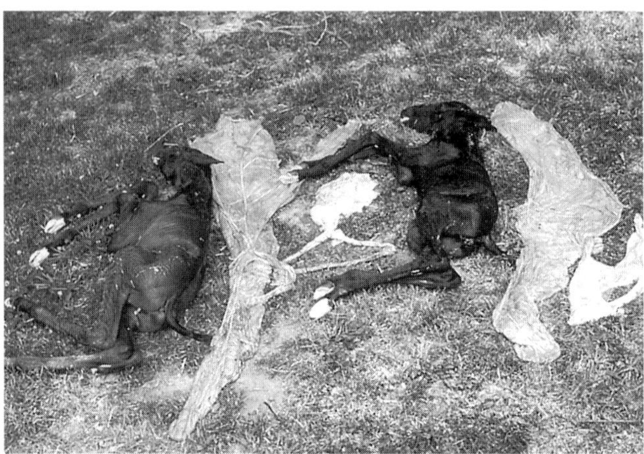

FIGURE 8-11. Aborted twins and their associated placentas.

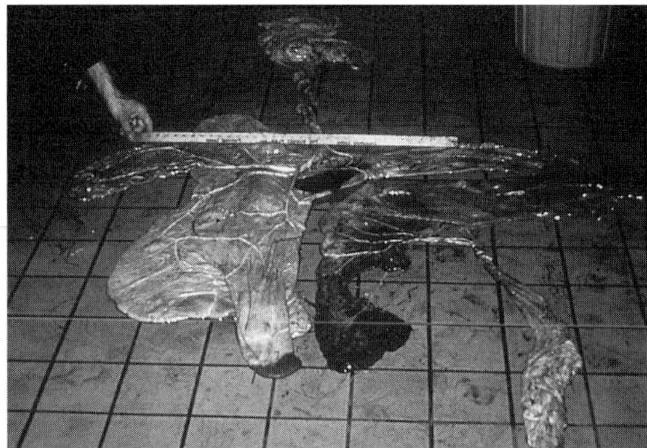

FIGURE 8-12. The placentas from this set of aborted twins occupied approximately equal portions of the uterus.

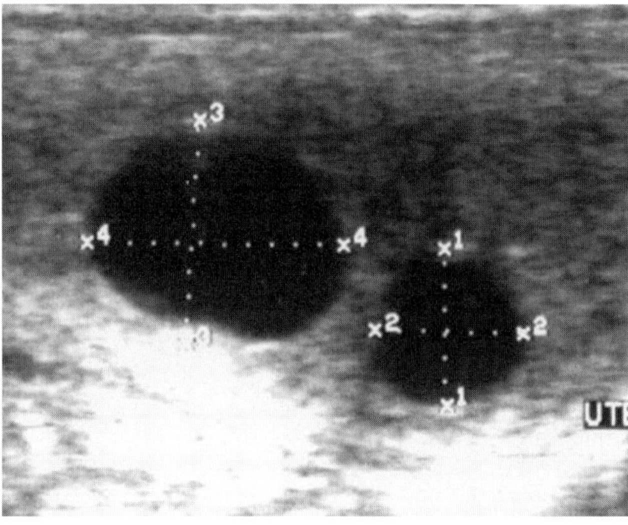

FIGURE 8-13. Transrectal ultrasonographic image of twin conceptuses located within the body of the uterus on day 15 postovulation.

would suspect, the incidence of twin conceptions varies with breed, being more common in those breeds with a higher incidence of multiple ovulations (e.g., Thoroughbreds have the highest incidence of multiple ovulations, approximately 15% to 25%). The double ovulations may be *synchronous* (occurring within 1 day of each other) or *asynchronous* (being more than 1 day apart). Synchronous ovulations (when more than one oocyte is fertilized) often produce twin conceptuses similar in size when examined by ultrasound, whereas asynchronous ovulations produce twin conceptuses that vary in size by up to several millimeters. Once twin conceptuses are present within the uterus, they migrate throughout both uterine horns and the uterine body (Figure 8-13) just as singleton conceptuses do. When the conceptuses become fixed in the same uterine horn at 16 to 17 days of gestation, they are referred to as *unilateral* (or *unicornuate*) *twins*. If, instead, each twin conceptus becomes fixed in a different uterine horn, they are referred to as *bilateral* (or *bicornuate*) *twins*. Mares are able to

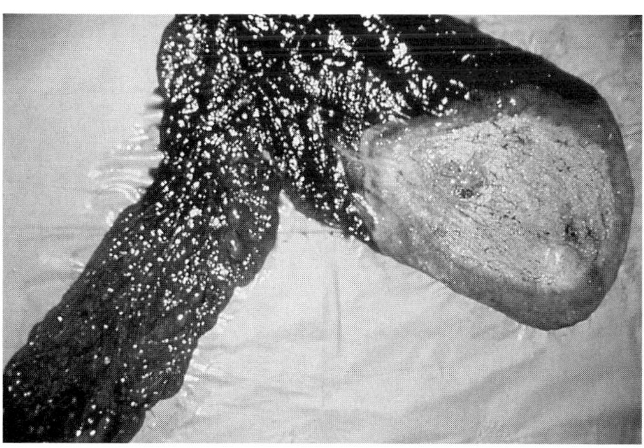

FIGURE 8-14. Avillous area of the placenta where a mummified twin prevented contact of the placenta with the endometrium, thereby yielding an area devoid of villi.

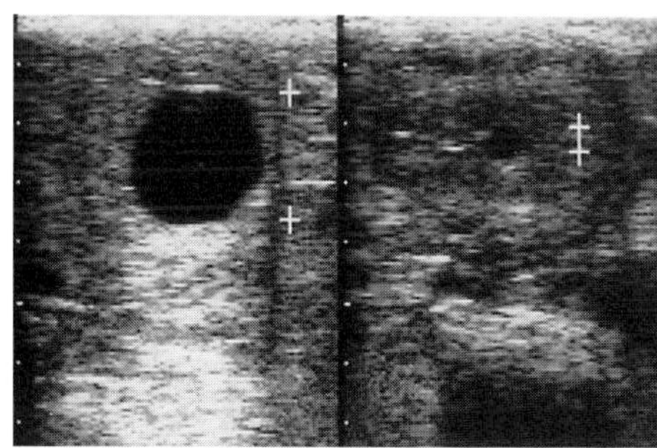

FIGURE 8-15. Ultrasonographic appearance of viable and nonviable twin conceptuses. The photograph was taken immediately after the conceptus on the right was manually crushed. A small amount of fluid remained in the luminal area where the conceptus was crushed.

spontaneously reduce unilateral twins to a singleton pregnancy with a high degree of efficiency (i.e., 75% of unilateral twins at 16 to 17 days of gestation will be reduced to a singleton pregnancy by 40 days of gestation). However, mares with a bilateral twin pregnancy or with a unilateral twin pregnancy beyond 40 days of gestation are likely to abort both twins late in gestation when placental contact with the uterus becomes insufficient to maintain fetal life. In some instances, one twin will die and become mummified, allowing the other twin to continue to develop and be maintained to term. The area of adjacent placental contact will be avillous as contact with the uterus is prevented (Figure 8-14).

The diagnosis of twins is generally thought to be best made at 14 to 15 days postovulation, before fixation, by transrectal ultrasound examination. Performing the examination at this time reduces the chances of missing the smaller twin if the twins arose from asynchronous ovulations (because one twin would be 1 to 2 days smaller in size and thus more difficult to detect than the other twin); yet it permits the diagnosis to be made before fixation when the twins conceptuses might become fixed in one uterine horn (making it extremely difficult to manually crush one twin without damaging the other). If twins are diagnosed and are not yet fixed, one twin can be crushed (per rectum) (Figure 8-15). Whether crushing of the smaller conceptus will improve the probability that the remaining conceptus survives to term is still a subject of controversy, but some workers recommend this practice. With experience, success rates are approximately 90% (i.e., 90% of pregnancies carried to term as singletons) when one twin is manually reduced at this stage of gestation. Mares that lose both pregnancies usually return to a fertile estrus within 2 weeks. The same technique (manual crushing) can be applied for perhaps 1 to 2 weeks longer with good success rates being expected if bilateral fixation of twins has taken place. However, manual crushing of one twin becomes progressively less successful (i.e., both twins are lost) the longer the pregnancy is allowed to survive before intervention. If both pregnancies are lost after endometrial cup formation (approximately days 36 to 40 of gestation), the mare usually will not return to fertile estrus until endometrial cups and supplementary corpora lutea spontaneously regress (e.g., 2 to 3 months later, depending on the gestational age at pregnancy loss). Even if supplementary corpora lutea are induced to regress by giving daily injections of prostaglandin $F_{2\alpha}$, the induced estrus is likely to be infertile until endometrial cups regress. Thus, if twins are not spontaneously or manually reduced to a singleton pregnancy before 35 days of gestation, prostaglandin is usually administered (a single injection is sufficient to induce abortion before endometrial cup stimulation of supplementary corpora lutea formation) to ensure that the mare will return to a fertile estrus in time to be rebred during the same breeding season.

Other methods of twin reduction to a singleton pregnancy, which have been used with limited success, include aspiration of vesicle contents through a needle inserted into the uterus per vagina (Figure 8-16), injection of the allantoic space or fetal heart (again, through a needle inserted into the uterus per vagina) with a toxic substance such as colchicine or potassium chloride solution, and fetal heart puncture later in gestation (beyond 100 days) through a needle inserted into the uterus and guided by use of transabdominal ultrasound.

To *induce abortion of twins* if they are detected between 40 and 110 days of gestation, multiple injections of prostaglandin $F_{2\alpha}$ (once daily for 4 to 5 days) are used. For pregnancies that do not respond to multiple injections of prostaglandin $F_{2\alpha}$ (typically those older than 110 to 120 days of gestation), the fetal membranes can be punctured transcervically and a toxic substance (such as dilute tamed-iodine solution) can be infused into the allantoic space. As with any method of induced abortion, reexamination at 1- to 2-day intervals is required to ensure that fetal death and expulsion of the fetuses and fetal membranes have occurred. Recently, South African workers proposed the use of prostaglandin E_2 for elective abortion in mares at 100 to 300 days of gestation. They instilled 0.5 to 1.5 mg of prostaglandin E_2 into the cervical canal, followed in 2 hours by manual dilation of

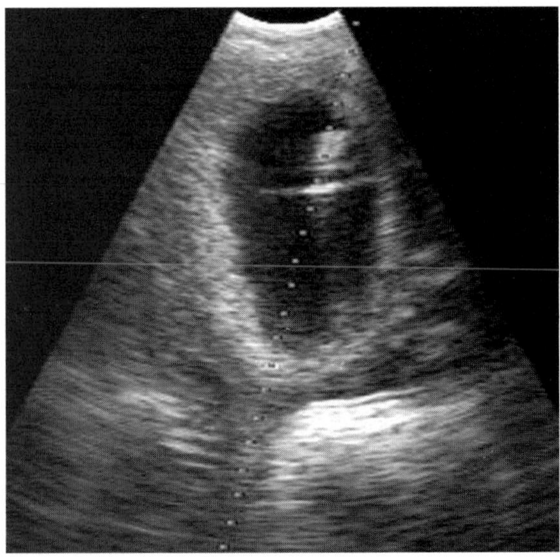

FIGURE 8-16. Image of a twin conceptus being reduced by ultrasound-guided transvaginal needle aspiration of allantoic fluid. The *dotted line* represents the direction the needle is expected to travel. A needle with an echogenic tip is used to facilitate visualization *(bright spot)* during the puncture procedure. When the needle is placed within the allantoic space, fluid is aspirated until the chorioallantois collapses.

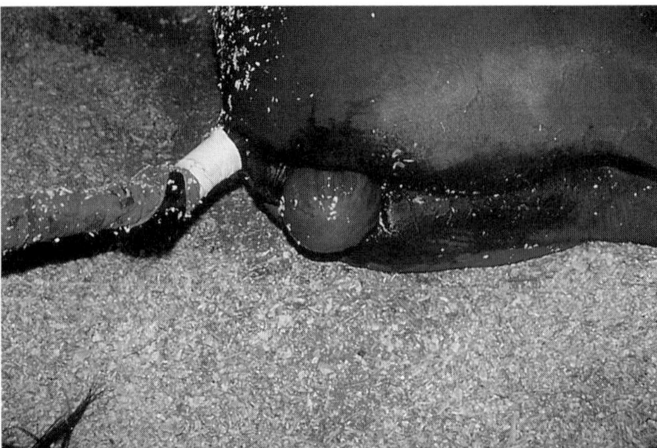

FIGURE 8-17. Chorionic surface of an unruptured placenta presented beyond the vulva as a result of premature placental separation.

the cervix to allow the hand to be passed into the uterus. The fetus and fetal membranes were then extracted, and no complications were seen.

Body Pregnancy

Occasionally the conceptus becomes fixed in the uterine body during early pregnancy (body pregnancy) rather than being fixed in the base of either uterine horn. Further growth of the conceptus continues, but this situation is thought to usually result in abortion later in gestation because of placental insufficiency. Placental insufficiency results from failure of the placenta to expand adequately into the two uterine horns. If a body pregnancy is detected after the period of embryonic mobility (i.e., after days 16 to 17 of gestation), the mare should be given a single injection of prostaglandin $F_{2\alpha}$ (or an analog) before day 35 of pregnancy to ensure an early return to estrus and rebreeding. Caution should be exercised because body pregnancy is uncommon, and a pregnancy that develops at the corpocornual junction (just cranial to the uterine body, which may appear to be a body pregnancy on cursory examination) will most likely proceed to term.

Premature Placental Separation

Premature placental separation occurs most commonly during birth. The chorion separates from the endometrium but the chorioallantois does not rupture to release allantoic fluid. Because gas exchange is impaired, the separation causes fetal hypoxia/anoxia that can contribute to weakness and dysmaturity *(dummy foal)* or even stillbirth. The condition is diagnosed by visualizing the reddish, velvet-like surface of the chorion bulging between the vulvar labia during birth (Figure 8-17). The chorioallantois should be manually ruptured or incised to allow the fetus to be delivered without the placenta being forced along with it. The fetus may already be compromised, so fetal delivery should be accomplished as soon as possible after the membranes are ruptured and allantoic fluid is released. Resuscitative procedures may be necessary, including administration of oxygen, to save the foal's life (see Chapter 11).

Premature placental separation sometimes also occurs in mid to late gestation with death of a fetal twin or impending abortion. The mare may begin to *lactate prematurely* in such cases. When fetal membrane separation during gestation is suspected, a thorough examination of the reproductive tract, including assessment of fetal well-being, should be performed (see Chapter 9). If abortion is imminent, assistance can be provided to ensure that the mare delivers the abortus without dystocia. If the cervix is closed and the fetus is alive, progestogen (altrenogest or progesterone) therapy has sometimes been used successfully to permit the pregnancy to be carried to term. If a fetal twin has died, it may mummify and be delivered at term with the other fetus.

Uterine Torsion

Uterine torsion occurs occasionally in pregnant mares, usually during mid to late term (5 to 9 months of gestation). Although it can occur in mares at term, it is much less common at this time. The cause is speculative, sometimes being thought to develop when a mare takes a sudden fall. The direction of the uterine twist can be either clockwise or counterclockwise (when viewed from the rear). Torsions less than 180 degrees seldom cause a problem. Torsions greater than 180 degrees are painful, creating a "low-grade, persistent colic" that is nonresponsive to analgesics (although some short-term relief may occur, abdominal pain returns). If the torsion restricts blood flow sufficiently, the uterus can become congested, friable, or even necrotic if left unattended. Unattended uterine torsions may lead to uterine rupture with loss of the fetus into the abdominal cavity. Alterations in blood flow caused by uterine torsion place the fetus at risk of hypoxia; if fetal death occurs, abortion usually follows in a few days to a week or more even if the torsion was corrected. In some mares in which uterine torsion is corrected and the fetus is alive when the mare is discharged from the hospital, abortion occurs 1 or 2 weeks later.

Uterine torsion is diagnosed by palpation of the genital tract per rectum. The direction of the twist is determined by following the broad ligaments to their respective ovaries (e.g., a clockwise torsion presents with the left broad ligament passing over the top of the uterus (and down if the torsion is greater than 180 degrees) to the right, while the right broad ligament passes underneath the uterus toward the left. The broad ligament passing over the top of the uterus is easier to locate than the ligament passing underneath the uterus. Because most uterine torsions in the mare do not involve the cervix or vagina, only occasionally can the diagnosis of a uterine torsion be confirmed by palpation per vagina (i.e., finding that the cranial vaginal vault is narrowed and twisted). Treatment of preterm uterine torsion involves one of three methods: (1) anesthetizing the mare and placing a board low in the flank to aid in maintaining pressure on the uterus while the mare is rolled in the direction of the torsion until it is corrected (in essence, the uterus and fetus are held in place while the mare is "unrolled" around them) (Figure 8-18); (2) performing a standing flank laparotomy, reaching under the uterus and lifting the fetus and uterus up and over into the torsion until it is corrected; and (3) performing a midventral laparotomy and either correcting the torsion through the incision or performing a cesarean section and then correcting the torsion. In all cases in which the fetus is not removed at the time of correction, the mare is at risk of having an abortion if severe fetal stress had occurred. Rolling the mare works best for torsions occurring earlier in gestation and is less likely to be successful in near-term or full-term uterine torsions.

Regardless of the method used to correct torsion, the position of the uterus should be ascertained after the mare recovers from anesthesia to ensure uterine torsion has not recurred. Additionally, fetal monitoring is indicated to ensure fetal death has not occurred.

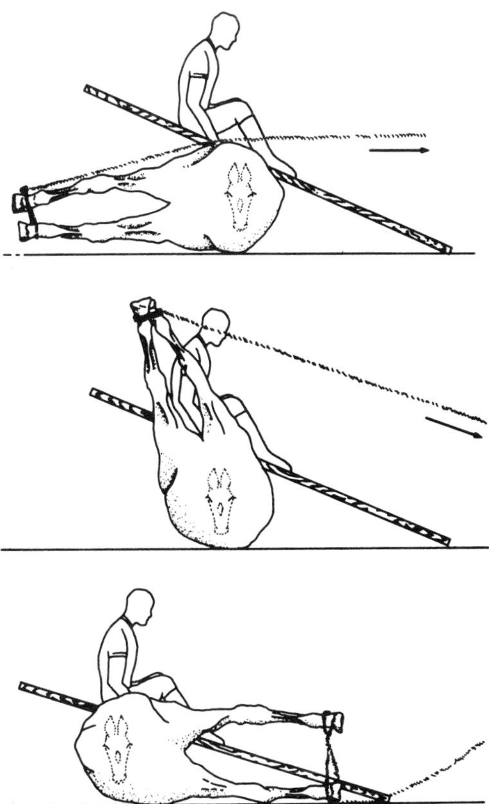

FIGURE 8-18. Illustration of the "rolling technique" used to correct uterine torsion in a preterm mare. **A,** The position of the mare, fetus, and plank before rolling; the direction of rolling is indicated *(arrow)*. **B,** Uterine and fetal position are maintained by applying weight on the plank during rotation; the direction is indicated *(arrow)*. **C,** The positions after a reduction of 180 degrees of uterine torsion. The procedure is repeated until the full extent of torsion has been corrected. (Modified from Bowen JM et al: Non-surgical correction of a uterine torsion in the mare. *Vet Rec* 99:496, 1976.)

Hydrallantois and Hydramnios

Hydrallantois is an uncommon condition that is thought to develop as a result of placental dysfunction (Figure 8-19). Excess allantoic fluid accumulates (as many as 100 to 200 liters or more), usually in mid to late gestation, overfilling the uterus. The condition generally develops over a period of a few days to 2 weeks. The mare is noted to have developed an extremely enlarged abdomen, predisposing her to rupture of the prepubic tendon. Hydrallantois is diagnosed by palpating (per rectum) the extremely enlarged, fluid-filled uterus. The uterus is sometimes so distended with fluid that it

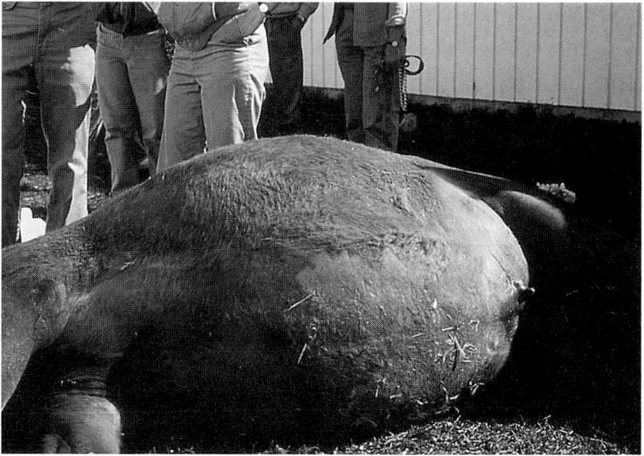

FIGURE 8-19. Hydrallantois apparent in a recumbent mare. The abdomen is greatly distended due to accumulation of excessive fetal fluids in the uterus.

is elevated to or above the level of the floor of the pelvis, and little else, including the fetus, can be palpated. *Hydramnios* is thought to be a more rare occurrence in the mare, but it has been reported. Uterine distension with hydramnios is reportedly less dramatic and may not develop as quickly. Reimer (1997) reported that transabdominal ultrasound examination may aid in making a diagnosis when excess accumulation of allantoic or amniotic fluid is unequivocally demonstrated. In a series of nine cases, she reported three in which fetal death had already occurred at the time of ultrasonographic diagnosis.

Because the fetus is usually nonviable, the treatment consists of inducing parturition to deliver the fetus and expel the fetal fluids from the uterus. Frazer (2000) reported that approximately 50% of fetuses are born alive, with euthanasia of the fetus being indicated because it is nonviable. If the mare is judged to be in such poor condition that she may enter shock as a result of the sudden loss of the tremendous volume of fluid, pretreatment with intravenous fluids and corticosteroids may be beneficial. The cervix should be manually dilated and the fetal membranes punctured to allow allantoic fluid to escape slowly for a period of time (perhaps ½ hour or more). Frazer (2000) suggested that siphoning of fluid through a catheter placed transcervically into the allantoic space may be required in some mares to gradually evacuate some of the excess fluid. If labor does not begin spontaneously, oxytocin can be administered. Texas workers recommend administering oxytocin in 5- to 20-U injections (intramuscularly or intravenously) given at 15-minute intervals, whereas Frazer (2000) suggests administering oxytocin in an intravenous drip at the rate of 1 U/min. Assistance should be given in fetal delivery, and after giving birth the mare should be encouraged to lie quietly for as long as possible before rising. Abdominal support wraps may be used for a period of time until abdominal muscle tone returns. The mare's condition should be monitored closely thereafter until danger of retained placenta, metritis, and laminitis is past. Uterine involution will be delayed, and rebreeding on foal heat should be discouraged. Anecdotal reports suggest that although fertility may be reduced during the season of occurrence, fertility in ensuing seasons is normal and the condition is unlikely to recur.

Ruptured Prepubic Tendon

A ruptured prepubic tendon sometimes occurs in aged mares having hydrallantois or those carrying a large fetus or twins. Sometimes before rupture of the tendon a very thickened, edematous plaque develops ventrally, extending from the udder to the xiphoid process. Rupture of the prepubic tendon results in loss of ventral abdominal support to the pelvis, so a typical "sawhorse stance" develops wherein the pelvis is tipped cranially and the feet are extended fore and aft. Support for the udder is lost, and it becomes swollen and congested (Figure 8-20). The affected mare is reluctant to move, and her condition rapidly deteriorates. Palpation per rectum reveals that the abdominal floor is falling away from the brim of the pelvis. If rupture has not occurred, and the objective is to save the mare, induction of parturition is indicated. Assistance with fetal delivery is likely to be required as the mare will probably have a weakened abdominal press. If the objective is to save the foal and the expected foaling date is near, sometimes support wraps and nursing care will permit the mare to maintain the foal until induced parturition can be performed at a time when foal survival is more likely. If the mare's life is spared, she should not be rebred if partial disruption of the prepubic tendon occurred, because rupture is likely to recur during the next gestation. A similar condition, which is handled in a similar manner, is *abdominal wall rupture* or *herniation*. However, with minor herniations, delivery of the fetus is often possible, and the hernia can sometimes be repaired surgically after the foal is weaned. The mare can then be rebred to carry a foal to term without recurrence of the hernia.

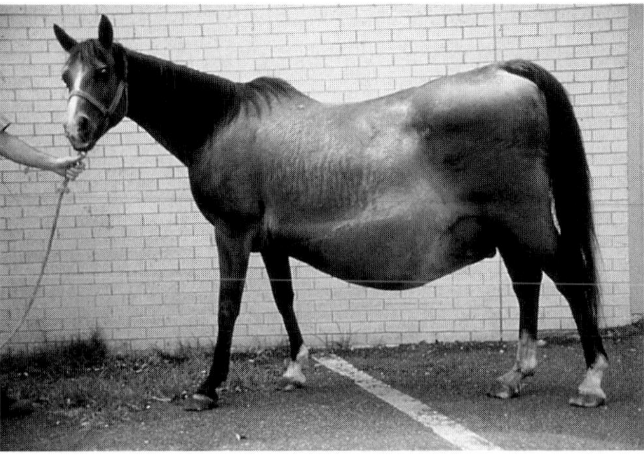

FIGURE 8-20. Mare with a sawhorse stance typical of a ruptured prepubic tendon caused by loss of ventral abdominal support, tipped pelvis, and elevated tail head. The udder is also swollen and congested.

Prolonged Gestation

In the mare, prolonged gestation (greater than 340 days) seldom results in birth of an oversize fetus that contributes to dystocia as occurs occasionally in the cow. Numerous reports exist of mares that deliver foals of normal size and viability after gestation lengths of 1 year or more. The causes of prolonged gestation are not known in the mare, but Belgium workers hypothesized that arrest of embryonic/fetal development sometimes occurs during early pregnancy (i.e., at 3 to 6 weeks of gestation). The arrested development has been postulated to sometimes last for 3 to 5 weeks, resulting in a corresponding delay in the interval to birth. However, this hypothesis remains unproved. The foals born from these prolonged gestations are normal. Another factor contributing to gestations longer than the expected 340 days is season. Mares conceiving early in the breeding season

(February and March) tend to carry the fetus longer than mares conceiving in late April and May. Regardless of the cause, induction of parturition should not be attempted unless the cardinal signs of fetal maturity and impending parturition are present. At present, adequate udder development and the presence of good-quality colostrum with a high calcium content are the best indicators that the fetus is mature and the mare is ready to deliver a live foal (see Chapter 9).

Pathologic prolonged gestation can occur in mares grazing *Acremonium*-contaminated fescue grass *(fescue toxicosis)*. The placenta is typically thickened, due partly to an increase in connective tissue, and stillbirth with the foal still encased in the fetal membranes may occur. Udder development is minimal *(agalactia)* in affected mares, presumably because of ergot alkaloids present in infested fescue that act as dopamine receptor agonists, which suppress prolactin production. Missouri workers recently demonstrated that pony mares affected with fescue toxicosis also had low circulating levels of relaxin, which were associated with placental disease and agalactia. Pennsylvania workers went further, documenting low circulating relaxin levels in mares with other forms of placental disease/insufficiency.

The condition is prevented by pasture management to control infestation by the fungus, supplemental feeding of nonfescue hay, and rotation of pregnant mares to a non-contaminated pasture for the last 3 months of gestation. Drugs used to stimulate prolactin production and overcome agalactia have included thyrotropin-releasing hormone (2.0 mg subcutaneously twice daily), reserpine (0.5 to 2.0 mg intramuscularly once every 2 days), and perphenazine (0.3 to 0.5 mg/kg orally twice daily). Missouri workers reported that treatment with a long-acting D_2-dopamine receptor antagonist (fluphenazine decanoate, 25 mg intramuscularly) 2 to 3 weeks before expected parturition increased circulating relaxin levels and decreased the incidence of fescue toxicosis-related problems in pony mares and their foals. The best results have been reported with the administration of the dopamine-D2 receptor antagonists sulpiride or domperidone. South Carolina workers demonstrated that domperidone (Equidone; 1.1 mg/kg administered orally once daily) before foaling reduced the incidence of dystocia, stillborn foals, retained placenta, and agalactia in gravid mares grazing *Acremonium*-contaminated fescue pastures. Beginning treatment 10 to 15 days before expected foaling gave better results than initiating treatment later, but treatment near or after foaling still appeared to reduce the incidence/severity of agalactia.

BIBLIOGRAPHY

Bain AM: Foetal losses during pregnancy in Thoroughbred mares: a record of 2,562 pregnancies. *NZ Vet J* 17:155-158, 1969.

Ball BA: Embryonic death in mares. In McKinnon AO, Voss JL, editors, *Equine reproduction*, pp 517-531. Philadelphia, 1993, Lea and Febiger.

Cross DL, Anas K, Bridges WC et al: Clinical effects of domperidone on fescue toxicosis in pregnant mares. *Proc Am Assoc Equine Pract* 45:203-209, 1999.

Dennis SM: Pregnancy wastage in domestic animals. *Comp Contin Educ Pract Vet* 3:S62-S70, 1981.

Frazer G: Hydrops, ruptures and torsions. *Proc Soc Theriogenol*, pp 33-38, 2000.

Ginther OJ: *Ultrasonic imaging and reproductive events in the mare*, pp 195-223, 253-285. Cross Plains, WI, 1986, Equiservices.

Ginther OJ. *Reproductive biology of the mare. Basic and applied aspects*, ed 2, pp 546-560. Cross Plains, WI, 1992, Equiservices.

McCue PM: Lactation. In McKinnon AO, Voss JL, editors, *Equine reproduction*, Philadelphia, 1993, Lea and Febiger.

Newcombe JR: Embryonic loss and abnormalities of early pregnancy. *Equine Vet Educ* April, 115-131, 2000.

Redmund LM, Cross DL, Trickland JR et al: Efficacy of domperidone and sulpiride as treatments for fescue toxicosis in horses. *Am J Vet Res* 55:722-729, 1994.

Reimer JM: Use of transcutaneous ultrasonography in complicated latter-middle to late gestation pregnancies in the mare: 122 cases. *Proc Am Assoc Equine Pract* 43:259-261, 1997.

Ryan P, Bennet-Wimbush K, Loch W et al: Effects of fescue toxicosis and fluphenazine on relaxin concentrations in pregnant pony mares. *Proc Am Assoc Equine Pract* 44:60-61, 1998.

Ryan P, Vaala W, Bagnell C: Evidence that equine relaxin is a good indicator of placental insufficiency in the mare. *Proc Am Assoc Equine Pract* 44:62-63, 1998.

Taylor TS, Blanchard TL, Varner DD et al: Management of dystocia in mares: uterine torsion and cesarean section. *Comp Contin Educ Pract Vet* 11:1265-1273, 1989.

Vanderwall DK, Squires EL, Brinsko SP et al: Diagnosis and management of abnormal embryonic development characterized by formation of an embryonic vesicle without an embryo proper in mares. *J Am Vet Med Assoc* 217:58-63, 2000.

9

Management of the Pregnant Mare

OBJECTIVES

While studying the information covered in this chapter, the student should attempt to:

1. Acquire a working understanding of procedures used to manage the pregnant and parturient mare.
2. Acquire a working understanding of procedures used to monitor fetal viability during gestation.
3. Acquire a working knowledge of the rationale and procedures for monitoring the mare for readiness for birth.
4. Acquire a working understanding of the birth process, including the three stages of labor.
5. Acquire a working knowledge of the events that occur in the early postpartum period of the normal foaling mare.

STUDY QUESTIONS

1. List the average duration of gestation in the mare, and discuss effects of season on gestation length.
2. Outline differences in nutritional needs for mares during early and late gestation and during lactation.
3. Outline a preventative health care program for pregnant mares on a broodmare farm.
4. Describe examination findings that indicate fetal well-being is at risk.
5. Describe the desirable characteristics of a foaling area or stall.
6. List changes that occur in the mammary gland and its secretions that are useful in predicting readiness for parturition in the mare.
7. Describe the progression of events occurring during the three stages of parturition in the mare.
8. Outline methods for inducing parturition in the mare.
9. Explain the economic pressure to breed mares on their "foal heat."
10. Describe the progression of events occurring during uterine involution and the return to a pregravid condition in the normal foaling mare.

Mares should be managed attentively during pregnancy to help ensure the birth of a strong, healthy foal with no injury incurred by the dam. Maintaining the mare in good health, being familiar with the signs of impending parturition, and preparing a foaling environment conducive to mare and foal health will increase the likelihood of obtaining a healthy foal. Although managerial programs are usually adapted to meet the special needs of individual mares or owners, certain strategies and methodologies are universally applicable. This chapter discusses routine care of the pregnant mare, methods for monitoring fetal viability, preparation of the mare for foaling, and the physiologic events of parturition to provide background for managing the mare at term and the birth process.

LENGTH OF GESTATION

The average duration of gestation in the horse is 335 to 342 days. Occasionally, viable term foals can be born as early as 305 days of gestation, but foals born before 320 days of gestational age are typically premature and nonviable. Some authors define abortion as the expulsion of the fetus before day 300 of gestation, and use the term *prematurity* to designate birth of an underdeveloped foal between days 300 and 320 of gestation. The student should realize use of these precise days for definition purposes can be misleading because gestation length is so variable in the horse. Certainly, foals can be delivered at >320 days of gestation that fit other criteria used to describe prematurity. *Dysmaturity,* on the other hand, designates birth of a full-term but immature and often undersized foal.

The duration of gestation is sometimes exceedingly long (≥360 days), with no untoward effects on the fetus or mare (i.e., the fetus is not oversized and is viable, and no increased risk of dystocia exists). These long gestational periods have been hypothesized (as yet unproven) to be due to the ability of the equine conceptus to undergo a period of arrested development during the first 2 months of gestation and then reinitiate growth and development.

There are seasonal effects on the duration of equine gestation, with mares due to foal in late winter and early spring carrying their foals approximately 5 to 10 days longer than mares foaling later in the breeding season (late spring or summer). This seasonal effect can partially negate efforts made to get mares pregnant early in the breeding season (February 15 or soon thereafter) and can be circumvented by exposing pregnant mares to artificial lighting regimens (beginning on December 1) identical to those used to initiate early ovulatory estrus in nonpregnant mares. Exposure of pregnant mares to artificial lighting systems can reduce gestation length by an average of 10 days.

Other factors that may influence gestational length in mares include sex of the foal, maternal nutrition, and environmental stresses. Ingested toxins (e.g., ergot alkaloids in contaminated fescue grass/hay) may also alter the length of gestation.

PREVENTIVE HEALTH CARE

Preventive health care measures recommended for pregnant mares include regular immunization for certain infectious diseases. Immunization of the pregnant mare serves two purposes: protection of the dam and eventual protection of the newborn foal. Antibodies produced in response to injected antigens are too large for diffusion across the placental barrier; nevertheless, the antibodies will be selectively concentrated in the colostrum and made available to the newborn foal at the time of nursing. If protection of the foal is of foremost concern, vaccine boosters should be administered approximately 3 to 4 weeks before the projected foaling date to optimize colostral antibody concentration against the disease of concern.

Selection of vaccines for immunization of pregnant mares depends on many factors, including expected exposure to the disease, economic constraints, and vaccine efficacy and safety. Therefore immunization programs should be tailored to meet the needs of individual mares or owners and to fit disease control measures used on farms where mares reside.

Equine Herpesvirus Abortion

Equine herpesvirus type 1 (EHV-1) is the primary form of equine herpesvirus that is associated with abortion. The virus has also been associated with perinatal foal mortality; rhinopneumonitis in foals, growing horses, and some adult horses; and encephalomyelitis in adult horses. The virus is distinct from EHV-4, which is the major cause of rhinopneumonitis in foals and is only rarely isolated from equine abortions.

EHV-1 infection is acquired by inhalation, with the virus attaching to, penetrating, and replicating in upper airway mucosal epithelial cells. If the local immune response fails to overcome the infection, the virus breaches the basement membrane to invade the lamina propria of the respiratory mucosa and infects T lymphocytes and endothelial cells. The resulting viremia disseminates virus throughout the body. Abortion is the result of ischemia caused by vasculitis of uterine vessels that disrupt the uteroplacental barrier. It is also thought that lymphocytes resident within the endometrium may transfer virus directly to uterine endothelium and result in abortion. This latter mechanism has been proposed to explain abortion in single mares in a group and abortions that occur many weeks or months after viremia.

Viral latency also occurs with EHV-1 infection, with periodic reactivation of latent virus resulting in asymptomatic shedding of the virus from the respiratory tract that may cause infection of in-contact horses. If local immunity has waned, reinfection with viremia can occur, again placing the fetus at risk. Although vaccinations do not eliminate preexisting latent EHV-1 infections, if they stimulate a sufficient local immune response to prevent shedding, transmission of virus to other in-contact animals may be prevented.

Timing and efficacy of vaccinations to protect against abortion associated with EHV-1 infection remain controversial. Pneumabort-K +1b (Fort Dodge Laboratories) is a killed-virus preparation approved for use to protect against EHV-1 abortions in mares, with administration recommended during the fifth, seventh, and ninth months of gestation. The vaccine should be administered to pregnant and nonpregnant mares at the same time. Rhinomune (Pfizer) is an attenuated live virus preparation approved for use to aid in preventing respiratory disease caused by EHV-1. Although the product label makes no claim that the drug provides protection against virus-associated abortion, it does state that no adverse reactions have been reported in pregnant mares vaccinated with this product and further recommends vaccination of pregnant mares after the second month of gestation and at 3-month intervals thereafter. Prestige II with Havlogen is a killed-virus preparation (Bayer Corporation) containing EHV-1, EHV-4, and equine influenza subtypes A1 and A2; the product label makes no claims concerning provision of protection against virus-associated abortion. Prodigy (Bayer Corporation) is a killed-virus preparation of EHV-1 labeled for the prevention of virus-associated abortion. Vaccination with this product is recommended at the fifth, seventh, and ninth months of gestation. Recommendations for how often booster vaccines are administered vary with the product used; however, herpesvirus vaccines typically do not stimulate long-lasting immune protection (even immunity resulting from natural infection wanes in 3 to 6 months) and thus boosters should be given at regularly scheduled intervals. Although the efficacy of vaccination in the face of an abortion outbreak caused by rhinopneumonitis is unknown, Pneumabort-K +1b is labeled for this use.

Research on changes in vaccine types/brands during gestation is lacking. Some practitioners feel that switching between different types or brands of vaccines during pregnancy leads to "vaccine breaks" in which EHV-1 infection-associated abortion is more likely. Until this phenomenon is studied, we caution against changing products during pregnancy in gestating mares.

A vaccination program cannot be the sole means relied on for prevention and control of abortion caused by EHV-1 infection because vaccination provides limited protection against viral shedding and the disease, and properly vaccinated mares will occasionally abort. One should use appropriate management procedures in concert with a vaccination protocol to reduce exposure of mares to the virus. Pregnant mares should be separated from the rest of the farm population. Permanent resident mares should not be allowed to have contact with transient boarders that normally reside elsewhere. Stress should be minimized to reduce the risk of activation of EHV-1 that may already be present in the mare. Mares that have aborted as a result of EHV-1 infection should be isolated from the rest of the herd. Additionally, all mares that have been in contact with aborting mares should be segregated from those not yet exposed to the virus, and booster vaccines may be administered to in-contact mares in an attempt to stimulate immunity. Strict hygienic measures should be instituted to minimize spread of infection to the rest of the mares on the premises.

Encephalomyelitis (Sleeping Sickness)

This insect-transmitted neurologic disease is caused by viruses of the Togaviridae family, of which eastern, western, and Venzuelan encephalomyelitis viruses are most pathogenic. Horses in endemic areas should be immunized with a suitable killed-virus vaccine before the mosquito season each year, which corresponds to the foaling season. Pregnant mares can be given booster vaccinations 1 month before parturition for maximal passive protection of the newborn foal.

Tetanus *(Clostridium tetani)*

Inclusion of *tetanus toxoid* should be mandatory in all vaccination programs because of the incidence and life-threatening consequences of tetanus in the dam and foal. Booster vaccines are given to pregnant mares 1 month before parturition.

Other Infectious Diseases

Immunization against other infectious diseases is sometimes desirable, depending on local risk factors such as endemic diseases, housing with horses of other ages, and contact with outside (nonresident) horses at risk of contracting transmissible infectious diseases such as *influenza, rabies, strangles, botulism, Potomac horse fever* and *West Nile Virus encephalitis*. Product labels should be examined because some products (e.g., FluAvert IN, Heska Corp.) caution against use in pregnant mares. Additionally, protection against *equine viral arteritis* may be required in some instances. Special precautions are necessary for use of this vaccine, and state and federal authorities may need to be contacted for approval of its use and guidelines for its administration. Equine viral arteritis vaccine, a modified-live virus vaccine (Arvac, Fort Dodge Laboratories), should not be administered to pregnant mares, and mares recently vaccinated with this product should be kept segregated from pregnant mares for a minimum of 2 to 3 weeks.

Other Preventive Measures

Regular *dental examination* and *floating* (smoothing the sharp enamel points off cheek teeth) at 6- or 12-month intervals enable proper grazing and chewing of feeds, which will help maintain body condition and prevent digestive upsets.

Regular *deworming* is second only to good nutrition for proper management. Discussion of the varied anthelmintics and programs for their use is beyond the scope of this chapter. However, many products effectively control exposure to internal parasites and eliminate parasitic infestations, and regularly scheduled use of anthelmintics as part of a health maintenance program is imperative. Deworming medications are *generally* considered safe for use during pregnancy unless otherwise indicated on the product label. A variety of dewormers are approved for use during pregnancy, including *ivermectin, pyrantel pamoate,* and *pyrantel tartrate. Thiabendazole, fenbendazole,* and *piperazine* have been used regularly throughout pregnancy with no known untoward effects. *Cambendazole* should not be used during the first 3 months of pregnancy. Always read the precautions on the package insert of anthelmintics before administering them to pregnant mares.

It is common practice to administer ivermectin to the broodmare on the day of foaling to minimize the parasitic load of *Strongyloides westeri*. The infective larvae of this parasite are transmitted to the foal by nursing beginning on about day 4 postpartum.

Any deworming program should be suited to the individual requirements of a farm or stable. Program success should be evaluated by examining feces at regular intervals to monitor parasitic egg levels. Sound pasture management (e.g., low stocking density, regular pasture rotation, and pasture harrowing) should be used in concert with deworming protocols to establish an effective antiparasitic program. An example of one health program, including a deworming schedule, for broodmares is presented in Table 9-1.

Nutritional Support

Proper nutritional support of the broodmare improves fertility and promotes normal growth and vigor of the developing fetus. The reader is referred to a recent review of nutrient requirements for gestating and lactating mares for a thorough discussion of feeding guidelines (Hintz, 1993). Pregnant mares should be kept in good *body condition* (body score of 6 to 7, based on a scoring system of 1 to 9). The best pregnancy rates are achieved in mares in good to fat condition. Fertility of thin mares is improved if they are gaining weight at the time of breeding. Mares should not be obese, because this has been reported to be associated with birth of weak, undersized foals. Specific nutrient requirements for gestating mares are available from the National Research Council (NRC) (Nutrient Requirements of Horses, 1989). In general, three different feeding programs are necessary for pregnant mares, with dietary requirements dictated by lactational status and stage of pregnancy. Digestible energy

TABLE 9-1

An Example of a Calendar for an Equine Herd Health Program for Pregnant Mares

January	Complete deworming* Equine rhinopneumonitis vaccine Tetanus toxoid *Streptococcus equi* vaccine
March	Deworming Equine rhinopneumonitis-influenza vaccine Rabies vaccine (before breeding)
May	Deworming Encephalomyelitis-influenza-tetanus vaccine†
July	Complete deworming* Equine rhinopneumonitis-influenza vaccine
September	Deworming Equine rhinopneumonitis vaccine
October	May want to repeat deworming every 30 days in the fall if using a seasonal program
November	Complete deworming* Equine rhinopneumonitis vaccine

*July and November dewormings include the administration of a botacide.
†Should be given before the mosquito season.

(DE) requirements for mares during the first 8 months of gestation are the same as for those for maintenance and gradually increase during late gestation over the maintenance requirement (1.11, 1.13, and 1.20 times maintenance requirements for 9, 10, and 11 months of gestation, respectively). Additional maternal nutrition during the last 3 months of pregnancy is required because 60% to 65% of fetal growth occurs during this time period. The growing fetus increasingly takes up abdominal space during this time; thus feeding of some grain and good-quality hay high in DE is necessary (perhaps as much as 0.5 to 1.0 kg of grain and 1 to 1.5 kg of hay per 100 kg of body weight). Because initial body condition is so important for optimizing fetal growth and mare lactation, constant monitoring of body condition should be done to ensure that dietary energy requirements are being met.

Mares in late gestation also need 44 g of crude protein per mcal of DE. A rule of thumb is to provide 9% to 10% of the total ration (on a dry matter basis) as crude protein during the last 3 months of gestation compared with 7% to 8% crude protein in the total ration during the first 8 months of gestation (Hintz, 1993). Alfalfa hay is a good source of protein for pregnant and lactating mares.

The primary minerals to be concerned with in rations for pregnant mares are calcium and phosphorus. The NRC recommends that calcium (in grams per day) in the total ration be fed at a rate of 1.90 × mcal DE, or approximately 0.2% and 0.4% of total rations for maintenance (first 8 months of gestation) and late gestation (last 3 months), respectively. To avoid osteochondrosis of the fetus, calcium should be added to the grain mixture rather than be fed ad libitum in a salt-mineral mix. Because legume hays are rich in calcium, feeding of alfalfa may preclude the need for calcium supplementation in the diet, whereas if grass hay is fed, the need for calcium supplementation may reach 0.6% of the grain mixture. Phosphorus content of the ration should be scrutinized closely so that mares in late gestation are fed a diet containing approximately 0.3%. However, phosphorus content should not exceed calcium content in the ration (Hintz, 1993). Recommendations for feeding of other minerals, including zinc, copper, manganese, iodine, and selenium, and for feeding of vitamins are discussed by the NRC. Finally, mares should be offered fresh clean water and salt ad libitum.

During the first 1 to 12 weeks of lactation, mares of light breeds produce milk equivalent to 3% of their body weight per day. Milk production is reduced to 2% of mare body weight per day later in lactation (i.e., 13 to 24 weeks). More nutrient drain on the mare occurs during lactation than during late gestation. Milk yield is markedly influenced by both water and feed consumption by the mare. The protein and energy contents of milk are markedly reduced by 12 hours postpartum, and then gradually decrease over the remainder of the lactation period. During the first 12 weeks of lactation, mares require approximately 70% more energy than for maintenance. This is reduced to a 48% increase over maintenance in late lactation. The dietary protein requirement is nearly 120% over maintenance during early lactation and is reduced to 60% over maintenance during late lactation. Calcium and phosphorus requirements are similar for pregnant and lactating mares (Hintz, 1993).

Monitoring Fetal Viability

Illness or injury can predispose the pregnant mare to fetal stress and abortion. Some pregnant mares develop genital discharges or precocious udder development with premature lactation that alerts the owner/manager to the possibility of abortion or premature delivery. Rarely, a mare may develop an overly large abdomen, which may cause the owner to worry about the possible presence of twins or hydrops of the fetal membranes. In such instances, examination of the mare's physical condition, uterine status, and viability of the fetus(es) is indicated.

The origin of genital discharges can usually be determined by speculum examination. It is important to perform this examination in an aseptic and expedient manner to avoid contaminating the vagina and cervix. Scanty mucopurulent discharges are most commonly caused by inflammation of the vulva or vestibulum, often from inadequate vulvar lip apposition, which can be corrected by Caslick's surgery (see Chapter 15). Purulent or brownish bloody discharge through a relaxed cervix should alert the practitioner to the probability of an impending abortion, and fetal viability should be assessed. Occasionally, older mares will develop urovagina caused by conformational changes associated with the enlarging pregnancy. Urovagina that cannot be controlled by improving body condition and exercise may require reconstructive surgery to prevent infection from ascending through an inflamed cervix (see Chapter 15). Rarely, bloody discharge (sometimes with clots of blood) occurs in aged pregnant mares because of hemorrhage from prolapsed subepithelial veins in the vulva or vagina (sometimes referred to as "vaginal hemorrhoids") (Figure 9-1). Bleeding from one of these vessels most often occurs on the cranial surface of the vestibular ring, which can be difficult to visualize without the use of a flexible endoscope. In most mares, treatment is not necessary because bleeding is minor and usually stops within a few days. Cauterization of affected vessels is usually effective, as is ligation.

To assess fetal viability during early gestation, transrectal ultrasonography can be performed to detect fetal movement, umbilical blood flow, and fetal heartbeat (Figure 9-2). The use of transrectal ultrasonography to assess these criteria is limited in more advanced gestations by the examiner's inability to see an image of the fetus. In advanced gestation, the fetus can be palpated per rectum to detect fetal movement, although the lack of fetal movement is no guarantee of fetal death. Transrectal ultrasonography has some value during more advanced gestation if the probe is placed in a position to view the caudal area of the allantochorion just cranial to the cervix. This technique is useful for detecting placental thickening, sometimes with separation and fluid accumulation between the endometrium and allantochorion (Figure 9-3). Minnesota and California workers suggested that a combined thickness of the uterine wall and allantochorion (referred to as the combined uterine-placental thickness, or CUPT) ≥8 mm between 271 and 300 days of gestation, ≥10 mm between 301 and 330 days of gestation, and ≥12 mm after 330 days

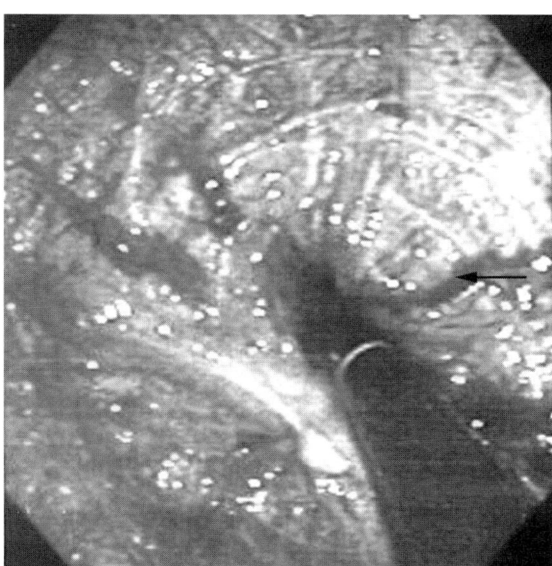

FIGURE 9-1. Prolapsed subepithelial veins ("vaginal hemorrhoids") beneath vaginal mucosa visualized through an endoscope. The endoscope has been turned 180 degrees to visualize the cranial surface of the vestibular ring. The arrow points to a vessel that has been bleeding.

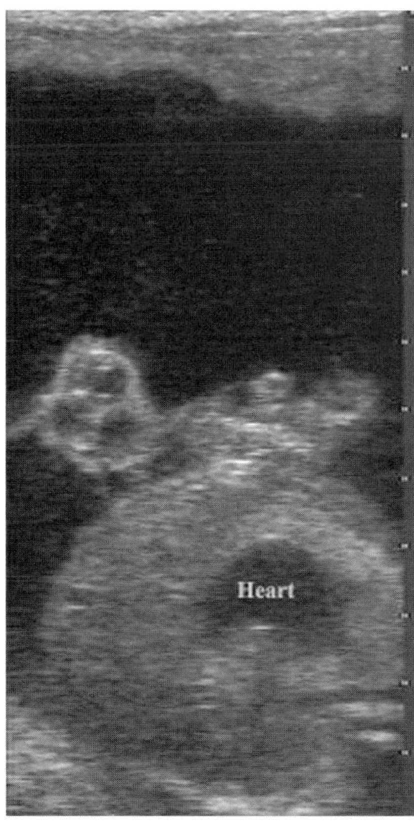

FIGURE 9-2. Transrectal ultrasonographic image of a fetus 3 months after breeding. Fetal movement and heartbeat were readily apparent. The distended heart is noted.

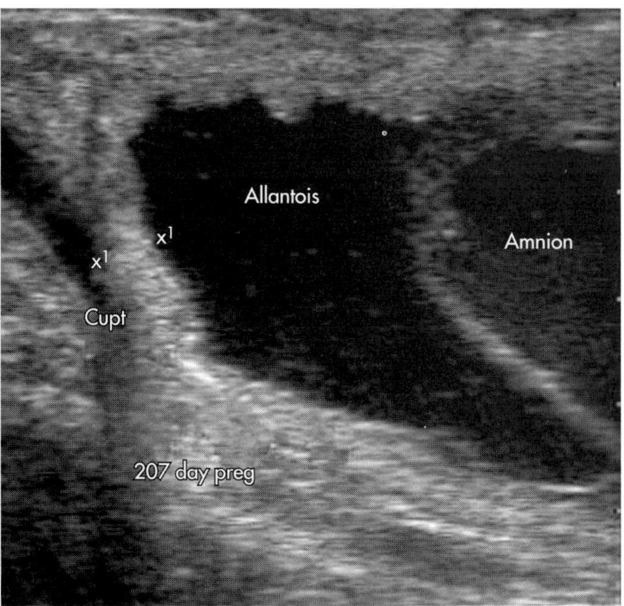

FIGURE 9-3. Transrectal ultrasonographic image obtained during assessment of uterine-placental thickness (combined uteroplacental thickness [CUPT] measured between cursors) in a mare at 207 days of gestation. The allantoic fluid (allantois) and amnionic fluid (amnion) is visible.

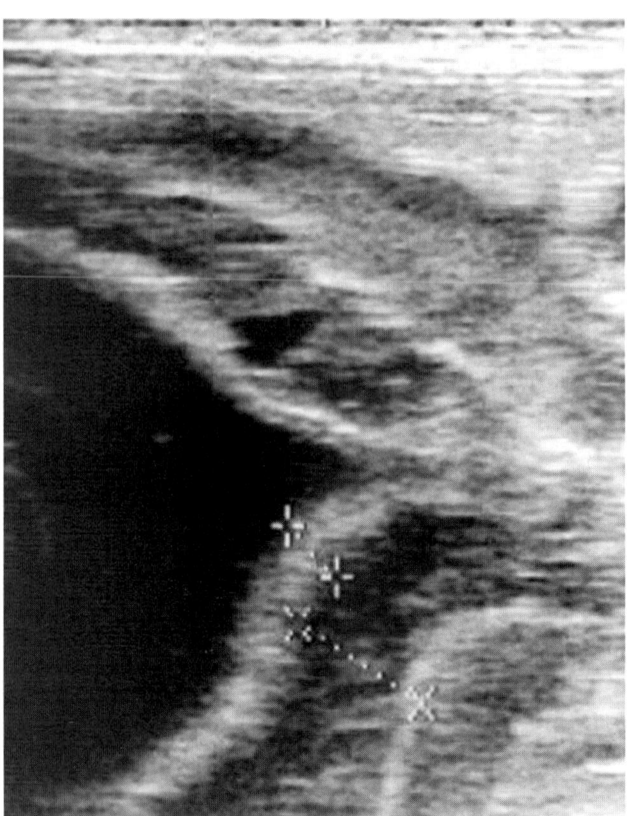

FIGURE 9-4. Transrectal ultrasonographic image of the caudal uterine body/cervix obtained during assessment of fetal well-being at 9 months of gestation. Premature udder development and cervical relaxation were apparent, and impending abortion caused by placental separation/placentitis was suspected. Fetal heart rate was normal. + - - - + represents chorioallantois; X - - - X represents an area of separation between the chorioallantois and endometrium. (Photo courtesy Dr. Jorge Colon, Equine Medical Associates, PSC, Lexington, KY.)

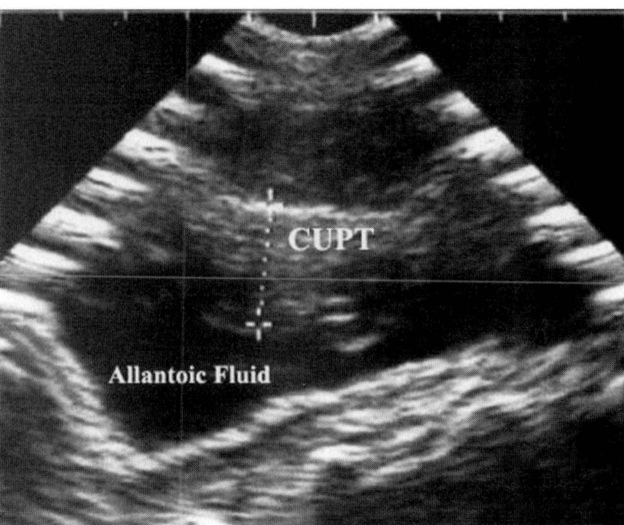

FIGURE 9-5. Transabdominal ultrasonographic image obtained during assessment of fetal well-being in a mare with premature udder development and lactation 4 weeks before her due date. Combined uteroplacental thickness (CUPT) was excessive (2 cm), and placental thickening and separation were apparent cranial to the cervix (Figure 9-4). Despite treatment with broad-spectrum antimicrobials, altrenogest, and flunixin meglumine, the foal was delivered 3 days later ("red-bag" delivery). Extensive chronic placentitis was evident throughout the placenta, which occupied more than 5 gallons and weighed more than 20 lb. (Photo courtesy Dr. Jorge Colon, Equine Medical Associates, PSC, Lexington, KY.)

of gestation is indicative of placental failure and pending abortion caused by ascending placentitis.

Transcutaneous ultrasonography, using 2.5- to 5-MHz sector or curvilinear probes, is a good method for evaluating the fetus, uterine fluids, uterus, and placenta of mares during mid to late gestation. Pennsylvania workers suggested using a depth setting of 27.5 to 30 cm for sector probes when the ventral abdomen is scanned. Doppler ultrasonography and M-mode echocardiography are especially useful for assessing fetal cardiac rhythm. Reimer (1997) described abnormal pregnancies identifiable during transcutaneous ultrasonography, including visible anomalies of the fetus (omphalocele or fetal ascites), excessive echogenic retroplacental fluid accumulations resulting in placental separation (Figure 9-4), thickening of the placenta from placentitis (Figure 9-5), hydrallantois, hydramnios, compromised twin pregnancies missed on earlier transrectal ultrasongraphic examinations (one or both dead), and fetal death. Determination of fetal heartbeat and cardiac rate is also useful for evaluating the fetus during late gestation. Florida and Pennsylvania workers determined that reduced fetal movement combined with failure of the fetal cardiac rhythm to substantially increase in response to fetal movements can be indicative of fetal hypoxic stress. Florida workers suggested that during late gestation equine fetuses should have a baseline heart rate of 60 to 92 beats/min that accelerates by 25 to 40 beats/min in the approximately 30-second period accompanying vigorous fetal movement. They also suggested monitoring fetal cardiac rhythm for periods of up to 10 minutes to evaluate fetal cardiac response during movement. Persistent bradycardia or tachycardia, particularly during more than one examination, has been associated with poor fetal outcome by several workers.

Unfortunately, even with the improved capability for monitoring fetal viability in the horse, methods for treatment that will improve outcome remain limited. For example, in the mare with precocious udder development and premature lactation—in which premature separation of the placenta or placentitis is suspected or confirmed and the fetus remains alive—treatment consists of administration of uterine tocolytics and progestogens, antiprostaglandins, and broad-spectrum antimicrobials. Monitoring of fetal viability is indicated at regular intervals until parturition, with the clinician being prepared to provide intensive care to a potentially dysmature foal. There is no doubt that the ability to monitor

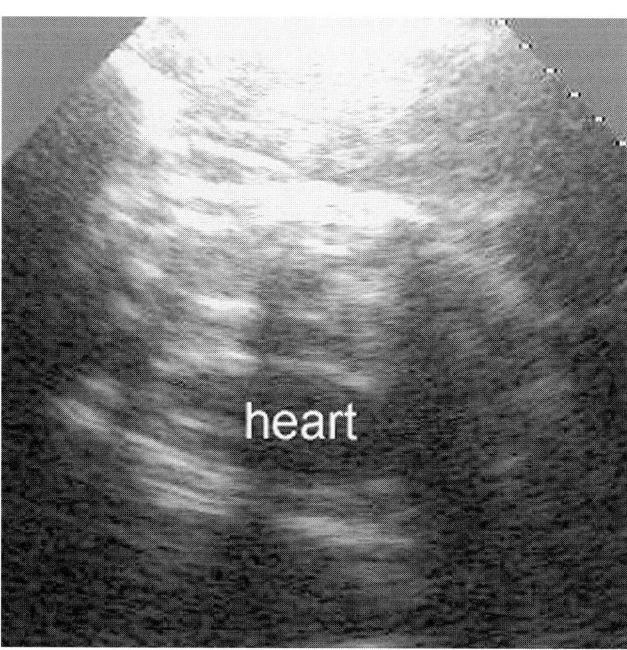

FIGURE 9-6. Transabdominal ultrasonographic image obtained during assessment of fetal well-being during advanced gestation. The mare had precocious udder development, and impending abortion was suspected. Twin fetuses were detected, with one being dead (no heartbeat) at the time of examination. The fetal thorax is visualized in this image (note "shadows" cast by ribs), with the anechoic structure being the heart.

fetal viability in some instances enables the clinician to better make a decision about whether to induce parturition by taking into account increasing fetal risk versus the capability of a foal to sustain extrauterine life. Transcutaneous ultrasonographic examination of the uterus and its contents improves the clinician's ability to make a proper diagnosis and justify induction of abortion/parturition when a dead fetus(es), twins (Figure 9-6), a prominent fetal abnormality, or hydrallantois is detected.

MONITORING AND PREPARING THE MARE FOR PARTURITION

Approximately 4 to 6 weeks before the date of expected foaling, the mare should be moved to a location that is clean and dry and that provides protection against inclement weather. Pasture is suitable if it is well drained, not overstocked, and has sheds or trees available in rainy, cold seasons. In cold climates, well-ventilated barns with clean, freshly bedded stalls are commonly used for housing mares overnight and during inclement weather. Moving mares to the area of foaling serves a variety of purposes. It allows the mares to become acclimated to the foaling premises and handling procedures. During this time, mares are exposed to organisms indigenous to the foaling area, thus providing them with the opportunity to develop antibodies to organisms that may be infectious. The antibodies are then transferred to the foal through the colostrum. Moving mares to such a location also allows closer, more frequent observation of the near-term mare. Because the mare is accessible, it is also an opportune time to provide immunization with appropriate vaccines.

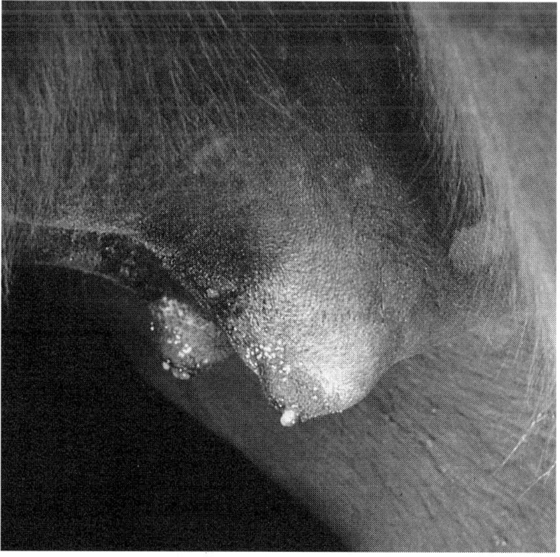

FIGURE 9-7. "Waxing" of the teat ends of a mare due to foal. Note that the udder is well developed and the teats are full. Waxing of the teat ends usually occurs 1 to 4 days before foaling.

Before foaling, the mare's udder should be cleansed and, if the mare has had the vulva sutured, it should be opened to prevent vulvar tearing at parturition. For indoor foaling, the mare should be placed in a large (14 by 14 feet), recently cleansed, well-bedded, and ventilated stall. When weather permits, the mare can be turned out for exercise in a small paddock or pasture during the day. During observation, particularly at night, care should be taken to avoid disturbing the mare.

During this last month before foaling, the mare should be examined regularly for physical changes that indicate nearness of delivery. Physical changes that occur as parturition nears include development of vulvar laxity and edema, scanty vulvar discharges, relaxation of pelvic ligaments, udder enlargement, and a change in the amount and character of mammary secretions. The most reliable indicator of impending parturition is a remarkable change in udder size and secretion. Mammary gland growth becomes quite apparent in the last month of gestation, particularly in the last 2 weeks. Filling of teats and changes in mammary secretion occur nearer to parturition. The udder typically becomes engorged within the last few days before foaling. The accumulation of a "waxy" secretion on teat ends (Figure 9-7), from early colostrum formation, usually occurs 1 to 4 days before foaling, but sometimes occurs as early as 2 weeks before parturition or not at all. Occasionally, milk will leak from teats of multiparous mares for several days to weeks before foaling, resulting in loss of colostrum.

Monitoring milk secretions is a valuable tool for predicting nearness of parturition. As parturition approaches, secretions change from thin, straw-colored fluid to milky white fluid. Eventually a thick, viscous fluid that is yellow to orange in color becomes apparent as colostrum formation occurs. Good-quality colostrum should contain >60 g of immunoglobulin G (IgG) per liter. Although not all mares produce yellow, viscous colostrum, a recent French study confirmed that yellow colostrum had a significantly higher IgG concentration than white colostrum, and viscous colostrum also appeared to contain more IgG than nonviscous colostrum.

The changing electrolyte contents of prefoaling udder secretions are related to fetal maturity and viability and thus to readiness for birth. Concentrations of minerals (particularly calcium and magnesium) in the prefoaling udder secretion increase, especially in the last 2 to 4 days before parturition. A number of methods can be used to measure calcium content in prefoaling udder secretions; these require that small samples be collected once or twice daily to monitor changes. When calcium concentrations exceeded 10 mmol/L as measured by atomic absorption spectrophotometry, 92% of mares (10 of 11) foaled spontaneously within 1 to 6 days (Peaker et al., 1979). The Predict-A-Foal Test Mare Foaling Predictor Kit (Animal Health Care Products) measures both calcium and magnesium concentrations (Figure 9-8). When 1 of five indicator squares change color with this test, the mare has only a 1% chance of foaling within the next 12 hours. When four of five test squares change color, the mare has a >80% chance of foaling within the next 12 hours. A colorimetric test kit (FoalWatch test kit available from CHEMetrics, Inc.) has been adapted to measure calcium carbonate concentrations in prefoaling udder secretions of mares (Ley et al., 1998). After diluting 1.5 ml of udder secretion with 9 ml of distilled water, Ley and associates used concentrations of calcium carbonate <200 ppm in the diluted sample as an indicator that most mares (99% probability) would not foal within 24 hours, whereas the predictive value that a mare would foal within 72 hours was 97% when calcium carbonate concentrations in secretions were >200 ppm. The majority of mares with colostrum testing results showing 300 to 500 ppm of $CaCo_3$ foaled within a short period of time.

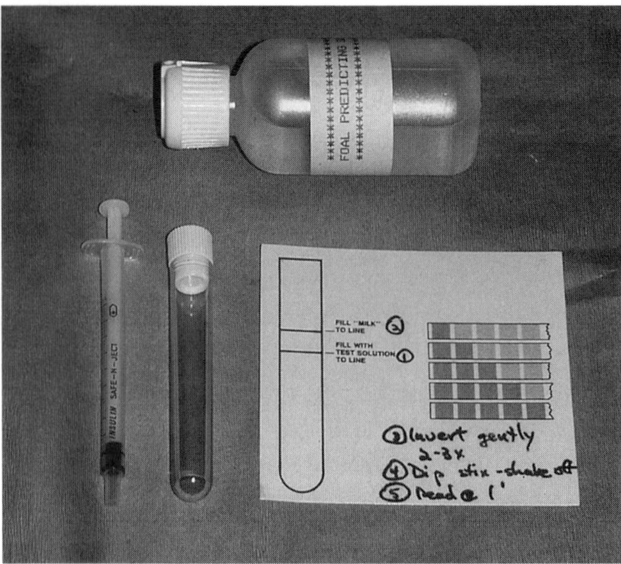

FIGURE 9-8. The "Predict-A-Foal" test uses an indicator test strip with succeeding squares changing color as calcium and magnesium contents increase in prefoaling udder secretions and the mare nears spontaneous parturition.

STAGES OF PARTURITION

Parturition, although it is a continuous process, has arbitrarily been divided into three stages for descriptive purposes. In mares, the **first stage of parturition** (or preparatory stage) usually requires 30 minutes to 4 hours. Shorter and less obvious signs may occur in multiparous mares. During the first stage, mares are restless and exhibit signs similar to those of colic (e.g., the mare may look back toward her flank, raise and switch her tail, urinate small quantities often, perspire, and lie down and get up repeatedly (Figure 9-9). This period is associated with uterine contractions of increasing intensity and frequency, as well as cervical dilation. Also during this stage, the cranial portion of the foal *rotates from a dorsopubic, through a dorsoilial, and eventually to a dorsosacral position*. The uterine contractions eventually push the foal's forefeet and muzzle with the surrounding chorioallantoic membrane into the dilating cervix.

When the determination has been made that the mare is in the first stage of labor, the tail should be wrapped and the perineal area scrubbed and dried. Late in this stage, the mare will lie down, roll from side to side, and stand up again (Figure 9-10). This activity may be very important in helping the fetus to reposition itself. As the fetus and fetal fluids

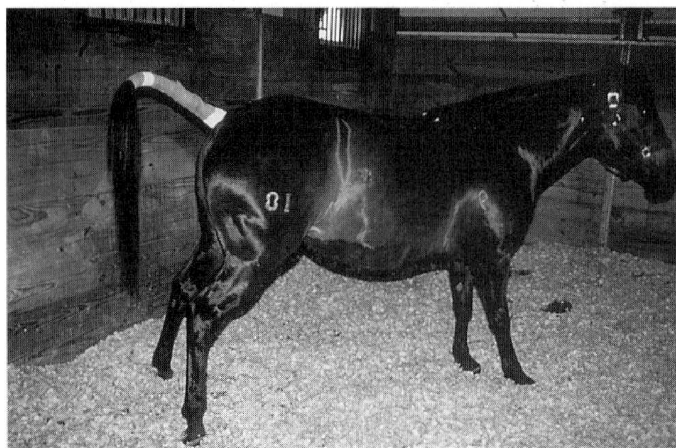

FIGURE 9-9. Mare in the first stage of labor. The tail has been wrapped and the perineal area and udder have been cleansed. The mare was sweating, stretching, lifting her tail, and urinating small quantities at periodic intervals.

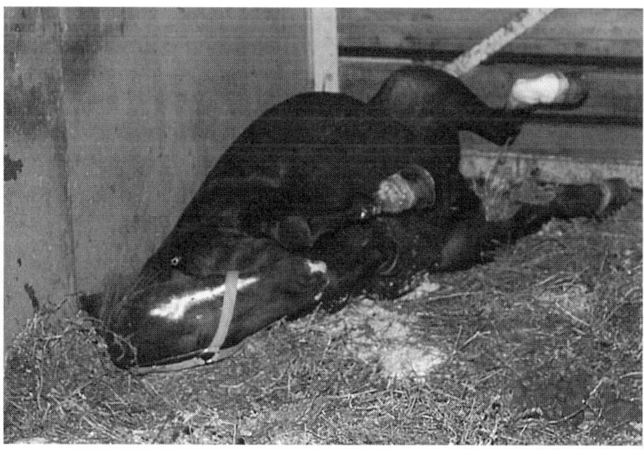

FIGURE 9-10. Pony mare in the first stage of labor. Regardless of the size of the stall used for foaling, a mare may get cast in a corner when rolling during this stage of labor. If the mare gets caught in a corner, she should be pulled away from the corners so she may rise again or so she will not attempt to deliver the foal against a wall or into a corner where delivery will be impeded.

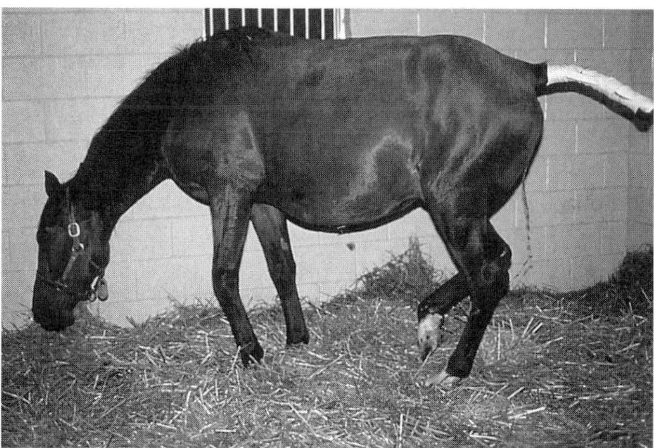

FIGURE 9-11. The chorioallantois has ruptured, and allantoic fluid escapes from the birth canal. The fluid may initially be released in a slow, almost undetectable stream or in a prominent stream that is obvious. This point marks entry into the second stage of labor.

(contained within the placenta) are forced against the cervix, cervical dilation progresses until the **chorioallantois** ruptures and several gallons of **allantoic fluid** escape from the genital tract (i.e., the "water breaks") (Figure 9-11). If the chorioallantois does not rupture and the velvety-red surface of the chorioallantois is presented at the vulva (see Figure 8-17), it should be immediately ruptured because this indicates the placenta is separating from the endometrium (i.e., **premature placental separation**) and fetal oxygenation will be impaired.

After cervical dilation is complete, the **second stage of parturition** usually ensues and the fetus passes into the birth canal. Fetal passage into the pelvic inlet elicits abdominal contractions and release of oxytocin from the neurohypophysis (posterior pituitary gland); these effects reinforce existing uterine contractions. The mare usually lies on her side and periodically *strains forcefully* during this active labor. The repeated abdominal press assists in fetal expulsion. Within 5 minutes after rupture of the chorioallantoic membrane, the **amnion** (the white, glistening membrane) is forced between the vulvar lips (Figure 9-12). As delivery progresses, first one forefoot and then the other will become visible with the soles of the hooves directed downward. The nose follows, with the head resting on the forelimbs at the fetlock or carpal level (Figure 9-13). It is not uncommon for the mare to rise when the forefeet are just being presented at the vulva, turn around, and then lie down again a few moments to minutes later and resume active straining. The most forceful contractions occur when the head and shoulders pass through the mare's pelvis (Figure 9-14). The

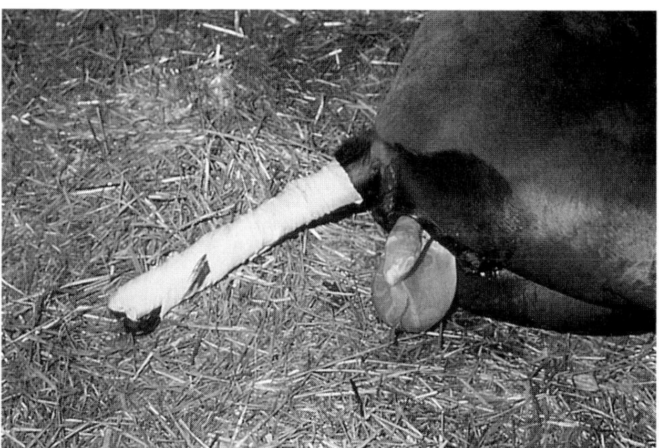

FIGURE 9-12. The white, glistening structure protruding from the vulva is the amnion, which contains the amnionic fluid. One foot is detectable within the amniotic cavity.

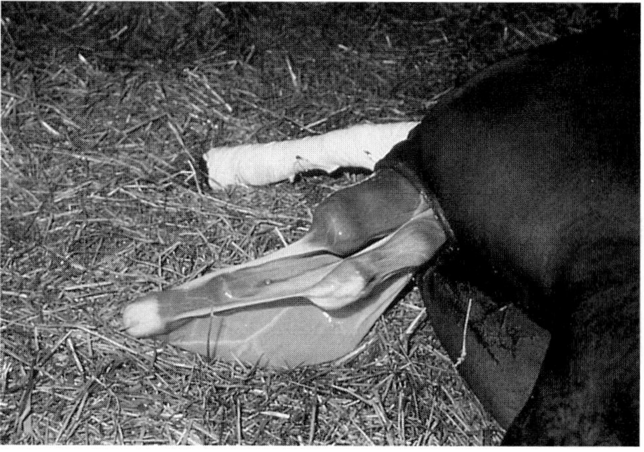

FIGURE 9-13. One foot precedes the other, with the soles of the feet directed downward, as the second stage of labor progresses. The muzzle of the foal is positioned at the carpus level. Because the amnion may remain intact at this point in delivery, some practitioners prefer to quietly enter the stall and remove the amnion from covering the foal's head to prevent suffocation.

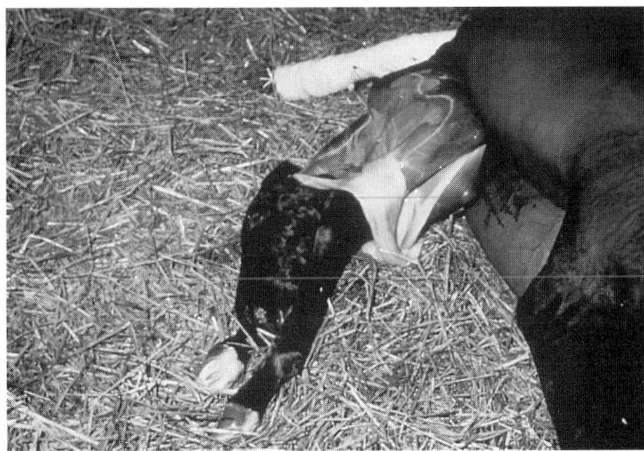

FIGURE 9-14. The head and shoulders of the foal have passed through the mare's pelvis. The amnion has been ruptured. The level of the shoulders represents the greatest cross-sectional diameter of the foal.

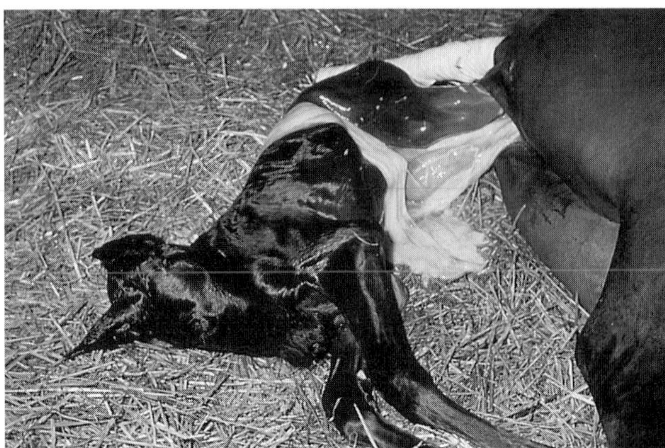

FIGURE 9-16. The foal's hips have been delivered through the maternal pelvis, and the foal's hindlimbs remain within the vagina. The exhausted mare usually rests for a period of time before rising.

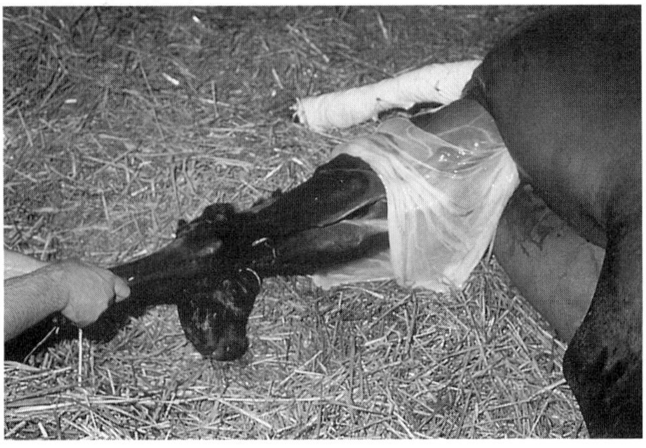

FIGURE 9-15. If traction must be applied during the dam's abdominal press, one foreleg should be pulled slightly in front of the other to ensure that one shoulder precedes the other during the foal's passage through the maternal pelvis, thereby reducing the effective diameter of the fetus at its shoulders.

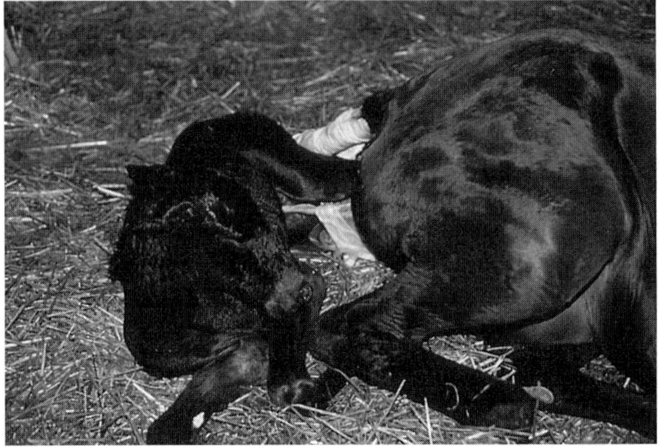

FIGURE 9-17. When possible, the umbilical cord should be left intact for a few minutes to ensure maximal blood flow from the placenta to the circulation of the newborn foal.

amnion usually ruptures at this point. If necessary, assistance can be provided at this time by gently pulling on the foal's forelimbs in synchrony with the mare's abdominal press (Figure 9-15). Once the foal's hips pass through the maternal pelvis, the mare usually rests for 15 or 20 minutes (Figure 9-16). If the foal has ruptured the amnion and cleared the fetal membranes, is breathing normally, and is able to struggle to a sternal position, the foal (and mare) need not be disturbed. Letting the umbilical cord remain attached during this time may result in return of blood from the placenta into the fetus (Figure 9-17). If the mare is disturbed, she may rise and rupture the cord prematurely. Under most circumstances, it is acceptable to let the cord break naturally when the mare stands or the foal attempts to rise. If manual separation is deemed necessary, the cord should be grasped with one hand on each side of the intended break point (e.g., the predetermined break site is seen on the umbilical cord as a pale strictured area 1 to 2 inches from the foal's abdomen) (see Figure 11-4). The thumb and forefingers are used to twist and pull the cord apart. Caution should be used to avoid placing undue tension on the cord attachment to the abdominal wall, and the cord should not be cut because this action may result in excessive hemorrhage or a patent urachus. The umbilical stump should be observed for hemorrhage, urine leakage, or swelling before being disinfected with 0.5% chlorhexidine (Nolvasan solution 2%, Fort Dodge Laboratories). A recent California study demonstrated that chlorhexidine was superior to 1% or 2% tamed iodine or 7% tincture of iodine in the ability to reduce numbers of bacteria without inducing tissue destruction of the foal navel. The *navel should be disinfected* several times for the first few days of life. An *enema* can also be given at this time to aid in prevention

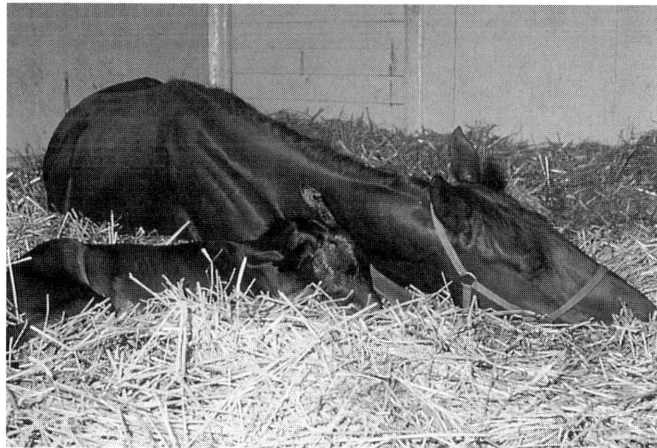

FIGURE 9-18. After the umbilical cord has been detached, the foal can be moved toward the mare's head. This procedure can aid in relaxing the mare and can also facilitate the bonding procedure between the mare and foal.

of meconial impaction. If the mare has not risen by this time, the foal can be moved near to the mare's head (Figure 9-18). This may reduce the likelihood of the mare stepping on the foal when rising. *Unnecessary disturbances should be avoided* to allow dam-foal interaction during the early postpartum period and permit the development of a strong bond between them. Guidelines for evaluation of the foal during the first 72 hours of life, including confirmation of sufficient transfer of immunoglobulins through ingestion of colostrum, are reviewed in Chapter 11.

Normally, the second stage of labor is explosive and short-lived; *delivery of the fetus usually occurs within 20 to 30 minutes*. If delivery is taking longer than this amount of time or if progression of delivery ceases, fetal position and posture should be assessed immediately (i.e., to ensure that **dystocia** is not a problem). The most common impediments to delivery are abnormalities in fetal posture, which must be corrected to facilitate delivery of a viable foal.

Stage three of parturition encompasses expulsion of the fetal membranes and uterine involution. When the mare rises or in the period immediately after birth when the mare is resting, the placenta can be tied to itself (Figure 9-19) so that it hangs just above the hocks to avoid being stepped on until it is passed. The *placenta is typically expelled within 30 minutes to 3 hours* after foaling. If the placenta is not passed by this time, treatment may be necessary to hasten its expulsion and avoid uterine trauma and infection. To prevent undue aspiration of air into the vagina when the mare attempts to stand, the use of temporary application of towel clamps has been advocated to appose vulvar labia. The authors do not find this procedure necessary except after some instances of dystocia when swelling and abrasion of tissues have occurred. Care should be taken to avoid incorporating placental tissue in the towel clamps if they are applied.

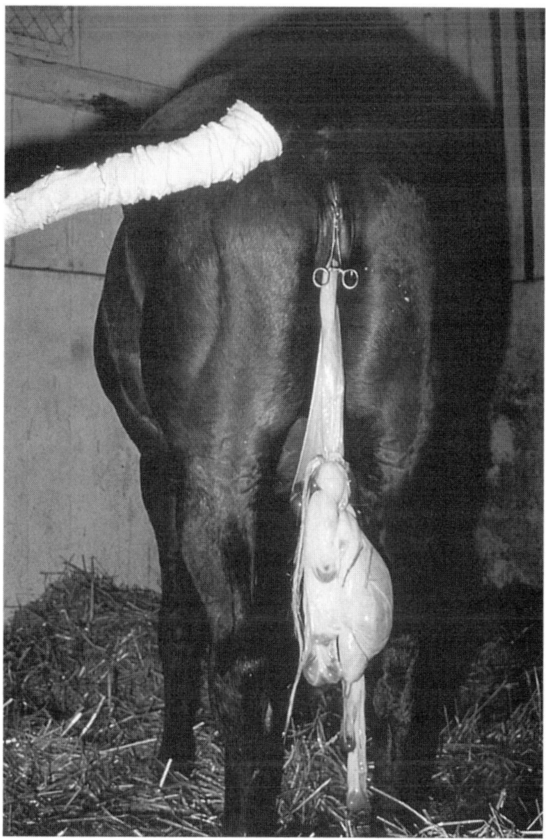

FIGURE 9-19. The placenta can be tied to itself so that it hangs at the level of the hocks when the mare stands. This will prevent the mare from stepping on the placenta until it is passed. The labia of the vulva can be temporarily apposed with towel clamps to minimize aspiration of air into the vagina when the mare rises after parturition.

INDUCED PARTURITION

Induction of parturition has been used in the mare for management of high-risk pregnancies, research, teaching, and convenience. Several drugs have been used to induce parturition in the mare. Regardless of which agent is used to induce parturition, it is crucial that the mare and fetus be ready for birth. Gestation should be at least 335 days in length. Adequate pelvic ligament and cervical relaxation should be apparent, and udder development and good-quality colostrum should be present (refer to guidelines given earlier to determine readiness for birth). Although parturition can be induced in mares with a nonrelaxed cervix (providing other signs of readiness for birth are apparent), the first stage of labor is prolonged. Texas workers have demonstrated that the prolonged first stage of labor is associated with an increased incidence of birth hypoxia and neontal maladjustment. In a subsequent study, the Texas workers demonstrated that placement of 2 mg PGE_2 in the external cervical os 4 to 6 hours before inducing parturition resulted in softening of the cervix and a shorter interval to delivery, which should decrease the chances of birth hypoxia and neonatal maladjustment. Whenever parturition is induced, if delivery is not progressive or is delayed once labor begins, prompt examination for dystocia is indicated.

Oxytocin is generally considered to be the drug of choice for inducing parturition in the mare. The drug has a rapid effect and usually results in delivery within 15 to 90 minutes after administration is begun. The patterns of induction are consistent and seem to have little untoward effect on the term foal. Various methods of oxytocin administration have been used to induce parturition, including (1) injection of 40 to 120 U (intramuscularly), (2) injection of 2.5 to 20 U at 15- to-20-minute intervals (intravenously, intramuscularly, or subcutaneously) until the second stage of labor ensues, and (3) intravenous drip of 60 to 120 U in 1 liter of saline at a rate of 1 U/min until the second stage of labor ensues.

Both natural and synthetic prostaglandins have also been used successfully for inducing parturition in the mare; however, the prostaglandin analogs are generally thought to produce more predictable responses with less risk to the foal. Fluprostenol (250 μg intramuscularly) has been reported to induce parturition only in mares in which the fetus is mature and capable of extrauterine life. However, this is not always the case, because some premature foals have been delivered after administration of fluprostenol. Additionally, the induction-parturition interval is more variable (1 to 6 hours) with fluprostenol than with oxytocin. Fenprostalene (0.5 to 1.0 mg subcutaneously; in 2 hours either repeat fenprostalene injection or initiate oxytocin administration) has also been used successfully to induce parturition in mares. When the two-injection scheme of fenprostalene is used, most mares delivered their foals within 2 to 4 hours after the first fenprostalene injection. When 2.5 U of oxytocin was administered intravenously at 15- to 20-minute intervals beginning 2 hours after the initial fenprostalene injection, mares delivered foals within 2 to 3 hours. However, neither fenprostalene nor fluprostenol is presently available in the United States.

THE POSTPARTUM PERIOD

Breeding on the First Postpartum Estrus

To realize optimum economic return in broodmares, management personnel must strive to maximize the number of foals produced per dam lifetime. The major constraint to achieving this goal in the mare is the relatively long gestation period, averaging 340 days, which permits only 25 days from parturition to conception to produce foals at yearly intervals. The pregnancy rate achieved by breeding during the first postpartum estrus ("foal heat") is often lower (e.g., 10% to 20% lower) than that achieved by breeding on subsequent estrous periods. However, failure to establish pregnancy by foal-heat breeding results in an 18-day drift toward a later conception and a corresponding delay in the foaling date the following year. Registry-derived time constraints that are placed on equine breeding seasons often result in barrenness in "late-foaling" mares. Failure to produce foals on a yearly basis culminates in irretrievable economic loss because of expenses for feed and housing, transportation, animal care, and non-productive breeding fees.

Uterine Involution

The decreased pregnancy rate associated with foal-heat breedings has been suggested to be caused by failure of the uterus, particularly the endometrium, to be completely restored to a pregravid state and therefore ready to support a developing embryo. Although a paucity of information is available on uterine involution and its relationship to fertility in the mare, changes that occur during the involution process have been studied. Vaginal exudate progressively decreases through the first postpartum ovulation, and the amount of fluid detected ultrasonographically in the uterine lumen decreases until it is nondetectable by day 15 postpartum. Uterine horns return to their pregravid size by day 32 postpartum, whereas involution of the endometrium occurs more rapidly. Resorption of microcaruncles is essentially complete by day 7 postpartum and the overlying luminal epithelium is intact by days 4 to 7 postpartum. Endometrial gland dilation is absent by day 4 postpartum and glandular activity increases, as indicated by taller epithelial cells with increased mitotic activity, to day 12 postpartum. The *endometrium usually has a normal pregravid histologic appearance by day 14 postpartum*. This is probably the reason for increased pregnancy rates in mares ovulating after 10 days postpartum when bred on foal heat, because embryo entry into the uterus occurs 5 to 6 days postovulation when intrauterine fluid is absent and the endometrium is restored. For a review of hormonal treatments to delay breeding of postpartum mares until uterine involution has taken place, refer to Chapter 4.

Factors responsible for uterine involution are not well understood. Uterine contractility probably plays an important role in rapidly reducing the postparturient uterus to its pregravid state. Concurrent with this decrease in uterine size, a significant amount of lochial fluid is discharged from the uterine lumen. The histologic character of the endometrium correspondingly reverts to a condition more conducive to embryonic support.

Examination of the Postpartum Mare

Routine examination of the postpartum reproductive tract of the mare is done when pathologic conditions are suspected and, in some instances, to provide information on which to base a decision to breed a mare on the first postpartum estrus. Procedures used for these purposes include inspection of the vulva and perineum, palpation of the genital tract per rectum, transrectal ultrasonographic examination of the genital tract, and examination of the vagina and cervix digitally or through a speculum. Knowledge of the characteristics of normal involution is necessary to accurately assess the status of the reproductive tract. The following is a listing of events that occur in the progression of uterine involution and return to ovarian cyclicity in the postpartum mare:

- **Placental passage:** normally within 3 hours after delivery of the foal.
- **Twelve to 24 hours postpartum:** marked decrease in uterine size; uterine discharge evident. The majority of uterine fluid is eliminated by 24 to 48 hours postpartum.
- **Three to 5 days postpartum:** usual time of thorough postpartum examination. Both uterine horns are palpable per rectum, the gravid horn is more enlarged than the nongravid horn, vulvar discharge ceases, blood-tinged discharge is noted at the external cervical os, and the external cervical os is hyperemic.
- **Five to 15 days post partum:** onset of first postpartum estrus (foal heat). The microcaruncles of the endometrium are no longer evident by day 7, the endometrium has a normal nonpregnant histologic appearance by day 14, the myometrium is still enlarged, the gravid horn is still more enlarged than the nongravid horn, a blood-tinged discharge may still be evident at the external cervical os, the external cervical os may still be hyperemic, and the cervix does not close from the time of parturition until after foal-heat ovulation occurs.
- **Foal heat (first postpartum estrus):** onset at 4 to 14 days. There may be a slight disadvantage in conception rate compared with breeding on subsequent heats but probably no difference in pregnancy loss rate. A consistent advantage to foal-heat breeding (18.5 days) is reduction of the interval from parturition to conception (25.3 versus 43.8 days open).
- **First postpartum ovulation:** 43% of mares ovulate by day 9, 93% ovulate by day 15, and 97% ovulate by day 20. Mares that ovulate after day 10 postpartum are reputed to have normal pregnancy rates (i.e., the same as mares that are bred for the first time on the second or later postpartum heats).
- **Twenty-five to 32 days postpartum:** onset of second postpartum estrus. The uterine horns have returned to pregravid size.

BIBLIOGRAPHY

Adams-Brendemuehl C: Fetal assessment. In Koterba AM, Drummond WH, Kosch PC, editors, *Equine neonatology*, Philadelphia, 1990, Lea and Febiger.

Hintz HF: Nutrition of the broodmare. In McKinnon AO, Voss JL, editors, *Equine reproduction*, Philadelphia, 1993, Lea and Febiger.

Ley WB, Parker NA, Bowen JM et al: How we induce the normal mare to foal. *Proc Am Assoc Equine Pract* 44:194-197, 1998.

Loy RC: Characteristics of postpartum reproduction in mares. *Vet Clin North Am Large Anim Pract* 2:345-358, 1980.

Macpherson ML, Chaffin K, Carroll GL et al: Three methods for oxytocin-induced parturition: effects on the neonatal foal, *Proc Ann Mtg Am Assoc Equine Practnr* 42: 150-151, 1996.

National Research Council: *Nutrient requirements of horses*. Washington DC, 1989, National Academy of Sciences, National Research Council.

Ousey J, Delcaux M, Rossdale P: Evaluation of three test strips for measuring electrolytes in mare's prepartum mammary secretions and for predicting parturition. *Equine Vet J* 21:196-200, 1989.

Peaker M, Rossdale PD, Forwyth IA et al: Changes in mammary development and the composition of secretion during late pregnancy in the mare. *J Reprod Fertil* 27(Suppl):555-561, 1979.

Reef VB, Vaala WE, Worth LT et al: Transcutaneous ultrasonographic assessment of fetal well-being during late gestation: a preliminary report on the development of an equine biophysical profile. *Proc Am Assoc Equine Pract* 42:152-153, 1996.

Reimer JM: Use of transcutaneous ultrasonography in complicated latter-middle to late gestation pregnancies in the mare: 122 cases. *Proc Am Assoc Equine Pract* 43:259-261, 1997.

Rigby S, Love CL, Carpenter K et al: Use of prostaglandin E_2 to ripen the cervix of the mare prior to induction of parturition. *Theriogenology* 50:897-904, 1998.

Roberts SJ: *Veterinary obstetrics and genital diseases, theriogenology,* ed 3, pp. 277-352. Woodstock, VT, 1986, SJ Roberts.

Rossdale PD, Ricketts SW: *Equine stud farm medicine,* ed 2, pp. 220-276. Philadelphia, 1980, Lea and Febiger.

Slater R: Immunologic control of viral and bacterial pathogens. *Proc Am Assoc Equine Pract* 46:10-20, 2000.

Troedsson MHT, Renaudin CD, Zent WW et al: Transrectal ultrasonography of the placenta in normal mares and mares with pending abortion: a field study. *Proc Am Assoc Equine Pract* 43:256-258, 1997.

10

Dystocia and Postparturient Disease

OBJECTIVES

While studying the information covered in this chapter, the student should attempt to:

1. Acquire a working understanding of maternal and fetal contributions to dystocia and those factors contributing to postparturient abnormalities in the mare.
2. Acquire a working knowledge of procedures used to diagnose and relieve dystocia in the mare.
3. Acquire a working knowledge of procedures used to diagnose and methodologies used to treat abnormalities of the postparturient period in the mare.

STUDY QUESTIONS

1. List equipment necessary to correct dystocia in the mare.
2. Describe procedures used to diagnose the cause of dystocia in the mare.
3. Define the following terms:
   a. dystocia.
   b. fetal presentation.
   c. fetal position.
   d. fetal posture.
   e. mutation.
   f. repulsion.
   g. delivery by traction.
4. Describe the more common obstetrical procedures used to correct dystocia in the mare by mutation and delivery by traction.
5. Describe proper treatment of the following postparturient abnormalities in the mare:
   a. retained placenta.
   b. metritis.
   c. laminitis.
   d. uterine prolapse.
   e. invagination of the uterine horn.
   f. uterine rupture.
   g. ruptured uterine or ovarian artery.
   h. other postparturient hemorrhages.

Dystocia and postparturient disease are uncommon in the mare; however, they may carry a guarded prognosis for life or future fertility in affected mares. Prompt, sound clinical management of dystocia, retained placenta, and other postparturient disorders can preserve the breeding potential of valuable mares.

☐ Dystocia

To better recognize dystocia, the processes and events of normal delivery must be well understood. Refer to Chapter 9 for a review of normal progression through the three stages of parturition. If either the first or second stage of parturition is prolonged or not progressing, dystocia is possible. Prompt veterinary examination is indicated to preserve the life of the foal and mare and to prevent injury to the mare's reproductive tract.

Obstetrical Equipment and Lubricant

High-quality, clean (preferably sterile) obstetrical equipment and lubricant should be readily available. Equipment should include, at a minimum, obstetrical chains or straps, obstetrical handles, a bucket, cotton or paper towels, tail wrap, and disinfectant soap (Figure 10-1). For the special equipment needed to perform a fetotomy, the reader is referred to Bierschwal and de Bois (1972).

When minimal obstetrical manipulations are required, we prefer to apply a small amount of polyethylene polymer powder (J-Lube, Jorgensen Laboratories) to the birth canal of the mare. The powder adheres to mucosal membranes, providing excellent short-term lubrication for extracting the fetus. Liquid lubricants (e.g., carboxymethylcellulose solution) provide good protection to the fetus and genital tract and can be pumped into the uterine lumen and around the fetus through a sterile stomach tube. Lubricant solution can be sterilized in gallon containers before use (by gas sterilization), or 0.5 to 1 tablespoon of chlorhexidine solution can be mixed with each gallon of lubricant as a disinfectant. Pumping lubricant into the uterine lumen provides some uterine distension that will

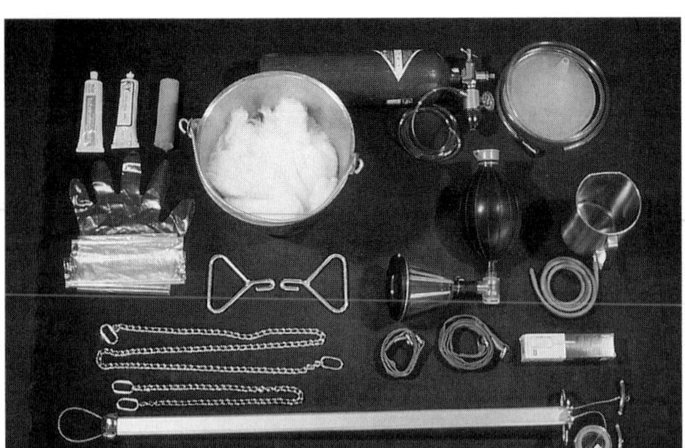

FIGURE 10-1. Obstetrical equipment. *Clockwise from upper left:* tubes of sterile lubricant, clean bucket containing cotton, oxygen bottle, and administration set, enema bucket and tube, Ambu bag, obstetrical straps, nasal catheter, fetatome, obstetrical chains and handles, and obstetrical gloves.

facilitate manipulation of the fetus. For fetotomy, petroleum jelly (Vaseline) can be applied to the fetus and birth canal to provide extra protection against physical injury during the procedure.

Examination of the Mare

If possible, the mare should be standing for the initial examination. The examination is done in a clean environment with good footing for the mare and veterinarian. The tail is wrapped and tied to the side, and the perineal area and rump are thoroughly scrubbed with an antiseptic soap and dried. If straining is a problem, the initial examination is made while the mare is being slowly walked. If necessary, a local anesthetic can be injected into the caudal epidural space to control straining. After the hair over the site of injection (usually Cy1-Cy2) is clipped, the skin is scrubbed and disinfected. Lidocaine (1.0 to 1.25 ml of 2% lidocaine per 100 kg of body weight) can then be administered in the caudal epidural space to provide perineal analgesia and control straining. The authors prefer to use a combination of xylazine (30 mg/454 kg of body weight), Carbocaine-V (2.4 ml of 2% mepivacaine hydrochloride per 454 kg of body weight), and sterile 0.9% NaCl solution (q.s. to 6.0 to 7.0 ml/454 kg of body weight) for epidural anesthesia. The rationale for use of this combination is that perineal analgesia is optimized while the risk of hind limb ataxia seen with higher doses of local anesthetics is lowered.

The hands and arms of the veterinarian are scrubbed with a disinfectant soap and then rinsed before entry into the birth canal. Sterile plastic sleeves can also be worn. The fetus is thoroughly examined to assess presentation, position, and posture, as well as the presence of any congenital abnormalities, such as contracted tendons, that might contribute to dystocia. An attempt is made to determine if the fetus is alive by stimulating reflex movements or by detecting a heartbeat or umbilical pulse if either the fetal thorax or umbilicus is within reach. Evidence of trauma that may indicate a previous attempt to deliver or allude to the duration of dystocia is noted.

For descriptive purposes, the student should be familiar with terms used to describe the fetus at the time of its entrance into the birth canal or pelvis. **Presentation** refers to the relationship of the spinal axis of the fetus to that of the dam—*longitudinal* or *transverse*—and the portion of the fetus entering the pelvic cavity—head *(cranial)* or tail *(caudal)* in longitudinal presentations or *ventral* or *dorsal* in transverse presentations. **Position** refers to the relationship of the dorsum of the fetus in longitudinal presentation or the head in transverse presentation to the quadrants of the maternal pelvis (sacrum, right ilium, left ilium, or pubis). **Posture** refers to the relationship of the fetal extremities (head, neck, and limbs) to the body of the fetus; they may be flexed, extended, or retained beneath or above the fetus. The normal presentation, position, and posture of the equine fetus during parturition are *cranial-longitudinal, dorsosacral,* with the *head, neck,* and *forelimbs extended.* Fetal *postural abnormalities* are the most common cause of dystocia in the mare. Equine fetuses are predisposed to postural abnormalities because of the long fetal extremities. Structural abnormalities of the fetus, such as hydrocephalus, may also result in dystocia. Caudal and particularly transverse fetal presentations are associated with a greatly increased incidence of fetal malformations (particularly contractures) that contribute to dystocia. Fetal death prevents the fetus from taking an active part in positioning for delivery, contributing to dystocia.

Accurate assessment of fetal presentation, position, and posture; the presence of fetal abnormalities; whether the fetus is alive; the condition of the genital tract; and the general condition of the mare is necessary to formulate a plan for delivery. Unless structural abnormalities of the fetus are present, *mutation and delivery by traction* are often possible. If dystocia is prolonged, the birth canal and uterus may become contracted, edematous, and devoid of fetal fluids, necessitating the choice of an alternate route of delivery.

Delivery by Mutation and Traction

Mutation refers to manipulation of the fetus to return it to normal presentation, position, and posture to facilitate delivery. To accomplish mutation, it is helpful to first *repel* the fetus from the maternal pelvis into the abdominal cavity (where more space is available for repositioning and correction of fetal malposture). Additional room can sometimes be gained by pumping 1 or 2 gallons of liquid lubricant into the uterine lumen and around the fetus. Deep intrauterine infusion of lubricants, however, is contraindicated for a live fetus in caudal presentation because the fetus may swallow or inhale the lubricant. To avoid uterine rupture, obstetrical manipulations must not be overvigorous. Repulsion is not attempted if the uterus is devoid of fetal fluids, dry, and contracted; an alternative form of delivery (cesarean section) is chosen.

In countries in which injectable clenbuterol (Solution Ventipulmin, Boehringer-Ingelheim) is available, slow intravenous administration of 0.17 to 0.35 mg/454 kg of body weight will induce uterine relaxation sufficient to permit safer repulsion and reposition of the fetus. Although this drug is antagonistic to the effects of $PGF_{2\alpha}$ and oxytocin, its use apparently does not result in an increased incidence of uterine prolapse or retained placenta. Clamping the dorsal vulvar labia for 6 to 8 hours after correction of dystocia with this drug may, however, be indicated to reduce the chance of prolapse.

Correction of Malposture

Regardless of presentation, the limbs of a fully grown fetus must be extended to permit passage through the birth canal. To correct **carpal** or **hock flexion,** the flexed carpus or hock is repelled out of the pelvis while traction is applied to the foot until it is fully extended. Traction can either be applied entirely by hand or be assisted by first placing an obstetrical chain or strap around the pastern and having an assistant pull on it while the other hand simultaneously repels the proximal portion of the limb. If adequate room is available, this procedure can sometimes be accomplished by introducing both arms into the birth canal. One hand should be cupped over the foot as it is brought outward to prevent uterine rupture when traction is applied on the distal end of a flexed limb.

Cranial presentations with *deviations of the head and neck* commonly lead to dystocia in mares. To correct **lateral** or **ventral head posture,** the fetus is repelled and the jaw or muzzle of the foal is grasped and pulled toward the pelvic inlet. To gain more room for this procedure, one forelimb can first be placed in carpal flexion after a chain is placed around the pastern. The chain is helpful for correcting the carpal flexion after the head is replaced in the pelvic inlet. Securing a snare around the lower jaw may aid one to correctly align the head and neck, provided minimal traction is applied. Alternatively, a loop of obstetrical chain can be secured to the head by placing it through the mouth and over the poll. Again, minimal traction should be applied and care should be taken to prevent damage to the uterus from incisors through a gaping mouth created by this technique.

When the fetus is presented normally (i.e., cranial longitudinal presentation, dorsosacral position, with the forelimbs, head, and neck extended), delivery can proceed. If the fetus is presented caudally, delivery can proceed after the hindlimbs are extended. Traction straps or chains can be placed around the fetal pasterns, with the eye of the straps on the dorsal aspect of the limbs. Some veterinarians prefer to place two loops on each limb, with the first encircling the distal cannon bone (immediately above the fetlock) and the second encircling the pastern (Figure 10-2). Traction is gradual and smooth, only being applied during the dam's abdominal press. With anterior-longitudinal presentation, traction is applied so one forelimb precedes the other until the shoulders travel through the birth canal.

Any impediments to delivery are corrected promptly to allow delivery to continue because the umbilicus may be compressed, thus restricting blood supply to the fetus. In caudal presentations, *rupture* or *impaction of the umbilicus* quickly leads to fetal anoxia, so delivery must be accomplished quickly to avoid fetal asphyxia.

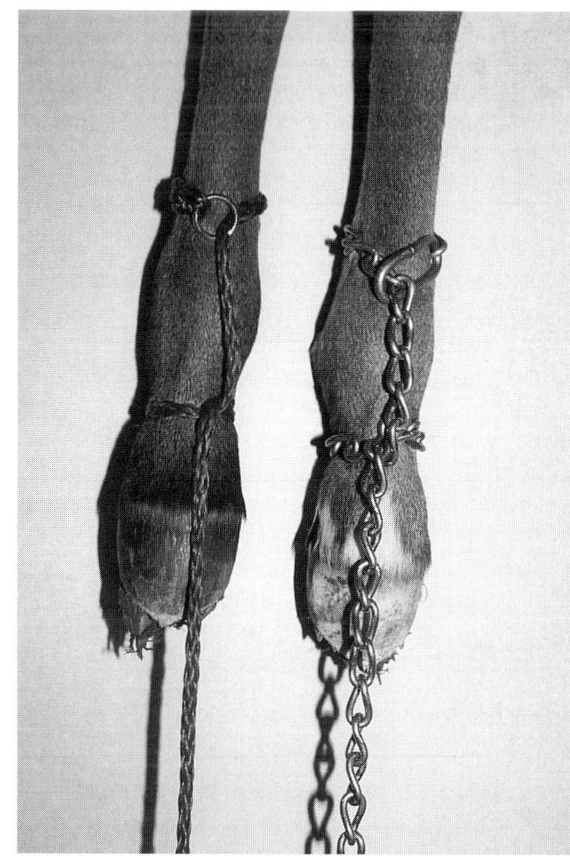

FIGURE 10-2. Obstetrical chain and strap, each placed with two loops on the forelimb with the first loop encircling the distal cannon bone above the fetlock and the second loop encircling the pastern.

If the fetus is in caudal presentation with bilateral hip flexion **(breech presentation)** or **transverse presentation,** the chances of delivery of a viable foal after dystocia are greatly reduced. The casual observer is often unaware that the mare is foaling in these cases because abdominal straining is often weak. Procedures for mutation and delivery by traction are reviewed by Roberts (1986).

If the dystocia cannot be corrected within 10 to 15 minutes by fetal manipulations with the mare standing, anesthetizing the mare may increase the chance of a successful delivery. After induction of anesthesia, the mare is positioned in dorsal recumbency, and the hindquarters are elevated with a hoist until the long axis of the mare is at a 30-degree angle to the floor or ground. If the mare is anesthetized in the field, placing the mare in a head-down position on an incline will often work as well. This procedure eliminates abdominal straining and increases the intra-abdominal space for easier manipulation of the fetus.

If the fetus is dead and cannot be delivered by mutation and traction, an alternative method of delivery must be chosen. **Fetotomy** may provide a more satisfactory alternative than cesarean section in such cases. When fetotomy is correctly performed, major abdominal surgery is avoided, resulting in a shorter recovery time for the mare and less aftercare than with cesarean section. The most common indication for fetotomy is to remove the head and neck of a dead fetus when manual correction of lateral or ventral head deviation is difficult. However, fetotomy should be avoided, if possible, in mares with protracted involution and fetal emphysema (because room to manipulate the fetus and fetatome are severely constrained), or if more than partial dismemberment (one or two cuts) of the fetus is required to avoid severe damage to the genital tract.

Cesarean section is indicated if attempts to deliver a foal per vagina jeopardize the foal or mare or are apt to impair the mare's subsequent fertility. Such situations include certain types of malpresentation; emphysematous fetuses; deformed fetuses; certain types of uterine torsion; and abnormalities of the dam's pelvis, cervix, or vagina. Extremely large foals or small dams might also require cesarean section for correction of dystocia. Refer to citations in the Bibliography for discussion of equipment, procedures, and techniques for performing percutaneous fetotomy and cesarean section.

Uterine Torsion

Uterine torsion occurs uncommonly in mares; however, it accounts for a significant percentage of serious equine dystocias. Uterine torsion occurs more commonly in preterm mares (5 to 8 months of gestation) than in term mares. Preterm mares with uterine torsion exhibit signs of intermittent, unresponsive colic. The condition is diagnosed by determining *displacement of the tense broad ligaments* by palpation per rectum. Identifying the ovaries is helpful in determining that "twisted" structures are indeed the uterus and broad ligaments. Diagnostic modalities are the same for preterm and term uterine torsion. The student is referred to Chapter 8 for discussion of diagnosis and treatment of uterine torsion in preterm mares (see Figure 8-11). It is quite rare for uterine torsion to occur at term with the cervix dilated. If the cervix is open, it may be possible to correct the torsion in a standing mare by grasping the fetus ventrolaterally with the arm resting on the pelvic floor and then rocking the fetus to impart momentum until it can be lifted upward and rotated into (opposite to) the direction of the uterine twist. If this method is successful, the fetus and uterus rotate into the normal position and the mare enters labor as soon as the cervix becomes fully dilated.

In many cases of uterine torsion, correction must be accomplished surgically. Surgical methods for correction of uterine torsion are described in citations in the Bibliography.

Postparturient Abnormalities

Retained Placenta

The fetal membranes are usually expelled 30 minutes to 3 hours after parturition. The placenta is considered to be *retained* if it is not expelled within 3 hours after birth of the foal. The percentage of postparturient mares with retained fetal membranes is reported to range from 2% to 10%.

The probability of retained placenta increases after dystocia, probably as a result of trauma to the uterus and myometrial exhaustion. Disturbance of the normal uterine contractions at parturition also might make retained placenta more likely. Retention is particularly likely if severe placentitis was present. Placental retention is more common in the nongravid uterine horn (Figure 10-3), perhaps because of a progressive increase in the degree of placental folding and attachment from the gravid horn to the nongravid horn. Partial placental retention is also more likely to occur in the nongravid uterine horn than in the gravid horn because the chorioallantoic membrane is thinner, resulting in easier tearing.

Disturbed uterine contractions might result from fetomaternal endocrine dysfunction, inadequate release of oxytocin, or inadequate response of the myometrium to oxytocin. The role of oxytocin in placental expulsion is attested to by prompt placental expulsion after oxytocin-induced parturition and by the failure of some mares with retained placenta to exhibit the characteristic abdominal discomfort typically associated with uterine contraction and placental expulsion in the early postpartum period.

A variable portion of the placenta may be exposed through the vulvar opening. Occasionally, the veterinarian is alerted to the possibility of retained placenta when no placenta is found after foaling. Aseptic intrauterine examination may reveal the presence of the placenta within the uterine cavity. Alternatively, part of the placenta may remain in the uterus and continue to initiate mild straining or colic after most of the placenta has been removed. For this reason, the fetal membranes should be examined to ensure that they are complete and that no portion remains in the uterus. Retention of portions of the placenta other than just the tip in the previously

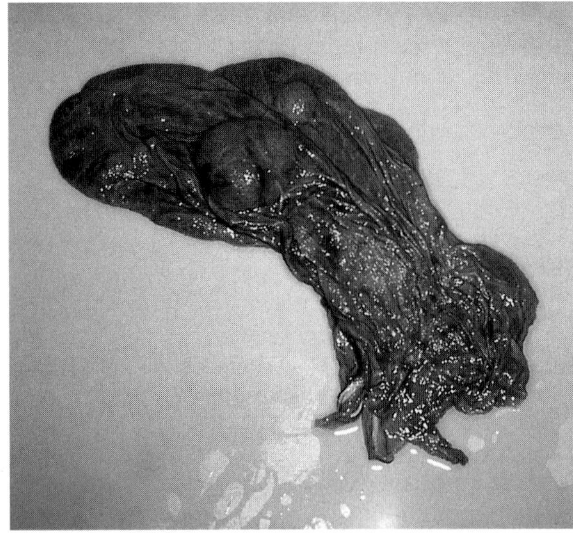

FIGURE 10-3. Tip of the placental horn typically retained in the uterus.

nongravid horn is also possible, so *thorough examination of both surfaces of the expelled chorioallantois* is necessary to detect less obvious missing portions. To facilitate examination, the chorioallantois can be filled with water (Figure 10-4). If the placenta is trampled, it may be impossible to determine whether remnants remain in the uterus.

Sequelae of retained placenta vary from none (particularly if mares are well managed and promptly treated) to the development of *metritis, septicemia* or *toxemia, laminitis,* and death. *Uterine involution is often delayed* even if mares do not develop these sequelae. Retained placenta with serious sequelae is reportedly more common in draft horses than in Thoroughbreds or Standardbreds, and mares with retained placenta after dystocia have a greater risk of developing toxic metritis and laminitis. Severe toxic metritis and laminitis after dystocia are believed to result from delayed uterine involution, increased autolysis of the placenta, and severe bacterial infection. In patients with toxic metritis after dystocia and retained placenta, the uterine wall becomes thin and friable or even necrotic. Absorption of bacteria and bacterial toxins probably follows loss of endometrial integrity and precipitates the peripheral vascular changes that lead to laminitis.

Various treatments for retained placenta in mares have been advocated. *Oxytocin therapy* (alone or in conjunction with other treatments) is the most common and apparently the most beneficial form of management. Recommended doses range from 20 to 60 U (smaller doses are given intravenously, whereas larger doses are given subcutaneously or intramuscularly) and doses can be repeated every 4 to 6 hours if the placenta is not passed. We prefer to inject 20 U intramuscularly to promote more physiologic (peristaltic-like) uterine contractions. Clinical signs of abdominal discomfort occur within a few minutes of injection and are usually followed by straining. Discomfort is more pronounced with large doses and might result from intense and perhaps spasmodic uterine contractions. A more physiologic, less intense response occurs during slow intravenous infusion of 30 to 60 U of oxytocin in 1 or 2 liters of normal saline over a 30- to 60-minute period. Occasionally, uterine prolapse can occur after oxytocin therapy, so care should be taken to observe for this potential complication. If not expelled shortly after injection of oxytocin, the placenta sometimes is expelled 1 or 2 hours later. The placenta can sometimes be extracted by applying *gentle traction* to the portion protruding from the patient's vulva. Mares that have undergone severe dystocia or that have aborted are less likely to respond.

If the chorioallantois is intact, *distension of the chorioallantoic cavity with 9 to 12 liters of warm, sterile water or saline solution* is an effective treatment for retained placenta (Figure 10-5). The opening of the chorioallantois is closed to contain the fluid. Stretch receptors are activated when the chorioallantois and uterus are distended, followed by endogenous release of oxytocin and separation of the chorionic villi from the endometrial crypts. Escaping fluid is forced back into the retained portion of the placenta until separation is complete and the placenta is expelled (usually 5 to 30 minutes). This treatment protocol can be used in conjunction with exogenous oxytocin therapy.

Other treatments that can be combined with oxytocin therapy include administration of systemic and local antibiotics, uterine lavage, exercise, and prophylactic measures to prevent laminitis (e.g., systemic administration of cyclooxygenase inhibitors or application of footpads). Whether intrauterine treatment should be continued after the fetal membranes have passed is a topic of controversy; use of such treatment is particularly questionable if contamination of the reproductive tract was minimal and placental passage after treatment was prompt.

The rationale for *uterine lavage* in mares that are at risk of developing metritis is to remove debris and bacteria from the uterus to reduce contamination and create a less favorable environment for bacterial growth. Purulent material and cellular debris that bind to and inactivate many antibiotics are also removed by uterine lavage. After disinfection of the perineal and vulvar areas, a sterilized or disinfected nasogastric tube is passed into the uterus. The hand is cupped around the end of the tube to prevent the uterus and any remaining placenta from being siphoned into its end (Figure 10-6). The uterus is gently

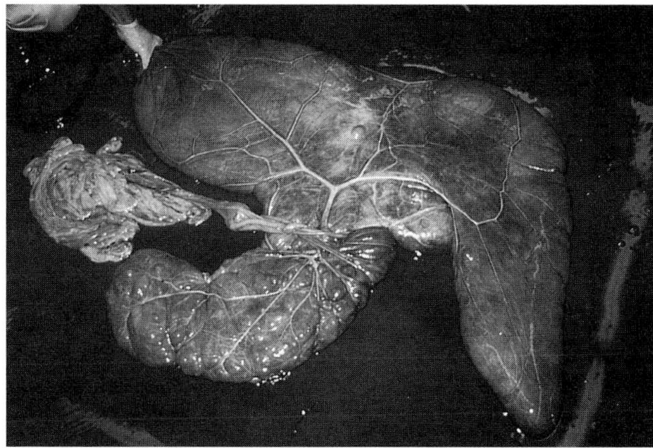

FIGURE 10-4. Expelled placenta is filled with water for examination.

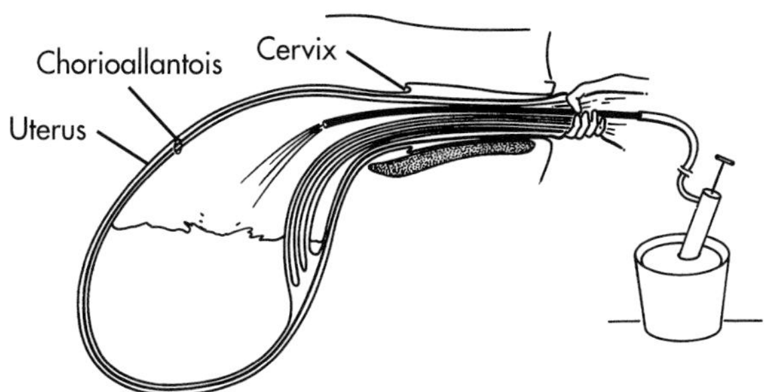

FIGURE 10-5. Distension of chorioallantoic cavity with fluid to promote expulsion of placenta. (Modified from Burns SJ, et al: Management of retained placenta in mares. *Proc Am Assoc Equine Pract* 23:381-390, 1977.)

lavaged with warm (40° to 42° C) physiologic saline (administered via a sterile or disinfected stomach pump) in 3- to 6-liter flushes until the effluent is relatively clear. If necessary, uterine lavage can be repeated on successive days until the initial effluent is free of purulent material and tissue debris.

If there is concern that the mare might develop septic or toxic metritis and laminitis, systemic and intrauterine antimicrobial therapy is indicated. *Intrauterine antimicrobial agents* are administered after evacuation of lavage fluid. Because antimicrobial agents infused into the uterus seldom reach acceptable levels anywhere except in the uterine lumen and endometrium, relatively high antibiotic doses are administered *systemically* to prevent or control the development of septicemia from uterine infection that might involve tissue deeper than the endometrium. The agents chosen should be compatible and should have *broad-spectrum activity* because a wide variety of organisms have been recovered from the postpartum uterus. The antimicrobial regimen must be effective against anaerobic bacteria and endotoxin-producing organisms.

If there is evidence of toxemia (e.g., neutropenia with toxic neutrophils in the peripheral circulation, elevated heart and respiratory rates, altered mucous membrane perfusion, or other circulatory disturbance), *cyclooxygenase inhibitors* such as flunixin meglumine should be administered. Cyclooxygenase inhibitors attenuate or prevent the circulatory disturbances associated with experimentally induced endotoxemia. Flunixin meglumine therapy is continued until there is no more danger of endotoxemia. The agent is usually given intravenously at a reduced dosage (0.025 mg/kg three times daily) to avoid potential adverse side effects.

Acute laminitis is a medical emergency, and treatment should commence as soon as possible. Many therapeutic regimens have been recommended for the treatment of laminitis. Refer to current equine medicine textbooks for discussion of various treatments for laminitis.

Uterine Prolapse

The uterus of the mare rarely prolapses. **Uterine prolapse** is more likely to occur immediately after parturition but sometimes occurs several days later. Conditions causing strong tenesmus (e.g., vaginal trauma) combined with uterine atony will predispose a mare to uterine prolapse.

Only one uterine horn may be prolapsed, or the uterine body may comprise the major portion of the exposed uterus. Uterine prolapse may be complicated by rupture of internal uterine vessels, shock, or incarceration and ischemia of viscera, leading to death. Additionally, damage to the prolapsed contaminated uterus predisposes the mare to development of tetanus.

Treatment of uterine prolapse is first focused on *control of straining*, either by administration of sedatives, caudal epidural anesthesia, or general anesthesia. In mares kept standing, the *uterus is lifted to the pelvic level* in an attempt to restore circulation, reduce congestion, and decrease traction on ovarian and uterine ligaments that causes pain (Figure 10-7). The uterus is gently cleaned with a disinfectant soap if it is grossly contaminated, and any placenta that remains attached is carefully removed. Bleeding vessels should be clamped and ligated. Uterine tears should be sutured, bringing serosal surfaces into contact. If the urinary bladder is distended, catheterization may be required before uterine replacement. Application of petroleum jelly to the endometrial surface is useful for protection against lacerations during massage and replacement. Placing the uterus inside two or three plastic garbage bags has been advocated to reduce the risk of puncturing or lacerating it during replacement (Figure 10-8). The garbage bags are removed as the uterus is pushed inside the vagina. *To avoid reprolapse, the uterus must be completely replaced.* Gently filling the uterus with warm saline may help to ensure complete replacement of uterine horns. Excess fluid is then siphoned off through a stomach tube. Small doses (10 to 20 U) of oxytocin are administered in an attempt to stimulate uterine contractions, and *intrauterine antibiotics* are given to control infection. Placing the mare in cross ties for 1 or 2 days has been advocated to reduce the chance of recurrence. *Suturing the vulva* will prevent pneumovagina and speed resolution of vaginal irritation, which might stimulate further straining. Broad-spectrum antibiotics are administered systemically to control infection. *Tetanus prophylaxis* is required. Other treatment is the same as that described for metritis.

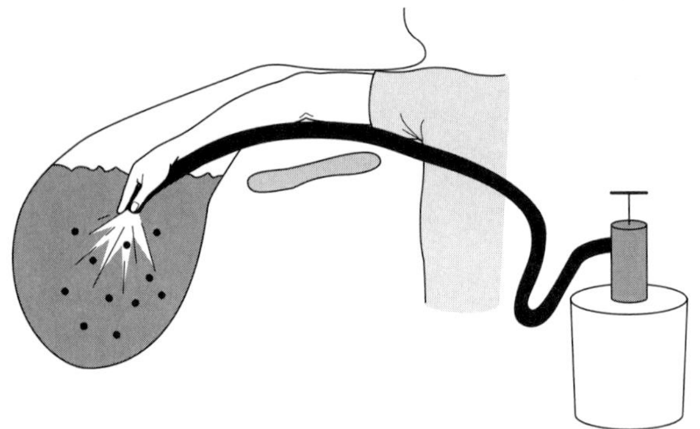

FIGURE 10-6. Technique used for lavage of the uterus of the postpartum mare. The hand should be cupped around the end of the tube to avoid injury to the uterus from the siphoning action.

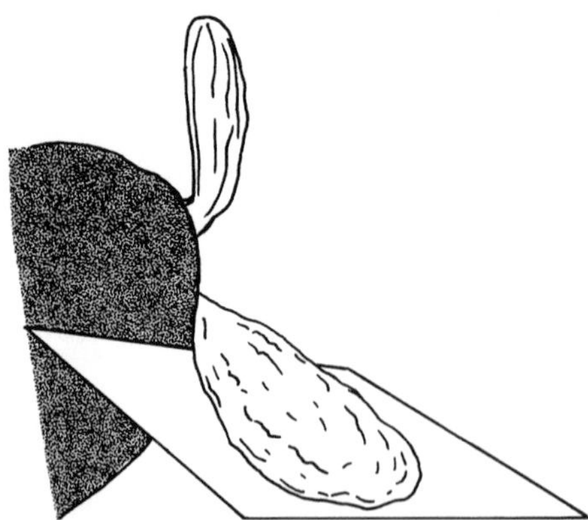

FIGURE 10-7. The prolapsed uterus is lifted to the pelvic level to restore circulation and reduce edema in preparation for replacement.

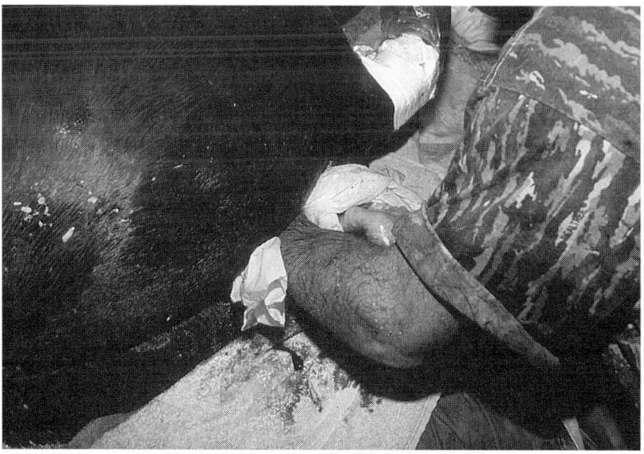

FIGURE 10-8. The prolapsed uterus is replaced after first covering the endometrium with petroleum jelly and then placing it inside clean plastic bags. The bags are removed as the uterus is pushed inside the vagina. This technique, described by Dr. Wendell Cooper, has been advocated to reduce the chances of lacerating the friable endometrium of the prolapsed uterus. The uterus should be completely replaced in its normal position to reduce the chance of reprolapse.

Invagination of Uterine Horn

An **invaginated uterine horn** is suspected when a postparturient mare has mild colic that is unresponsive to analgesics. The invagination is sometimes associated with a placenta that remains attached to the tip of the uterine horn, being partially inverted as a result of traction. Palpation per rectum may reveal a short, blunted uterine horn and tense mesovarium (Figure 10-9). Intrauterine examination will typically reveal the dome-shaped, inverted tip of the horn projecting into the uterine lumen. The placenta may be incarcerated in the intussuscepted horn. Rarely, with advanced invaginations, a reddish-black discharge will be associated with necrosis of the inverted uterus.

Treatment involves *replacement of the uterine horn* to its normal position, which may require manual removal of the placenta. The mare is sedated to control straining. To digitally separate the placenta, it is carefully twisted at the vulvar opening while simultaneously an attempt is made to manually separate the chorion from the endometrium. The portion of the placenta protruding from the vagina will have to be severed if manual separation cannot be accomplished safely. This reduces the weight pulling on the tip of the uterine horn, permitting it to return to its normal position. The invaginated portion of the uterine horn is gently kneaded inward to its normal position. If the examiner's arms are too short to reach or fully correct the invagination, a clean bottle can be inserted into the affected horn and used to gently push against the invaginated horn to aid in its reduction. Infusion of 1 to 2 gallons of warm, sterile water has also been used to facilitate complete replacement of the inverted uterine horn. Aftercare is the same as that described for metritis. If a portion of the placenta was left within the uterus, daily uterine lavage and intrauterine treatment are necessary until the portion of the placenta left within the uterus is expelled.

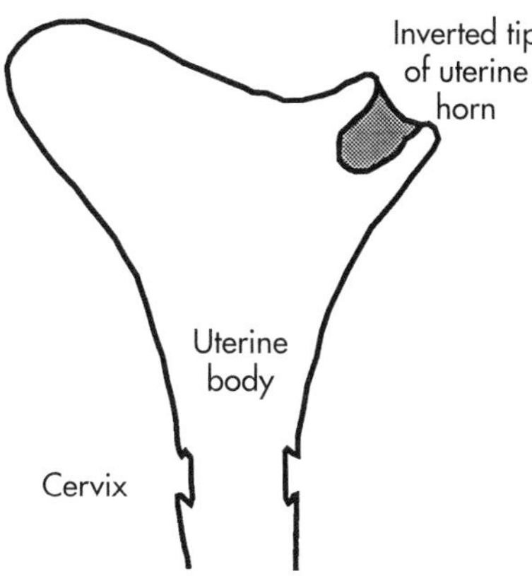

FIGURE 10-9. An invaginated uterine horn. Palpation per rectum reveals a short, blunted uterine horn and tense mesovarium.

Uterine Rupture

Rupture of the uterus occurs predominantly during the second stage of labor. The cause of the rupture is usually unknown, or it may result from dystocia. In rare instances the fetus may be found free in the abdominal cavity, particularly if uterine torsion was present. Many ruptures occur during fetal manipulation to correct dystocia (Figure 10-10). The uterus may also rupture during overly vigorous treatment in the postparturient period (e.g., during uterine lavage).

A number of uterine ruptures are detected in mares after seemingly normal deliveries, usually in the tip of the previously gravid uterine horn. Wisconsin researchers used radiography to monitor fetal changes in position during delivery and demonstrated that the caudal portion of the fetus completed its rotation to a dorsosacral position as the fetal abdomen passed through the birth canal. The hindlimbs to the level of the fetlocks remained encased in the gravid horn during this rotation, and straightening of the hindlimbs was a forceful process when the fetal stifles engaged the pelvic inlet. Perhaps this forceful extension of the hindlimbs explains the occasional uterine rupture in the end of the gravid horn of mares with seemingly uneventful deliveries. When rupture of the tip of the gravid horn occurs, close examination of the expelled placenta may reveal a corresponding rupture in this area of the placenta.

Hemorrhagic vaginal discharge may be present after uterine rupture. Acutely, hemorrhage (and pain) from the torn uterine wall may result in signs of circulatory shock, including pale mucous membranes, elevated heart and respiratory rate, sweating, and extremities that are cold to the touch. Unless the hemorrhage is severe, a large decrease in the packed cell volume is seldom seen at this time. If the uterine rupture remains undiagnosed and untreated, the mare will gradually develop signs of colic, and rapidly become depressed and febrile (within 24 hours). Although exsanguination is un-

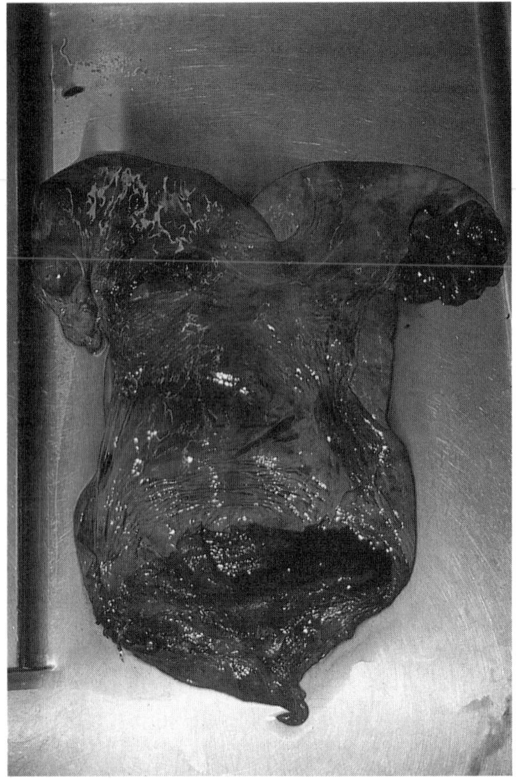

FIGURE 10-10. Transverse uterine rupture in the uterine body that was discovered after dystocia was relieved. Note that a rupture in the tip of the previously gravid uterine horn is also present.

common, blood loss may be sufficient to result in anemia and pale mucous membranes within 12 to 24 hours. Elevated white blood cell counts with degenerative left shifts due to peritonitis eventually develop.

Dorsal uterine tears can sometimes be identified per rectum. Signs of discomfort may be elicited during palpation of the rupture. Careful palpation of the internal surface of the uterus per vagina is more likely to result in identification of a rupture. However, the large size of the postpartum uterus makes evaluation of the entire uterus impossible. Abdominocentesis provides evidence for *intra-abdominal hemorrhage,* even with some partial-thickness tears when diapedesis and peritoneal contamination occur. An undetected, full-thickness uterine tear culminates in *septic degenerative peritonitis,* which can be confirmed by abdominocentesis. On occasion, viscera may herniate through the uterine rent and be found within the uterine cavity, the vagina, or beyond the vulvar opening.

Immediate treatment for hemorrhagic shock or dehydration is instituted. The best treatment for saving both the life and breeding potential of the mare is laparotomy and surgical repair of the uterine rupture. This is best accomplished using a ventral midline approach with the mare under general anesthesia. After uterine closure, the abdominal cavity is lavaged to reduce contamination. If the mare's general condition makes her a poor risk for anesthesia, conservative treatment is used, consisting of administration of 1 to 3 mg of ergonovine maleate intramuscularly every 2 to 4 hours (to contract smooth muscle in the uterus and uterine vessels), systemic administration of broad-spectrum antibiotics and flunixin meglumine, and intravenous replacement of fluids and electrolytes. Abdominal lavage can be performed to reduce contamination. Conservative treatment is most likely to be successful with small, dorsally located uterine tears, but the risk of development of fatal peritonitis is great. After either primary closure of the uterine tear or conservative treatment, the uterus should be massaged per rectum at 3- to 5-day intervals to break down adhesions that may form. Tetanus prophylaxis and additional treatments to prevent laminitis are also indicated.

Internal Hemorrhage

Rupture of the utero-ovarian or uterine artery, within the broad ligament, sometimes occurs at parturition or shortly thereafter. Rarely, the artery ruptures before parturition. *External iliac artery rupture occurs less often.* Right utero-ovarian or middle uterine artery rupture occurs more commonly than left utero-ovarian artery rupture. Age-related (i.e., mares >10 years of age) degenerative changes in vessel walls, including aneurysms, predispose these mares to vascular rupture. Vascular rupture may also occur with uterine prolapse or torsion.

The affected mare may show signs of severe, unrelenting colic, with profuse sweating and *evidence of hemorrhagic shock* (pale mucous membranes, low packed cell volume, increased pulse and respiratory rate, sweating with cold extremities, weakness, and prostration). Alternatively, the mare may fail to show signs of pain, with hemorrhage being controlled within the broad ligament. A *hematoma,* usually 20 to 30 cm in diameter, may be detected in the broad ligament of the uterus during routine prebreeding examination of mares in which hemorrhage has been restricted to this area.

Treatment of severe hemorrhage associated with rupture of uterine, utero-ovarian, or iliac arteries is often unsuccessful. The mare should be confined in a darkened stall to prevent activity and excitement. The added excitement associated with possible therapeutic methods such as blood transfusion and the administration of drugs may raise the mare's blood pressure enough to exacerbate bleeding, causing the broad ligament to burst and death to occur. Analgesics, such as flunixin meglumine (0.5 to 1.0 mg/kg intravenously) and butorphanol tartrate (0.02 to 0.04 mg/kg intravenously) may be administered to control the pain associated with distension of the broad ligament. Corticosteroids can be administered to combat shock. Rupture of the broad ligament with intra-abdominal hemorrhage will usually lead to rapid extravasation and death. Intra-abdominal hemorrhage can be confirmed by abdominocentesis.

Some mares with evidence of intra-abdominal hemorrhage have survived after treatment for hemorrhagic shock. The mare's circulatory status should be evaluated to determine whether whole blood transfusion or plasma expansion therapy will be necessary. Changes in laboratory parameters (e.g., a packed cell volume <15%, a hemoglobin concentration

<5 mg/dl, and a plasma protein concentration <4 mg/dl) are indicative of marked blood loss and deficient oxygen-carrying capacity. If these changes are seen, transfusion should be considered. The clinician should remember that when marked quantities of whole blood are lost, laboratory values supporting the need for transfusion often lag behind clinical signs of hypovolemic blood loss. Therefore when clinical signs of hypovolemic blood loss (e.g., tachycardia, weak pulse, pale mucous membranes, weakness, and depression) are present, whole blood transfusion should be strongly considered. Guidelines for collection of blood from a suitable donor and for administering blood to the affected mare are discussed in textbooks.

Administration of *naloxone hydrochloride* has been advocated for treating rupture of the uterine or utero-ovarian artery in mares. Endogenous opioids may be released during hemorrhagic shock, and naloxone, a narcotic antagonist, should block their effects. The rationale for this theory is predicated on the finding that the administration of naloxone attenuated some of the cardiovascular responses associated with experimentally induced shock in horses. Thus naloxone has been proposed to have potential therapeutic value for shock treatment. Apparently, naloxone antagonizes the actions of endogenous opioids mobilized by pain or stress and involved in the regulation of blood pressure by the central nervous system. The naloxone (8 to 20 mg) is administered intravenously to the mare that has already been placed in a darkened, quiet stall. Whether this treatment is superior to simply placing the mare in the same type of quiet environment, with or without the administration of other drugs, is not known.

An antifibrinolytic drug, *aminocaproic acid,* has also been used to control hemorrhage (e.g., with ruptured uterine arteries or incision sites of cesarean sections). This drug inhibits factors that promote clot lysis, thereby reducing secondary hemorrhage.

We do not generally recommend that the foal be separated from the mare unless it is necessary to protect it from inadvertent injury by the colicky mare. If it is necessary to remove the foal from the dam, steps should be taken to ensure that the foal's nutrient and passive immunity needs are met.

Hematomas that remain contained within the broad ligament regress gradually over a few weeks. Some hematomas may remain palpable as firm uterine enlargements for several months or, occasionally, longer. Such uterine hematomas may be detected per rectum during prebreeding examination of mares in which no postpartum problems were suspected. Ultrasonographically, the consolidating hematoma will appear more echolucent than the rest of the uterus, with echodensities being dispersed throughout the clot (Figures 10-11 and 10-12). The hematoma will become palpably more firm and progressively more echodense as fibrous tissue organizes.

Some investigators suggest that there may be an increased likelihood of recurrence of vascular rupture with fatal hemorrhage at the subsequent parturition. However, a number of practitioners from large breeding farms report that affected mares are generally fertile once the hematomas regress, and affected mares that are rebred usually deliver subsequent foals without recurrence of hemorrhage.

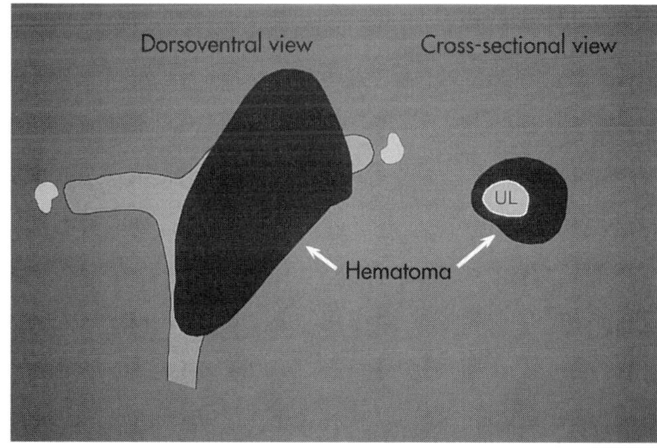

FIGURE 10-11. Drawing of uterine hematoma discovered during postpartum examination of the uterus of a mare, illustrating the extent of the surrounding hematoma.

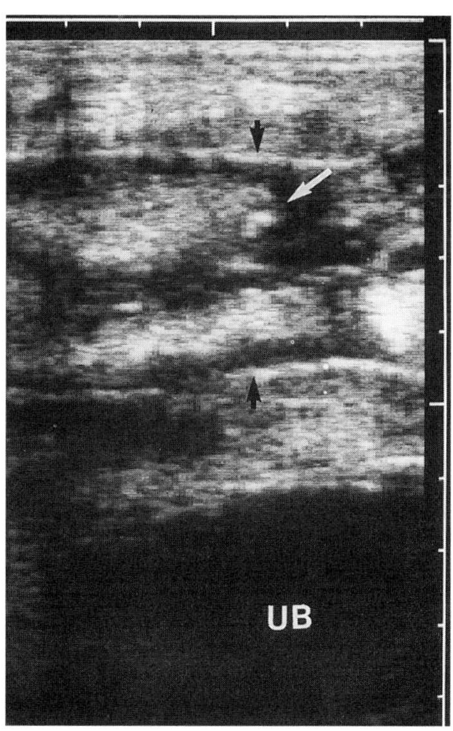

FIGURE 10-12. Transrectal ultrasonographic appearance of the hematoma depicted in Figure 10-11: margins of the uterine wall *(black arrows)*; lumen of the body of the uterus *(UB)*; clotting blood is becoming echogenic *(white arrows)*.

Other Postparturient Hemorrhages

Hemorrhagic vulvar discharge may originate from lacerations in the birth canal or from internal uterine trauma. Forceful, premature removal of fetal membranes may induce intrauterine hemorrhage. Hemorrhage may be profuse if a large blood vessel in the cervix, vagina, or vulva is ruptured. Alternatively, hemorrhage may be extravaginal (resulting in perivaginal hematoma) or intraperitoneal if the ruptured blood vessel is located retroperitoneally. The mare may become anemic, but usually will survive.

Slight hemorrhage does not require treatment. Profuse hemorrhage originating from blood vessels identified per vagina can often be clamped and ligated. If bleeding vessels cannot be identified, 1 to 3 mg of ergonovine maleate is injected intramuscularly to stimulate contraction of uterine and arterial muscles in an effort to control the hemorrhage. Oxytocin (20 to 40 U) can be administered intramuscularly to stimulate uterine contractions but does not cause contraction of muscular elements in the vasculature. If intrauterine or intravaginal hemorrhage cannot be controlled, packing the uterus or vagina with long strips of cotton sheets lubricated with petroleum jelly may be beneficial. The sheets should be removed 1 to 2 days later. Sequential measurements of red blood cell count, packed cell volume, and plasma protein concentration should be obtained to monitor blood loss. Supportive therapy, including use of broad-spectrum antibiotics to control infection and perhaps whole blood transfusion, is administered as required. Lacerations in the vagina should be sutured if possible. Repair of cervical lacerations must be delayed until uterine involution is complete. Vaginal stenosis may result from intrapelvic/perivaginal bleeding.

BIBLIOGRAPHY

Bierschwal CJ, de Bois CHW: *The technique of fetotomy in large animals.* Bonner Springs, KS, 1972, VM Publishing.

Ginther OJ: Equine pregnancy: physical interactions between the uterus and conceptus. *Proc Am Assoc Equine Pract* 44:73-104, 1998.

Roberts SJ: *Veterinary obstetrics and genital diseases, theriogenology,* ed 3, Woodstock, VT, 1986, SJ Roberts.

Rooney JR: Internal hemorrhage related to gestation in the mare. *Cornell Vet* 54:11-17, 1964.

Rossdale PD, Ricketts SW: *Equine stud farm medicine,* ed 2, Philadelphia, 1980, Lea & Febiger.

Vandeplasssche M: The pathogenesis of dystocia and fetal malformation in the horse. *J Reprod Fertil* 35(Suppl):547-552, 1987.

Vandeplassche M, Spincemaille J, Bouters R: Aetiology, pathogenesis and treatment of retained placenta in the mare. *Equine Vet J* 3:144-147, 1971.

Vandeplassche M, Spincemaille J, Bouters R et al: Some aspects of equine obstetrics. *Equine Vet J* 4:105-109, 1972.

11

Routine Management of the Neonatal Foal

OBJECTIVES

While studying the information covered in this chapter, the student should attempt to:

1. Acquire a working understanding of procedures for evaluating the newborn foal.
2. Acquire a working understanding of the need for colostrum acquisition by the newborn foal, techniques for administering colostrum to foals, and techniques for testing for failure of passive antibody transfer to foals.
3. Acquire a working understanding of techniques for caring for the umbilical cord of the foal at the time of parturition and for preventing meconial impaction.

STUDY QUESTIONS

1. Describe the procedure for performing a physical examination of a newborn foal and include expected normal findings.
2. Describe the procedures for testing foals for passive antibody transfer failure and methods for administering colostrum to foals to avoid this condition.
3. Describe the procedures used for treating passive antibody transfer failure in foals.
4. Describe the techniques involved in caring for the umbilical cord of the newborn foal.
5. Describe the clinical signs of meconium impaction in foals, methods used to differentiate meconium impaction from other causes of colic or straining in newborn foals, and methods for administering enemas to prevent this condition.

The neonatal period is a vulnerable segment of foal development. The transition from a protected, intrauterine existence to a state of relative independence is subject to a myriad of interferences. The vast array of potential inherent defects and environmental assaults can be devastating to the viability of the newborn foal and in turn can lead to significant losses for the horse industry. Equine practitioners should be well versed in all aspects of neonatal care to properly assist broodmare owners in managing newborn foals.

The managerial recommendations described herein are arranged in a chronologic sequence that can be applied to foals on a large broodmare farm. The order of events often is altered, especially on smaller farms where a veterinarian is not present during parturition to evaluate foals in the first few hours of life.

The chronologic span of the neonatal period is not defined uniformly; descriptions vary by as much as several weeks. The most critical part of neonatal development occurs within the first 4 days of life, when the newborn foal attempts to establish somatovisceral homeostasis. This chapter discusses general management guidelines for the immediate postnatal period. Application of basic management principles during the immediate neonatal period can prevent many problems that might result from birthing or environmental insults.

EVALUATION OF RESPIRATORY AND CARDIAC FUNCTION

Airway clearance and the establishment of a normal respiratory-cardiac rhythm are crucial. When the amnion envelops the mouth and the nostrils at birth, it should be removed to prevent asphyxiation (see Figure 9-13). Excessive fluid in the nasal cavity can be partially removed by stripping the nostrils with the fingers and thumb. If necessary, gentle suction also can be applied.

Fetal passage through the birth canal promotes thoracic compression and resultant expulsion of fluid from the upper airway. If a cesarean section is performed, the newborn is apt to need additional assistance to remove these contents effectively. The foal can be placed in lateral recumbency in a well-bedded location with the forequarters in a lower plane than the hindquarters, facilitating dependent drainage of fluid. Some practitioners hold the foal up by the hindlegs for a short period of time to promote better fluid evacuation; this procedure should be brief because abdominal viscera compress the diaphragm and limit the ability of the foal to expand its lungs. The foal is dried with a towel or blanket and

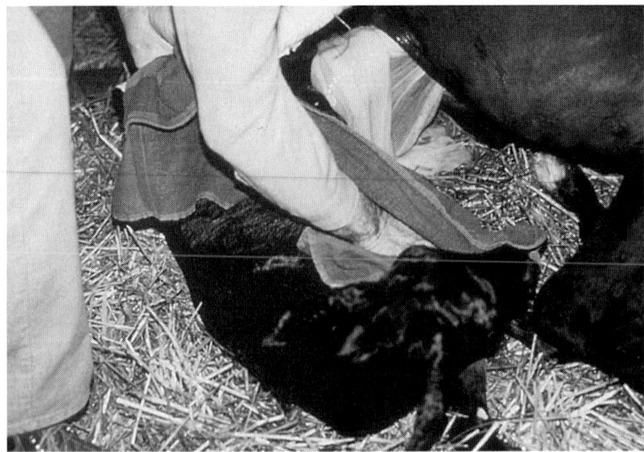

FIGURE 11-1. Respiratory activity can be stimulated by briskly rubbing the newborn foal with a towel.

rubbed briskly to stimulate respiratory activity (Figure 11-1). The rate and intensity of the heart beat/peripheral pulse should be evaluated (refer to "Physical Examination" later in this chapter).

VIABILITY ASSESSMENT AND RESUSCITATION PROCEDURE

The practitioner should look for signs of a strong, vigorous animal. Weak or immature foals are more vulnerable to stressful influences of the extrauterine environment and thus require more intensive care to maximize their chances for survival.

The degree of neonatal stress and birth asphyxia can be evaluated in the newborn foal using a modification of the Apgar scoring system used in human neonatology (Table 11-1). The observations listed for the modified *Apgar scoring system* should be made 1 and 5 minutes after delivery. In infants, the 1-minute score correlates directly with umbilical cord blood pH and is an index of intrauterine asphyxia. The 5-minute Apgar score correlates more with the infant's eventual neurologic outcome.

Although the Apgar score has had limited use in equine neonatology, the criteria presented here provide a rational set of guidelines for evaluating the degree of neonatal asphyxia and for determining whether resuscitative measures are indicated. Early signs of asphyxia include increased rate and depth of respiration followed by a period of gasping and primary apnea. With *severe asphyxia,* the respiratory center becomes progressively depressed and is no longer responsive to sensory and chemical stimuli. The gasping episodes become weaker, and bradycardia develops, followed by a stage of secondary apnea.

Foals exhibiting signs of *mild to moderate asphyxia* (Apgar score 4 to 6) should be given moderate stimulation that includes brisk rubbing of the foal's back and sides with a dry towel, postural drainage in conjunction with gentle thoracic coupage, limb manipulation, and stimulation of the inside of the nares to elicit a sneeze or a cough. The induced cough helps to move secretions out of the lower airways. The neck should be gently hyperextended and the oropharynx cleared of mucus or amniotic fluid to ensure a patent airway. *Suctioning of the oropharynx and the trachea* can be performed with a 10 French suction catheter (Regu-Vac R, Becton Dickinson). It is important that one preoxygenate the foal (12 L/min through a catheter) before applying suction to avoid causing respiratory distress, cardiac arrhythmias, or cardiac arrest. Prolonged periods of suction should also be avoided because they can decrease arterial oxygenation. Suction (vacuum set at 80 to 120 mm Hg) should be applied only during withdrawal of the catheter from the airway.

Placing the foal in sternal recumbency (Figure 11-2) helps decrease dependent lung atelectasis, thus minimizing the ventilation-perfusion inequalities created by prolonged lateral recumbency. Supplemental oxygen (humidified) can be delivered via a nasal cannula or a facemask at a flow rate of 5 to 10 L/min. A nasal cannula should be passed in the ventral meatus to the approximate level of the medial canthus of the

TABLE 11-1

Modified Apgar Scoring System for Evaluating Foals 1 to 5 Minutes after Birth

	Assigned Values*		
Observation	**0**	**1**	**2**
Heart and pulse rate	Undetectable	<60 beats/min	>60 beats/min
Respiration (rate and pattern)	Undetectable	Slow, irregular	60 breaths/min, regular
Muscle tone	Lateral recumbency, limp	Lateral recumbency, evidence of some muscle tone	Able to maintain sternal recumbency
Nasal stimulation (with straw)	Unresponsive	Grimace with mild rejection	Cough or sneeze

From Martens RJ: Pediatrics. In Mansmann RA, McAllister ES, Pratt PW, editors: *Equine medicine and surgery,* ed 3, vol 1. Santa Barbara, CA, 1982, American Veterinary Publications.

*A value of 0, 1, or 2 is assigned for each of the four observations. Total score: 7 to 8 = normal; 4 to 6 = mild to moderate asphyxia; 0 to 3 = severe asphyxia.

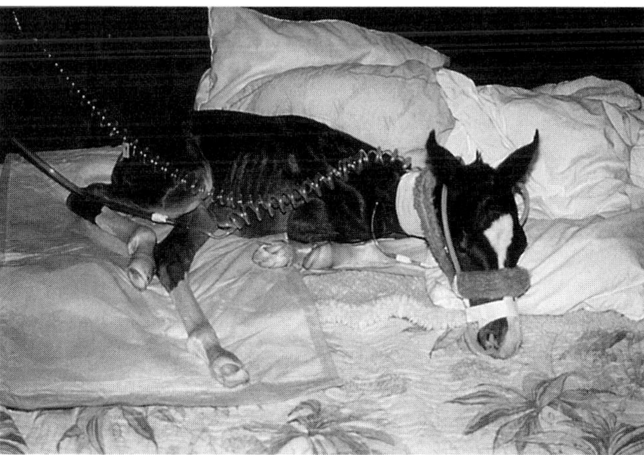

FIGURE 11-2. This premature (born at 315 days of gestation) foal was unable to maintain sternal recumbency and was propped up on its sternum to decrease dependent lung atelectasis. Supplemental oxygen is being delivered via a nasal cannula.

eye. A tight-fitting facemask requires a reservoir bag and adequate oxygen flow rates to prevent rebreathing of exhaled gases. Loose-fitting facemasks result in lower inspired oxygen concentrations but still require a minimum oxygen flow rate of 10 liters/min to prevent build up of CO_2 in the mask. Sternal recumbency, tactile and sensory stimulation, a judicious suction technique, and oxygen supplementation are sometimes sufficient therapy for foals with asphyxia/hypoxia.

Foals suffering from *severe asphyxia* (Apgar score 0 to 3) require rapid, aggressive intervention to stimulate and support ventilation. Manual *mouth-to-nose resuscitation* can be accomplished by the clinician using both hands to occlude one of the foal's nostrils and the mouth and then breathing rhythmically into the foal's patent nostril to expand its lungs. Assisted ventilation is probably best performed with an endotracheal tube directly attached to a ventilator, an oxygen demand valve (Hudson oxygen demand valve II, H. S. Osborn), or a 1-liter nonrebreathing resuscitation bag (Lifesaver II manual resuscitator, A. J. Buck and Son) (Figure 11-3).

Oral intubation of the trachea can be done in emergency situations if short-term ventilation is all that is necessary. *Nasotracheal intubation* is better tolerated for prolonged periods. Inert plastic or silicone rubber endotracheal tubes with high-volume, low-pressure cuffs (Aire-Cuf, Biovana Surgical) are preferred to minimize tracheal mucosal damage. A breathing rate of 20 to 30 breaths/min should be maintained. Excessive ventilatory pressure can result in overinflation with alveolar rupture and pneumothorax. Visual assessment of the foal's thorax is used to assess needed tidal volume.

Because the *acidosis* associated with terminal apnea usually is metabolic and respiratory in nature, administration of intravenous isotonic (1.3%) sodium bicarbonate solution at an initial dose of 2 mg/kg may help to correct the metabolic component. Administration of alkaline solutions without first

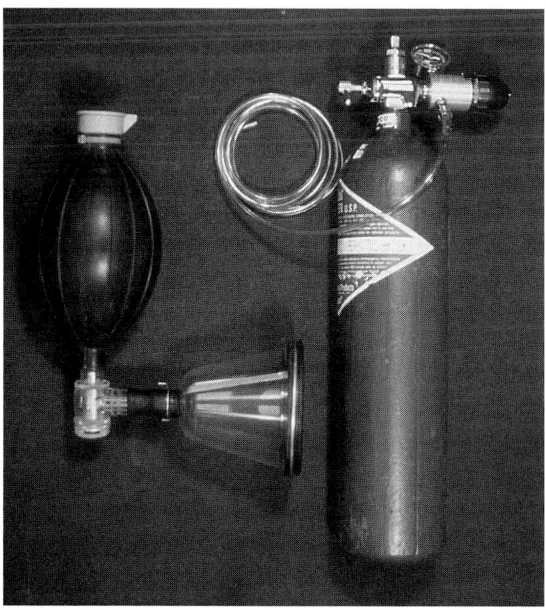

FIGURE 11-3. A resuscitation bag, mask, and small oxygen tank with attached nasogastric tubing is shown. This equipment should be readily available at the time of parturition to help prevent hypoxia in newborn foals.

ensuring that *adequate ventilation* is present can worsen the acidosis becauses sodium bicarbonate is converted to carbon dioxide and retained when poor ventilation-perfusion exists. Large volumes of hypertonic sodium bicarbonate solutions should be avoided—their use has been associated with hypernatremic and hyperosmotic states and with increased incidence of cerebrovascular accidents, especially in infants.

The ultimate outcome of severe, untreated asphyxia is *myocardial* and *cerebral hypoxia,* resulting in death. Irreversible brain damage usually occurs after approximately 5 minutes of complete asphyxia. Therefore the recognition and accurate, rapid treatment of asphyxia is vitally important.

Some parameters used to assess neonatal viability are presented in Table 11-2. There is much normal variation in the period during which these behavioral events occur.

TABLE 11-2

Normal guidelines used to assess neonatal viability

Adaptive Response	Time Elapsed Since Birth
Normal respiratory and cardiac rhythms	Within 1 min
Righting reflexes established	Within 5 min
Suck reflex established	Within 5 min
Attempts to stand	Within 30 min
Ability to stand unassisted	Within 60 to 120 min
Nurses from udder	Within 60 to 180 min

Modified from Rossdale PD, Ricketts SW: *Equine stud farm medicine,* ed 2, Philadelphia, 1990, Lea & Febiger.

INTERPRETATION OF CLINICAL LABORATORY DATA

Analysis of whole blood and serum from all newborn foals is customary on many well-managed broodmare farms. Thus proper interpretation of the laboratory results is reviewed here.

Normal hematologic, blood gas, and serum chemistry values for the newborn foal are cited in veterinary literature. Hematologic parameters of the newborn foal change during the first 2 weeks of life. Because of the shortened life span of erythrocytes in fetal and neonatal foals, the number of red blood cells peaks at term and then decreases during the next 10 days.

There is a relatively abrupt decrease in packed cell volume, hemoglobin concentration, and number of erythrocytes within the first 12 to 24 hours postpartum. The high hemoglobin concentration and packed cell volume at birth are attributed to the presence of peripheral vasoconstriction in animals immediately after birth, which offers physiologic protection against shock, cold, and excessive blood loss from the umbilicus. After parturition, there is a gradual release from this vasoconstriction, and circulatory volume increases with a concomitant drop in packed cell volume, number of erythrocytes, and hemoglobin concentration.

The increased leukocyte count during the first 24 hours after birth primarily results from an increase in the number of mature neutrophils, which can continue during the next 3 days. The finding of >10% band cells suggests underlying disease. The lymphopenia present at birth might result from immature lymphatic organs or from the response to endogenous steroid release during parturition. Lymphocyte numbers should continue to rise in early postnatal life. *Premature foals tend to have lower numbers of leukocytes and neutrophils.* Eosinophils, basophils, and monocytes are low in number or absent in the newborn foal. Neutrophil counts <4000/mm^3 or >12,000/mm^3, band neutrophil counts >50/mm^3, toxic changes in neutrophils, and fibrinogen concentrations >600 mg/dl help to predict infection (Brewer and Koterba, 1990).

Concentrations of serum electrolytes remain relatively constant during the postnatal period. Liver enzyme concentrations generally are higher in neonates than in adults. The increased serum liver enzyme activity in foals is attributed to a relative increase in hepatic mass (as a percentage of total body weight) in the newborn and to a higher rate of enzyme production and release. The level of alkaline phosphatase is higher in foals up to 3 to 5 months of age because of osteoblastic activity of bone.

The *dark yellow serum of newborn foals* reflects increased postpartum bilirubin levels. An increase in the indirect bilirubin concentration accounts for the hyperbilirubinemia. Lower concentrations of glucuronyl transferase in the neonatal liver result in a slower conjugation of bilirubin during the first 5 days after birth. Bilirubin concentrations should approach adult values by 2 weeks of age. The bilirubin concentration is generally increased in foals with neonatal isoerythrolysis and may be of value in diagnosing this condition when anemia, pallor, and tachypnea are present in newborns.

Serum creatinine concentrations during the neonatal period often are greater than adult values. This difference in creatinine levels probably reflects the initial immaturity of the renal transport and filtration systems. A markedly elevated serum creatinine concentration has been associated with both prematurity and neonatal maladjustment syndrome. Monitoring of creatinine levels is necessary when drugs with a potential for renal toxicity, such as aminoglycosides, are administered to foals.

The blood glucose level of presuckle foals usually is lower than that in adults but increases after suckling. Sepsis or insufficient energy intake should be suspected in foals with low blood glucose concentrations and the clinician should be aware of the need for closer monitoring of nursing activity, the possible presence of agalactia, and the need for additional testing or examination for septicemia. Hypoglycemia can be treated by administering 5% to 10% dextrose solutions intravenously.

Interpretation of clinical laboratory data must be done with an understanding of the normal physiologic and biochemical adaptations that occur in the neonate. A precise history of peripartum events and a careful physical examination always should precede the interpretation of laboratory data.

PHYSICAL EXAMINATION

A thorough, systematic physical examination should be performed on every foal during the first day of life. Before actual physical examination, the clinician should begin by observing the foal from a distance to assess its alertness and behavior, ability to rise, coordination and strength, desire and willingness to nurse, and overall attitude. Rectal temperature should always be determined and is normally 99.5° to 100.5° F (37.5° to 38.5° C). When rectal temperature is below 98.5° F, hypothermia should be suspected. When rectal temperature exceeds 101.5° F, infection should be suspected.

The actual physical examination should be systematic, beginning at the head and progressing to the hindquarters. It should yield prompt recognition of various maladies, including cleft palate, entropion, fractured ribs, umbilical or inguinal hernias, and limb abnormalities.

The foal's degree of maturity should be assessed. Signs suggesting prematurity include low birth weight, general weakness, inability to stand, decreased ability to suck and maintain body temperature, silky haircoat, floppy ears, soft lips, and increased passive range of limb motion with a decreased pastern slope. A premature foal also can have immature organ systems (e.g., pulmonary, endocrine, gastrointestinal, renal, immune, and hematopoietic system) and therefore requires close observation and monitoring with appropriate supportive care.

Neurologic Examination

A brief neurologic examination should be performed; it includes a systematic evaluation of general behavior, mentation, cranial nerve function, posture, gait, coordination, and spinal reflexes. A normal newborn foal is aware of and responsive to its environment soon after birth and demonstrates close bonding behavior with the dam. Certain physiologic differences between the neonate and the adult should be acknowledged—equine neonates normally have limb hyperreflexia, resting extensor hypertonia, crossed extensor reflexes, hypermetric gait, base-wide stance, intention movements, and an absence of menace response. Neurologic abnormalities should be recognized, identified as to cause (e.g., developmental, infectious, or secondary to vascular accidents within the central nervous system), and treated accordingly.

Cardiovascular System Examination

Evaluation of the cardiovascular system begins with examination of the visible mucous membranes, which should be pink and moist with a capillary refill time of 1 to 2 seconds. The jugular veins should not be distended but should fill readily when occluded at the thoracic inlet. *Jugular pulsations* reflect normal pressure changes within the right atrium and the thorax and should not extend beyond the level of the point of the shoulder. The apex beat—easily palpated over the left fifth intercostal space in the ventral third of the thorax—should be evaluated for intensity and for the presence of murmur-associated thrills.

Arterial pulses should be strong and readily palpable in the extremities, indicating adequate peripheral perfusion. Percussion of the left hemithorax outlines a normal area of cardiac dullness extending from the fourth intercostal space just below the point of the shoulder to the sternum at the sixth intercostal space. There is a smaller area of cardiac dullness over the right third and fourth intercostal spaces.

Auscultation of the heart base requires a general knowledge of the anatomic location of the four heart valves. Foals generally have loud heart sounds on auscultation because of their thin body walls and small size. The most commonly reported murmur in newborn foals is associated with blood flow through a *persistent patent ductus arteriosus* and is characterized by a continuous machine-like murmur that is loudest over the left heart base. The diastolic component of the murmur often is localized over the left third or fourth intercostal space, whereas the systolic component might be heard easily over the entire heart base. Continuous murmurs associated with a patent ductus arteriosus disappear in some normal foals by 24 hours of age and are considered abnormal if present beyond 4 days of age. Pulmonary hypertension can reduce the intensity of the diastolic component.

The *heart rate* of the foal is 40 to 80 regular beats/min initially but increases to 150 beats/min when the foal struggles to rise. It then falls to a rate of 70 to 95 beats/min. *Sinus tachycardia* can be associated with stress, excitement, fever, hypovolemia, or sepsis. *Bradycardia* can occur with hyperkalemia, hypertension, or increased intracranial pressure.

Respiratory System Examination

The respiratory rate, effort, and pattern should be examined carefully in the resting foal before handling. The rate decreases from a mean of 75 breaths/min at birth, to 50 breaths/min at 1 hour, and to 34 breaths/min at 12 hours. Lung sounds in the young foal typically are louder, harsher, and easier to hear than in the adult. The auscultation of *moist rales* in the neonate can stem from fluid accumulation in the lungs that has not yet dissipated completely. Decreased or absent lung sounds can be associated with lung *atelectasis* or *consolidation* related to lung immaturity or pneumonia.

Because auscultation alone is not the most accurate means of detecting pulmonary pathologic problems in the foal; other respiratory parameters should be monitored closely. *Increased rate and effort of breathing* in an unstressed foal are early indications of possible lung disease. Nonrespiratory factors such as fever, high environmental temperatures, metabolic acidosis, pain, excitement, hypotension, and neurologic disease also can result in tachypnea. *Mucous membrane color* should be evaluated but is not a reliable indicator of oxygenation because cyanosis usually is not observed until the partial pressure of arterial oxygen reaches very low levels. Chest radiographs and measurement of arterial blood gases are critical diagnostic aids in the workup of a foal with possible abnormal respiratory function.

Upper airway obstruction or abnormality can be another cause of moderate to severe tachypnea in the newborn. There should be equal airflow from each nostril. Congenital anomalies associated with respiratory distress in newborn foals include bilateral choanal atresia, subepiglottic cyst formation, abnormal function and conformation of the larynx and the arytenoid cartilages, and tracheal malformations. Severe upper airway obstruction requires emergency tracheotomy.

Gastrointestinal System Examination

The gastrointestinal system can be evaluated grossly by auscultation of the abdomen for normal borborygmi and by careful observation to document the passage of dark, pasty meconium followed by softer, tan-colored feces associated with a milk diet. Absence of manure passage might indicate meconium retention or impaction or congenital anomalies such as *atresia ani* and *atresia coli*. The abdomen should be palpated to determine whether abnormal amounts of gas or fluid are present. Abdominal distension accompanied by colic can herald a variety of gastrointestinal disorders, including peritonitis, abnormal gut motility associated with enterocolitis, intestinal volvulus or intussusception, and gastrointestinal ulceration with or without perforation.

The size and consistency of the umbilicus should be evaluated. Careful abdominal palpation will identify the presence of other congenital anomalies, including *umbilical, inguinal*, or *scrotal hernias*. Small hernias usually close spontaneously.

Daily manual reduction of the hernia or bandaging of the area can hasten resolution of the defect. All hernias require regular monitoring because intestinal strangulation can occur; this usually requires prompt surgical intervention.

Genitourinary System Examination

The genital tract should be examined to identify the foal's sex and look for the presence of possible congenital defects. In males, the scrotum and the inguinal region should be palpated for the presence of the testicles. The *testes often are within the scrotum at birth but might not descend for several weeks.* Observation of normal micturition decreases the likelihood of *uroperitoneum* in the newborn. Urine specific gravity in normal nursing foals usually is quite dilute.

Musculoskeletal System Examination

During examination of the musculoskeletal system, all the joints, the bones, and the surrounding soft tissues should be palpated for signs of trauma, distended joints, and flexor or angular limb deformities.

Ophthalmic Examination

An ophthalmic examination is best performed in a dark stall. The eyes of the newborn foal are open at birth with clear corneas. The pupils are circular and large, with a sluggish pupillary light reflex. Closer scrutiny of the chambers, the lens, and the fundus requires knowledge of normal adult and neonatal equine fundic anatomy.

The practitioner must not confuse pathologic processes with normal findings such as the Y-sutures of the lens or the hyaloid artery, both of which invariably are present in the newborn foal. The Y-suture of the anterior lens is inverted. The remnants of the fetal hyaloid artery—viewed as a fine, dark line—are visible, attached to the posterior lens capsulae and floating freely in the vitreous body. Occasionally, this artery traverses the vitreous body to its posterior attachment at the optic nerve. The remnant usually degenerates as the foal ages. Persistent strands of pupillary membrane occasionally are observed in the midiris region.

Congenital cataracts are the most common congenital ocular defect in the foal. Cataracts associated with persistent hyaloid vasculature and Y-suture lines are of minor importance. Complete cortical and nuclear congenital cataracts are more serious and can cause partial or complete loss of vision.

Scleral, subconjunctival, or *conjunctival hemorrhage* usually is associated with rupture of the conjunctival or episcleral vessels resulting from compressive or blunt trauma during birth. This type of hemorrhage should resolve without treatment in 1 or 2 weeks. If *hyphema* is present, a topical mydriatic agent should be used to prevent synechia formation. Occasionally, petechial and ecchymotic hemorrhages in this area can herald a generalized bleeding disorder resulting from *disseminated intravascular coagulation* or endothelial damage associated with *septicemia.*

The normal cornea should be clear, with a smooth, intact epithelial surface. *Entropion,* although relatively uncommon in normal foals, can result in corneal irritation, keratitis, and ulceration, producing blepharospasm and lacrimation in the affected eye. Mild forms of entropion often are self-limiting. Temporary, nonabsorbable, vertical mattress sutures placed ventral to the lower lid margin usually correct the entropion; secondary corneal disease should be treated concurrently with topical antibiotics and a mydriatic agent as indicated. Hypotonia, corneal edema, miosis, hypopyon, and aqueous flare resulting in a green-yellow glow in the anterior chamber are characteristic signs of *uveitis.* Uveal inflammation usually is secondary to foci of infection elsewhere in the body and might result from bacteremia or septicemia.

Examination of Mare's Udder

Before the foal is allowed to nurse, the *udder should be washed and checked* for the presence of *colostrum* and for evidence of *agalactia, mastitis,* nonfunctional teats, or other malformations. The udder should be inspected routinely for signs of *abnormal distension,* which can be the first sign of decreased sucking and possible illness in the foal. The blood glucose level can be checked to ensure that adequate suckling is taking place. A low blood glucose level should alert the clinician to the possibility of insufficient dietary energy ingestion.

CARE OF THE UMBILICAL CORD

The umbilical cord of the foal is intact as the foal emerges from the birth canal. To ensure maximum blood flow from the placenta into the newborn's circulation, *the cord should remain attached for several minutes.* The foal may be deprived of up to 1.5 liters of blood by premature separation of the umbilical cord. One study, however, suggests that this is not the case. Under most circumstances, it is *acceptable to let the cord break naturally.* This usually occurs when the mare or the foal attempts to rise. A *predetermined break site* is easily identifiable on the umbilical cord approximately 1 to 2 inches from the body wall (Figure 11-4).

If *manual separation* is necessary, the clinician should grasp the cord on each side of the intended break point and then twist and pull (from the placental side of the umbilicus) with the thumb and the forefingers to effect separation. Precautions must be taken to prevent undue tension on the ventral abdominal wall during this procedure. The *cord should not be severed with a sharp instrument* because this is more likely to result in excessive hemorrhage from the umbilical stump and possibly in a patent urachus (Figure 11-5). The umbilical stump should be observed after rupture for location of the break and for evidence of hemorrhage, urine, or abnormal swelling. The elastic, muscular walls of the two umbilical arteries allow prompt, prolonged constriction of the umbilical stump when it is separated through stretching. Failure of umbilical vessels to close when the cord breaks

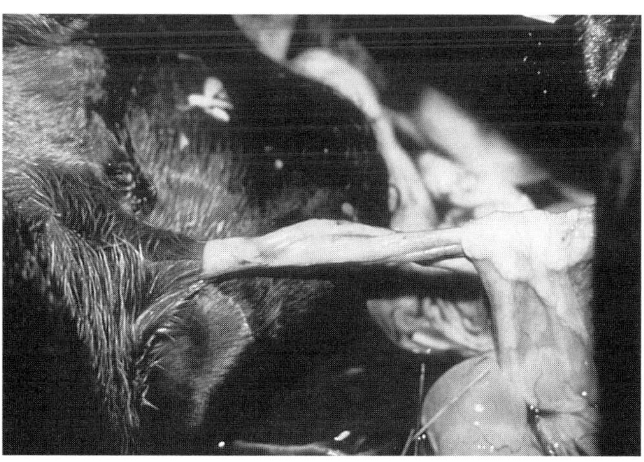

FIGURE 11-4. The usual break point of the foal's umbilicus is indicated by the pale, strictured area. If manual separation is necessary, the cord is grasped on each side of the intended break point. The cord is twisted and pulled until separated, taking care to avoid undue tension on the ventral abdominal wall.

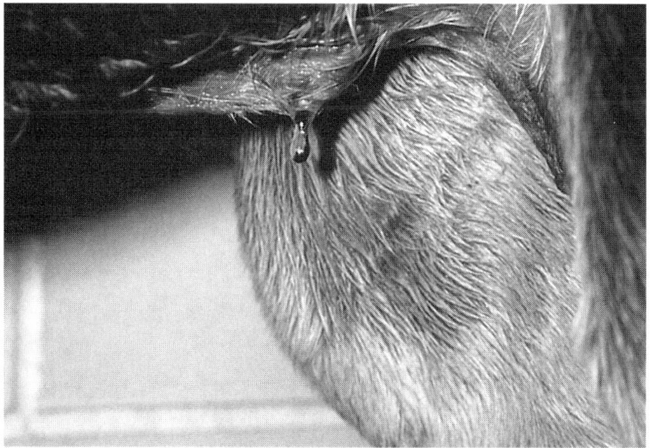

FIGURE 11-5. A moist umbilical stump with urine discharge is present in this foal with a patent urachus.

can lead to excessive blood loss, hemoperitoneum, and/or hypovolemic shock.

If hemorrhage is a problem, digital pressure should be applied to the stump for 30 to 60 seconds. If bleeding persists, an umbilical clamp or sterile, nonabsorbable ligature can be applied to the distal end of the stump, with removal in 6 to 12 hours. Prevention or treatment of shock may necessitate whole blood transfusion. Cardiovascular stabilization must preclude any surgical procedure requiring general anesthesia. In all cases, the *umbilical stump ("navel") should be submerged without delay in a suitable disinfectant* to minimize the opportunity for infectious organisms to ascend through the umbilical cord. A California study demonstrated that 0.5% chlorhexidine solution (Nolvasan solution is 2% chlorhexidine) is superior to 1% or 2% Betadine solution or to 7% tincture of iodine for killing bacteria and preventing adverse umbilical tissue

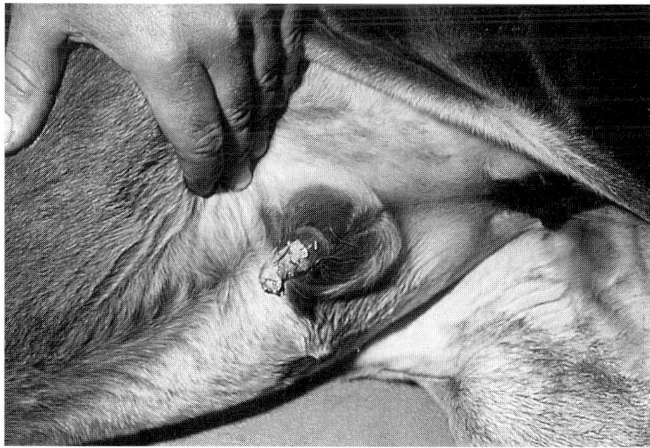

FIGURE 11-6. Omphalitis in a foal, as depicted by swelling at the base of the umbilical cord and reddening and necrosis of the tip of the umbilical stump.

destruction in newborn foals. Disinfectant should be applied twice daily for 3 to 4 days. Contact of disinfectant with the abdominal wall or the thighs must be avoided because it can have an irritating effect on these areas. The umbilical stump should be evaluated daily for signs of *omphalitis* (including moistness, reddening, and swelling) (Figure 11-6), abscesses, or a patent urachus. If the umbilical region becomes abscessed or necrotic, it should be surgically removed. Under normal circumstances, the umbilicus appears as a dried stump 24 hours after birth. The dried umbilical stump usually falls off when the foal is between 1 and 2 weeks of age and the urachus remains sealed. In compromised neonates, the urachus may become patent *(patent urachus)* and drain urine when the stump falls off. In such cases the umbilicus remains moist because of continuous urine dribbling. Patent urachus can also be congenital. Broad-spectrum antibiotics should be administered until urachal closure occurs because of the threat of ascending infection. If concurrent umbilical infection is not present, patent urachus will often resolve spontaneously or with conservative therapy (e.g., mild cauterization applied 1 to 3 cm up into the urachal lumen two to three times per day for several days). If the urachus does not close, resection of the umbilical remnants and correction of urachal patency should be accomplished surgically.

Many umbilical infections can be detected by close examination of the umbilical stump and body wall. Palpation is sometimes helpful, but the absence of palpable abnormalities does not rule out infection of the umbilical vessels. Ultrasonography of the abdominal wall and umbilicus should be performed when fever of unknown origin, chronic unthriftiness or changes in the complete blood count (e.g., neutrophilia or hyperfibrinogenemia) suggest infection.

DAM-FOAL INTERACTION

Unnecessary disturbances to the dam and the foal during the immediate postnatal period should be avoided. Dam-foal

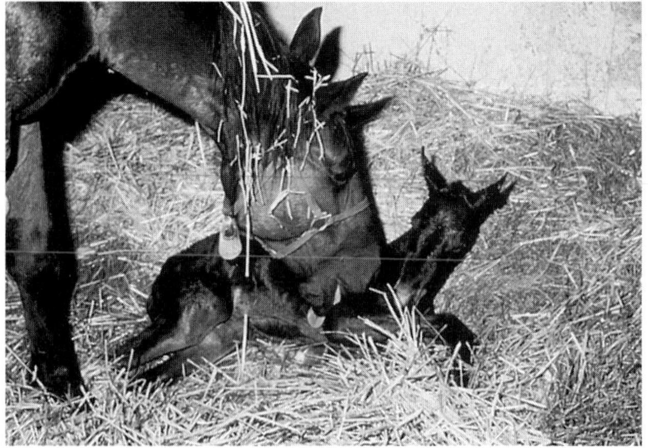

FIGURE 11-7. Interaction between the mare and newborn foal is very important to the establishment of a bond between them. Efforts should be made to avoid disturbing the mare or foal during this bonding period.

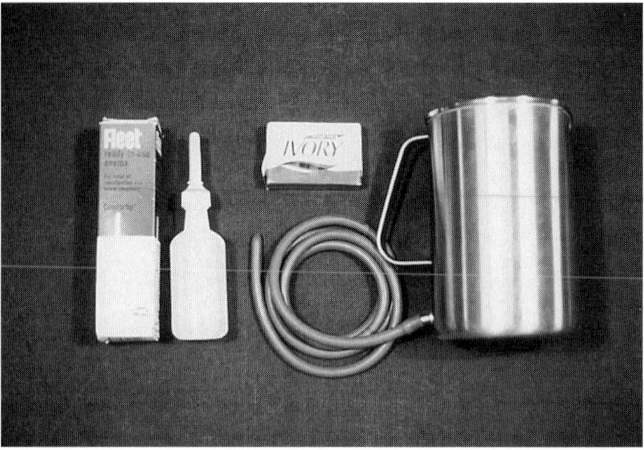

FIGURE 11-8. A commercially available phosphate enema and equipment commonly used for administering a warm, soapy water enema, including an enema bucket and soft rubber tubing.

interaction (sniffing, licking, and touching) is essential to the establishment of the bond between them (Figure 11-7). Interference during this period increases the likelihood of foal rejection by its dam, especially in nervous primiparous mares.

GIVING ENEMAS

Foals often exhibit *meconial impactions* in the immediate postnatal period. *Meconium* consists of glandular secretions, swallowed amniotic fluid, and cell debris; it is dark brown to black in color and is present either in pasty consistency or as firm pellets. Meconium occupies the lumen of the rectum and the colon in the full-term fetus and, under normal circumstances, is not expelled until after birth (in utero stress can lead to meconial staining of amniotic fluid, fetal membranes, and the fetus). As the newborn foal passes meconium, fecal consistency changes to less tenacious, lighter brown material. Masses of meconium often are quite firm and large, resulting in various degrees of constipation and dyschezia in the first few days of postnatal life. Routinely giving enemas to newborn foals tends to reduce the rate of occurrence of meconial impaction. The most commonly used types of enemas are 1 to 2 pints of warm, mild, soapy water, given by gravity flow through soft rubber tubing, or commercially available phosphate enemas (Figure 11-8).

Extreme care should be taken during enema administration to prevent undue rectal trauma and perforation. Most instances of clinically apparent meconial impaction respond favorably to repeated enemas, often in conjunction with orally given fluids containing mineral oil. Few impactions require surgical intervention.

ANTIBIOTIC INJECTIONS

The use of a single, prophylactic injection of antibiotics to guard against infection is a topic of controversy. Proponents contend that it serves in a protective capacity when the foal is at a vulnerable stage and is exposed to a variety of organisms in the immediate environment and cite data that the leading cause of illness in neonatal units is bacterial infection (septicemia due most commonly to Gram-negative bacteria). Adversaries assert that indiscriminate use of antibiotics can potentiate problems by prompting the development of antibiotic-resistant microorganisms. Madigan (1997) contends that short-term (48 to 72 hours) administration of broad-spectrum antibiotics (e.g., 20,000 U of procaine penicillin per kilogram of body weight intramuscularly every 24 hours and 6.6 mg of gentamicin per kilogram of body weight intramuscularly every 24 hours) is a prudent and effective, yet safe, means to treat exposure from bacteria across the gut wall in the newborn foal at risk of developing septicemia.

We do not recommend the prophylactic use of antibiotics in newborn foals except under extenuating circumstances (e.g., for foals born and raised in filthy environments, for foals with delayed ingestion of adequate colostrum and milk during the first few hours of life when indiscriminate active absorption of large molecules through the open gut may occur, when extensive placentitis is apparent during examination of the expelled fetal membranes, or for foals with complete or partial failure of passive antibody transfer). The clinician should make clients aware that proper hygiene, colostrum intake, and management cannot be replaced by prophylactic antibiotic administration.

Because no single physical examination or laboratory test finding confirms the presence of septicemia, a sepsis score was developed by Brewer and Koterba (1990) to aid in diagnosing this condition. The scoring system ranks (0 to 4) neutrophil count, band neutrophil count, toxic changes of neutrophils, fibrinogen level, glucose level, immunoglobulin content, scleral petechiation or injection, rectal temperature, gestation length at birth, and other physical and historical data into an overall score. High and low scores were >90%

and >85% accurate in predicting the presence or absence of sepsis, respectively. If infection is suspected, administration of broad-spectrum antibiotics should be initiated immediately. The spectrum of activity of the antimicrobials chosen should include effectiveness against Gram-negative organisms most commonly associated with septicemia and against Gram-positive organisms sometimes involved in neonatal infections. A combination of ampicillin (20 to 25 mg/kg of body weight intravenously every 6 hours) and amikacin (15 mg/kg of body weight intravenously every 24 hours) is used by some practitioners. Aseptically obtained blood cultures to identify organisms associated with neonatal septicemia, as well as their antimicrobial sensitivity patterns, are useful for selecting antibiotics for use. If blood samples are collected for culture, sampling should occur before administration of the antibiotics.

VITAMIN INJECTIONS

Routine neonatal vitamin (A, D, and E) injections are a prescribed procedure in some veterinary practices. The value of this policy is equivocal, however, unless specific deficits in maternal nutrition can be determined. An inadequate ration might interfere with the nutritional needs of the dam and the developing fetus. If the dam's diet is not adjusted according to the increased demands of late pregnancy, frank deficiencies may evolve.

Vitamin A

Adequate maternal vitamin A levels can be maintained by providing green pasture or green hay in the diet because β-carotene, a vitamin A precursor, is present in the chlorophyll of green plants. With increasing maturity and long-term storage of hay, β-carotene content decreases to negligible levels. Vitamin A supplements therefore are required when overmature pasture or long-stored hay is the sole source of the vitamin. Neither β-carotene nor the alcohol form of vitamin A crosses the placenta during gestation but rather both become concentrated in the colostrum. The newborn foal therefore requires ample colostrum to ensure satisfactory vitamin A levels. When given to the dam via oral or parenteral routes, the ester form of vitamin A crosses the placenta and contributes to fetal hepatic stores of vitamin A.

Vitamin D

Vitamin D deficiency is unlikely to develop unless a horse is confined continually to a stable with no exposure to sunlight. Vitamin D can be acquired by two mechanisms, both of which depend on exposure to ultraviolet light. Consumption of sun-cured hay provides the horse with vitamin D_2, which then is converted to a functional metabolite in the body. Direct exposure to sunlight also supplies a horse's vitamin D requirements, because the solar irradiation converts 7-dehydrocholesterol in the skin to vitamin D_3, which then is accessible for use.

Vitamin E

Absolute vitamin E deficiency has not been documented in horses. Relative vitamin E deficiency can exist if the diet is high in polyunsaturated fatty acids because the vitamin's antioxidant function can be hindered by rancidification of these oils. *Selenium* exerts a synergistic role with vitamin E in protecting tissues from oxidation damage. In areas in which selenium-deficient soils produce selenium-deficient feedstuffs, dam and foal vitamin E-selenium supplementation is required.

If vitamin supplementation is chosen, recommended doses of vitamins A, D, and E (as intramuscular injections) in the newborn foal are as follows: vitamin A, 250,000 to 500,000 IU; vitamin D, 25,000 to 50,000 IU; and vitamin E, 50 to 100 IU. Excessive amounts of vitamins A and D, as well as of selenium, can produce toxic effects. Vitamin E is considered to be nontoxic and actually is believed to provide additional immune protection against infectious diseases when given in increasing amounts.

NEONATAL VACCINATION

Protection of the newborn against specific infectious diseases should be provided by dam immunization in late gestation (booster immunizations with inactivated antigens 4 to 6 weeks before parturition). If the foal is not protected against indigenous pathogens through passively acquired immunity, neonatal vaccination can be provided when indicated and available. If low circulating levels of colostrum-derived tetanus antitoxins are suspected in the foal, tetanus antitoxin should be given to ensure protective levels during the first few weeks of life. However, the passive protection provided by antitoxin administration is short-lived. The practitioner must recognize that vaccinal response of foals varies by infectious agent and product used; however, he or she should also abide by the directions and precautions that accompany the vaccines.

In foals receiving adequate colostral protection from appropriately vaccinated broodmares, Wilson (1999) recommended that vaccination against equine herpesvirus 1 and 4 could begin at 4 months of age; vaccination against tetanus, western equine encephalitis, and eastern equine encephalitis could begin at 6 months of age; and vaccination against influenza could begin at 9 months of age. He recommended that vaccination against other potential pathogens (e.g., strangles, rabies, and equine viral arteritis) be included in the foal immunization program when conditions of significant risk exist.

Current recommendations for active immunization of foals may change as more information on interference of colostrum-derived maternal antibodies with response to many vaccinal antigens becomes available. Foals from vaccinated mares usually respond poorly to active immunization against common vaccinal antigens begun at 3 months of age, even when repeated boosters are given. Most investigators agree that a more consistent response occurs if vaccines are not administered before 6 months of age and if three (rather than two) doses of the vaccine are given. Of additional concern with early vaccination is the finding that vaccination of foals against influenza before 6 months of age may induce tolerance that results in a poor response to vaccine administration later in life. In high-risk situations, particularly when colostral immunoglobulin transfer was poor, beginning vaccine administration at 3 months of age may be justified.

COLOSTRUM ACQUISITION

Although the equine fetus appears to be immunocompetent at midgestation, at birth it is virtually devoid of circulating antibodies, except for small amounts of immunoglobulin (Ig)M. The newborn foal adapts to the environment by producing its own antibodies, but these autogenous immunoglobulins are not evident for 1 to 2 weeks postpartum and do not attain protective levels for as long as several weeks. Assurance that the neonate receives and absorbs an adequate supply of immunoglobulins therefore is of paramount importance. The passive immunity obtained via colostrum will protect the newborn for several weeks while its own immune system is developing.

It is essential that a foal receives colostrum early in the first few hours of life. Absorption of intact antibodies through the intestinal epithelium of the newborn is a transient event lasting approximately 24 hours. The efficiency of this process begins to decline approximately 6 to 8 hours after birth. Colostrum deprivation beyond this period increases the likelihood of a partial failure of passive immunoglobulin transfer to the foal. It is beneficial for all newborn foals to *receive good quality colostrum within 2 hours after birth* to maximize intestinal absorption of antibodies.

Colostrum can be delivered by bottle to newborn foals that are weak and unable to rise. When the suck reflex is absent, giving colostrum via nasogastric intubation is indicated. A foal that is unable to nurse the dam (resulting from dam agalactia, maternal death at parturition, foal rejection by the dam, or foal abnormalities such as neonatal maladjustment syndrome) should receive colostrum before placement on a receptive foster mare or hand-feeding of mare milk or milk replacer.

A minimum of *1.5 to 2 liters of high-quality colostrum* currently is believed necessary to achieve a high postingestion serum level of passively obtained immunoglobulins. The newborn foal fed via bottle or nasogastric tube should receive colostrum at hourly intervals, with a maximum volume of 1 pint per feeding (Figure 11-9). Mares should be immunized properly during pregnancy and should be moved to the foaling premises 4 to 6 weeks before parturition to ensure high colostral levels of antibodies against the diseases of greatest concern to the equine population of the geographic location.

The *immunoglobulin content of colostrum* can be determined accurately but requires a tedious processing technique. Such verification is not routinely necessary but can be useful for evaluating colostrum to be stored or colostrum of questionable quality. Experimentation suggests that the *specific gravity of colostrum* is closely correlated with immunoglobulin content (>3000 mg/dl; specific gravity >1.06); specific gravity of colostrum therefore might be a quick, reliable field test (>1.06 is desirable; determined by a *colostrometer* available from Jorgensen Laboratories) (Figure 11-10). Sticky consistency typically indicates colostrum with a high IgG concentration, but it is difficult to determine the approximate immunoglobulin content of colostrum based on the color of the sample. However, thick, yellow-orange colostrum tends to have a higher IgG content than white, milky-appearing colostrum.

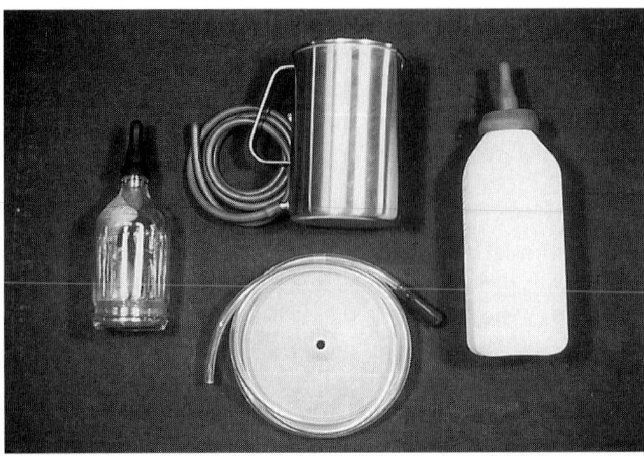

FIGURE 11-9. Colostrum can be fed to foals by using either a bottle and nipple or by nasogastric intubation with an attached funnel. Enema buckets with attached tubing also work well for this purpose if properly cleaned before use.

If a source of fresh colostrum is not available, an alternative should be readily obtainable. The most feasible alternative is frozen equine colostrum from the same farm or a nearby farm or veterinary hospital. For such cases, colostrum from a mare is hygienically collected and stored at –20° C (–4° F) for future use. Colostrum preserved in this way maintains its antibody activity for at least 1 year. When needed, the frozen colostrum is thawed and warmed to body temperature by placing the receptacle in a warm (35° to 37° C) waterbath.

Only colostrum from the first postpartum milking should be used as an antibody source, because it has the highest concentration of immunoglobulins; immunoglobulin content rapidly diminishes with subsequent milkings. A maximum of 1 pint of colostrum should be removed from a *single* mammary gland of the donor mare at parturition. Attendants then should be certain that the foal nurses from the other mammary gland to ensure adequate ingestion of colostrum. Alternatively, some managers prefer not to milk out one teat until the foal has suckled.

Lyophilized equine IgG is an alternative to fresh or frozen equine colostrum. Foals require a dose of 40 to 60 g to elevate serum IgG concentrations to 400 to 1000 mg/dl. Serum or plasma can also be administered orally, but 6 to 9 liters may be needed to obtain a satisfactory serum IgG concentration in the foal.

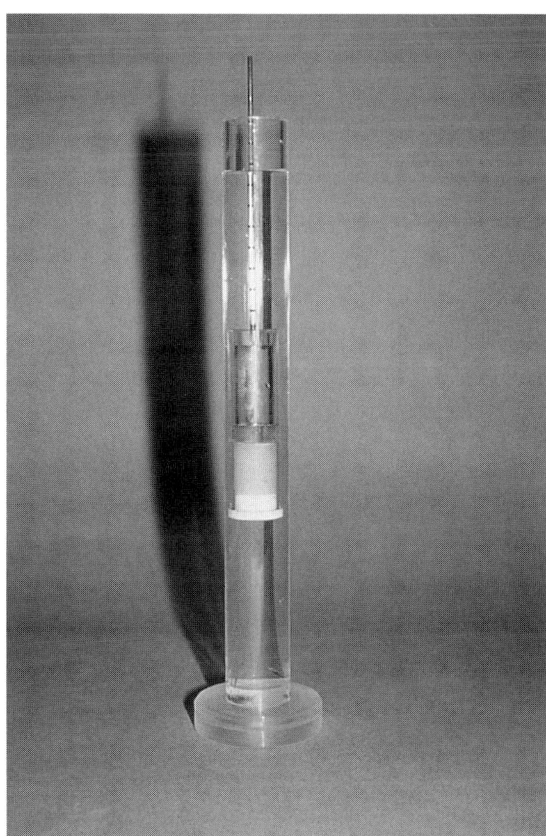

FIGURE 11-10. This colostrometer is used to measure the specific gravity of colostrum. The specific gravity of colostrum is highly correlated with immunoglobulin concentration.

Colostrum and colostrum substitutes should be free of antierythrocyte antibodies (especially against the Aa and Qa blood group antigens) to prevent *neonatal isoerythrolysis.* The mare's serum can be tested (ideally during the last month of gestation) for the presence of antierythrocyte antibodies; if present, the colostrum should be discarded. An alternative source of antibodies will have to be supplied to the foal (either colostrum tested against the foal's RBC using the jaundiced foal agglutation test or preferably serum or plasma known to not contain antierythrocyte antibodies [see treatment for failure of passive antibody transfer]).

The practitioner also should document that all foals have received an adequate amount of passively obtained antibodies by determining serum immunoglobulin levels at 16 to 24 hours of age.

FAILURE OF PASSIVE ANTIBODY TRANSFER

Passive antibody transfer failure is a primary underlying cause of infection in newborn foals. One study demonstrated that approximately one quarter of all foals receive inadequate levels of passively obtained antibodies. The condition of such foals is precarious because they are not fully capable of warding off infectious assaults in the early weeks of life. Because the equine placenta does not permit transplacental transfer of maternal antibodies, the *presuckle foal is virtually agammaglobulinemic.*

At birth, the foal is capable of autogenous antibody synthesis against environmental antigens; however, a time lapse of several days is required for these actively obtained antibodies to be detected in the circulation. Protective levels of the antibodies might not be reached for weeks. The foal therefore relies entirely on passive immunity obtained through the colostrum as a defense against pathogens for the first weeks of life.

Colostrum acquisition by the foal is a time-dependent process. The antibody concentration of colostrum is depleted quickly after the first nursing and drops to negligible levels by 24 hours postpartum. Furthermore, the intestinal wall of the foal is permeable to these antibodies for only approximately 24 hours. With adequate passive antibody transfer, the serum antibody levels of the foal should be approximately equal to those of its dam by 24 hours of age. From this time, passive protection is gradually eliminated (through immunoglobulin catabolism) concurrent with a steady rise in active immunity. Because the half-life of IgG reportedly is 3 weeks, passive protection reaches low levels by 6 to 8 weeks of age. Active immunization cannot be maximally stimulated until the titer of passive immunity is relatively low. Thus foals reach a vulnerable stage in total immune status at approximately 1 to 2 months of age, during the transition to complete autogenous antibody protection. Because intestinal absorption of immunoglobulins is most expedient during the first few hours after birth and drops steadily thereafter, there are many potential opportunities for partial or complete failure of passive antibody transfer.

Causes

Causes of passive transfer failure can include the following: (1) weak, sick, or rejected foals receiving an insufficient quantity of colostrum during the crucial 24 hours before the antibody absorptive function of the small intestine has ceased; (2) dysmaturity or prematurity, resulting in foals that are too weak to nurse; (3) premature parturition, resulting in insufficient time for the mammary gland to concentrate antibodies for passive transfer through the colostrum; (4) low colostral IgG content in mares with no evidence of premature lactation, premature parturition, or subnormal serum IgG levels (the cause of this dysfunction in mammary gland antibody-concentrating ability remains uncertain); and (5) depressed antibody absorptive capacity of the foal's intestinal mucosa in the early hours of the postnatal period. Stress to the mare or the foal during the perinatal period is postulated as one mechanism behind intestinal malabsorption of antibodies. Increased endogenous steroid production, induced by stress, is believed to arrest intestinal absorption of immunoglobulins prematurely in other species.

Categories

Several gradations of passive transfer failure can occur. For practical purposes, two basic categories have evolved—partial failure of passive transfer (200 to 400 mg of IgG per deciliter of serum) and complete failure of passive transfer (<200 mg of IgG per deciliter of serum). Studies have demonstrated that rate of occurrence and severity of illness are proportional to the amount of passive immunoglobulin deprivation. Approximately 25% of foals in the partial failure category become ill, whereas 75% of foals in the complete failure category contract infectious diseases. Few foals become ill when the serum level exceeds 400 to 800 mg/dl.

Detection

Early detection of passive transfer failure is an essential element in managing the disorder because prompt treatment helps alleviate encroaching infectious complications. If practical, performing diagnostic tests to determine IgG concentrations in foal blood at 8 to 12 hours of age can facilitate early detection of failure of passive transfer; this permits oral administration of high-quality colostrum in an attempt to correct the immunodeficiency. Antibody absorption effectively nears completion at 18 to 24 hours of age; if the IgG concentration is low at this time, intravenous supplementation with plasma will be required. A variety of kits are available for determination of the serum immunoglobulin concentration. Commonly used diagnostic kits are the single radial immunodiffusion test, the zinc sulfate turbidity test, the enzyme-linked immunosorbent assay (ELISA), and the glutaraldehyde coagulation test.

Radial Immunodiffusion Test. The single radial immunodiffusion test uses equine IgG antisera and therefore is specific for measuring the IgG class of immunoglobulin. The test kit can be prepared by the practitioner or purchased commercially (Kit for the Quantitative Determination of Horse Immunoglobulin G, Miles Laboratories). Accuracy is the primary advantage of this diagnostic technique. The test requires approximately 24 hours to perform. The commercially available test kit consists of agar gel plates, each of which can accommodate several samples for testing. The plates should be used only once; therefore the cost per test sample increases as fewer samples are incorporated into the test plate.

Zinc Sulfate Turbidity Test. The zinc sulfate turbidity test is based on precipitation of salts created by the chemical combination of heavier globulins and trace metal ions. It can be interpreted by visual assessment or by spectrophotometry. Visual assessment offers the advantage of quick results (within 30 to 60 minutes) for a rough estimate of immunoglobulin protection. A precipitate gives the mixture a turbid appearance when the serum IgG concentration is at least 400 to 500 mg/dl, thus implying adequate IgG transfer. The degree of turbidity is directly proportional to the concentration of serum IgG. A more quantitative study is permitted when the absorbance of the mixture is determined using a spectrophotometer. The optical density of the sample is compared with a standard curve obtained by using serial IgG dilutions of standardized serum. The zinc sulfate turbidity test is not specific for IgG but rather measures total immunoglobulin levels. Test results can be altered by sample hemolysis, carbon dioxide in the zinc sulfate solution, and time of interpretation; therefore steps should be taken to prevent misinterpretation. Test kits can be fabricated at a veterinary hospital or obtained commercially (Equi-Z, Veterinary Medical Research and Development, Inc.). The procedure and necessary materials for the test are described in the literature.

ELISA. A kit for ELISA (CITE Foal IgG Test, AgriTech Systems, Inc.) is commercially available and offers prompt, semiquantitative measurement of serum IgG concentration. Test results can be obtained within 10 to 20 minutes of venipuncture. Results of this test compare favorably with those of the single radial immunodiffusion test and the zinc sulfate turbidity test.

Glutaraldehyde Coagulation Test. The glutaraldehyde coagulation test is relatively new. The test is based on cross-linkages formed by glutaraldehyde with basic proteins, resulting in formation of insoluble complexes. A stock solution of 25% glutaraldehyde is diluted to 10% with deionized water, and 50 μl of this solution is added to 0.5 ml of test serum in a tube. The tube contents are examined at 5- to 10-minute intervals for evidence of coagulation. A positive reaction is evident as a solid gel that does not move when the tube is tilted. A positive reaction in <10 minutes is equivalent to >800 mg of IgG per deciliter, and a positive reaction between 10 and 60 minutes is equivalent to >400 mg of IgG per deciliter. The major advantage of the test is its low cost ($0.25/test), and the major disadvantage is the time required to obtain results (i.e., the blood sample must be allowed to clot to obtain serum, and 60 minutes is required to get final results). A glutaraldehyde coagulation test is commercially available from Veterinary Dynamics.

Treatment

Treatment measures for failure of passive antibody transfer vary depending on the stage of detection and the degree of immunoglobulin deprivation. If transfer failure is suspected before 12 hours of age, giving colostrum orally is indicated. *The foal should receive 500 ml of fresh or frozen/thawed colostrum at hourly intervals until a total intake of 1.5 to 2 liters is achieved.* To minimize the likelihood of neonatal isoerythrolysis or transfusion reactions, all colostrum must be checked for *antierythrocyte alloantibodies* before being given. Ideally, the IgG content of frozen colostrum is predetermined to ensure its quality.

If passive antibody transfer failure is detected more than 12 hours after birth, the foal should receive a plasma transfusion. The donor's plasma should be screened for compatibility with the foal's plasma. The ideal donor is Aa and Qa negative with no alloantibodies to these blood group antigens. Depending on the IgG level of the foal and donor plasma, a plasma dose guideline is *20 to 50 ml of plasma per kilogram of body weight.* This dose reportedly increases the foal's IgG content to 30% of that of the donor. Measurements for serum IgG should be repeated after transfusion because some foals might require a total of 2 to 4 liters of plasma to attain satisfactory immunoglobulin levels.

Because frozen (–20° C) plasma is thought to remain viable for several months to years, it may be advantageous to collect several liters of plasma from a universally compatible donor, determine the plasma IgG content, and then freeze it until needed. Properly immunized horses on the same premises that would have antibody production against antigens indigenous to the area should be used. Plasma for transfusions also is available through commercial laboratories (Foalimmune, Lake Immunogenetics; Equine Plasma, Veterinary Dynamics, Inc.). These products are generally screened for anti–red blood cell antibodies and certain immunoglobulins against a variety of equine diseases. Specific guidelines for plasma collection are reported in the literature.

A healthy foal older than 3 weeks with 200 to 400 mg of IgG per deciliter of serum probably should not be given a plasma transfusion because this passively obtained antibody protection would hinder active immune development. Such foals should be monitored carefully, however, and placed in a clean, environmentally suitable area to minimize exposure to pathogens.

Prevention

Prevention of passive transfer failures consists of good management. All foalings should be attended, and the foal should receive colostrum by 6 hours of age. Routine serum evaluation of foals before 16 to 24 hours of age is necessary to check for adequate immunoglobulin transfer. If an inadequate circulating level of IgG is confirmed, appropriate therapeutic steps should be taken. Additional supportive measures for foals with passive transfer failure include isolation in a clean, protected, well-ventilated environment and antibiotic therapy when necessary.

BIBLIOGRAPHY

Brewer BD, Koterba AM: Development of a scoring system for the early diagnosis of equine neonatal sepsis. *Equine Vet J* 20:18-22, 1990.

Koterba AM: Physical examination. In Koterba AM, Drummon WH, Kosch PC, editors, *Equine clinical neonatology,* Philadelphia, 1990, Lea & Febiger.

LeBlanc MM: Immunologic considerations. In Koterba AM, Drummon WH, Kosch PC, editors, *Equine clinical neonatology,* Philadelphia, 1990, Lea & Febiger.

Madigan JE: Method for preventing neonatal septicemia, the leading cause of death in the neonatal foal. *Proc Am Assoc Equine Pract* 43:17-19, 1997.

Madigan JE: Physical exam of the neonate. In Madigan JE, editor, *Manual of equine neonatal medicine,* Woodland, CA, 1987, Live Oak Publishing.

McClure JJ: The immune system. In McKinnon AO, Voss JL, editors, *Equine reproduction,* Philadelphia, 1993, Lea & Febiger.

Traub-Dargatz JL: Postnatal care of the foal. In McKinnon AO, Voss JL, editors, *Equine reproduction,* Philadelphia, 1993, Lea & Febiger.

White SC: The use of plasma in foals with failure of passive transfer. *Proc Am Assoc Equine Pract* 35:215-218, 1989.

Wilson WD: Vaccination programs for foals and weanlings. *Proc Am Assoc Equine Pract* 45:254-263, 1999.

12

Semen Collection and Artificial Insemination

OBJECTIVES

While studying the information covered in this chapter, the student should attempt to:

1. Acquire a working knowledge of procedures used for collection of semen from stallions.
2. Acquire a working knowledge of proper breeding management of stallions and semen processing and handling techniques, used in artificial insemination programs.

STUDY QUESTIONS

1. Discuss advantages and disadvantages of artificial insemination programs compared to natural breeding programs for horses.
2. Describe important components of a breeding shed to be used in an equine artificial insemination program.
3. Give advantages and disadvantages of the commonly used equine artificial vaginas.
4. Describe the technique for preparing an artificial vagina for semen collection in the stallion.
5. List the advantages of using a breeding phantom for semen collection.
6. Describe the role of semen extenders and temperature in maintaining equine spermatozoal viability in vitro.
7. Discuss the proper insemination dose (number of spermatozoa and insemination volume), insemination timing, and insemination technique for artificial insemination in the mare.

Proper application of artificial insemination (AI) in an equine breeding program can dramatically improve operating efficiency and increase the availability of sires to the general public. This chapter addresses advantages and disadvantages of AI programs and provides a detailed description of the techniques involved.

Few breed registries in the United States do not currently permit the use of AI (e.g., the Jockey Club [Thoroughbreds] and the Standard Jack and Jennet Registry of America). The allowances and limitations regarding storage and transport of semen vary considerably among the breed registries that permit the use of AI. One should contact specific breed registries before instituting an AI program to determine restrictions that might limit registration of foals produced.

ADVANTAGES AND DISADVANTAGES

AI offers numerous advantages over natural mating. For instance, dividing an ejaculate into several insemination doses permits more efficient use of stallion semen, provided the stallion has normal fertility. Accordingly, the number of mares that a stallion can impregnate during a breeding season or calendar year may be increased several-fold. The availability of stallion semen to mare owners is likewise increased within those breed organizations whose bylaws permit preservation and transport of stallion semen. Addition of antibiotics to semen extenders for AI minimizes venereal transmission of bacterial diseases to the mare where the stallion serves as a carrier. Transmission of potential pathogens from mare to stallion can also be reduced. Semen extenders contain supportive and protective factors for spermatozoa that may improve the pregnancy rates of certain stallions. Using a breeding phantom for collection of semen reduces the risk of breeding injuries. Collection of semen with an artificial vagina also allows scrutiny of semen quality before insemination and assists in early detection of problems that may adversely affect the fertility of stallions.

Certain disadvantages are inherent to AI programs. The success of such programs requires heightened knowledge and skill on the part of the stallion manager because ejaculated spermatozoa are very susceptible to environmental injury. Improper semen collection, handling, processing, and insemination technique can lower pregnancy rates. Expenses related to the purchase of necessary equipment and supplies for AI can increase overhead costs of the breeding program. However, expenses incurred on a per mare basis are usually decreased because of the multiple inseminations possible with a single ejaculate. Another disadvantage is the somewhat increased risk of human injury during the process of semen collection with an artificial vagina. Therefore, proper training of persons involved in the semen collection process is essential.

Semen Collection

The semen collection procedure is an essential part of the AI program. Facilities and equipment that permit safe and efficient collection and handling of the semen are discussed.

Artificial Vagina Selection

A properly constructed and prepared artificial vagina (AV) increases the efficiency of semen collection in AI programs and optimizes the quality of ejaculated semen. Several well-designed AVs are available. Each type has distinct attributes and peculiarities, so AV selection is based on specific requirements and personal preference. AVs have also been homemade by users to meet their specific needs. When contemplating the purchase of an equine AV, one should consider initial costs and maintenance costs, durability, weight, temperature maintenance, and spermatozoal losses incurred during semen collection.

Missouri Model Artifical Vagina. The Missouri model AV (Figure 12-1) (NASCO, Ft. Atkinson, WI) probably is the most widely used AV in the United States. It is composed of a double-walled rubber liner containing a permanently sealed water chamber and a leather carrying case. This AV is relatively inexpensive, lightweight, and easy to assemble and clean. It has fairly good heat retention, and because the glans penis should be beyond the water jacket at the time of ejaculation, internal temperature of the AV may exceed the 45° to 48° C spermatozoal tolerance threshold without causing heat-related injury to ejaculated spermatozoa. This property can be advantageous for stallions that prefer higher temperatures. This AV is equipped with an air valve so that it can be pressurized with water alone or with air and water to reduce its weight. Because the liner is made of heavy rubber and the water chamber is permanently sealed, there is little chance of water leakage contaminating the semen sample during collection.

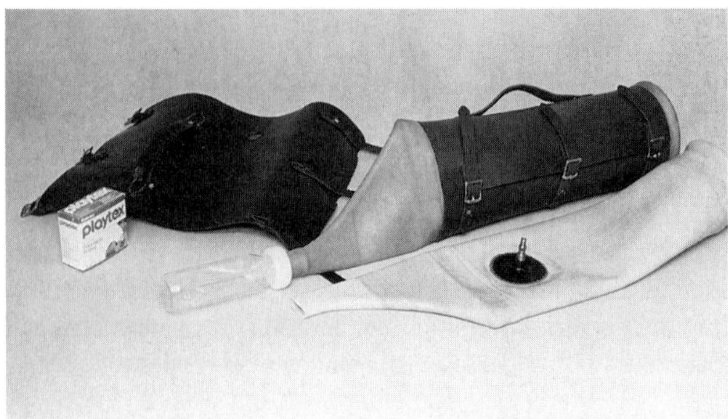

FIGURE 12-1. Missouri model artificial vagina: leather carrying case, double-layered latex rubber water jacket with attached latex rubber cone, bottle adapter, and collection bottle with semen filter inside. Disposable bottle liners (shown) can be used inside most collection bottles. (From Varner DD, Schumacher J, Blanchard TL, Johnson L: *Diseases and management of breeding stallions,* p. 118. Goleta, CA, 1991, American Veterinary Publications.)

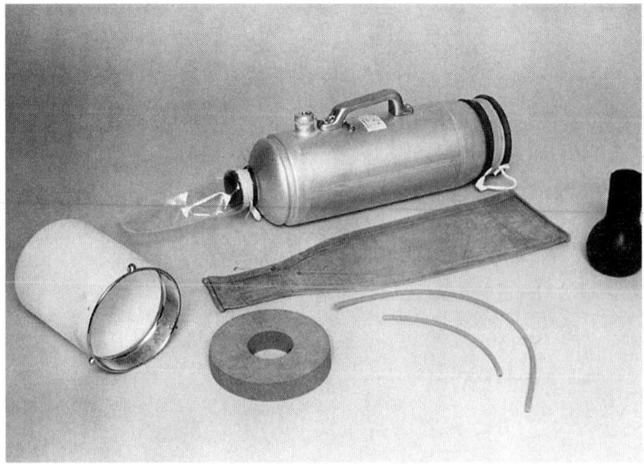

FIGURE 12-2. Japanese model artificial vagina: aluminum case with rigid handle, latex rubber liner, rubber bands for attaching the rubber liner to the aluminum case, collection bag and attached rubber band, insulating receptacle for the end of the artificial vagina, and rubber cushion (doughnut) for placement at the inside front of artificial vagina. The black rubber attachment can be used around the collection bag if desired. (From Varner DD, Schumacher J, Blanchard TL, Johnson L: *Diseases and management of breeding stallions,* p. 119. Goleta, CA, 1991, American Veterinary Publications.)

Japanese (Nishikawa) Model Artificial Vagina. The Japanese (Nishikawa) model AV (Figure 12-2) (Scott Medical Supply, Hayward, CA) is composed of a small, rigid aluminum case and a single rubber liner, so it is lightweight and easy to maneuver. The AV is easy to assemble and clean. Another attribute of this AV is the direct attachment of a semen receptacle to the aluminum casing. This design permits the ejaculate to be discharged directly into the receptacle, allowing only minimal contact of semen with the rubber liner. The liner must be secured tightly to the aluminum case with rubber bands before water is added to the chamber between the liner and aluminum case. Water can leak out if this seal is not tight, reducing AV pressure and increasing the risk of water contamination in the ejaculate. The liner should be checked for defects before use because pinpoint holes in the rubber liner can develop, resulting in water leakage into the AV lumen.

Colorado Model Artifical Vagina. The original Colorado model AV is composed of two independent rubber liners and a heavy plastic case covered by a leather collar. It is more cumbersome to use than the previous two AVs but offers good heat retention. In addition, it has two rubber liners between the water chamber and the AV lumen, thus greatly reducing the likelihood of water contamination of the semen sample. Because the water jacket of this AV is longer than the penis, the temperature must be carefully regulated to prevent undue heat damage to ejaculated spermatozoa.

CSU Model Artificial Vagina. The CSU model AV (Figure 12-3) (Animal Reproduction Systems, Chino, CA) and Lane

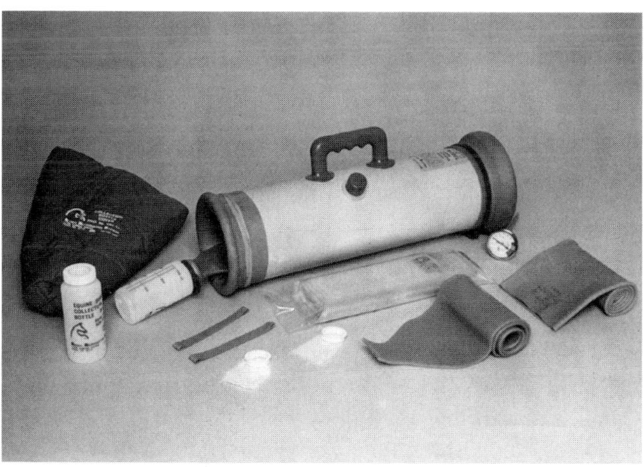

FIGURE 12-3. CSU model artificial vagina: rigid plastic case and handle with padded ends, outer latex rubber liner that forms the water jacket, inner latex rubber liner and cone, collection bottle and filter, and insulating bag for placement over the end of assembled unit. (From Varner DD, Schumacher J, Blanchard TL, Johnson L: *Diseases and management of breeding stallions,* p. 120. Goleta, CA, 1991, American Veterinary Publications.)

model AV (Lane Manufacturing, Denver, CO) are modified versions of the original Colorado model. Both models are lighter than the original and have a rigid handle to facilitate AV manipulation. These versions have the advantages described above for the Colorado model and come with an assortment of accessories, including several AV liners, semen filters and collection bottles, a thermometer to monitor internal temperature of the AV, and an insulated protector cone to cover the semen receptacle during the semen collection process.

Polish Model Artificial Vagina. The Polish model AV (Figure 12-4) was designed as an open-ended AV for collection of only the spermatozoa-rich fraction of the ejaculate from breeding stallions. This method of semen collection increases spermatozoal concentration and, likewise, reduces the contribution (volume) of seminal plasma in ejaculates. The first three jets of an ejaculate contain 75% to 80% of the spermatozoa present in total ejaculates; yet seminal volume is reduced more than 50%. The result of this semen-fractionation step is a significant increase in spermatozoal concentration, sometimes exceeding 0.6 to 1×10^9 spermatozoa/ml. The technique is considered useful for in vitro semen preservation programs, because the spermatozoal concentration can be increased without centrifugation, and toxic influences of seminal plasma on spermatozoal viability may be diminished. Collection of semen by this method reduces contamination of ejaculates: by bacteria from the exterior of the penis; by urine from stallions affected by urospermia; and by blood from stallions with a penile injury. Removal of the coned end of the Missouri model AV or shortening of the CSU model AV will work well for this purpose. The glans penis is allowed to protrude from the AV, and semen is collected as it "spurts" from the urethra through a funnel system attached to semen receptacles, through urethral prosthetic devices attached to a bag, or by catching semen in individual cups.

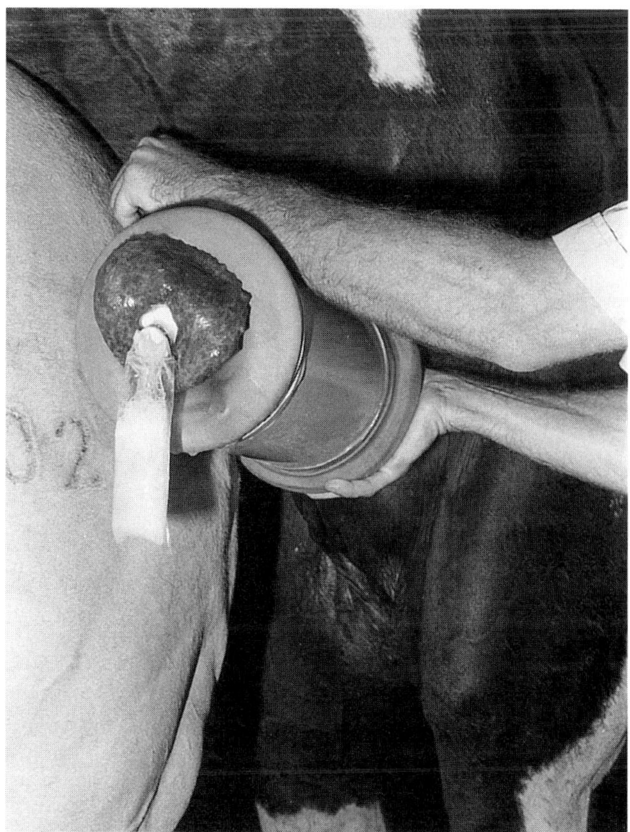

FIGURE 12-4. A modification of the Polish model artificial vagina (open-ended AV) is being used to collect semen from a stallion. The AV is open at either end, permitting penile protrusion and collection of fractions of the ejaculate. The fractions ("spurts" or "jets") of the ejaculate can either be caught in hand-held containers or by placing a prosthetic device attached to a sterile collection bag on the distal urethral process. (From Varner DD, Schumacher J, Blanchard TL, Johnson L: *Diseases and management of breeding stallions,* p. 122. Goleta, CA, 1991, American Veterinary Publications.)

Artificial Vagina Maintenance

All AV components that come in contact with ejaculated semen must be nonspermicidal. Reusable items must be cleansed properly to render them chemically clean, then dried, and, if possible, sterilized between uses. Soaps or disinfectants should not be used to clean AV liners, because the residue can be toxic to spermatozoa during subsequent semen collections. Used rubber AV liners should be cleaned with hot running water soon after use. If smegma within a used AV is allowed to dry before cleaning, the chore becomes more difficult. Cleaned rubber liners can be submerged in ethyl or isopropyl alcohol for 0.5 to 24 hours for disinfection followed by air drying in a dust-free cabinet. Any of the latex rubber liners can be gas sterilized with ethylene oxide, as long as an adequate "air out" period is allowed (i.e., 48 to 72 hours). Sterile, nontoxic disposable equipment should be used when possible to avoid chemical contamination of ejaculates or horizontal transmission of disease. Plastic disposable AV liners, with or without attached semen receptacles, are commercially available for the AVs described earlier. This equipment helps ensure a clean, nontoxic method of semen collection. Unfortunately, some stallions do not readily accept AVs fitted with a disposable plastic liner rather than a reusable rubber liner.

Preparation of Artificial Vaginas for Semen Collection

Immediately before semen collection is attempted, the water jacket of the AV is usually filled with 45° to 50° C water to provide an internal AV temperature of 44° to 48° C (Figure 12-5). Providing an AV temperature above that of the body seems to aid in penile stimulation during copulation. Spermatozoa can be permanently damaged, however, by contact with surfaces above 45° C. As mentioned above, the luminal temperature of a Missouri model AV can exceed 45° C without damaging spermatozoa, provided that the glans penis protrudes beyond the water jacket when ejaculation occurs. Occasionally, some stallions may respond more favorably to semen collection with an AV if its luminal temperature is 50° to 55° C.

Luminal pressure of the AV should be adjusted to provide uniformly good contact around the penis, without interfering with penile penetration. Proper AV pressure accommodates expansion of the penis to full erection. It is important to fully insert the penis into the AV during the first penile thrust and then maintain the penis in this fully inserted position; otherwise, the glans penis will dilate and may be too large to permit full penile penetration into the AV. The result would be extended contact of ejaculated semen with the AV liner en route to the semen receptacle or ejaculatory failure from inadequate penile stimulation. Both temperature and water pressure in the AV should be maintained relatively constant during semen collection to promote consistent stallion performance and maximal spermatozoa harvest.

The inner surface of the AV should be lubricated with a sterile, nonspermicidal lubricant before penile insertion. The collection receptacle (Figure 12-6) should be maintained at body temperature during semen collection and transport to the laboratory to prevent cold shock to the spermatozoa before they are placed in a protective extender. Semen should also be protected from light.

To maximize the number of spermatozoa available from each semen collection, an appropriate filter should be

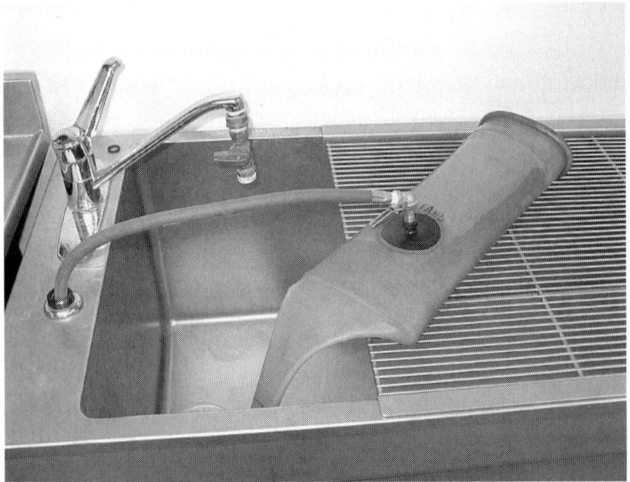

FIGURE 12-5. Filling a Missouri model AV with hot (45° C) water. An air nozzle attachment has been placed on the water hose and connects to the air/water valve inserted into the AV. This system avoids water spillage during the filling procedure. A dial thermometer *can be* placed within the lubricated AV to monitor temperature.

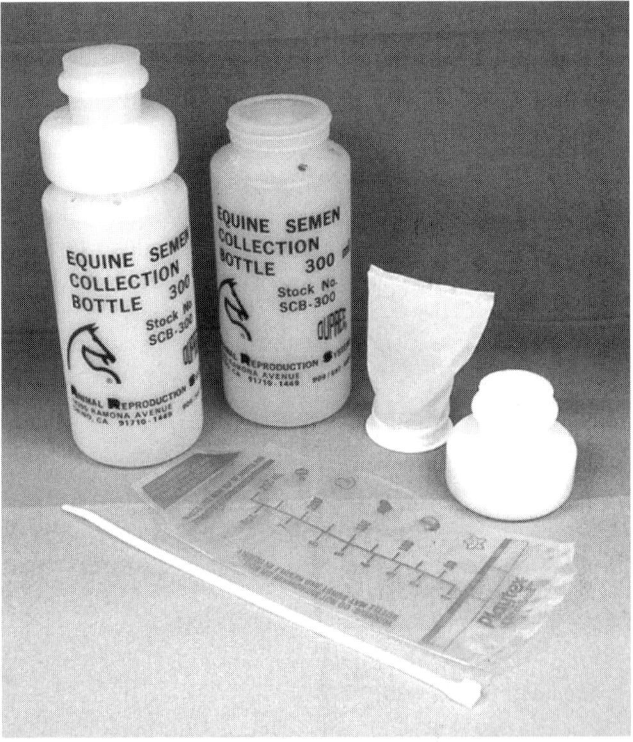

FIGURE 12-6. An efficient semen collection receptacle modified for use with the Missouri model AV. Vent holes have been punctured around the neck of the equine semen collection bottle (Animal Reproduction Systems) to allow semen to freely enter the disposable baby bottle liner (Playtex Products, Inc., Westport, CT) placed inside the bottle. The plastic bottle adapter (NASCO) has been modified to permit attachment of the large semen collection bottle and is screwed onto the bottle top after the nylon mesh gel filter (Animal Reproduction Systems) has been inserted into the top of the bottle with the baby bottle liner inserted. This bottle adapter then fits into the latex coned-end of the Missouri model AV. If the attachment is loose, a plastic snap-tie can be used to prevent the assembled receptacle from detaching during the semen collection process. Finally, a collection bottle cover (Animal Reproduction Systems) is attached over the bottle by a drawstring when the AV is fully assembled. The insulated cover protects the semen against cold shock and light damage.

incorporated into the AV. The filter allows most of the gel-free (but spermatozoa-rich) fractions to pass into the seminal receptacle but traps the gel (which is presented in the final fractions of an ejaculate). Although some spermatozoa inevitably are trapped in the gel and filter, more would be lost if the semen were filtered *after* collection of the combined gel and gel-free portions or if the gel were aspirated from the gel-free portion with a syringe. Nylon micromesh filters (Figure 12-6) are superior to polyester matte filters for separating gel from gel-free fractions because they are non-absorptive and do not trap as many spermatozoa. The filter with its contained gel should be removed immediately upon collection of the semen to prevent seepage of gel into the gel-free portion of the ejaculate.

Use of Condoms for Semen Collection

A condom (Figure 12-7) is a poor alternative to an AV for semen collection but may be the only viable option if the stallion will not breed an AV or if an AV is unavailable. Stallions most reluctant to breed an AV are those that have never bred before and those accustomed to breeding mares by natural service. The quality of semen collected in a condom is inferior to that obtained with an AV because of the marked contamination of the sample with bacteria and debris from the exterior of the penis.

Preparation of Stallion Mount

Semen collection using an AV ordinarily is performed by allowing the stallion to mount a mare or breeding phantom. In certain situations, however, stallions have been trained to ejaculate using an AV or manual stimulation while standing on the ground (Figure 12-8). To train a stallion for ground collection, the stallion is teased to erection, and the penis is washed and dried. The stallion is approached by the collector from the left shoulder, and the AV is placed on the stallion's penis. The AV is pushed toward the base of the penis to encourage thrusting. Stallions usually ejaculate after 5 to 10 pelvic thrusts. If the stallion does not ejaculate after the first attempt, the procedure is repeated until successful.

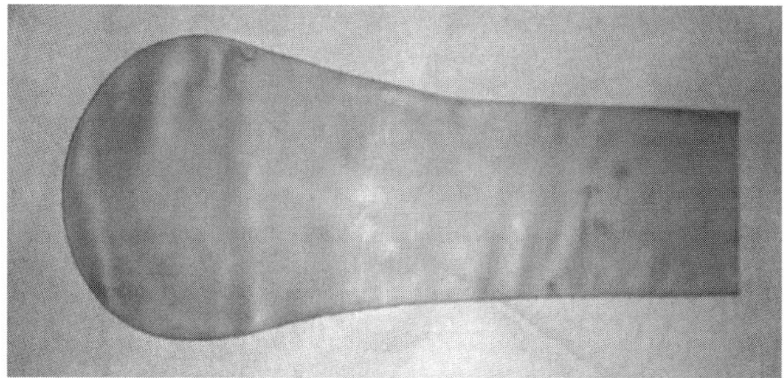

FIGURE 12-7. A stallion condom (NASCO) can be placed onto the stallion's penis before the stallion is permitted to breed a mare in estrus. After ejaculation and dismounting, the condom is removed, and semen is poured through a filter to remove gel and extraneous debris before processing the semen.

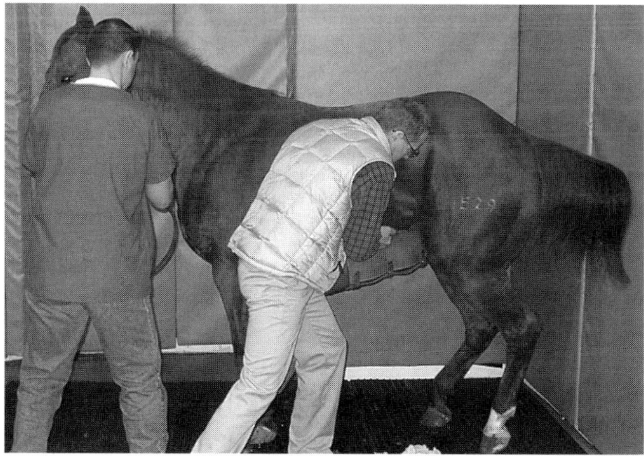

FIGURE 12-8. Collection of semen from a stallion standing on the ground (i.e., unmounted on a mare or phantom). Many stallions can be trained to ejaculate in such a manner, eliminating the need for a mount source.

As an alternative for ground collection, some practitioners prefer to use thin plastic mitts or rectal sleeves instead of an AV. The mitt is loosely placed on the penile shaft with 6 to 8 inches hanging beyond the end of the glans. Excess air is expelled from the mitt, and gentle pressure is applied to the glans penis to stimulate thrusting until ejaculation occurs. Application of hot compresses (6-inch squares of folded towels dipped in 50° to 55° C water, squeezed to remove excess water from the compress), with one hand on the glans penis and one hand on the base of the penis, is often helpful in stimulating pelvic thrusting and ejaculation. A consistent, uniform method to which each individual stallion responds should be adopted. A modification of this technique can be used for chemical ejaculation (Figure 12-9). Chemical ejaculation is most often used by the authors for stallions with ejaculatory problems associated with neurologic or musculoskeletal disorders that preclude mounting.

For standard semen collection protocols with the stallion mounted on a mare, either gonad-intact or ovariectomized mares can be used. Intact mares should not be used unless they are exhibiting strong signs of behavioral estrus. Ovariectomized mares generally are considered more appropriate than intact mares for daily semen collection activities because they are predictable and can be used anytime. Mares should be selected as candidates for ovariectomy based on their degree of receptivity to a stallion while in estrus as intact mares. Ovariectomized mares rarely require exogenous hormonal therapy to display behavioral signs of estrus. When needed, 1 to 2 mg of estradiol cypionate (Upjohn, Kalamazoo, MI) can be given intramuscularly to intensify signs of behavioral estrus in ovariectomized mares. This regimen does not induce estrus in intact mares with a functional corpus luteum.

Mares should be physically restrained before the stallion is allowed to mount. Leg hobbles and a twitch on the muzzle can be applied to mares (Figure 12-10). Rarely is tranquilization needed. If a mare's reactions to an approaching stallion are

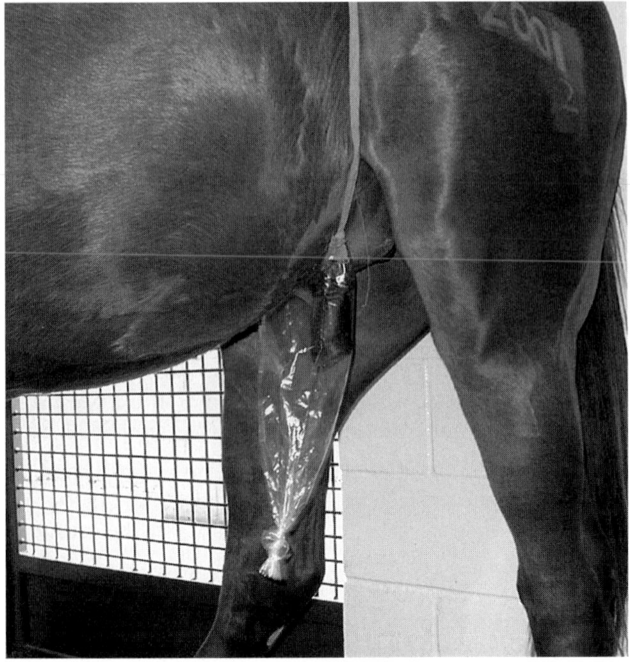

FIGURE 12-9. Use of a thin plastic mitt (or rectal sleeve) for collection of semen from a stallion standing on the ground. Hot compresses can be used to apply pressure to the glans penis and base of the penis to stimulate thrusting and ejaculation. In this particular stallion, the mitt has been hung over the penis for semen collection by chemical ejaculation. After sedating the stallion with detomodine, the stallion is left undisturbed until ejaculation occurs. Semen collected in this manner is highly concentrated and of low volume.

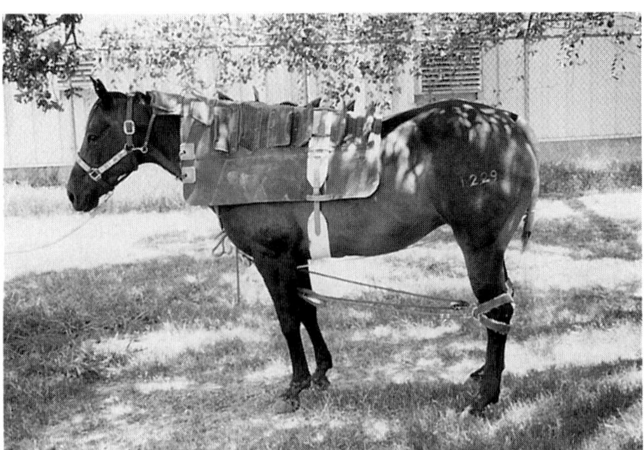

FIGURE 12-10. Ovariectomized mount mare in breeding hobbles; the tail is wrapped and a protective cape is fitted to protect the withers and neck of mare while the stallion is mounted.

unknown or unpredictable, it is wise to allow a "teaser stallion" (with a breeding shield attached to prevent inadvertent breeding; Pinkston's Turf Goods, Lexington, KY) to mount the mare to test the mare's response before permitting a more valuable stallion to mount for semen collection. If the mare reacts unfavorably, an alternative mount source should be used. It is equally important that the stallion not be allowed to savage the mare during breeding. This behavior usually can be controlled with a chain shank passed through the stallion's mouth (Figure 12-11). Muzzles can be fastened to the halter of stallions if excessive biting cannot be controlled by other methods. If necessary, a leather breeding shroud can be secured around the neck of the mount mare so that the stallion bites this apparatus rather than the mare during breeding.

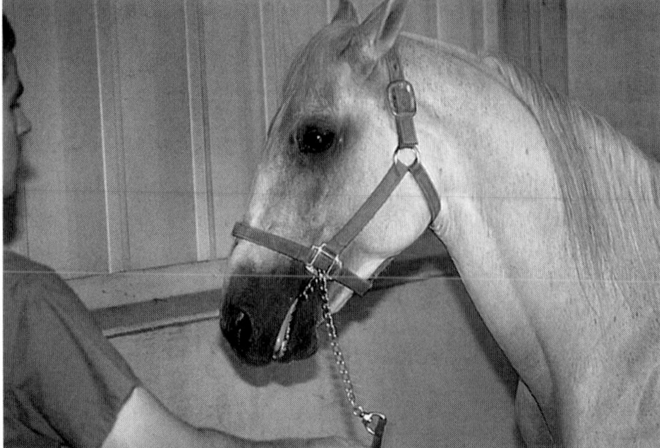

FIGURE 12-11. Chain shank placed through stallion's mouth to facilitate restraint during breeding.

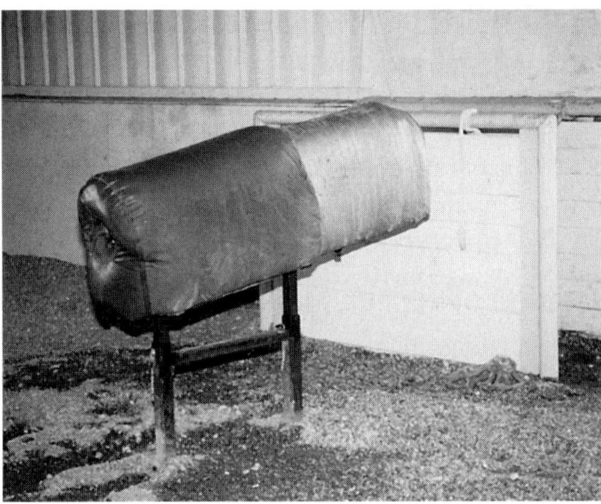

FIGURE 12-12. A commercial model of a breeding phantom (or dummy) commonly used for collection of semen from stallions.

For most stallions, semen collection can be enhanced by use of a breeding phantom, or dummy (Figures 12-12 and 12-13). Although additional training will be required to teach a stallion to mount one of these devices, they offer several advantages over an estrous or ovariectomized mount mare for semen collection. Breeding phantoms eliminate variability in the mount source, thereby allowing a more consistent semen collection protocol. They also greatly reduce the likelihood of stallion injury during semen collection and mare injury resulting from the vicious biting of some stallions. Stallions with rear limb or back maladies can mount a stationary breeding phantom more easily than a live mare. The

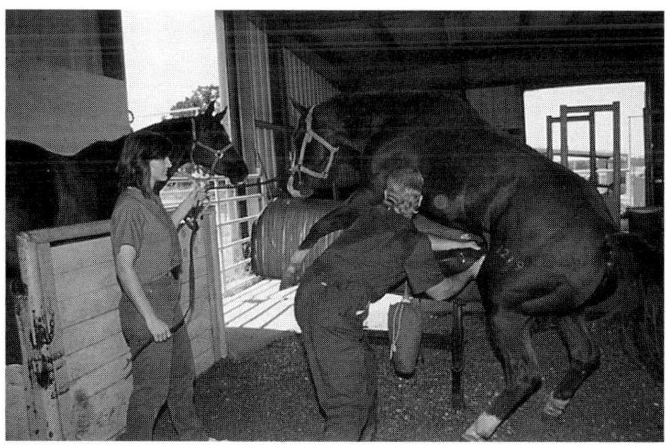

FIGURE 12-13. Collection of semen from a stallion mounted on a breeding phantom. The stimulus mare is placed in front of the breeding phantom in this breeding shed.

height of the phantom can be adjusted to accommodate the stallion. In addition, the phantom can be thoroughly cleaned between mounts, thereby minimizing horizontal transmission of disease.

The size, shape, and composition of *breeding phantoms* are quite diverse, ranging from padded hot-water tanks to sophisticated structures with mounted AVs and hydraulic controls for adjusting the height. Desirable elements of a dummy include the following:

- Adjustable height, with midheight slightly shorter than the average height of the breed involved.
- Width sufficient to permit the stallion to grasp the dummy firmly with the forelegs (total width, including padding, usually should be 22 to 24 inches).
- Adequate padding with an overlying cover that is durable, nonabrasive, and easy to clean.
- A stand with a centrally placed upright support to prevent injury to the stallion's hindlimbs or feet during collection.
- Installation in an area free of obstructions, with space for a live mare to stand adjacent to the dummy.

Most stallions readily accept the phantom as a mounting device. The novice stallion is trained by placing a mare alongside the phantom. The stallion is allowed to tease the mare over the end of the phantom. This stimulates mounting behavior in the stallion, but the stallion is diverted so that he mounts the phantom rather than the live mare. Very little training is required in most instances. Sometimes a mare in estrus must be close to the phantom to stimulate the stallion to mount it. Once trained, some stallions do not require the presence of an estrous mare to mount the phantom. When properly constructed, breeding phantoms greatly improve the efficiency and safety of semen collection in the stallion.

General Semen Handling Techniques

Immediately after its collection, semen should be quickly transported to the laboratory while minimizing physical trauma, exposure to light, cold shock, or excessive heat. All materials that come in contact with the semen (including the semen extender) should be prewarmed to body temperature (37° to 38° C). If an in-line filter was not fitted in the AV when semen was collected, the semen should be poured through a nontoxic filter to remove any gel or extraneous debris. The gel fraction of an unfiltered ejaculate can also be removed by careful aspiration with a syringe. Loss of spermatozoa is greater with the latter two methods than with an in-line, nylon, micromesh filter (Animal Reproduction Systems), which is contained within the AV bottle. Spermatozoal concentration, volume and color of the gel-free semen, and the percentage of progressively motile spermatozoa should be determined and recorded (Figures 12-14 through 12-18).

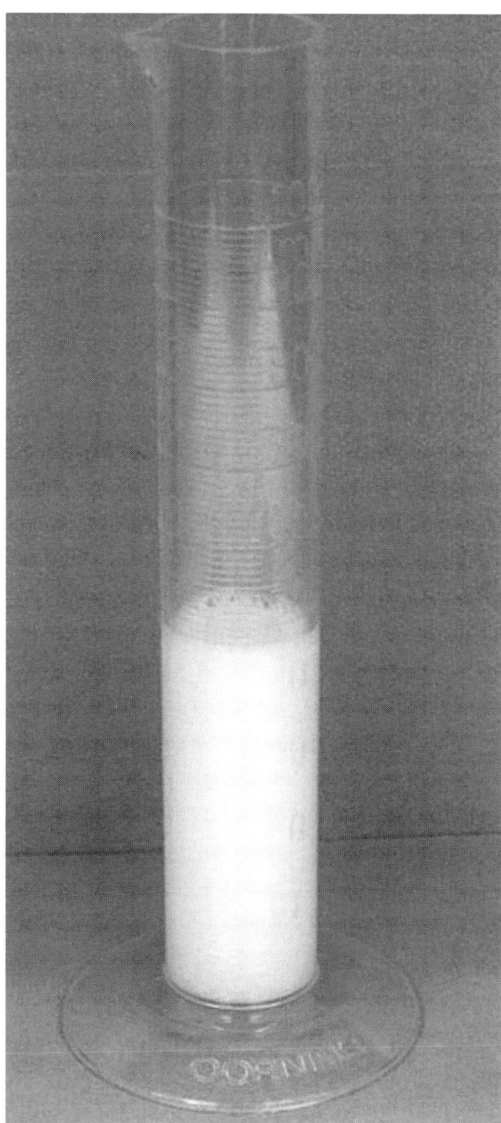

FIGURE 12-14. Measuring filtered raw semen volume in a graduated cylinder.

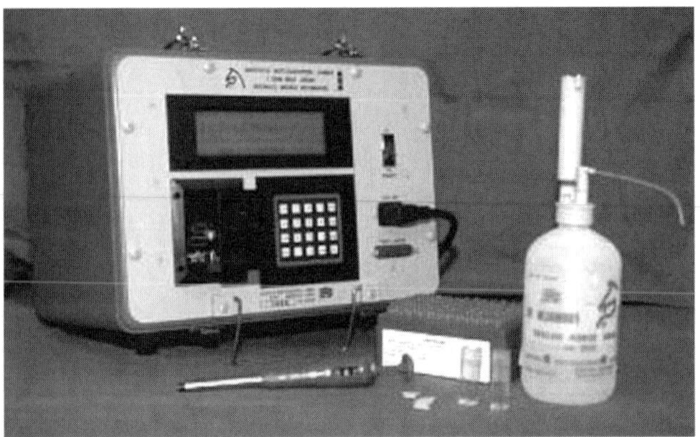

FIGURE 12-15. Determining the spermatozoal concentration of raw semen using a Densimeter (Animal Reproduction Systems). After the Densimeter is standardized for 100% transmittance through a diluent-loaded cuvette, 180 µl of mixed gel-free raw semen is pipetted into the cuvette. The top of the cuvette is covered, and the cuvette is gently rotated to mix the semen evenly in the diluent. The cuvette is placed into the Densimeter, the door is closed, and the spermatozoal concentration in the raw semen is read on the screen of the instrument. This machine can also be used to determine the volume of raw semen required to inseminate one mare, after the percentage of progressive spermatozoal motility has been entered.

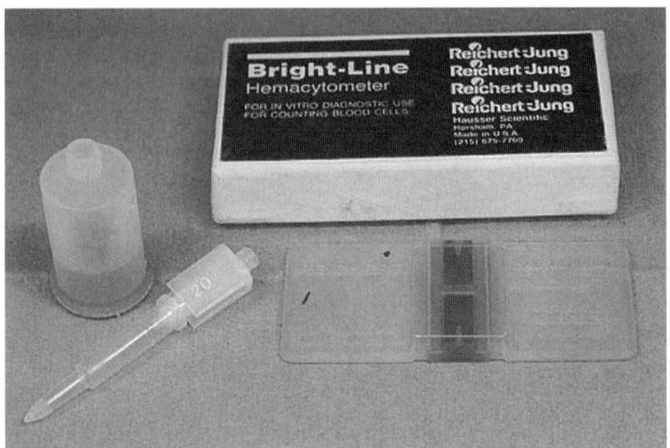

FIGURE 12-16. The spermatozoal concentration of semen (raw or extended) can be determined using a hemocytometer counting chamber (catalog no. 02-671-5; Fisher Scientific, Pittsburgh, PA) and the white blood cell/platelet Unopette system with 20-µl pipettes (catalog no. 13-680). The raw semen is gently mixed, and the pipette is loaded with the semen. The semen in the loaded pipette is aspirated into the diluent within the Unopette and mixed. The pipette is reversed, and the diluted semen is expressed into the cover-slipped hemocytometer chamber, allowing 5 min for spermatozoa to settle. A phase-contrast microscope is used to enumerate the number of spermatozoa in one of the nine large squares on the hemocytometer grid. This procedure is repeated on the other side of the hemocytometer, and the two counts are averaged. The averaged count represents the number of spermatozoa (in millions) per milliliter of raw semen.

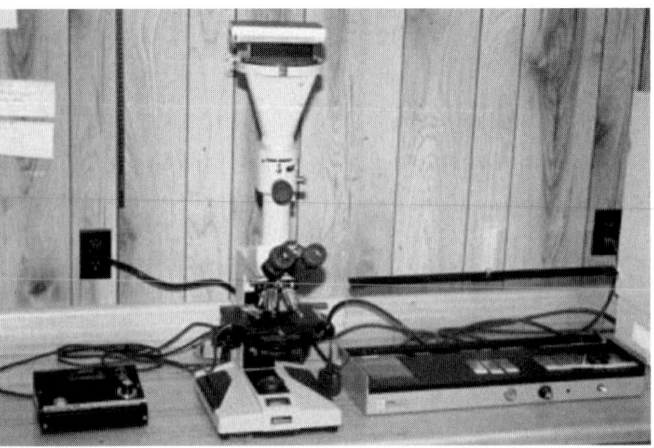

FIGURE 12-17. Raw semen is diluted with prewarmed extender for spermatozoal motility assessment using a phase-contrast microscope with a warming stage. The percentage of spermatozoa moving in a rapid, linear manner represents the percentage of progressively motile spermatozoa in the ejaculate.

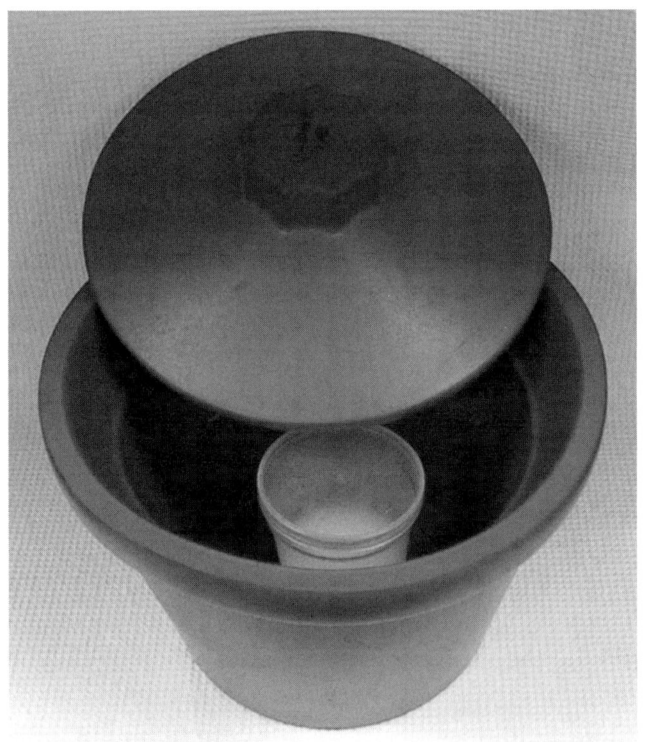

FIGURE 12-18. After semen is extended, it should be removed from the incubator and kept in a light-shielded insulated environment maintained at room temperature (22° to 25° C) until mares have been inseminated (preferably within 1 to 2 hours).

Whether the semen is to be used immediately or preserved, it should always be mixed with an appropriate extender within a few minutes after collection to maximize longevity of spermatozoal viability. An initial semen/extender dilution ratio of 1:1 to 1:2 is generally adequate if semen will not be stored (at room temperature, protected from light) for more than 1 to 2 hours before insemination. Warmed extender can also be placed in the semen receptacle before collection so that the spermatozoa come in contact with this supportive medium immediately after ejaculation. This procedure is seldom necessary except for the occasional stallion whose spermatozoa are found to benefit from immediate placement in a semen extender (i.e., stallions whose seminal plasma seems to depress longevity of spermatozoal motility or otherwise interfere with fertility). To obtain accurate measurements of spermatozoal concentration in extended semen with a spectrophotometer or densimeter, the extenders must be optically clear. If the extender used is not optically clear, a hemocytometer must be used to quantify spermatozoa in the extended ejaculate or, ideally, a small aliquot of raw (undiluted) semen can be procured for quantification of spermatozoal concentration using a spectrophotometer or densimeter.

Properly formulated semen extenders improve spermatozoal survival during the interval between collection and insemination. The most commonly used equine semen extenders are milk based (Table 12-1). Some milk-based extenders are available commercially (Table 12-2). Addition of appropriate antibiotics to semen extenders will aid elimination of bacteria, which invariably contaminate the semen sample during its collection. Polymixin B sulfate (200 to 1000 U/ml), crystalline penicillin (1000 to 1500 U/ml), gentamicin sulfate (100 to 1000 µg/ml), amikacin sulfate (100 to 1000 µg/ml), and ticarcillin (100 to 1000 µg/ml) are commonly used antibiotics. When gentamicin or amikacin are used in extenders, sodium bicarbonate should be added to adjust the pH of the extender. An extender pH range from 6.6 to 7.2 may optimize spermatozoal motility while avoiding premature capacitation of spermatozoa, particularly during cool storage. Texas workers suggest that a combination of potassium penicillin G (1000 U/ml) and amikacin sulfate (1000 µg/ml) in a milk-based semen extender may optimize longevity of spermatozoal motility while providing good broad-spectrum antibacterial activity.

TABLE 12-1

Commonly Used Equine Semen Extenders

Name	Formula*
Kenney extender	1. Mix nonfat dry milk solids (2.4 g) and glucose (4.9 g) with 92 ml of denionized water. 2. Add crystalline penicillin G (150,000 U) and crystalline streptomycin sulfate (150,000 µg) or gentamicin sulfate (100 mg) mixed with 2 ml of 7.5% sodium bicarbonate.
Modified Kenney extender (TAMU formula)	1. Mix nonfat dry milk solids (24 g), glucose (26.5 g), and sucrose (40 g) with 907 ml of deionized water. 2. Add potassium penicillin G (1,000,000 U) and amikacin sulfate (1 g). 3. Buffer to pH 6.8-6.9
Skim milk extender	1. Heat 100 ml of nonfortified skim milk to 92°-95° C for 10 minutes in a double boiler. Cool. 2. Add polymyxin B sulfate (100,000 U).
Cream-gel extender	1. Dissolve 1.3 g of unflavored gelatin in 10 ml of sterile deionized water. Sterilize. 2. Heat half & half cream to 92°-95° C for 2-4 minutes in a double boiler. Remove scum from surface. 3. Mix gelatin solution with 90 ml of heated half & half cream (100ml total volume). Cool. 4. Add crystalline penicillin G (100,000 U), streptomycin sulfate (100,000 µg), and polymyxin B sulfate (20,000 U).
Modified cream-gel extender	1. Heat half & half cream (1 pint) to 85°-92° C in a glass flask in a double boiler for 10 minutes. Remove scum from surface. 2. Dissolve 6 g of unflavored gelatin in 40 ml of 5% dextrose and heat to 65° C in a water bath. 3. Add hot gelatin solution to cream and allow to cool covered to 35°-40° C. 4. Add potassium penicillin G (1,000,000 U) and/or amikacin sulfate (0.5 g).

*Many different antibiotics and antibiotic dosages have been used with these basic extenders, including potassium penicillin G (1000-2000 U/ml), streptomycin sulfate (1000-1500 µg/ml), polymyxin B sulfate (200-1000 U/ml), gentamicin sulfate (100-1000 µg/ml), amikacin sulfate (100-1000 µg/ml), or ticarcillin (100-1000 µg/ml). Use of gentamicin sulfate or amikacin sulfate may require the addition of sodium bicarbonate to adjust the pH of the extender to 6.8-7.0. The extenders can be stored in small packages at −20 °C and thawed immediately before use.

TABLE 12-2

Some Commercially Available Equine Semen Extenders*

Trade Name	Manufacturer	Comments
E-Z Mixin	Animal Reproduction Systems 14395 Ramona Ave. Chino, CA 91710	Available with choice of different antibiotics
Skim Milk Extender	Lane Manufacturing Co. 2045 S Valentia St., Unit 1 Denver, CO 80231	Available with or without antibiotics
Kenney Skim Milk Extender	Har-Vet, Inc. 219 S. McKay Ave. Box 39 Spring Valley, WI 54767	Available with or without antibiotics
Kenney Extender	Hamilton Research, Inc. P.O. Box 2099 South Hamilton, MA 01982	Available without antibiotics
Dr. Kenney Ready Mix Extender	Equine Breeders Services 1102 "S" Street Penrose, CO 81240	Available with or without antibiotics
Next Generation Universal Stallion Semen Extender	Exodus Breeders Supply 5470 Mt. Pisgah Road York, PA 17406	Available with or without antibiotics

* No endorsement of products is intended.

Artificial Insemination

Insemination Timing and Breeding Frequency

In many AI programs, mares are inseminated every other day, beginning on the second or third day of estrus, until ovulation is detected or until the mare no longer exhibits signs of behavioral estrus. When semen from fertile stallions is used, acceptable pregnancy rates can sometimes be obtained when mares are inseminated within 72 hours before ovulation. Rarely will daily, or twice daily, inseminations result in improved pregnancy rates, except for occasional stallions with short spermatozoal viability in ejaculated semen. Limiting the number of inseminations improves the overall efficiency of the breeding program and reduces the risk of iatrogenic contamination of the mare's reproductive tract. Reduction of uterine contamination is especially important when mares with an increased susceptibility to uterine infections are bred. Ideally, regular genital tract examinations should be performed to more accurately predict time of expected ovulation so that the number of inseminations required is minimized. For most stallions, the *goal should be to inseminate each mare once within 48 hours prior to ovulation*. If a mare has not ovulated after being bred 48 hours previously, the mare should be inseminated again.

Although good fertility has been reported when mares were bred after ovulation, postovulation breeding requires further study before it can be recommended as a routine practice. For example, Wisconsin workers reported that mares bred 0 to 6 hours postovulation had normal pregnancy rates (similar to mares bred 1 to 3 days before ovulation) and did not experience increased embryonic death rates. Mares bred 6 to 12 hours postovulation had normal pregnancy rates but suffered an increase in embryonic losses. Mares bred 12 to 24 hours postovulation suffered both lower pregnancy rates and higher embryonic losses than mares bred before ovulation or within 6 hours after ovulation.

Insemination Dose (Number of Spermatozoa)

Typically, mares in an AI program are inseminated with 250 to 500 million progressively motile spermatozoa. Insemination of mares with 500 million progressively motile spermatozoa will help ensure that acceptable pregnancy rates are achieved by allowing some margin for error in semen evaluation and handling when conditions are less than optimal. If semen is carefully handled and from a highly fertile stallion, the insemination dose can sometimes be reduced to 100 million progressively motile spermatozoa without reducing fertility. Reducing insemination doses to <100 million progressively motile spermatozoa is not recommended. For example, Texas workers recently achieved reduced pregnancy rates per cycle (30%) when using only 20 to 60 million progressively motile spermatozoa in an insemination volume of 4 ml.

Another study revealed that mares inseminated with 50 million motile spermatozoa had a lower overall pregnancy rate (38%) than did mares inseminated with 500 million motile spermatozoa (75%).

Insemination Volume

The number of spermatozoa in an insemination dose appears to be more critical than the volume of the inseminate. Although smaller or larger volumes can be used successfully, typical insemination volumes for extended equine semen range from 10 to 30 ml. When timed closely with ovulation, insemination of frozen/thawed semen in volumes as low as 0.5 ml has resulted in pregnancies. Large insemination volumes are not advantageous because much of this volume may be lost through the mare's dilated cervix after insemination.

Often, only a small number of mares are to be inseminated with an ejaculate, so it is commonly diluted with extender with the total volume being equally divided among the mares to be bred. When a large number of mares are to be inseminated with a single ejaculate, insemination volume (IV) can be calculated by dividing the desired number of progressively motile spermatozoa per insemination (PMS dose) (e.g., 100 to 500 million) by the product of the spermatozoal concentration in the extended semen (SC) and the percentage of progressively motile spermatozoa in the ejaculate (%PM, expressed as a decimal):

$$\text{IV (ml)} = \frac{\text{PMS dose}}{\text{SC} \times \text{\%PM}}$$

Insemination Procedure

Sterile, nontoxic disposable equipment is recommended for AI procedures (Figure 12-19). Syringes with nonspermicidal, plastic plungers (Air-Tite, Vineland, NJ) are preferable for AI because some rubber plungers may possess spermicidal properties. Individual stallion variation seems to exist regarding spermatozoal sensitivity to the toxic effects of syringes with rubber plunger tips. Toxic effects are apparent in semen from some stallions with as little as 1 minute of contact with some syringe plungers. Washing and sterilization of syringes does not appear to affect spermatozoal motility; therefore, properly prepared syringes may be reused as a cost-saving and ecologically sound approach to horse breeding.

Insemination of the mare should be performed in accordance with the minimum contamination techniques described by Kenney and coworkers (1975). The mare should be adequately restrained with her tail wrapped and diverted either to the side or over her rump. The perineal area is thoroughly scrubbed and rinsed, paying particular attention to the vulva. Any dirt or fecal material within the caudal vestibule should be removed during the washing process to prevent contamination of the upper reproductive tract during insemination. Two to three scrubs with soap or a surgical scrub are recommended, followed by thorough rinsing to eliminate residual soap that may be spermicidal or irritating to mucous membranes.

To inseminate a mare, a sterile shoulder-length plastic sleeve is first placed over the arm used for insemination. The tip of a 20- to 22-inch insemination pipette is then positioned in the cupped hand and a small amount of sterile, nonspermicidal lubricant is applied to the back of the hand. The covered hand and insemination pipette are passed into the cranial vaginal vault where the index finger identifies and penetrates the cervix. The insemination pipette is then advanced through the cervix to the mid-body of the uterus. A syringe containing extended semen is attached to the insemination pipette, and the semen is slowly deposited into the uterine lumen (Figure 12-20). An alternative, but equally satisfactory, method of insemination is to pass the insemination pipette through the cervix using a lighted speculum preplaced in the vagina (Figures 12-21 and 12-22).

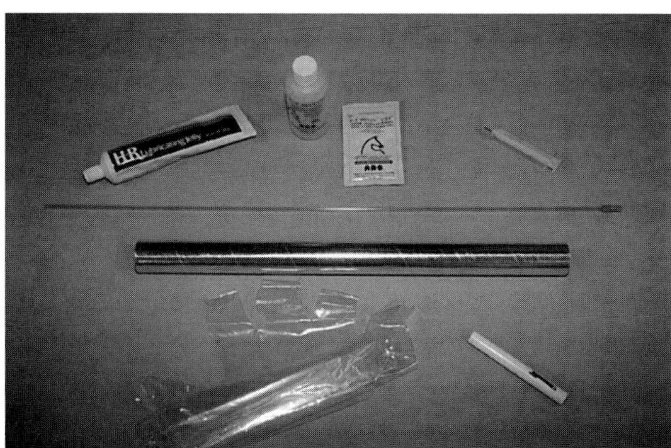

FIGURE 12-19. Equipment commonly used for artificial insemination of horses using fresh semen. *Clockwise from upper left:* sterile, nonspermicidal lubricant; semen extender; sterile nontoxic syringe; insemination pipette; disposable vaginal speculum; pen-light for illuminating cervix through speculum; and plastic sleeve.

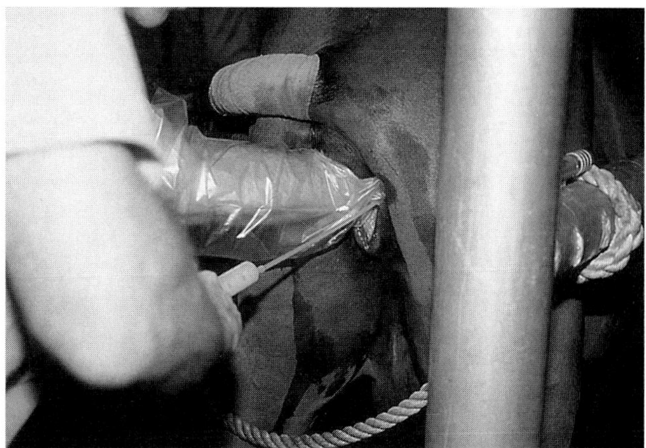

FIGURE 12-20. To perform artificial insemination, a pipette is carried in a lubricated, gloved hand into the cranial vagina and guided through the cervix into the uterine body where the extended semen is slowly deposited.

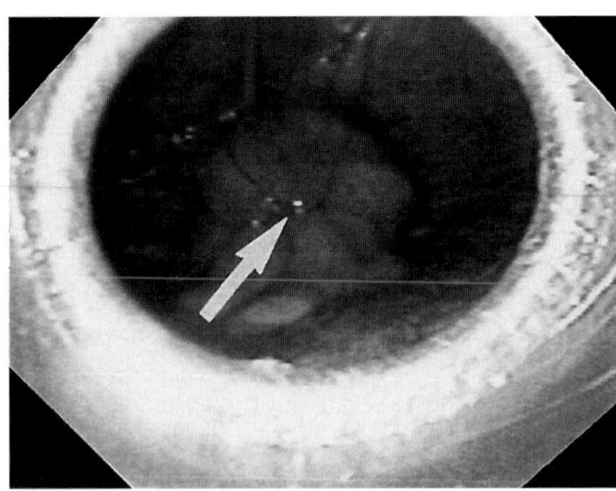

FIGURE 12-21. A sterile, disposable vaginal speculum and light can be used for artificial insemination of horses. The external os of the cervix is positioned at the end of the speculum as shown in this photograph.

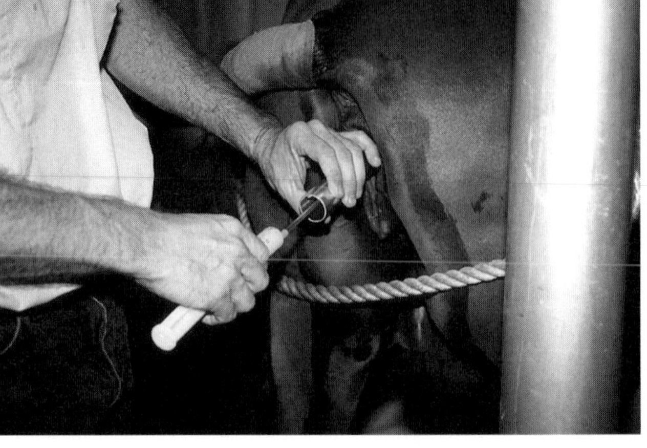

FIGURE 12-22. Photograph illustrating insemination through a vaginal speculum. The pipette has been passed through the cervix (shown in Figure 12-21), and the syringe is attached for insemination.

General Considerations

Semen from the stallion is normally delivered directly to the protective confines of the mare's reproductive tract at the time of breeding; therefore, if one plans to collect semen for in vitro storage and transport, it is necessary to first become fully aware of the vulnerability of spermatozoa to the external environment. Spermatozoa are very sensitive to many environmental factors, including temperature, light, physical trauma, and a variety of chemicals.

SUMMARY

Artificial insemination is an effective technique for improving the use of stallions in breeding programs. When proper semen handling and insemination procedures are used, optimal pregnancy rates are attainable. When AI techniques are used for mares and stallions with marginal fertility, pregnancy rates are sometimes improved over those achieved with natural mating.

BIBLIOGRAPHY

Brinsko SP, Varner DD: Artificial insemination and preservation of semen. *Vet Clin North Am Equine Pract* 8:205-218, 1992.

Forney BD: How to collect semen from stallions while they are standing on the ground. *Proc Am Assoc Equine Pract* 45:142-144, 1999.

Kenney RM, Bergman RV, Cooper WL et al: Minimum contamination techniques for breeding mares: techniques and preliminary findings. *Proc Am Assoc Equine Pract* 21:327-336, 1975.

McDonnell SM, Love CC: Manual stimulation collection of semen from stallions: training time, sexual behavior and semen. *Theriogenology* 33:1201-1210, 1990.

Varner DD, Schumacher J, Blanchard TL et al: *Diseases and management of breeding stallions.* Goleta, CA, 1991, American Veterinary Publications.

Woods J, Bergfelt DR, Ginther OJ: Effects of time of insemination relative to ovulation on pregnancy rate and embryonic-loss rate in mares. *Equine Vet J* 22:410-415, 1990.

13

Examination of the Stallion for Breeding Soundness

OBJECTIVES

While studying the information covered in this chapter, the student should attempt to:

1. Acquire a working understanding of the anatomy and physiology of the reproductive organs of the stallion.
2. Acquire a working understanding of how abnormalities of the reproductive organs, general physical soundness, or sexual behavior can adversely affect stallion fertility.
3. Acquire a working understanding of procedures used for evaluation of a stallion for breeding soundness.

STUDY QUESTIONS

1. Describe the objective of a breeding soundness examination of a stallion.
2. List procedures that should be performed during a breeding soundness examination of a stallion.
3. Describe the anatomy of the normal reproductive tract of a stallion, including the prepuce, penis, scrotum and its contents, vas deferens, and accessory sex glands.
4. List potential venereal pathogens that may be transmitted by stallions.
5. Describe procedures used for evaluating semen quality of stallions, including but not limited to:
   a. gross evaluation of semen.
   b. spermatozoal concentration.
   c. semen volume.
   d. number of sperm in ejaculate.
   e. semen pH.
   f. spermatozoal motility.
   g. spermatozoal morphology.
6. Summarize minimal criteria that should be met for a stallion to be classified as a satisfactory breeding prospect.

OBJECTIVE

The objective of a breeding soundness examination is to determine whether a stallion has the mental and physical faculties necessary to deliver semen that contains viable spermatozoa but no infectious disease to the mare's reproductive tract at the proper time, ensuring the establishment of pregnancy in a reasonable number of mares bred per season. The examiner not only *evaluates the quality and quantity of ejaculated spermatozoa* but also tests the *libido* and *mating ability* of a stallion, attempts to recognize *congenital defects* that may be transmissible to offspring and/or decrease a stallion's fertility, identifies *infectious diseases* that may be transmitted venereally, and searches for any other lesions that may reduce a stallion's longevity as a sire.

A record that summarizes results of the breeding soundness examination should be provided to the owner of the stallion after completion of the examination. An example of a type of form used for this purpose is shown in Figure13-1.

HISTORY AND IDENTIFICATION

Collection of historical information about a stallion is an indispensable part of a breeding soundness examination. This information should be gathered in a methodical unassuming manner to ensure completeness and avoid inaccuracies. Possible environmental and heritable causes for the admitting problem should be addressed, and previous modes of therapy for an existing problem should be investigated when applicable. A historical review of stallions to be examined for breeding soundness should include their present usage, previous breeding performance, results of prior fertility evaluations, illnesses, injuries, and medications and vaccinations, with explicit information about previous and current reproductive management and medical programs.

Positive identification of the stallion, often considered a mundane procedure, is an integral part of the examination process, especially when sale of the horse is involved. Identification of a stallion must be accurate to avoid any ambiguity in identity at a subsequent date. Name, age, breed, and

Stallion Information:
Name: ____________ Case #: ____________
Age: ________ Breed: ____________ Color: ________
Lip Tattoo #: __________ Registration #: __________
Markings / Brands: ____________________

Present Breeding Status:
☐ Sexually rested ☐ Actively breeding
☐ At daily sperm output (DSO)
Intended Use: ____________________

Owner / Agent: ____________________
Address: ____________________
Telephone: ____________________
Facsimile: ____________________
Referring Veterinarian: ____________________
Address: ____________________
Telephone: ____________________
Facsimile: ____________________

History: ____________________

Physical Breeding Condition: ____________________

External Genital Examination: Method(s) Used: ☐ Palpation ☐ Ultrasound ☐ Calipers ☐ Other ________

- Testis: Left Right
  - L x W x H (cm): ________ ________
  - Volume (cm^3): ________ ________
  - Consistency: ________ ________
- Epididymis: ________ ________
- Spermatic Cord: ________ ________
- Other Findings: ____________________

A

- Prepuce/Penis: ____________________
- Scrotum: ____________________
- Total Testicular Volume (cc): ____________________
- Actual sperm # ejaculated at DSO ($x10^9$): ____________
- Estimated sperm # ejaculated at DSO ($x10^9$) (method): ________
- Predicted DSO based on testicular volume ($x10^9$): ________
- Spermatogenic efficiency (%): ____________
- Sperm output/gram testis/day at DSO ($x\ 10^6$): ________

Internal Genital Examination: ☐ Performed ☐ Not performed
Methods(s) Used: ☐ Palpation ☐ Ultrasound ☐ Other ________

	Left	Right		Left	Right
● Inguinal Ring (size):	________	________	● Ampulla :	________	________
● Vesicular Gland:	________	________	● Prostatic Lobe:	________	________

Behavior and Breeding Ability:

Temperament	Libido	Erection	Mounting	Intromission	Ejaculation

Culture and Sensitivity:
☐ Pre-Wash Penile Shaft: ____________________
☐ Pre-Wash Fossa Glandis: ____________________
☐ Post-Wash Urethra: ____________________
☐ Post-Ejaculate Urethra: ____________________
☐ Semen: ____________________
☐ Other (__________): ____________________

Other Examination Findings: ____________________

Additional Diagnostic Tests:

Test	Date Performed	Result

FIGURE 13-1. Example of a stallion breeding soundness evaluation form.

Semen Evaluation	Ejaculate 1	Ejaculate 2	Ejaculate 3
Collection Time / Collection Method:			
Number of Mounts / Time to First Mount (minutes):			
Volume (ml) - gel-free / gel:			
Gross Appearance:			
Seminal pH (method) / Seminal Osmolarity(method):			
Initial Motility (% total / % progressive[velocity]) ☐ Raw			
(Vel.. = 0-4 or microns/sec) Method used: _________ ☐ Extended			
Concentration (x 10^6/ml) - Method used: ____________________			
Total Number of Sperm (x 10^9):			
Total Number of Sperm x % Progressively Motile (x 10^9):			

Sperm Morphology: ☐ Buffered Formol Saline ☐ Phase Contrast Microscopy ☐ Bright Field Microscopy ☐ Differential Interference Microscopy ☐ Stain: ____________________ ☐ Other: ____________________

	Ejaculate 1	Ejaculate 2	Ejaculate 3
% Normal			
% Abnormal Heads			
% Abnormal Acrosomes			
% Tailless Heads			
% Proximal Droplets			
% Distal Droplets			
% Abnormally-Shaped Midpieces			
% Bent Midpieces			
% Bent Tails			
% Coiled Tails			
% Premature (Round) (Germ Cells)			
% Other Abnormalities: ________________________________			
Total Number Sperm x % Morphologically Normal (x 10^9)			

Longevity (Viability) Test: Reported as Storage Time (Hours) / Motility (Total/Progressive[Velocity])

	Ejaculate 1	Ejaculate 2	Ejaculate 3
Raw at __ °C:			
__________________ Extender at __ °C: (dilution = _______)			
__________________ Extender at __ °C: (dilution = _______)			

Comments:____

Classification as Breeding Prospect: ☐ **Satisfactory** ☐ **Questionable** ☐ **Unsatisfactory**

B

☐ See attached letter

Signature: ________________________________

registration number of the stallion are recorded, in addition to identifying marks, such as a lip tattoo, hide brands, color markings, and hair whorls. When possible, photographs of the stallion should be taken for permanent identification.

GENERAL PHYSICAL EXAMINATION

Although a breeding soundness examination focuses on the genital health of stallions, general physical condition cannot be ignored. An assessment of general body condition is done first. Particular attention should be given to abnormalities that will affect mating ability (e.g., lameness or back problems) or that are potentially heritable (e.g., cryptorchidism, parrot mouth, or wobbler syndrome). All abnormalities are recorded. Examination of the various body systems (respiratory, cardiovascular, digestive, nervous, urinary, ophthalmic, and musculoskeletal) can be cursory, although abnormalities should be noted and pursued diagnostically if the potential exists for interference with breeding ability or fertility. Common laboratory tests (Coggins test, hematologic analysis, serum chemistry, urinalysis, and fecal egg counts) can support physical examination findings in determining the general health of a stallion.

PHYSICAL EXAMINATION OF REPRODUCTIVE TRACT

Knowledge of normal genital anatomy is essential to a competent physical examination of the stallion's reproductive tract. A thorough physical examination of both external and internal genital organs always should be incorporated into procedures for predicting stallion fertility.

External Genitalia

The preferred method to allow close inspection of the penis (Figure13-2) is to stimulate penile tumescence through exposure of the stallion to a mare in estrus. This procedure also permits assessment of sexual behavior, including erection capability. Manual extraction of the penis from the prepuce for examination is difficult and usually met with resistance from the stallion. In shy stallions, the penis can often be visualized from a distance while the horse urinates. Urination can sometimes be stimulated by placing the horse in a freshly bedded stall; shaking the bedding may increase the horse's urge to urinate. Tranquilization (acepromazine or xylazine) elicits penile prolapse, making the penis accessible; however, tranquilizers, especially those that are phenothiazine-derived (e.g., acepromazine), can cause *penile paralysis* or *priapism* and, therefore, should not be used indiscriminately. Additionally, tranquilizers will probably render the horse ataxic and interfere with mounting when collection of semen is attempted.

The penis may require cleansing before its inspection (Figure 13-3), because epithelial debris mixed with secretions from the preputial glands accumulates in the preputial cavity

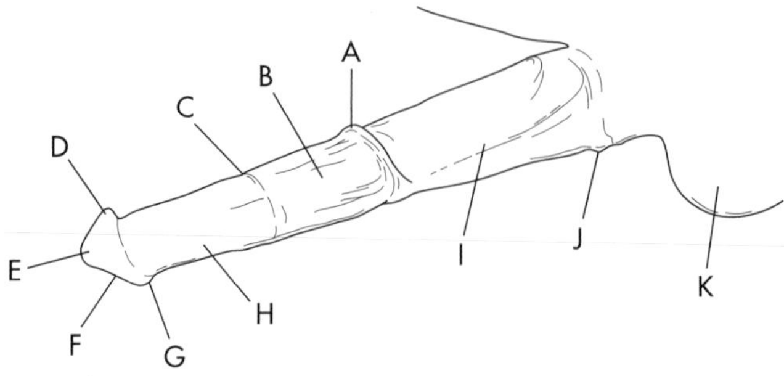

FIGURE 13-2. Structures of the stallion's penis and prepuce: *(A)* preputial ring, *(B)* internal lamina of the internal prepuce, *(C)* attachment of the internal lamina of the internal prepuce to the penis, *(D)* corona glandis, *(E)* glans penis, *(F)* urethral process, *(G)* collum glandis, *(H)* free portion of the penile body, *(I)* external lamina of the internal prepuce, *(J)* preputial orifice, and *(K)* scrotum. (From Varner DD, Schumacher J, Blanchard TL, et al: *Diseases and management of breeding stallions.* St Louis, 1991, Mosby.)

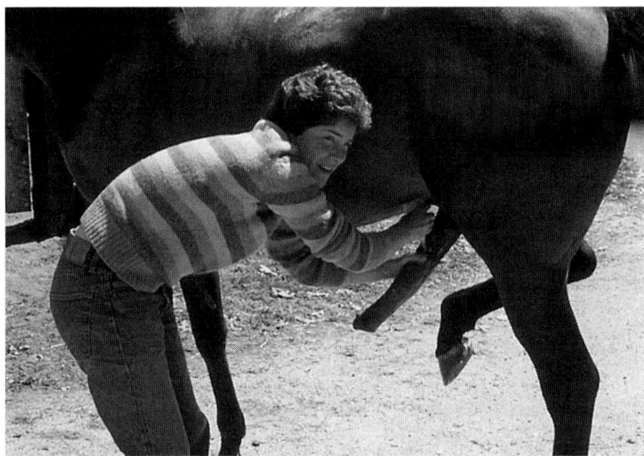

FIGURE 13-3. Cleansing the shaft of the penis of a stallion. Generally only warm tap water and clean paper towels are needed to wash a stallion's penis. Soaps or disinfectants are not usually used to avoid displacement of normal flora.

and on the exterior of the penis when it is unattended. The root and proximal body of the penis are buried in tissue, thereby limiting the examination to the exposed body and glans. The penis should be examined thoroughly, and any palpable or visual lesions should be recorded. Because the fossa glandis and urethral process are partially concealed, particular attention should be given to these areas (Figure 13-4). Common penile lesions include those of traumatic origin as well as vesicles/pustules of equine coital exanthema, habronema granulomas, squamous cell carcinomas, and papillomas.

During penile tumescence, the prepuce also is readily available for examination. The skin of the prepuce should be thin and pliable, with no evidence of inflammatory or proliferative lesions. Developmental abnormalities of the penis and prepuce are rare.

The scrotum (Figure 13-5) of the stallion should be thin and elastic, with a distinct neck. The scrotum and its contents

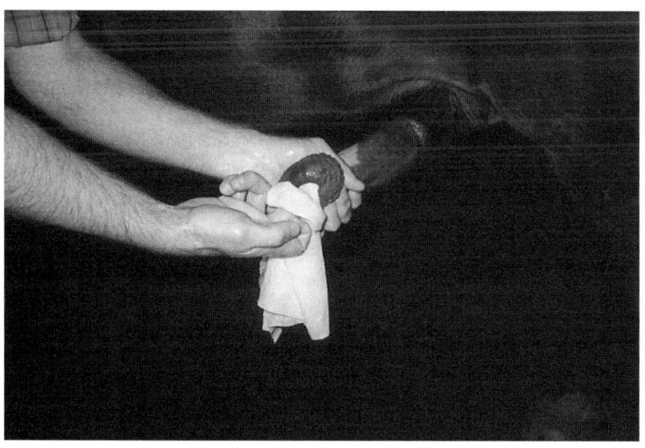

FIGURE 13-4. Cleansing the fossa glandis and urethral process of a stallion's penis.

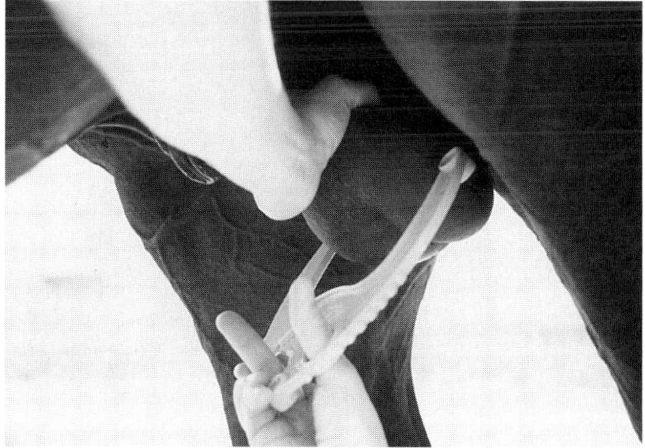

FIGURE 13-6. Measurement of scrotal width using calipers. The testes are gently held in the bottom of the scrotum while the widest measurement across both testes is taken.

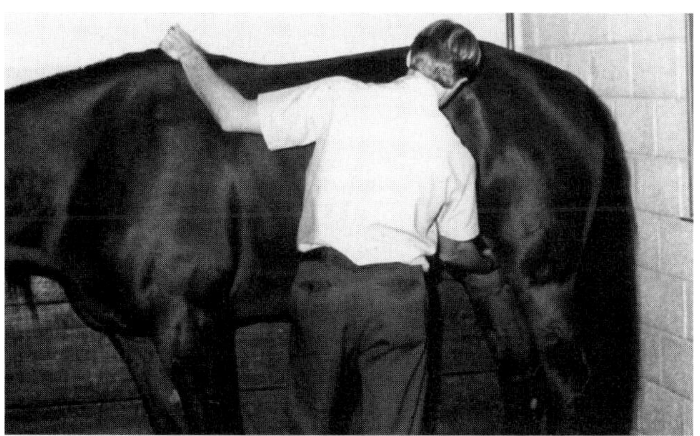

FIGURE 13-5. Palpation of the external genitalia of a stallion for identification of abnormalities. (From Varner DD, Schumacher J, Blanchard TL et al: *Diseases and management of breeding stallions.* St Louis, 1991, Mosby.)

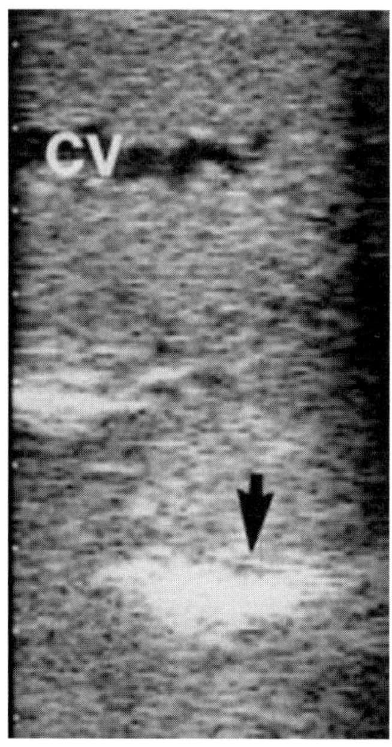

FIGURE 13-7. Transcrotal ultrasonographic image of stallion testes. The anechoic area in the near testis is the central vein. The *arrow* points to a hyperechoic area of the far testis. At castration, the testes were degenerated and the hyperechoic area was fibrous tissue with some calcification.

are normally pendulous (except during cold weather because of contractions of the tunica dartos) but may be drawn toward the body during palpation because of voluntary contractions of the cremaster muscles. Both testes and attached epididymides should be freely movable within their respective scrotal pouches. Size, texture, and position of each testis always should be determined as part of a breeding soundness examination. Testicular size correlates highly with daily spermatozoal production, so this measurement helps predict a stallion's breeding potential. Testes of mature (≥4 years of age), fertile stallions generally are approximately 4.5 to 6 cm in width, 5 to 6.5 cm in height, and 8.5 to 11 cm in length; the total scrotal width (largest measurement taken across both testes and the scrotal skin) (Figure 13-6) generally is approximately 9.5 to 11.5 cm. Transcrotal ultrasonographic examination, including accurate measurement of size, can provide useful information about the normality of the scrotal contents (Figures 13-7 and 13-8). When length, width, and height of each testis are measured in centimeters, testicular volume (in milliliters) can be estimated using the formula for an ellipsoid (volume = 0.5233 × width × height × length). Volume should be computed for each testis, and the two volumes are added together to provide total testicular volume. Testicular volumes can be compared against averages established for horses of a similar age to give the examiner an impression of whether the testes are small or not (Table 13-1). The total testicular volume (TV) can also be used to predict daily sperm output (DSO) with the following formula:

$$\text{DSO (billions of sperm/day)} = (0.024 \times \text{TV}) - 1.26.$$

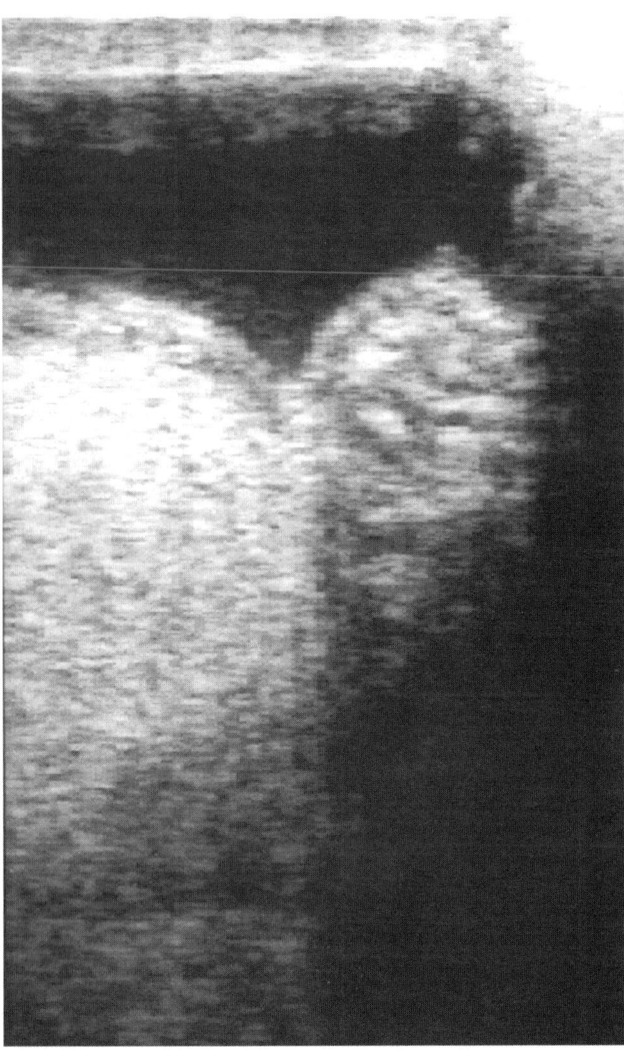

FIGURE 13-8. Lateral to medial longitudinal ultrasonographic image of the caudal half of the testis. The tail (cauda) of the epididymis is located at the right of the testis. The epididymis and testis are surrounded by fluid (hydrocele).

TABLE 13-1

Average Total Testicular Volumes for Horses of Different Ages

Age (yr)	Total Testicular Volume (ml)
1.0	50
1.5	71
2.0	95
2.5	119
3.0	167
4-5	272
6-12	313
13-20	306

Modified from Johnson L, Thompson DL Jr: *Biol Reprod* 29:777-789, 1983; and from Johnson L et al: *J Reprod Fertil* 44(Suppl):97, 1987.

When predicted DSO is significantly less than actual DSO, low spermatogenic efficiency due to testicular dysfunction is probably present.

In addition to its use to obtain accurate testicular measurements, ultrasonography can be used to detect intratesticular masses and intrascrotal fluid accumulations and to examine the cavernous spaces of the penis (see Chapter 16). Ultrasonography is also a useful adjunct to examinations made per rectum (e.g., for evaluation of the accessory genital glands or abdominal/inguinal exploration for an undescended testis in a stallion suspected of being a cryptorchid).

Both testes should be oval, with a smooth regular outline and a slightly turgid, resilient texture. The position of each testis within the scrotum can be determined accurately by palpation of the attached epididymis. The caudal ligament of the epididymis, a remnant of the gubernaculum, remains palpable during adult life as a small (~1 cm) fibrous nodule adjacent to the epididymal tail which, itself, is attached to the caudal pole of the testis. Therefore, this remnant serves as a landmark for determining testicular orientation within the scrotum. The epididymis normally is palpable in its entirety as it courses over the dorsolateral surface of the testis; however, its borders sometimes are difficult to identify.

Exploration of the spermatic cord is possible via palpation through the neck of the scrotum, although its specific contents often are not definable. Transcrotal ultrasonographic examination can also be used to visualize these structures. Spermatic cords should be of equal size and uniform diameter (2 to 3 cm). Acute pain in this area usually is associated with inguinal herniation or torsion of the spermatic cord. Inguinal herniation can usually be confirmed by ultrasonography, which reveals some degree of hydrocele (anechoic fluid accumulation between parietal and vaginal tunics) with hyperechoic gut wall patterns, in which fluid within the bowel lumen is sometimes visible. Transrectal palpation/ultrasonography of internal inguinal ring(s) will confirm the herniation. Torsion of the spermatic cord can result in congestion of the affected testis (palpably turgid and slightly hyperechoic) with thickening and engorgement of the spermatic cord due to vascular obstruction (see Chapter 16).

Internal Genitalia

The internal genital organs (Figure 13-9) can be examined by palpation per rectum. Adequate restraint is of paramount importance to this procedure. Minimal but effective restraint is the key to a safe examination and varies from stallion to stallion. The disposition of the stallion should be determined at the onset, and the examination should be canceled if the risk factor is high. Such precautions will protect both the stallion and operator from severe injury. Before the examination, stallions should be placed in stocks, if available. Ideally, the stocks should be equipped with a solid rear door to help prevent leg extension if the stallion decides to kick. The height of the door should be level with the mid-gaskin region of the stallion's hindquarters. Higher doors can damage the operator's

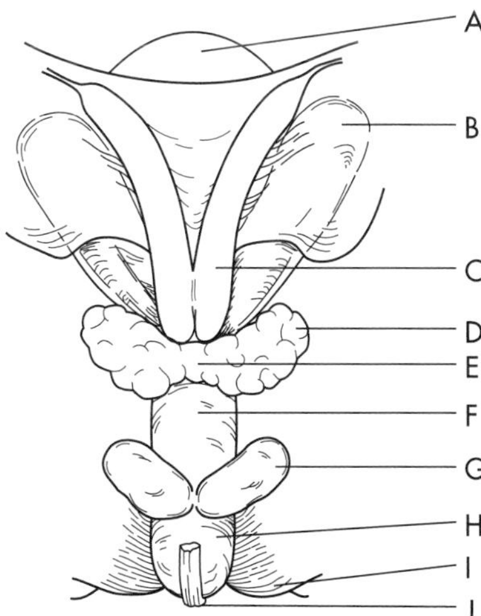

FIGURE 13-9. Accessory genital glands of the stallion (dorsal view): *(A)* bladder, *(B)* right vesicular gland, *(C)* right ampulla, *(D)* right lobe of the prostate gland, *(E)* isthmus of the prostate gland, *(F)* urethralis muscle, *(G)* right bulbourethral gland, *(H)* bulbospongiosus muscle, *(I)* right ischiocavernosus muscle, and *(J)* retractor penis muscle. (Modified from Varner DD, Schumacher J, Blanchard TL et al: *Diseases and management of breeding stallions.* St Louis, 1991, Mosby.)

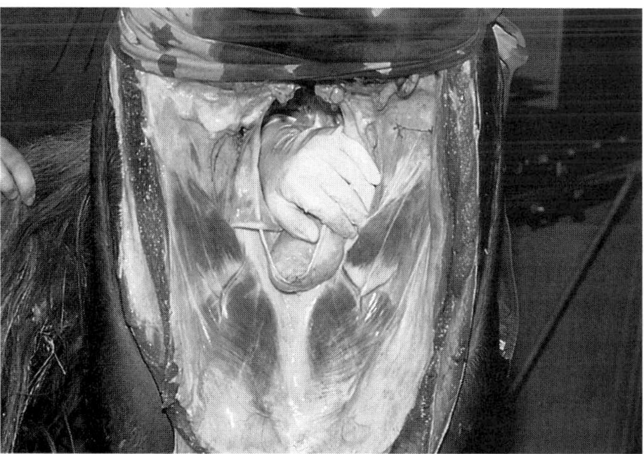

FIGURE 13-10. Palpation of the vaginal rings per rectum. The rectum has been removed to facilitate visualization.

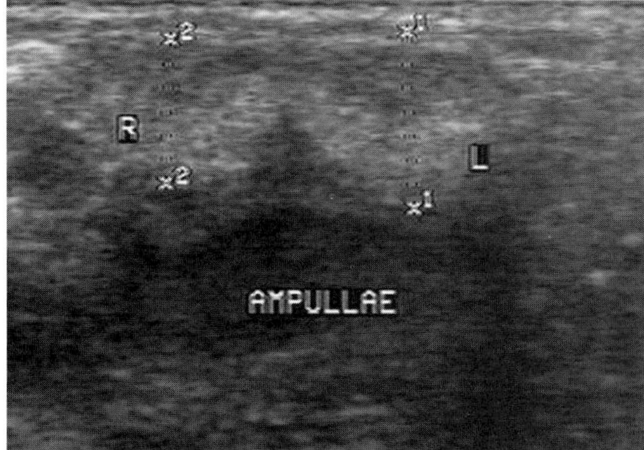

FIGURE 13-11. Transrectal transverse-oblique ultrasonographic image of the ampullae of a stallion. In some stallions, the lumen is visible as an anechoic central area within the ampullae.

arm if a stallion squats abruptly while the operator's arm is in the rectum. Lower doors permit the stallion to kick over this barrier. Poorly designed doors do not protect the examiner and increase the likelihood of unnecessary injury to the stallion. If necessary, a twitch also can be placed on the stallion's muzzle for additional restraint. Tranquilization may be required to adequately restrain an anxious stallion. Remember, over-restraint can be as dangerous to the stallion and operator as under-restraint.

The hand should be well lubricated, and all manure in the rectum and distal colon should be removed before evaluation of pelvic and abdominal structures is attempted. The two vaginal rings (abdominal orifices of the inguinal canals) are palpable as slit-like openings ventrolateral to the pelvic brim (Figure 13-10). The deferent duct and pulse of the testicular artery usually can be detected at the opening. The site is evaluated for size as well as for evidence of adhesions or herniation of viscera. The diameter of the opening is normally 2 to 3 cm. A larger opening may predispose the stallion to inguinal herniation or scrotal hydrocele. Some of the accessory genital organs (i.e., the *ampullae,* and bilobed *prostate gland*) are also readily detected by palpation per rectum and by transrectal ultrasonography (Figures 13-11 through 13-13). Lesions of the accessory genital glands, however, are uncommon in stallions.

OBSERVATION OF LIBIDO AND MATING ABILITY

Excellent semen quality in a breeding prospect is inconsequential unless that stallion also has the desire and ability to deliver the semen to the mare's reproductive tract or an artificial vagina. Sexual behavior can be evaluated by bringing the stallion in contact with a mare in estrus. Typically, a stallion with good libido shows immediate and intense desire for the mare, manifested by restlessness, pawing, vocalization, and intimate precopulatory activity, such as sniffing, licking, and nipping the mare; exhibition of the "Flehmen" reaction (curling of the upper lip, primarily a response to sniffing of the mare's genitalia or urine); and development of an erection (Figure 13-14). The onset, intensity, and duration of this courtship phase are affected by the stallion's genetic makeup, learned behavior (through both positive and negative experiences), seasonal variation, and disease. A common cause for reduced or arrested libido in stallions is mismanagement, especially overuse or repetitive abusive punishment for expression of sexual interest. Length of the courtship phase and number of mounts required for ejaculation tend to increase in winter compared with summer. The physiologic mechanisms of stallion sexual behavior are not well understood but

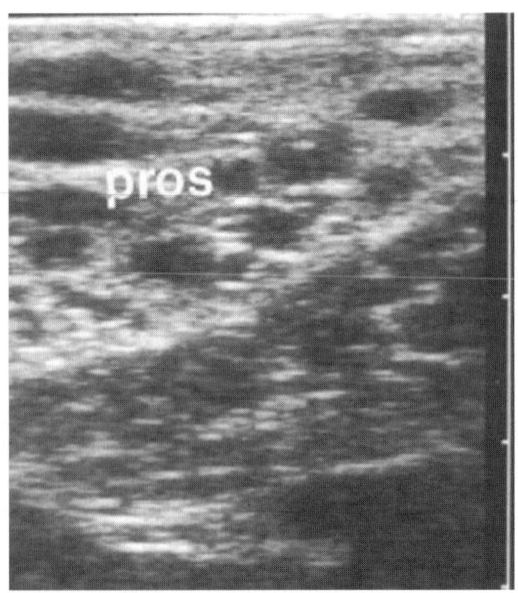

FIGURE 13-12. Transrectal longitudinal image of the right prostatic lobe of a stallion. Acini are visible within the prostate.

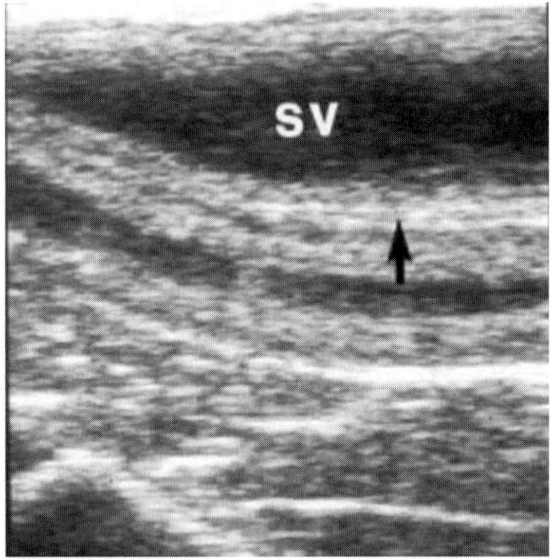

FIGURE 13-13. Transrectal longitudinal image of the right seminal vesicle of a stallion. The stallion was teased to a mare in estrus before examination to ensure that the seminal vesicle would fill with gel. Unless this procedure is used, the seminal vesicle is often difficult to palpate or visualize by ultrasonography. The ventral border of the seminal vesicle is denoted by the *black arrow.*

involve an intricate relationship between endocrine and neural systems.

The ability of a stallion to copulate normally (develop an erection, mount without hesitation, insert the penis, provide intravaginal thrusts, and ejaculate) should be assessed before the stallion is considered to be a satisfactory prospect for breeding. The most common physical abnormalities associated with inability to mount are hindlimb lameness (e.g., degenerative arthritis of the hock or stifle or even chronic laminitis). The etiology of erection and/or ejaculatory failure, unrelated to psychologic malfunction, can be difficult to determine. Penile injuries, spinal cord lesions, and idiopathic organic dysfunctions can lead to impotence. For a thorough discussion of sexual behavior or ejaculatory dysfunction, the student is referred to McDonnell (1992a, 1992b).

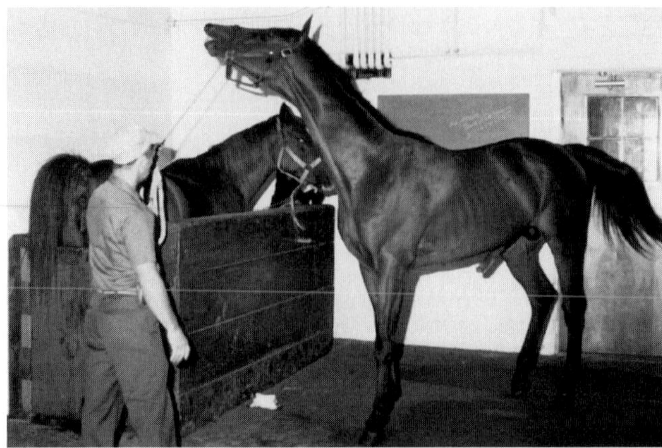

FIGURE 13-14. Exposure of a stallion to a mare in estrus, resulting in penile erection, vocalization, and display of the "Flehmen" reaction. (From Varner DD, Schumacher J, Blanchard TL et al: *Diseases and management of breeding stallions.* St Louis, 1991, Mosby.)

EXAMINATION FOR VENEREAL DISEASE

Several pathogenic microorganisms are transmitted by sexual contact, including bacteria, viruses, and protozoa. The role of fungi and *Chlamydia, Mycoplasma,* and *Ureaplasma* spp. in venereal disease is unknown but is not considered to be significant. Depending on the etiologic agent involved, venereal disease may manifest itself through overt clinical signs in the stallion or, more commonly, "infected" stallions may be asymptomatic carriers.

Bacterial Genital Infections

Superficial bacterial colonization of the equine prepuce, penis, and distal urethra results in unavoidable contamination of the mare's reproductive tract during coitus. A variety of environmental bacteria can be isolated from these sites, many of which contribute to the normal nonpathogenic bacterial flora of healthy stallions. These commensal bacteria tend to prevent overpopulation of the external genitalia with potentially harmful organisms (*Klebsiella pneumoniae* or *Pseudomonas aeruginosa*). Mismanagement of breeding stallions (through repeated penile washings with soaps or disinfectants or poor selection and upkeep of bedding) may convert the bacterial population on the surface of the penis from a mixed group of harmless bacteria to a population teeming with potential pathogens. The external genitalia of some stallions harbor large numbers of these opportunistic bacteria despite the lack of evidence for precipitating factors. The organism that causes contagious equine metritis, *Taylorella equigenitalis,* represents the only known bacterium capable of consistently producing venereal disease in horses. The stallion serves as a lesionless carrier of this disease, harboring the bacteria on its external genitalia, with subsequent horizontal transmission to the mare's reproductive tract at breeding.

Internal Genital Infections. Internal genital infections in the stallion are rare. Such infections are sometimes associated with hemospermia. Accumulation of leukocytes and the inciting bacteria in ejaculates is typical for stallions with internal genital infections.

Documentation of a bacterial infection depends on serial isolation of a pathogen, preferably in large numbers and in relatively pure culture. The exception is culture of *T. equigenitalis,* for which a single isolation is considered diagnostic (tests for *T. equigenitalis* must be conducted only at designated stations and by an accredited veterinarian under the direction of a state or federal veterinarian). To identify organisms on the exterior of the penis or prepuce, swabs of these areas should be taken for bacteriologic culture before one scrubs the penis to obtain urethral swabs. Ideally, specimens should be retrieved from the fossa glandis, urethral sinus, free portion of the penile body, and folds of the external prepuce to provide an overall perspective of the microbial population. The stallion should be placed near a mare in estrus to achieve an erection and facilitate procurement of these samples for culture.

If one is to gain insight into the cause of a possible infection of the internal genital tract, the penis and prepuce of the stallion should be washed meticulously with a surgical scrub before collection of appropriate samples for culture. Particular attention is given to removal of debris and organisms from the glans penis and fossa glandis. A thorough rinse should follow the scrub, and the procedure should be repeated twice. After the final rinse, the penis is dried thoroughly to ensure that the urethral orifice has not been contaminated. Briskly rubbing the glans penis during the washing process usually stimulates voluminous secretion of clear fluid (the presperm fraction of ejaculate), originating from the urethral and/or bulbourethral glands, into the urethral lumen. This procedure helps remove any bacterial contaminants that may have gained access via the external urethral orifice from the urethral lumen. Some of this fluid may be collected for culture and cytologic examination if an infection of the urethra or bulbourethral glands is suspected. A cotton swab is inserted 3 to 5 cm into the distal urethra to procure a sample for bacterial culture before semen collection (pre-ejaculate swab) (Figure 13-15).

After collection of semen, the distal urethra is swabbed again immediately upon removal of the penis from the artificial vagina; the urethral opening should not be contaminated before or during the swabbing process. Semen also can be sampled for bacteriologic culture, realizing that the semen has passed through the artificial vagina contaminated by the surface of the stallion's penis during thrusting. Collection of semen using an open-ended artificial vagina (Figure 13-16) minimizes contamination of the semen with organisms still residing on the exterior of the penis. Swabbings of semen collected into sterile containers using the open-ended artificial vagina are less likely to be contaminated and thus are more likely to yield meaningful cultures.

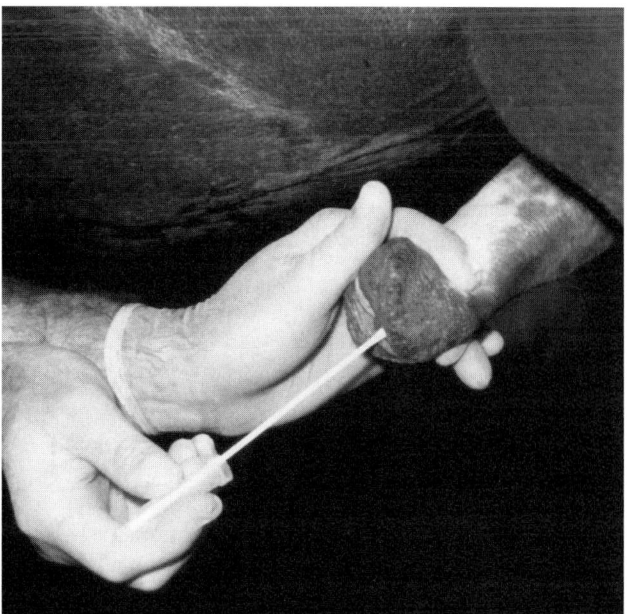

FIGURE 13-15. To obtain a urethral culture, the distal tip of the glans penis is first deflected dorsally with a thumb to allow better exposure of the urethral orifice for swab insertion. This procedure is performed immediately before (pre-ejaculatory swabbing) and immediately after (postejaculatory swabbing) ejaculation to screen for potential internal genital infections. (From Varner DD, Schumacher J, Blanchard TL et al: *Diseases and management of breeding stallions.* St Louis, 1991, Mosby.)

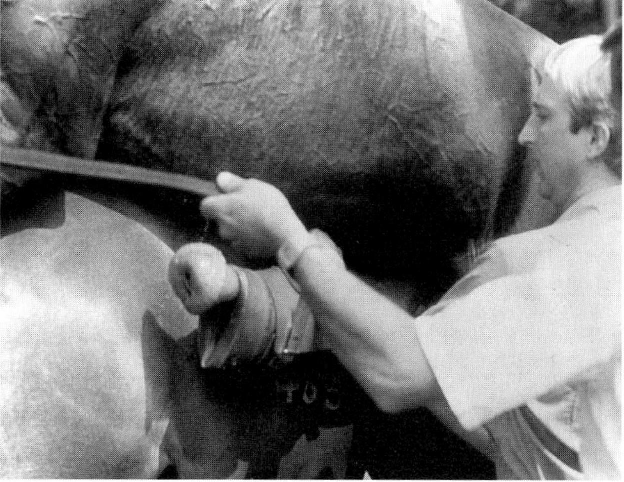

FIGURE 13-16. Collection of semen with an open-ended artificial vagina effectively reduces contamination of semen with microorganisms on the surface of the penis. Semen can be collected in sterile containers using a funnel or urethral prosthetic device. (From Varner DD, Schumacher J, Blanchard TL, et al: *Diseases and management of breeding stallions.* St Louis, 1991, Mosby.)

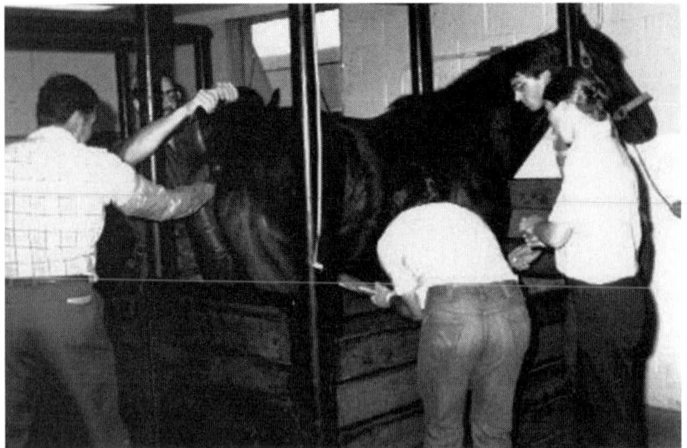

FIGURE 13-17. A sterile 100-cm flexible catheter has been passed into the pelvic urethra of this stallion. One examiner determines, by palpation per rectum, where to place the catheter tip and then expresses the fluid from each seminal vesicle in turn by using downward pressure with the digit(s)—first from the blunt end and progressing toward the apical end, where the duct opening is located in the seminal colliculus. Fluid is collected through the catheter from each seminal vesicle in turn, which can also be examined further for evidence of infection (Photo courtesy Dr. Wendell Cooper.)

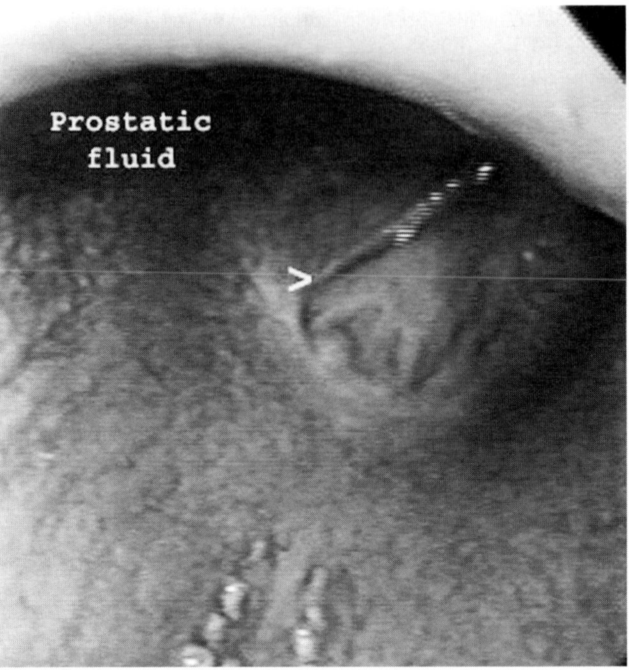

FIGURE 13-18. Endoscopic visualization of prostatic gland fluid being expressed per rectum. Fluid can be collected through a catheter passed through the biopsy channel of the endoscope or through a urinary catheter passed just into the pelvic urethra as described in the text.

Vesicular gland fluid can be collected selectively for culture by first teasing the stallion vigorously to distend the lumen of these bladder-like glands with secretions. After aseptic preparation of the penis and distal urethra, a 1- × 100-cm sterile catheter with an inflatable cuff is passed into the urethra to the level of the seminal colliculus (origin of the excretory ducts of the vesicular glands). The cuff is inflated, and the fluid in each vesicular gland is expressed manually per rectum for collection and study (Figure 13-17). Secretions from the prostate gland, ampullae, and ductus deferens may be cultured by swabbing semen collected in the first "spurt" or "jet" of an ejaculate using an open-ended artificial vagina, because this fraction of the ejaculate contains secretions originating primarily from these sites. Alternatively, the prostate and bulbourethral glands can be identified by transrectal ultrasonographic examination. After each gland is identified, the probe is retracted 2 to 3 inches while the digits are used to apply pressure to the gland of interest. Fluid expressed from the gland (Figure 13-18) can be retrieved through a preplaced catheter, and the gland can be immediately rescanned to confirm that fluid was expressed.

Infections originating from the epididymides or testes usually induce changes that are palpable through the scrotum. Additionally, the incriminating organism usually can be recovered from the semen, along with inflammatory cells recognized on cytologic examination of stained semen smears.

Viral Genital Infections

The two known venereal diseases attributed to viruses are equine coital exanthema, which is caused by equine herpesvirus 3, and equine viral arteritis, which is caused by a togavirus.

Equine Coital Exanthema. Equine coital exanthema, typically diagnosed by physical examination, produces characteristic blisters on the penile body and prepuce (Figure 13-19) that subsequently form pustules that ulcerate, and eventually resolve in 2 to 4 weeks. The clinical disease is self-limiting, and fertility is not affected unless lesions are painful enough to interfere with breeding. Venereal transmission to mares is common during the active stage of the infection and results in similar lesions on the external genitalia of the mare (Figure 13-20). To avoid transmission of the virus, breeding can be delayed until lesions have healed.

Equine Arteritis Virus. Equine arteritis virus can cause a generalized illness 1 to 10 days after infection that is characterized by fever, lymphopenia, edema of the limbs, stiffness of gait, periorbital swelling with conjunctivitis and lacrimation, nasal discharge, maculopapular skin rash, edema of the scrotum and prepuce of the stallion and occasionally the mammary gland of the mare, abortion in the mare, and rarely a fulminating interstitial pneumonia in neonatal foals. Many strains of the virus are nonpathogenic. The disease is of special interest to stallion managers because acutely or chronically infected stallions can transmit the virus to susceptible mares during breeding (even by artificial insemination with cooled or frozen semen). Infected mares are then capable of transmitting the virus by the respiratory route to other susceptible mares they contact. Abortion may occur during or shortly after the febrile period in affected mares, but it may also occur in

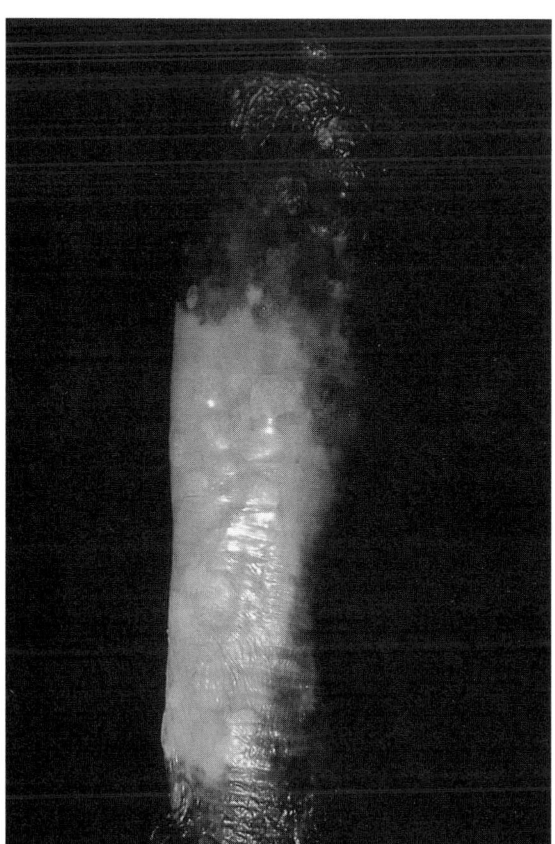

FIGURE 13-19. Lesions (vesicles) of coital exanthema, caused by equine herpesvirus 3 on the penile body of a breeding stallion.

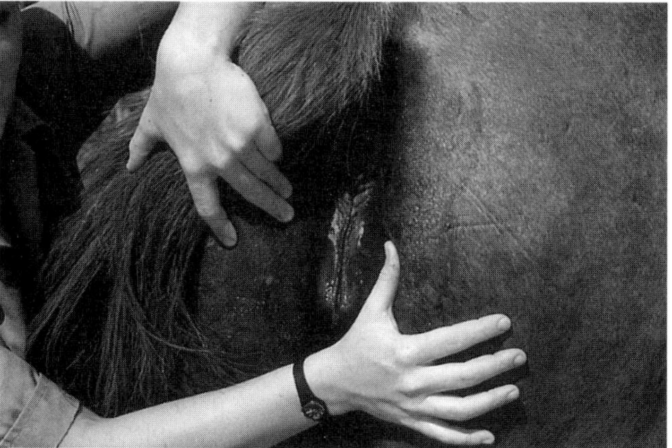

FIGURE 13-20. More chronic lesions (pustules) of coital exanthema on the vulvar and perineal area of a mare. This mare had been pasture bred during an equine herpesvirus 3 outbreak and was confirmed to be pregnant 35 days at the time this photograph was taken.

exposed susceptible mares that display only mild or no premonitory clinical signs. The venereal mode of transmission is considered a major pathway for dissemination of the virus.

Stallions infected with the equine arteritis virus can remain long-term asymptomatic carriers, with viral sequestration in the genital tract (particularly in the ampulla and vas deferens) and shedding in the semen (the spermatozoa-rich portion of ejaculate is laden with virus). The venereal route appears to be the sole means of virus transmission from chronically infected stallions. Diagnosis of the disease in a stallion presumed to be a carrier is based on isolation of the causative virus from ejaculated semen or, alternatively, development of serum neutralization antibodies in seronegative mares that are bred to the suspect stallion. Health regulatory officials should be contacted for discussion and supervision of diagnosis/management of equine arteritis virus carrier or shedder stallions, which necessitates immunization of seronegative mares with a modified live-virus tissue culture adapted product (ARVAC, equine arteritis vaccine, Fort Dodge Laboratories, Inc.) before breeding. Mares confirmed to be seronegative for equine arteritis virus are vaccinated. Vaccinated mares must be isolated from all other horses for 3 weeks to prevent infection of in-contact horses with the vaccinal virus. After isolation requirements are met, vaccine-induced seroconversion is confirmed by repeating the blood test, and the mare can then be mated to the shedder stallion.

Protozoal Genital Infections

Trypanosoma equiperdum, the organism causing dourine, is the only protozoan known to produce venereal disease in horses. The disease, which is presently not seen in the United States, is characterized initially by edematous swelling of the external genitalia, attendant mucopurulent discharge from the urethra, formation of 2- to 10-cm diameter urticarial cutaneous plaques, and progressive emaciation, sometimes in conjunction with penile paralysis. Diagnosis is based on a complement fixation test and isolation of trypanosomes from the urethral exudate, blood, or urticarial plaques. Treatment is possible but generally impractical, and euthanasia is recommended.

COLLECTION OF SEMEN

Accurate assessment of semen quality depends heavily on proper semen collection techniques. Ejaculated semen is very susceptible to environmental influences, so mishandling of semen samples before evaluation negates their value for representing a stallion's innate fertility. The reader is referred to Chapter 12 for discussion of semen collection techniques and procedures.

EVALUATION OF SEMEN

To enhance the reliability of a semen evaluation, it should be performed in a thorough, methodical manner by an experienced person in an adequately equipped laboratory. Both routine and in-depth diagnostic tests are available and are selected based on time, availability of specialized equipment, and economic constraints of the stallion owner. Routine tests include gross evaluation of the sample, determination of semen volume and spermatozoal concentration (to calculate total sperm number), and assessment of spermatozoal motility and morphology. More involved tests performed on selected stallions include chemical analysis of seminal plasma (including assay of alkaline phosphatase), electron microscopic study of spermatozoal ultrastructure, a sperm chromatin structure assay, and various spermatozoal function tests (e.g., membrane integrity and the ability of spermatozoa to undergo the acrosome reaction).

Gross Evaluation of Semen Quality

The gel is separated from the gel-free fraction of the ejaculate in the laboratory by aspiration into a syringe if a filter was not placed in the artificial vagina to perform this function during semen collection. Filtration also helps to remove extraneous debris (e.g., smegma, hair, and dirt) from the gel-free semen. The volume of gel-free semen is measured, and the color and consistency of the sample are noted. Although volume, by itself, is seldom an important determinant of fertility, it is used in calculation of total sperm number in an ejaculate. Consequently, accurate measurement of volume is essential. The filtered gel-free semen can be poured into 100-ml graduated cylinders to accurately measure volume. Semen volume can be increased by excessive precopulatory teasing, but the total sperm number in the ejaculate usually remains unchanged. Ejaculate volume is affected by season (e.g., smaller volumes produced in winter compared with summer) and sexual preparation time (i.e., prolonged teasing increases accessory sex gland secretions, which increase volume and decrease spermatozoal concentration in the ejaculate). The gel-free portion of an ejaculate contains the majority of spermatozoa, so the gel fraction usually is discarded after its volume is recorded without measurement of its spermatozoal content. Gross evaluation of the semen sample provides a rough estimate of its spermatozoal concentration and permits detection of color changes that may be associated with blood, urine, or purulent material in the ejaculate.

SPERMATOZOAL CONCENTRATION

An accurate measurement of spermatozoal concentration is critical because total sperm number in an ejaculate is derived by multiplying spermatozoal concentration by semen volume. An imprecise estimate of spermatozoal concentration produces a corresponding inaccurate calculated sperm number in an ejaculate. Such errors can produce misleading judgments and should be avoided. Spermatozoal concentration of the gel-free semen can be determined using a hemacytometer (Bright-Line Hemacytometer, Hausser Scientific) (see Figure 12-16). Advantages of hemacytometer counting to determine spermatozoal concentration include the following: it is a direct method for counting spermatozoa visually identified under a microscope; discoloration of the sample does not affect accuracy of the count; and equipment expense is minor. Disadvantages of hemacytometer counting include the counting takes a long time and variability due to dilution and loading errors is common. For routine hemacytometer counting of spermatozoa, we use the platelet/white blood cell Unopette system (Becton-Dickinson) with 20-μl capillary pipettes (see Figure 12-16). The capillary pipette is filled with semen, which is transferred to the Unopette (providing a 1:100 dilution). After thorough mixing, both sides of the cover-slipped hemacytometer chamber are loaded, and a few minutes are allowed for spermatozoa to settle on the hemacytometer grid. The number of spermatozoa within one of the nine large squares are counted (Figure 13-21), and this number is multiplied by 1 million to provide the number of spermatozoa per milliliter in the semen sampled. Both sides of separately loaded hemacytometer chambers should be counted and averaged. If the counts vary considerably, the dilution and loading procedures should be repeated, and the sample should be counted again.

Hemacytometer counting of spermatozoa can be replaced by determination of spermatozoal concentration with a spectrophotometer or densimeter (Animal Reproduction Systems) (Figure 13-22). Besides the densimeter, other automated systems that use optical density to estimate spermatozoal concentrations are commercially available (e.g., SpermCue from Minitube of America, Inc., the model 10 sperm counter from Hamilton Research, and Micro-Reader I from I.M.V.). These instruments allow faster measurement of spermatozoal concentration, and their accuracy is good if spermatozoal concentration is not exceedingly high (>300 million/ml) or low (<100 million/ml), and the ejaculate is free of debris, blood, purulent material, or premature germ cells. Mixing semen

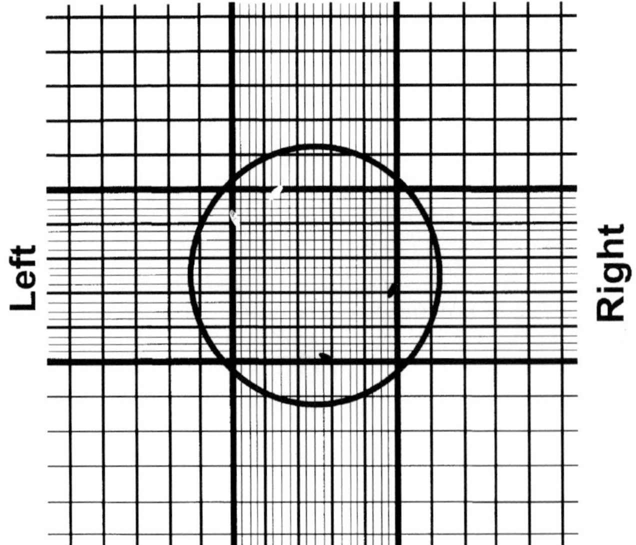

FIGURE 13-21. Illustration of the hemacytometer grid used for counting sperm. Nine large squares are present, with additional cross-hatched dividing lines within the center and central squares. All sperm present within the large center square are counted. For sperm heads lying on the lines, only those sperm heads lying on the upper and left lines are included in the count and not those lying on the lower or right lines.

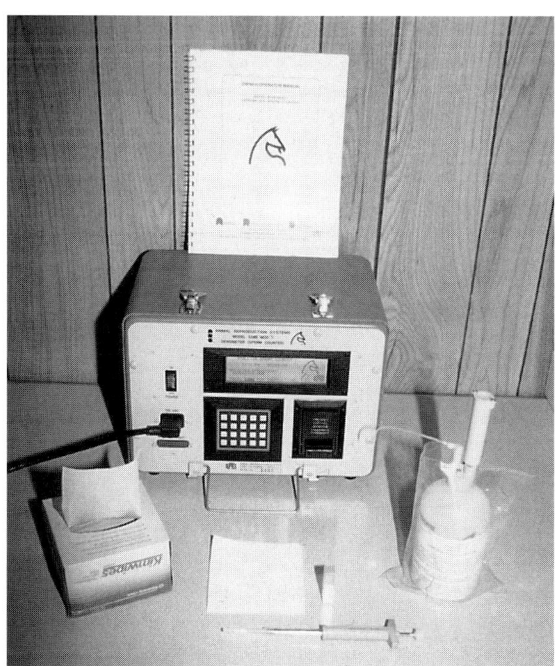

FIGURE 13-22. A densimeter (with accessories) is commercially available (Animal Reproduction Systems) for estimation of spermatozoal concentration in raw, gel-free stallion semen. The instrument can also be used to determine the volume of semen to use as an insemination dose after the percentage of progressively motile spermatozoa has been entered.

with an extender that is not optically clear before measuring spermatozoal concentration will produce erroneous measurements with instruments that measure optical density. Dilution factors are automatically taken into account when commercially available optic density measuring systems are used (the exception is the SpermCue, which requires no dilution of the raw semen).

Total sperm number, calculated as the product of spermatozoal concentration and semen volume, is one of the more important measurements used in estimating a stallion's fertility. Total sperm number per ejaculate is subject to seasonal variation but also is affected by numerous other factors that include rate of occurrence of ejaculation, age, testicular size, spermatogenic efficiency (i.e., number of sperm produced per unit of testis), size of extragonadal spermatozoal reserves, and various forms of reproductive disease. Total sperm number in ejaculates obtained from mature stallions typically ranges from 4 to 12 billion, but may exceed 15 to 20 billion in sexually rested stallions. For stallions ejaculating low numbers of spermatozoa, an accurate estimation of actual *DSO* is advised. This usually requires determination of number of spermatozoa present in ejaculates collected once daily for 7 to 10 days. After extragonadal spermatozoal reserves are stabilized (requiring approximately 4 days of once daily semen collection for stallions with smaller testes and 5 to 6 days of once daily semen collection for stallions with larger testes), the numbers of spermatozoa recovered in ejaculates obtained on each of 3 consecutive days are averaged to provide the estimate of DSO. The stallion can be expected to ejaculate approximately this number of spermatozoa each day when he is used for repeated breeding. DSO varies with season (reaching the highest values in the summer and lowest values in the winter), age, testis size, and testicular health.

SEMINAL pH

The pH of gel-free semen should be determined using a properly calibrated pH meter, preferably within 1 hour after semen collection. Measurements obtained using pH paper are less precise than those derived with a meter, so this method of pH determination should be used only as a last resort. The pH of normal semen is slightly basic, with a reported range of 7.2 to 7.7. Season of the year, rate of occurrence of ejaculation, and spermatozoal concentration can affect the pH of normal stallion semen. An abnormally high semen pH value can be associated with contamination of the ejaculate by urine or soap or with inflammatory lesions of the internal genital tract.

SPERMATOZOAL MOTILITY

Spermatozoal motility generally reflects the viability of a sperm population. A positive relationship between spermatozoal motility and fertilizing capacity has been demonstrated in many species, although this correlation is not absolute. Several different instruments and methods have been developed for objective assessment of equine spermatozoal motility, including time-lapse photomicrography, frame-by-frame playback videomicrography, spectophotometry, and computerized analysis (Figure 13-23). Computerized motility analysis provides a number of objective measures of spermatozoal motion characteristics taken from tracks of large numbers of sperm, including percentage of motile sperm, percentage of progressively motile sperm (i.e., above a preset cutoff for speed and direction of movement), amplitude of lateral head displacement during forward movement, average path velocity in micrometers per second, and curvilinear velocity in micrometers per second. Subjective assessment of spermatozoal motility by visual estimation, using a microscope equipped with *phase-contrast* optics and a *warming stage,* is acceptable when personnel are experienced in analysis of spermatozoal motility.

Visual assessment of spermatozoal motility should include *total spermatozoal motility* (percentage of spermatozoa exhibiting motility of any form), *progressive spermatozoal motility* (percentage of spermatozoa which exhibit rapid, linear movement), and *spermatozoal velocity* (on an arbitrary scale of 0 [immotile] to 4 [rapidly motile]). For example, a motility of 75/70 (4) would indicate that 75% of sperm were motile and 70% of sperm were progressively motile, moving rapidly across the microscopic field. Rapid progressive spermatozoal motility generally is considered to be the most credible gauge

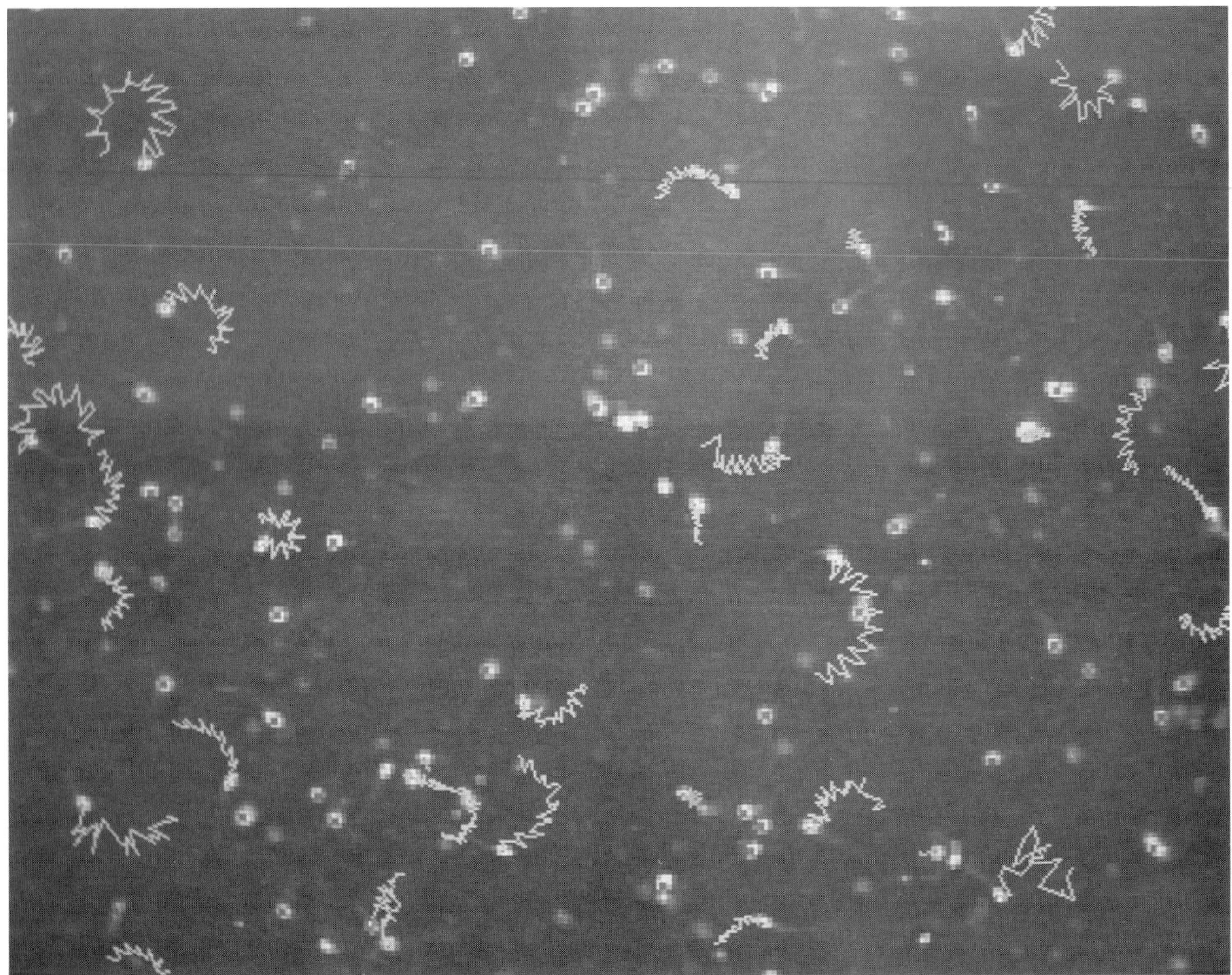

FIGURE 13-23. Image obtained from a Hamilton-Thorn computerized motility analyzer during assessment of spermatozoal motility. The computer-identified tracks of moving sperm analyzed over a short time span are shown.

of spermatozoal motion for predicting the fertilizing capacity of a semen sample.

Both the initial spermatozoal motility and the longevity of progressive spermatozoal motility should be assessed and recorded. Initial spermatozoal motility of raw (undiluted) semen samples can be estimated as a control for testing the possible detrimental effects of semen extenders on spermatozoal motility. Accuracy and repeatability of the spermatozoal motility evaluation is improved markedly by diluting the semen in an appropriate extender before analysis (see Tables 12-1 and 12-2). Warmed (37° C) nonfat dry skim milk-glucose extender serves this purpose well, because it supports spermatozoal motility and does not interfere with microscopic visualization of the spermatozoa. To standardize the spermatozoal motility testing protocol, all semen samples should be diluted with extender before analysis. We prefer to dilute sperm to a standard concentration of 25 million sperm/ml for motility assessment. One advantage of using a standard concentration of extended semen is to condition the viewer to seeing sperm at a consistent concentration among all stallion ejaculates evaluated. This concentration of sperm diluted in extender has also been shown to maximize both immediate spermatozoal motility and the longevity of spermatozoal motility.

The longevity of spermatozoal motility can be determined on raw semen samples stored at room temperature (20° to 25° C) and on samples diluted in extender (preferably to a final spermatozoal concentration of 25×10^6 sperm/ml) and stored at room temperature or refrigerated (4° to 6° C). The longevity of spermatozoal motility is enhanced by dilution of semen with extender and refrigerated storage. The Society for Theriogenology guidelines for evaluating the semen of prospective breeding stallions recommends that at least 10% progressive spermatozoal motility be maintained in raw and extended semen samples maintained in a light-shielded environment at room temperature for 6 and 24 hours, respectively.

The relationship between longevity of spermatozoal motility in samples maintained at room temperature is questioned by many investigators, whereas there is less dissension concerning the value of determining the longevity of the motility of cooled spermatozoa when processed ejaculates are used for breeding with cooled, transported semen.

SPERMATOZOAL MORPHOLOGY

The morphology (structural appearance) of spermatozoa is typically examined using a light microscope at 1000× magnification (under oil immersion). Standard bright-field microscope optics can be used to examine air-dried semen smears provided that appropriate stains are used in slide preparation. Specific stains for sperm include those developed by Williams and Casarett. General purpose cellular stains (e.g., Wright's, Giemsa, and hematoxylin-eosin) also have been used to accent both germinal and somatic cells in semen smears. Background stains (e.g., eosin-nigrosin and India ink) probably are the most widely used stains because of their ease of use (Figure 13-24). Visualization of the structural details of sperm can be enhanced by fixing the cells in buffered formol-saline or buffered glutaraldehyde solution and then viewing the unstained cells as a wet mount with either phase-contrast (Figure 13-25) or differential interference-contrast microscopy (Figure 13-26). Sperm fixation also is simplified by this method and the incidence of artifactual changes is reduced compared with that seen with stained smears. In one Texas study, droplet and midpiece abnormalities were underestimated in semen smears stained with eosin-nigrosin and examined under oil immersion with light microscopy compared with samples of the same ejaculates fixed in 2% buffered formol-saline and examined under oil immersion by phase-contrast microscopy.

At least 100 spermatozoa should be evaluated for evidence of morphologic defects. The type and incidence of each defect

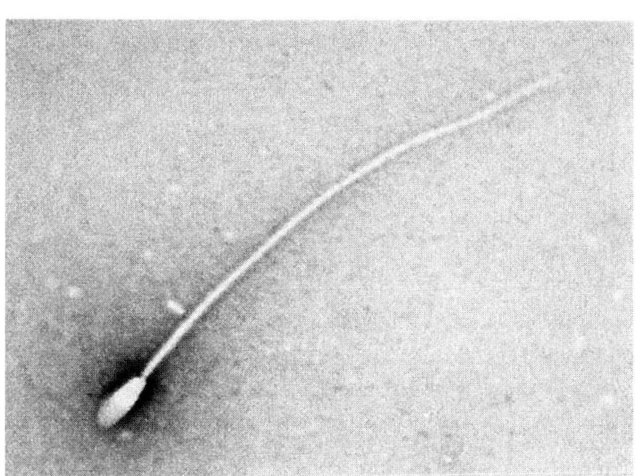

FIGURE 13-24. A normal equine spermatozoa prepared for morphologic evaluation by mixing a drop of semen with a drop of eosin-nigrosin stain, smearing this mixture along a slide, allowing it to air dry, and examining the smear under oil immersion using a light microscope.

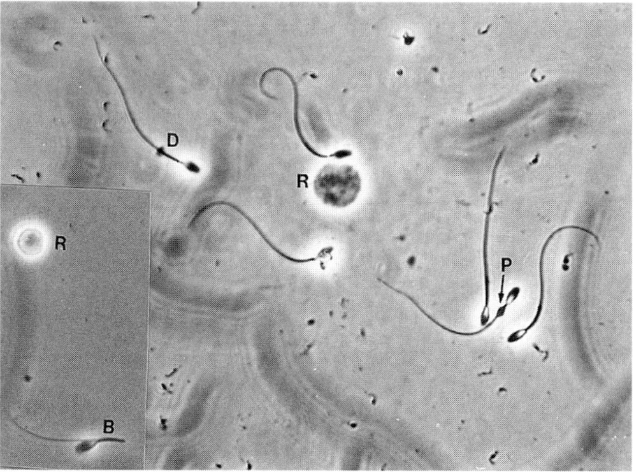

FIGURE 13-25. Equine spermatozoa fixed in 2% buffered formol-saline solution and examined on a wet mount slide preparation under oil immersion using a phase-contrast microscope. Morphologic defects of these sperm include distal protoplasmic droplets *(D)*, reversed or bent tails *(B)*, proximal cytoplasmic droplets *(P)*, and round spermatogenic cells *(R)*. (From Blanchard TL et al: Testicular degeneration in large animals: identification and treatment, *Vet Med* 86:537, 1991.)

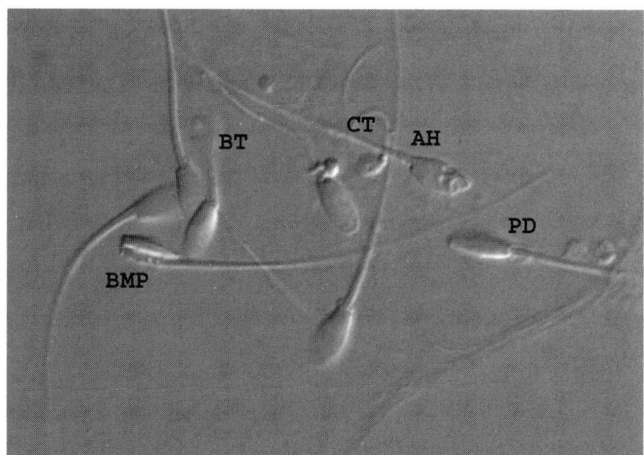

FIGURE 13-26. Equine spermatozoa fixed in 2% buffered formol-saline solution and examined on a wet mount slide preparation under oil immersion using a differential interference contrast microscope. The morphologic defects of these sperm include proximal protoplasmic droplets *(PD)*, reversed or bent tails *(BT)*, coiled tails *(CT)*, bent midpiece *(BMP)* and abnormal heads *(AH)*.

(Figure 13-27) should be recorded. Abnormalities in spermatozoal morphology traditionally have been classified as primary, secondary, or tertiary. *Primary morphologic abnormalities* are considered to be associated with a defect in spermatogenesis and, therefore, are of testicular origin. *Secondary morphologic abnormalities* are considered to be created in the excurrent duct system. *Tertiary morphologic abnormalities* are

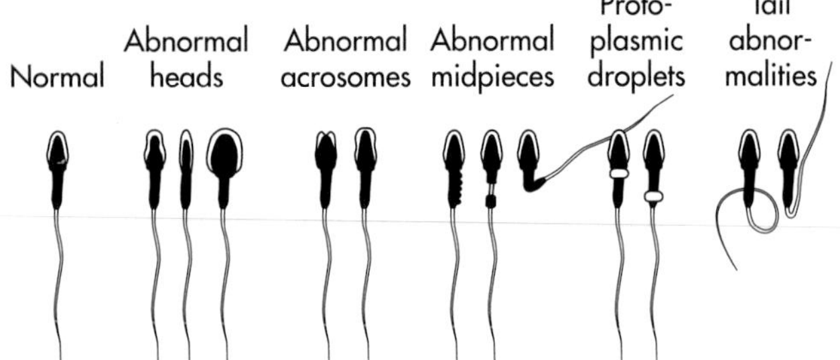

FIGURE 13-27. Drawing of morphologically normal and abnormal spermatozoa. (From Blanchard TL, Varner DD: Evaluating breeding soundness in stallions. II. Semen collection and evaluation, *Vet Med* February: 144, 1996.)

considered to develop in vitro as a result of improper semen collection or handling procedures.

The current trend is to record the numbers of specific morphologic defects, such as detached heads, abnormal heads, knobbed acrosomes, proximal and distal protoplasmic droplets, bent or irregular midpieces, and bent or coiled tails. This method of classification is considered superior to the traditional system because it reveals more specific information about a population of sperm while avoiding erroneous assumptions about the origin of these defects, which is often unknown. Some morphologic abnormalities (e.g., detached heads) can be primary, secondary, or tertiary in nature, thereby introducing the possibility of error when this classification system is used exclusively. Another example would be osmotic shock, which can cause bending of the tail that might be construed as a secondary defect rather than as a tertiary morphologic abnormality.

The value of spermatozoal morphologic studies in predicting the fertility of a stallion is met with a degree of skepticism, because some stallions can have many spermatozoal abnormalities; however, good pregnancy rates can be achieved when they are bred with good management conditions. Conversely, some stallions exhibit decreased fertility even though the percentage of morphologically normal sperm in their ejaculates is high (based on light microscopic studies). It is assumed that morphologically abnormal sperm do not have a negative influence on normal sperm. Therefore, the *total number of morphologically normal sperm* in ejaculates may provide more information regarding the fertility of a stallion than the percentage of morphologically abnormal sperm.

CHEMICAL ANALYSIS OF SEMINAL PLASMA

Adverse effects of some stallion's seminal plasma on their sperm have been demonstrated. Excess seminal plasma present in dilute ejaculates may damage sperm and has been shown to adversely affect the longevity of spermatozoal motility and sperm chromatin structure in cool-stored semen. Centrifugation and removal of excess seminal plasma followed by extension of the spermatozoal pellet in dried skim milk extender before cooling has been shown to improve spermatozoal motility and %COMP alpha-t of sperm chromatin structure assays in ejaculates of stallions with "poor cooling" semen. Adding seminal plasma from stallions with high post-thaw spermatozoal motility to ejaculates from stallions with low post-thaw spermatozoal motility enhanced both the post-thaw spermatozoal motility and membrane integrity of these stallions.

Despite increasing work on the potential adverse effects of seminal plasma on stallion sperm, the factors present in seminal plasma that cause problems remain unknown. Chemical analyses of equine seminal plasma have been reported, but the relationship of the various components of seminal plasma to spermatozoal fertilizing capacity has not been established. One study revealed that electrolyte concentration, total protein concentration, or specific protein composition of seminal plasma does not provide good predictive information regarding post-thaw motility of cryopreserved spermatozoa.

The alkaline phosphatase activity of seminal plasma can be determined. It is one important assay that can be performed on seminal plasma that is of practical use. The sources of alkaline phosphatase are primarily the testes and epididymides. Turner (1996) suggested that seminal plasma alkaline phosphatase activity <100 U/L results from failure of testicular/epididymal secretions to reach the ejaculate and values >2500 U/L confirm complete ejaculation with normal contribution of the testes and epididymides to the ejaculate. This test is useful for evaluating stallions producing azoospermic ejaculates (e.g., no sperm in the ejaculate with high alkaline phosphatase activity indicates a testicular problem with formation of sperm, whereas no sperm in the ejaculate with low alkaline phosphatase activity indicates either failure to ejaculate or testicular/epididymal products not entering the ejaculate, which may occur with blockage of the excurrent duct system).

TRANSMISSION ELECTRON MICROSCOPIC EXAMINATION OF SPERMATOZOA

Light microscopy affords limited magnification and, therefore, limited appraisal of spermatozoal morphology. This obstacle can be overcome by use of scanning and/or transmission electron microscopic techniques. Although expensive, these two microscopic methods offer high-resolution detail and permit closer examination of spermatozoal morphology. Subtle morphologic alterations, inapparent with light microscopy, often can be identified easily by electron microscopic analysis. Scanning electron microscopy offers three-dimensional visualization of entire spermatozoa (Figure 13-28). Transmission electron microscopy permits cross-sectional viewing of spermatozoa and reveals their ultrastructure in detail (Figure 13-29). Both electron microscopic techniques may be economically justifiable diagnostic aids in selected circumstances.

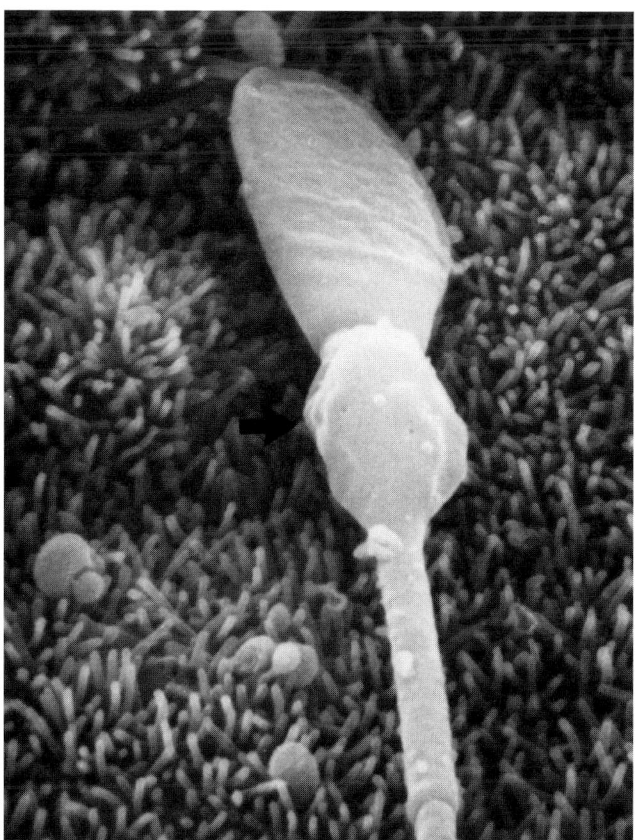

FIGURE 13-28. Scanning electron micrograph of an equine spermatozoan from an efferent ductule. Note the proximal cytoplasmic droplet *(arrow)*. (Photo courtesy Dr. Larry Johnson. From Varner DD, Schumacher J, Blanchard TL et al: *Diseases and management of breeding stallions.* St Louis, 1991, Mosby.)

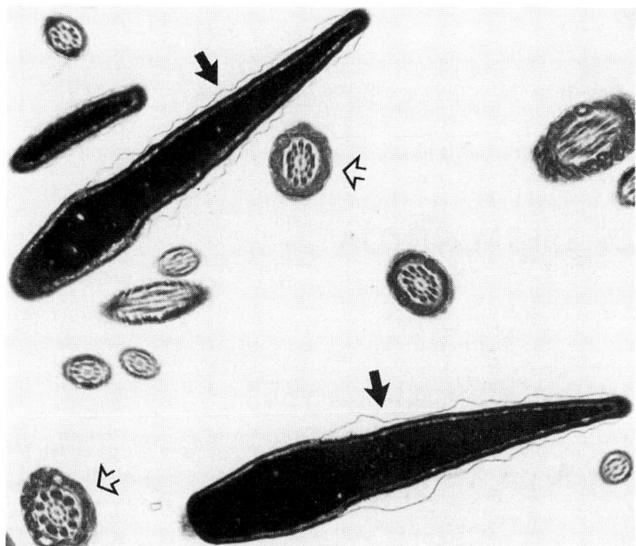

FIGURE 13-29. Transmission electron micrograph of stallion spermatozoa, demonstrating the head *(solid arrows)* and flagellar *(open arrows)* components. (Photo courtesy Dr. Larry Johnson. From Varner DD et al: *Diseases and management of breeding stallions.* St Louis, 1991, Mosby.)

EVALUATION OF THE ABILITY OF SPERMATOZOA TO UNDERGO THE ACROSOME REACTION

Ejaculated sperm are not immediately capable of fertilizing an oocyte. Instead, they must undergo final maturational changes within the reproductive tract of the mare. Two of these events (thought to be accomplished in the mare's oviduct) are completion of capacitation and the acrosome reaction. The acrosome reaction culminates in fusion (and shedding) of the spermatozoal plasma membrane and outer acrosomal membrane, which allows acrosomal contents to be released and thus aid in penetration of the vestments of the oocyte and fusion with the oocyte's plasma membrane. These changes are necessary for fertilization to occur.

There are substances known to induce the acrosome reaction in vitro, which can be used in a variety of assays to quantitate the percentage of sperm that have reacted. Texas workers used a 3-hour incubation of ejaculated sperm with the ionophore A23187 (Calbiochem) and determined the percentage of sperm undergoing an acrosome reaction by transmission electron microscopy (Figures 13-30 and 13-31). Using this assay they noted that some highly subfertile stallions with otherwise normal semen quality apparently produce sperm incapable of undergoing the acrosome reaction. California workers used progesterone to initiate the acrosome reaction in ejaculated sperm and determined that subfertile stallions

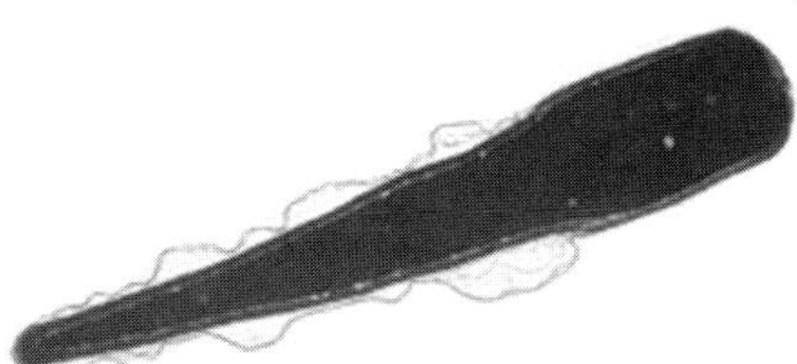

FIGURE 13-30. Transmission electron micrograph of a sagittal section through the head of a stallion spermatozoan before incubation with calcium ionophore to induce acrosome reaction. No vesiculation of the outer acrosomal and plasma membranes is present (i.e., the spermatozoan has not undergone the acrosome reaction).

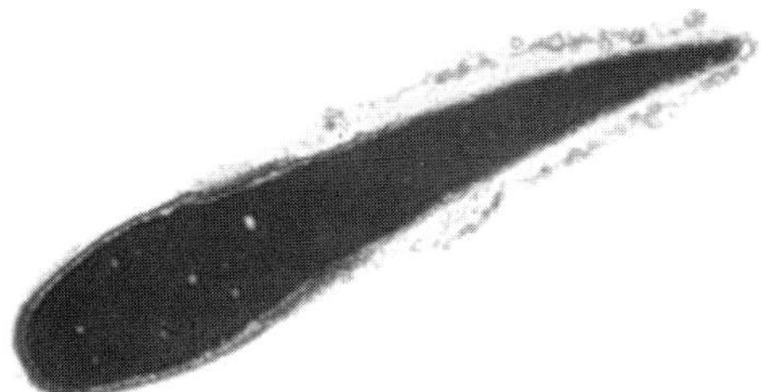

FIGURE 13-31. Transmission electron micrograph of a sagittal section through the head of a stallion spermatozoan after 3 hours of incubation with calcium ionophore to induce acrosome reaction. Vesiculation of the outer acrosomal and plasma membranes is present (i.e., the spermatozoan has undergone the acrosome reaction).

had sperm with decreased ability to undergo the acrosome reaction compared with sperm of fertile stallions. At present, practitioners must work with research laboratories to have an acrosome reaction assay performed.

URETHRAL ENDOSCOPY

Urethral endoscopy generally is reserved for use in stallions with *hemospermia* or those with suspected specific *urethral, bladder,* or *vesicular gland* lesions. Use of a flexible endoscope is recommended because it easily negotiates the ischial arch when passed via the urethral orifice, avoiding the need for subischial urethrotomy. To permit easy passage through the urethral lumen, the endoscope should have a maximum outside diameter of 10 mm. A working length of 100 cm permits access to the bladder lumen if the penis is not fully erect. Proper preoperative disinfection of equipment is critical. Endoscopic examination of the urethra and bladder may reveal mural and luminal abnormalities undetectable by other means. Urethral pathologic entities detectable by endoscopic examination include inflammation, ulcerations, lacerations (see Chapter 16), fistulae, strictures, growths, calculi, and foreign bodies. Cystitis, bladder calculi, and bladder tumors also may be revealed, as may lesions of vesicular adenitis.

RADIOGRAPHY

Radiographic techniques have been used effectively in the stallion to evaluate *patency of the urethra and ductus deferens.* Contrast or double-contrast radiography also may be useful for evaluation of the corpus cavernosum penis. Urethrograms (contrast and double-contrast radiography of the urethral lumen) have been used to diagnose urethral strictures and ulcerations, space-occupying lesions, and urethral fistulae. Contrast radiography has been used to detect bilateral luminal obstructions of the ductus deferens, which cause azospermia. A contrast radiographic study of the corpus cavernosum penis also may be useful to evaluate the *patency of the corpus cavernosum penis* after chronic penile paralysis or priapism.

CHROMOSOMAL ANALYSIS

Cytogenetics has become an increasingly popular area of clinical reproduction analysis in stallions. Oftentimes, the etiology of infertility and reduced fertility in the stallion is not disclosed by conventional diagnostic methods; therefore, investigators are relying more heavily on chromosomal studies to isolate genetically derived causes for such problems. Karyotyping permits scrutiny for numeric and/or structural changes in chromosome composition that could affect reproductive performance. Pennsylvania workers karyotyped 62 fertile, subfertile, and infertile stallions and identified chromosomal defects (including mosaicism with sex or autosomal deletions or duplications) in 18 of these stallions (Kenney et al., 1991). To perform karyotying, a cytogenetics laboratory needs aseptically obtained blood samples shipped at room temperature overnight. In some instances, the cytogeneticist may request that an aseptically obtained skin biopsy be placed within a tube that contains aseptically obtained whole blood and transported at room temperature overnight, which will facilitate culture of fibroblasts to improve the karyotyping capability.

A flow-cytometric procedure has been developed to evaluate the structural integrity of sperm chromatin. The potential of the *sperm chromatin structure assay* for predicting fertility has recently been evaluated in stallions with encouraging results. This assay system measures the susceptibility of sperm nuclear DNA to acid denaturation in situ. The extent of denaturation is determined by flow cytometry, measuring the red and green fluorescence emitted from acid-treated sperm stained with the metachromatic dye acridine orange. Green fluorescence is emitted upon laser excitation when the stain is intercalated into the native (stable), double-stranded DNA; red fluorescence is emitted when the stain is bound to denatured, single-stranded DNA. The extent of sperm chromatin acid denaturation is negatively correlated with fertility. The COMPα_t value (percentage of abnormal cells outside the main population) is calculated after large numbers (>5000) of sperm are counted (Figures 13-32 and 13-33), and in one Pennsylvania study it was found to be 16% in fertile stallions (seasonal pregnancy rate of 86%) and 41% in very subfertile stallions (seasonal pregnancy rate of 38%). Stallions with a COMPα_t value between 16% and 41% often experience lesser reductions in fertility. The sperm chromatin structure assay requires freezing of semen (usually raw) on dry ice or in liquid nitrogen, followed by transport frozen to an appropriate laboratory.

Equine antisperm antibody tests have been developed to assess the potential role of these antibodies in the infertility of stallions and mares. Antisperm antibodies are hypothesized to interfere with spermatozoal transport and/or gamete interaction, resulting in fertilization failure and perhaps even early embryonic death. There is some suggestion that damage to the testis, particularly degeneration, may culminate in the formation of antibodies against the sperm as a result of disruption of the blood-testis barrier. At present, no commercial laboratories offer these tests.

HORMONAL ANALYSES

The goal of reproductive endocrine assessment in stallions is to detect which components in the *hypothalamic-pituitary-gonadal* system might be contributing to abnormal reproductive function. The hypothalamus secretes *gonadotropin hormone-releasing hormone (GnRH),* which stimulates the pituitary gland to secrete *follicle-stimulating hormone (FSH)* and *luteinizing hormone (LH),* which in turn stimulate their respective target cells in the testis. The primary effect of LH is to indirectly promote spermatogenesis by stimulating Leydig

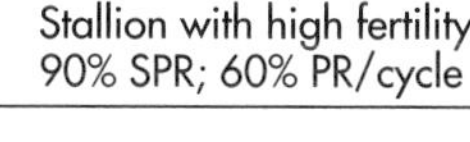

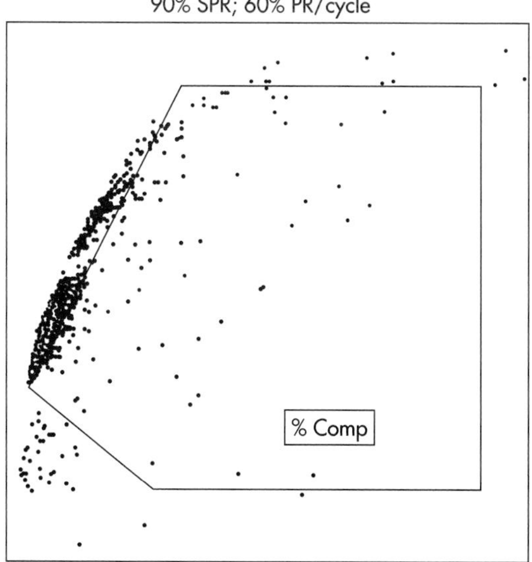

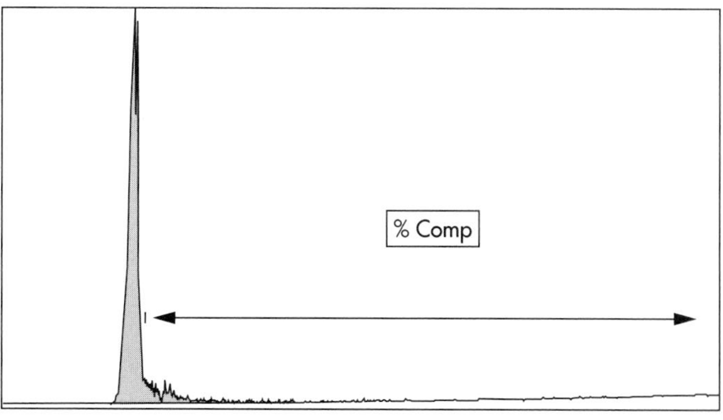

FIGURE 13-32. Sperm chromatin structure assay cytogram *(left)* of a fertile stallion's sperm stained with acridine orange and measured by flow cytometry. Green fluorescence is on the *y*-axis and red fluorescence in on the *x*-axis. A corresponding α_t frequency histogram with the number of cells on the *y*-axis is presented on the *right*. The cells in the region denoted by the *arrow (↔)* are denatured and fall outside the main (normal) population; they are termed the COMPα_t cells.

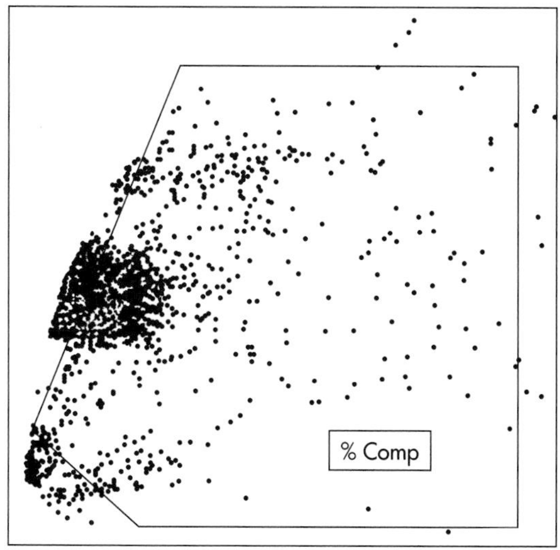

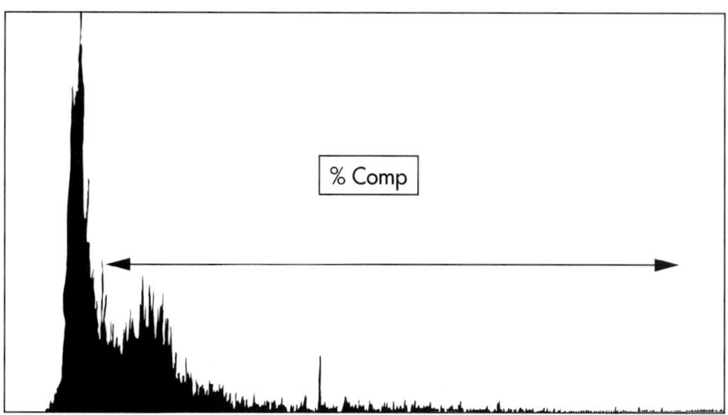

FIGURE 13-33. Sperm chromatin structure assay cytogram *(left)* of a subfertile stallion's sperm stained with acridine orange and measured by flow cytometry. Green fluorescence is on the *y*-axis and red fluorescence is on the *x*-axis. A corresponding α_t frequency histogram with the number of cells on the *y*-axis is presented on the *right*. The cells in the region denoted by the *arrow (↔)* are denatured and fall outside the main (normal) population; they are termed the COMP alpha-t cells.

cells in the testicular interstitium to produce testosterone. Stallion Leydig cells also produce large amounts of estrogens, most of which are conjugated. High concentrations of intratesticular testosterone are thought to be necessary for spermatogenesis to proceed normally. Testosterone feedback to the brain primarily inhibits LH secretion. Sertoli cells within the seminiferous epithelium initiate and maintain spermatogenesis in response to testosterone and FSH. Sertoli cells also produce the protein hormone inhibin (which decreases pituitary gland secretion of FSH) and the protein hormone activin (which increases pituitary gland secretion of FSH). Although research is improving our understanding of more intricate endocrine control of spermatogenesis in horses and other species, clinicians can effectively use this endocrine

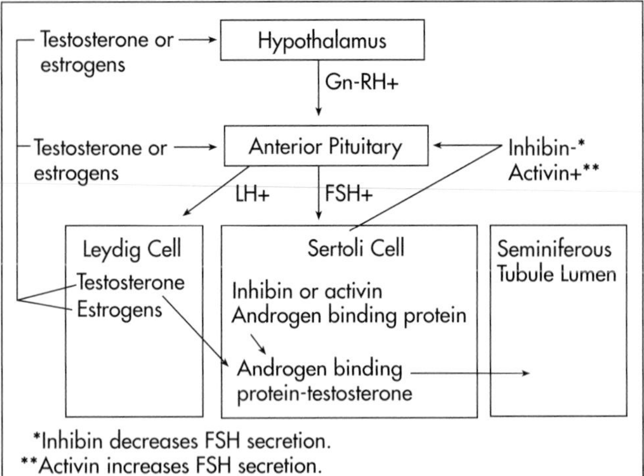

FIGURE 13-34. A proposed model for reproductive hormone feedback control in a stallion. An elevated testosterone level in the bloodstream feeds back on the hypothalamus and anterior pituitary gland to suppress discharge of GnRH and thus LH, causing Leydig cells to produce less testosterone. As testosterone levels in the blood decline, the inhibiting effect of a high testosterone level on release of GnRH and LH will be removed, permitting bursts of secretion to occur. In this model, estrogens are assumed to be produced primarily by the Leydig cells and to have a negative feedback effect similar to that of testosterone. Circulating FSH acts directly on Sertoli cells, which secrete the protein hormones inhibin and activin. When the FSH level is high, inhibin secretion will rise, causing a subsequent decrease in the amount of FSH secreted by the anterior pituitary gland. As FSH secretion declines, activin secretion will rise and cause a subsequent increase in FSH secretion by the anterior pituitary gland. Testosterone and FSH concentrations must be adequate to stimulate a Sertoli cell environment conducive to spermatogenic cell support and development. (From Blanchard TL, Varner DD: Evaluating breeding soundness in stallions. IV. Hormonal assay and testicular biopsy, *Vet Med* April: 358, 1996.)

control model (Figure 13-34) when attempting to diagnose an endocrine abnormality associated with subfertility or infertility in stallions.

The reader should note, however, that an endocrinologic basis for reproductive malfunction in stallions has not been firmly established. An exception is the administration of exogenous testosterone or anabolic steroids, both of which adversely affect spermatogenesis. One unrefuted application of a hormonal assay is to aid in diagnosing cryptorchidism in horses without scrotal testes. In cryptorchids, baseline concentrations of testosterone and/or estrogens are often elevated, and a two- or threefold increase in testosterone concentration in response to administration of 10,000 U of human chorionic gonadotropin (hCG) *(hCG stimulation test)* indicates the presence of testes.

It has been postulated that an abnormally high plasma concentration of FSH, sometimes accompanied by a high plasma concentration of LH, indicates testicular degeneration in older stallions. Conversely, a low plasma LH concentration has been associated with poor fertility in young stallions. Some investigators also contend that low libido or impotence in stallions may be related to low plasma concentrations of LH and estradiol-17β in the presence of normal testosterone values. Contradictory reports indicate that stallions with low plasma concentrations of LH and estradiol-17β can have excellent libido and semen quality. When collecting blood samples for hormone assays, one should remember that most hormones are released into the bloodstream in a pulsatile fashion; therefore, assays of single blood samples may not be truly representative of the endocrine status of the stallion. We recommend hourly collection of heparinized blood samples from 9 am through 1 pm, because this is the time when gonadotropin and testosterone concentrations normally peak in the stallion. Plasma is harvested and kept chilled, and equal volumes of plasma from each sampling are pipetted into five separate tubes (i.e., each representing a pooled sample from the 4-hour sampling), which are frozen and shipped overnight to the endocrine laboratory. The pooled samples should more closely represent a true average (i.e., "smooth out" the peaks) for each hormone assayed. Separate pooled samples are submitted because not all assays may be performed on a given day, and thus samples do not have to be thawed and refrozen. For this type of baseline screening, we request assays of LH, FSH, estradiol, testosterone, and inhibin in the pooled plasma samples. Poor semen quality is sometimes associated with low estradiol and inhibin concentrations and high FSH concentration in stallions with abnormal testicular function. On occasion, low testosterone and/or high or low LH concentration(s) will also exist.

To pursue whether the endocrine anomaly is associated with hypothalamic, pituitary, or testicular abnormality, hormone stimulation tests can be performed. Intravenous administration of 5 to 25 µg of GnRH to normal stallions typically stimulates LH release (≥50% increase) in 15 to 30 minutes, followed by testosterone release (≥100% increase in 1 to 2 hours) (Figure 13-35). We recommend obtaining

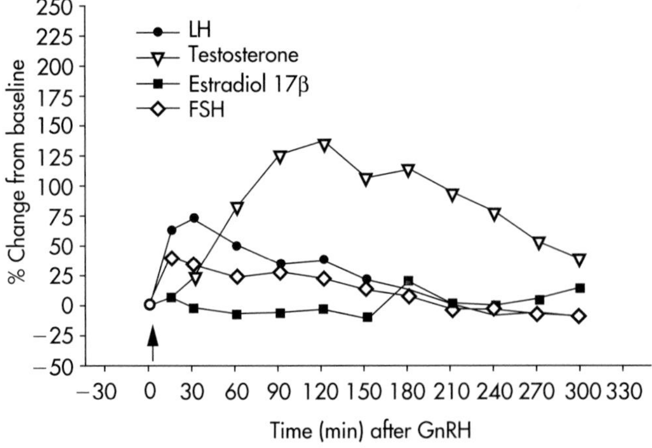

FIGURE 13-35. Results of intravenous administration of 15 µg of GnRH to a group of eight reproductively normal stallions. The *arrow* represents the time of GnRH administration.

samples before administration of GnRH, and at 15, 30, 60, and 120 minutes thereafter. Only LH and testosterone assays need to be performed on GnRH stimulation tests. If LH and/or testosterone response is inadequate, the stimulation can be repeated with larger doses (50 to 250 µg) of GnRH to determine if the pituitary and testicular Leydig cells are capable of responding. Roser (1995) proposed that hCG stimulation testing should be done to determine if an abnormality exists at the testicular level. Blood samples are collected before drug administration, then 10,000 U of hCG is administered intravenously, and blood samples are collected 1, 2, and 48 hours later for testosterone assay. Testosterone concentrations should reach 3 to 6 ng/ml in 1- to 2-hour samples and may reach 9 to 12 ng/ml in 48-hour samples from stallions with a normal Leydig cell response. Failure of significant testosterone secretion to occur would confirm that a primary testicular endocrine abnormality exists (most likely due to atrophied Leydig cells).

TESTICULAR BIOPSY

Although testicular biopsy has been recommended by some investigators as an innocuous diagnostic procedure for stallion infertility, we do not endorse it for routine use. Postoperative complications, such as sperm granuloma formation or intratesticular hemorrhage and an attendant increase in intratesticular pressure, could cause irreparable interference with spermatogenesis. However, biopsy provides the only method for directly assessing testicular tissue parameters (e.g., hormone concentrations, stages of spermatogenesis, sperm production rates, and the presence of space-occupying lesions) and therefore provides useful information in some circumstances.

An aspiration biopsy is potentially less damaging than a punch biopsy but usually will not offer useful information about spermatogenesis. Aspiration biopsy may help in differentiation among causes of testicular enlargement, such as neoplasia, trauma, or septic orchitis. To provide a better sample of tissue for histologic interpretation, we prefer to use a spring-loaded biopsy instrument (e.g., Bard Biopty biopsy instrument, C. R. Bard, Inc.). Similar disposable biopsy instruments are also available (14 to 18 gauge). The technique can be performed using profound sedation with the horse standing; local anesthesia of the scrotum is unnecessary. The scrotum is disinfected and the sterile biopsy instrument is pushed through the scrotal skin and fascia just through the outer tunica albuginea in the mid-region of the cranial one third of the testis. The testis is held firmly, the instrument is triggered, and the needle is withdrawn. The tissue is transferred to Bouin's, paraformaldehyde, or glutaraldehyde (fixative), left for 24 hours, transferred to alcohol, and processed for staining. Sufficient testicular tissue is present in biopsy specimens procured in this manner to evaluate whether qualitatively normal spermatogenesis is occurring (Figure 13-36). Pronounced testicular degeneration or the failure of spermatogenesis to proceed to sperm formation is also easily determined.

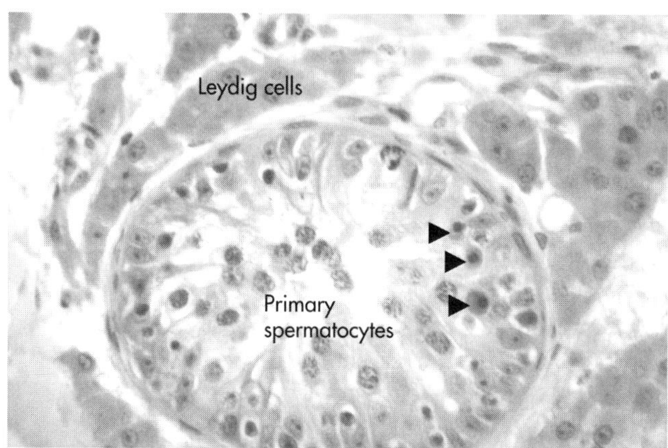

FIGURE 13-36. A representative testicular biopsy specimen procured using the Bard Biopty Biopsy Instrument (C. R. Bard, Inc.) from a stallion with azoospermia. The specimen was stained with periodic acid Schiff-hematoxylin. Spermatogenesis was not proceeding to completion and several degenerating germ cells *(arrowheads)* were noted.

INTERPRETATION OF FINDINGS—BREEDING SOUNDNESS EXAMINATION

An inherent drawback of a stallion fertility (or breeding soundness) examination is imprecision due to the biologic nature of the specimens under consideration. Even though the examination process has scientific merit, precision is impossible. In addition, factors other than innate stallion fertility, including mare fertility and management procedures, markedly influence pregnancy and foaling rates for a given stallion and often are difficult to control or assess.

The purpose of a fertility examination is to estimate a stallion's capability as a sire. Ideally, the testing process should produce sufficient information about a stallion to permit approximation of the number of mares to which that stallion can safely be booked during a breeding season. An indispensable ingredient in this formulation is the stallion's estimated daily sperm output (DSO). Numerous other factors also must be considered before a reasonable judgment can be made about a "stallion book."

Stallions typically are classified as *satisfactory, questionable,* or *unsatisfactory breeding prospects.* The categorizations are usually predicated on a stallion's ability to produce a seemingly low season pregnancy rate of 60%, but this percentage coincides with conditions for payment of fertility insurance the first year that insured stallions stand at stud. This pregnancy rate assumes that the stallion breeds a standard number of mares (e.g., 40 to 45 mares by natural service or 120 to140 mares by artificial breeding during a typical breeding season of 135 to 150 days). It is now known that most normal stallions can produce satisfactory pregnancy rates with even larger books of mares. An additional stipulation is that the stallion will be bred to mares of normal fertility under good management conditions. Specific criteria that must be met before a prospective breeding stallion can be appropriately classified are discussed in depth in the Society for Theriogenology's *Manual for Clinical Fertility Evaluation of the Stallion.* The reader should refer to this official manual for a thorough discussion of the subject.

In general, to be classified as a satisfactory breeding prospect, stallions must be free of undesirable, potentially heritable defects, behavioral disorders, or transmissible diseases (venereal or otherwise); possess no physical traits that would interfere with mating ability, semen quality, or sperm output; and ejaculate $\geq 1 \times 10^9$ progressively motile, morphologically normal spermatozoa in the second of two ejaculates collected 1 hour apart after 1 week of sexual rest.

BIBLIOGRAPHY

Blanchard TL, Kenney RM, Timoney PJ: Venereal disease. In Blanchard TL, Varner DD, editors, *Stallion management. Vet Clin North Am Equine Pract* 8:191-203, 1992.

Blanchard TL, Varner DD, Miller C et al: Recommendations for clinical GnRH challenge testing of stallions. *J Equine Vet Sci* 20:678-682, 686, 731-737, 2000.

Hurtgen JP: Evaluation of the stallion for breeding soundness. In Blanchard TL, Varner DD, editors, *Stallion management. Vet Clin North Am Equine Pract* 8:149-166, 1992.

Kenney RM, Evenson DP, Garcia MC et al: Relationships between sperm chromatin structure, motility, and morphology of ejaculated sperm, and seasonal pregnancy rate. *Biol Reprod Monogr* 1:647-653, 1995.

Kenney RM, Hurtgen JP, Pierson H et al: *Manual for clinical fertility evaluation of the stallion,* pp 1-100. Hastings, NE, Society for Theriogenology, 1983.

Kenney RM, Kent MG, Garcia MC et al: The use of DNA index and karyotype analyses as adjuncts to the estimation of fertility in stallions. *J Reprod Fertil* 1991;44(Suppl):69-75.

McDonnell SM: Normal and abnormal sexual behavior. In Blanchard TL, Varner DD, editors, *Stallion management. Vet Clin North Am Equine Pract* 8:71-90, 1992.

McDonnell SM: Ejaculation: physiology and dysfunction. In Blanchard TL, Varner DD, editors, *Stallion management. Vet Clin North Am Equine Pract* 8:57-70, 1992.

Meyers SA: Diagnosis of subfertility in stallions: evaluation of sperm function. *Proc Soc Theriogenol* 271-277, 1996.

Pickett BW et al: *Procedures for collection, evaluation and utilization of stallion semen for artificial insemination.* Colorado State University Experiment Station Animal Reproduction Laboratory General Series Bulletin, 1987.

Pickett BW et al: *Management of the stallion for maximum reproductive efficiency. II.* Colorado State University Experiment Station Animal Reproduction Laboratory General Series Bulletin, 1989.

Roser J: Endocrine profiles in fertile, subfertile, and infertile stallions: testicular response to human chorionic gonadotropin in infertile stallions. *Biol Reprod Monogr* 1:661-669, 1995.

Turner RM: Alkaline phosphatase activity in stallion semen: characterization and clinical implications. *Proc Am Assoc Equine Pract* 42:284-293, 1996.

Varner DD, Schumacher J, Blanchard TL et al: *Diseases and management of breeding stallions,* pp 61-96. St Louis, 1991, Mosby.

Varner DD, Brinsko SP, Blanchard TL et al: Subfertility in stallions associated with spermatozoal acrosomal dysfunction. *Proc Am Assoc Equine Pract* 47:221-228, 2001.

14

Semen Preservation

OBJECTIVES

While studying the information covered in this chapter, the student should attempt to:

1. Acquire a working understanding of the advantages and disadvantages of breeding with transported, cooled or frozen equine semen.
2. Acquire a working understanding of techniques and procedures used to process equine semen for cooling or freezing and to manage/breed mares with cooled or frozen equine semen.

STUDY QUESTIONS

1. List the ingredients in semen extenders that protect equine spermatozoa against cold shock.
2. Discuss desirable cooling rates for minimizing damage to spermatozoa in extended equine semen.
3. List the steps (in order) to be followed to prepare equine semen for cooling and shipment in an Equitainer.
4. List the steps (in order) to be followed to freeze equine semen.
5. Discuss mare management procedures that will optimize pregnancy rates when breeding with
   a. transported, cooled semen.
   b. frozen semen.

EQUINE SEMEN PRESERVATION: COOLED AND FROZEN SEMEN

Most equine breed registries within the United States condone pregnancies achieved by artificial insemination. Many of the registries also permit artificial insemination with cooled and/or frozen semen. Before embarking on an artificial insemination program, particularly with cooled or frozen semen, it is imperative that one obtains the current regulations for the breed registry of interest because regulatory allowances may change without widespread notification.

Transported, cooled semen is being used increasingly for breeding in the United States. Outside the United States, preserved semen has been used on a large scale for artificial insemination in China, where more than 100,000 mares have been inseminated with transported frozen or liquid semen in recent years. In European countries, preserved semen is used predominantly for warmblood, draft, and Standardbred breeds.

Spermatozoa are sensitive to many environmental factors, including temperature, light, physical damage, and a variety of chemicals. Cold-shock damage to spermatozoa is attributed to temperature-induced lipid structural changes in the plasma membrane.

Cooling of extended semen for transport is generally successful if the initial quality of the semen is good, a proper storage technique is used, and insemination is not delayed beyond 24 hours. For some stallions, good pregnancy rates can be obtained with semen stored for 48 to 72 hours before insemination.

Currently, frozen preservation of stallion spermatozoa yields poorer results than cool storage and is also far less successful than frozen preservation of spermatozoa from dairy bulls. Direct extrapolation of techniques used to freeze bull semen has yielded discouraging results with stallion semen, an outcome probably related to compositional differences between the spermatozoa of the two species. Research has revealed that spermatozoa of dairy bulls are unusually resistant to the effects of cryopreservation. This phenomenon is probably attributed to years of careful selection of bulls with spermatozoa capable of surviving the freezing and thawing processes, a mindset not followed in horse-breeding circles.

The economic incentives for improving techniques of semen preservation in stallions are becoming increasingly evident, as major breed registries now permit its use. Previously, limited financial support for research in this field had slowed progress in development of superior methods for preserving stallion semen, be it in cooled or frozen form. Advancements now being made in this area may lead to more prolonged storage intervals for cooled semen and successful cryopreservation of semen from a larger percentage of stallions.

GENERAL CONSIDERATIONS

Preservation of semen begins with the actual collection process. To ensure that spermatozoal quality is optimized, semen should be collected as described in Chapter 12. Regardless of the technique of semen preservation to be used, it is important that semen be placed in a suitable extender within a few minutes after its collection from the stallion. To maximize success with preserved semen, one should screen for ejaculates of poor quality. If the quality of fresh stallion semen is poor (see Chapter 13) or if fertility achieved by breeding with fresh semen is poor, it is highly unlikely that successful results can be obtained by breeding with preserved semen.

Figure 14-1 provides an example of a processing form to be sent with the transported, cooled semen as a method of quality control. Copies of this form can be kept in a log book for the stallion owner to help maintain accurate records of mares being bred.

COOLED SEMEN

Extended semen from fertile stallions can oftentimes be stored in a cooled state for hours to days before insemination without a significant reduction in pregnancy rate. Guidelines for maximizing the longevity of spermatozoal viability in vitro follow.

Dilute Semen with a High-Quality Extender

Semen extenders contain protective ingredients that permit survival of spermatozoa outside the reproductive tract. Lipo-

Stallion Information: Name: Breed: Lip tattoo #: Registration number: Markings/Brands:	Owner/Agent: Name: Address: Telephone: Facsimile:
Processor Information: Name: Address: Telephone: Facsimile:	Referring Veterinarian: Name: Address: Telephone: Facsimile:

Semen information:

•Date and time of semen collection:
•Volume of raw gel-free semen (cc):
•Concentration of raw gel-free semen (x 10^6/ml):
•Semen extender used:
•Antibiotic used:
•Dilution ratio:
•Sperm concentration of extended semen (x 10^6/ml):
•Initial spermatozoal motility (Total/progressive):
•Initial spermatozoal velocity (0-4):

•Date and time of semen shipment:
•Volume of extended semen shipped (cc):
•Total sperm number shipped (x 10^9):
•Total number of progressively motile sperm shipped (x 10^9):

•Recommended volume/insemination(cc):
•Number of insemination doses shipped:

Signature Date

FIGURE 14-1. An example of an equine cooled semen transport form to accompany transported semen.

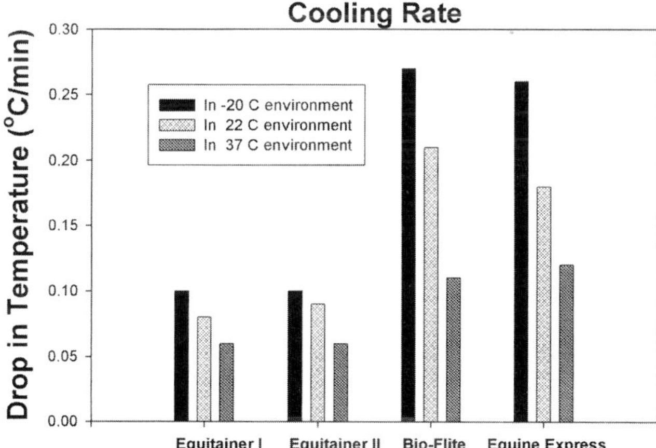

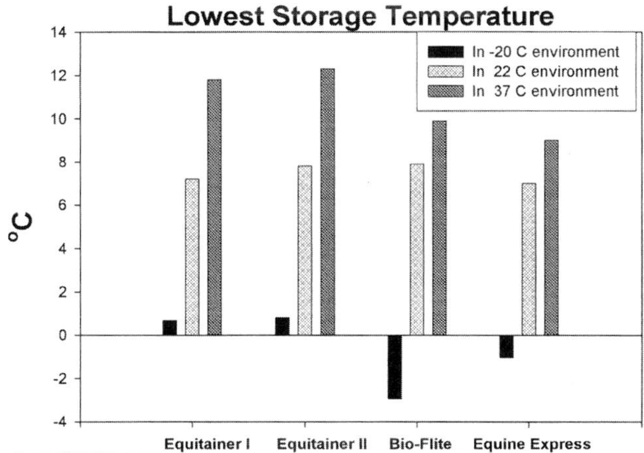

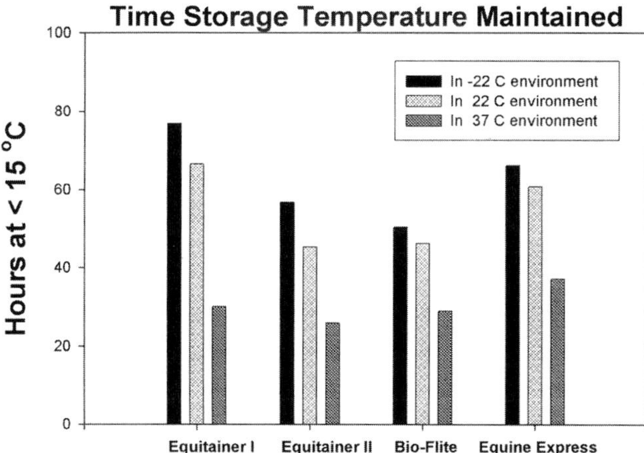

FIGURE 14-2. Effect of storage container on internal temperature when exposed to three different ambient storage conditions. Tests were performed on 40-ml volumes of extended semen. All extended semen was packaged according to manufacturer's recommendations. Containers were initially stored for 6 hours to mimic environmental conditions during shipment (i.e., in a freezer [–20° C] to mimic airline transport at high altitudes or ground transport in cold climates; at room temperautre [20° C] to mimic ground transport in mild climates; and in an incubator [37° C] to mimic ground transport in hot climates). Containers in freezers for 6 hours were then moved to room temperature for the remainder of the storage period.

proteins, such as those contained in milk or egg yolk, protect spermatozoa against cold shock by stabilizing cellular membranes. Metabolizable substrates, such as glucose, provide a plentiful source of energy for spermatozoa. Antibiotics are added to extenders to retard or eliminate growth of bacterial organisms. The osmotic pressure and pH of extenders can be adjusted to maximize spermatozoal survival. The osmolality of milk-based extenders should be between 300 and 400 mOsmol/L, with 350 mOsmol/L considered to be optimal. The pH of semen extenders can probably range from approximately 6.7 to 7.2 without affecting the longevity of spermatozoal viability during storage, but a pH of 6.7 to 6.9 may optimize spermatozoal track linearity (i.e., a computerized motility assessment measure of the straightness of spermatozoal movement). Extenders may be home-made formulations (Table 12-1) or commercially available preparations (Table 12-2). Nonfat dried milk solids-glucose (NFDMS-G) extender maintains better spermatozoal motility of cooled semen than does heated skim milk extender, although fertilizing capacity may not differ between the two extenders. The NFDMS-G extender also maintains cooled spermatozoal motility better than a sucrose-bovine serum albumin extender. No conclusive studies have been done to determine whether cream-gel or egg yolk-based extenders are more or less desirable than milk-based extenders either for enhancing spermatozoal viability or fertility of cooled equine semen. Milk-sugar extenders are the most popular formulations in the United States, and milk-based extenders are more commonly used worldwide than are egg yolk-based extenders.

The proper selection of antibiotics to include in the semen extender will enhance the viability of stored semen. A combination of amikacin sulfate (1 mg/ml) and potassium penicillin G (1000 U/ml) was shown in one Texas study to be effective for controlling bacterial growth and optimize spermatozoal motility of stored semen. This antibiotic combination has also yielded excellent fertility in breeding trials. One may wish to compare antibiotics for inclusion in semen extender because variations among individual stallions may exist. The objective of using the antibiotic(s) is to eliminate all bacterial growth while not hampering spermatozoal viability. Antifungal drugs may be needed to control fungal growth if the storage temperature exceeds 10° to 12° C.

Ideally, semen should be mixed with a prewarmed (37° C) extender within 2 to 15 minutes after ejaculation. A minimum ratio of 1:1 (extender to semen) is recommended for immediate inseminations. If semen is to be stored for a period 2 to 4 hours or longer before insemination, greater dilution (i.e., a higher extender to semen ratio) is usually required. A *final concentration of 25 to 50 million spermatozoa/ml in extended semen generally maximizes spermatozoal survivability in vitro.* To maximize spermatozoal survival, a minimum of 1:4 (1 part semen to 4 parts extender) dilution should be obtained to ensure that the final seminal plasma concentration in extended semen is ≤20%. For dilute ejaculates (<100 million sperm/ml), it may be necessary to centrifuge the semen, remove excess seminal plasma, and resuspend the spermatozoa in extender to ensure that no more than 20% seminal plasma remains in the extended semen.

Cool Semen to Refrigerated Temperature for Storage

Extended semen should be promptly removed from the incubator (37° C) because extensive cellular death will occur within a few hours if spermatozoa are maintained at this temperature. Cooling extended semen to 4° to 6° C for storage is superior to storage at room temperature (i.e., 20° to 25° C) for breeding 1 to 2 days later. The longevity of spermatozoal viability is probably improved by storage at near refrigeration temperature compared with storage at higher temperatures because of a corresponding reduction in metabolic activity. Spermatozoal fertilizing capacity is often maintained for 24 to 48 hours or longer when extended semen is stored at refrigerated temperature. Normal fertility has been reported after refrigerated storage of semen for periods of 72 to 96 hours. If semen is stored at room temperature, fertility is often reduced after 12 to 24 hours. Studies are currently being conducted to determine if warmer temperatures (10° to 15° C) are superior to cooler temperatures (4° to 6° C) for storing stallion semen.

When stallion semen is prepared for transport and subsequent artificial insemination, a rapid change to temperatures of less than 18° to 20° C cause spermatozoa to undergo cold-shock damage. Currently, only *passive* cooling/transport systems are commercially available for use with stallion semen. *Passive cooling systems* generate *variable* rates of cooling (i.e., cooling rates become progressively slower as semen temperature is reduced). Cooling rates may also vary according to environmental temperatures, initial temperature of semen, and volume of extended semen being cooled (Figure 14-2). Interpretation of results of studies using extended stallion semen in passive cooling systems originally suggested that an initial cooling rate of –0.3° C/min was desirable for maximizing spermatozoal viability. This cooling rate is

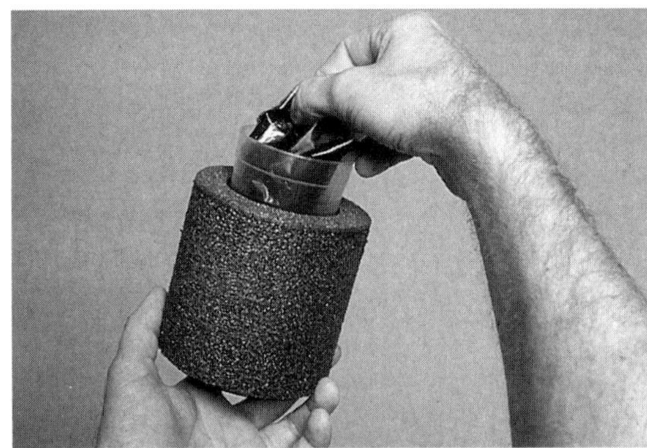

FIGURE 14-4. Placement of a prewarmed (37° C) ballast bag into the cup in the isothermalizer of the Equitainer. Each ballast bag contains 60 ml of diluent, and one or two ballast bags are used to bring the total volume of liquid placed into the isothermalizer to 120 to 170 ml, an amount necessary to ensure that the proper cooling rate is established for the extended semen.

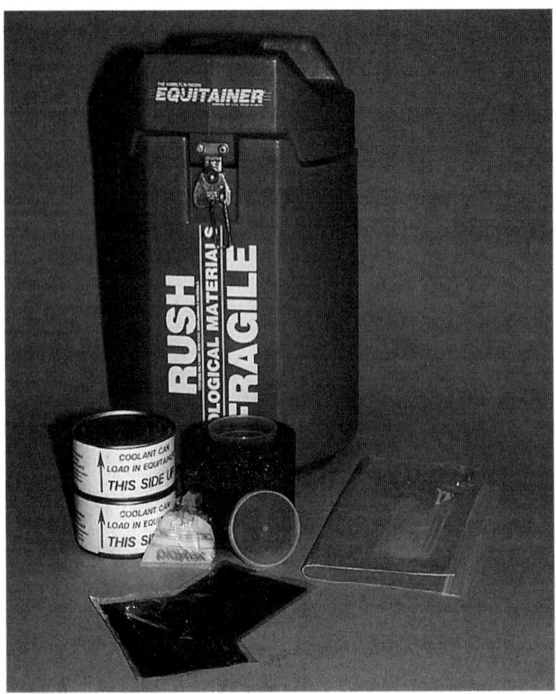

FIGURE 14-3. Components of the Equitainer semen cooling/transport system: thermal container, coolant cans, cup and isothermalizer, plastic bag, and ballast bags.

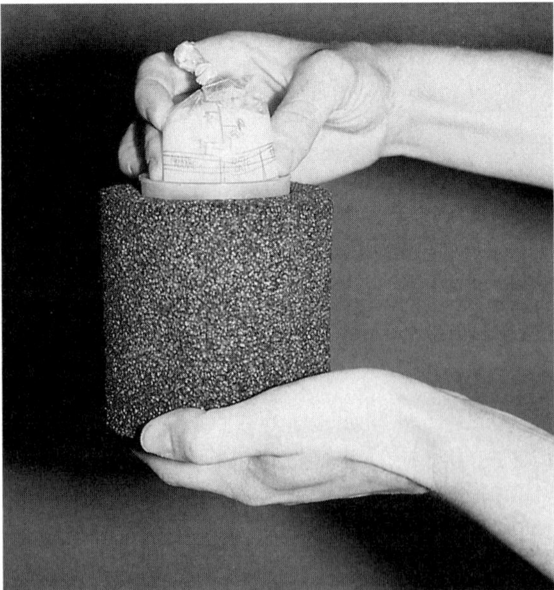

FIGURE 14-5. Placement of a double-bagged extended semen sample into the cup inside the isothermalizer of the Equitainer. Residual air has been expressed, and bags have been sealed with tightly wrapped rubber bands.

achieved by using the Equitainer or Equitainer II (Hamilton Research, South Hamilton, MA). Cooling rates from 20° to 8° C are thought to be critical for stallion spermatozoal survival and are currently recommended to be in the range of –0.1° to –0.05° C/min to maximize the maintenance of spermatozoal motility. Once cooled, storage temperatures of 4° to 6° C have been shown to be superior to temperatures of 0° to 2° C when spermatozoal motility was examined after 48 hours.

Commercial systems for semen storage, such as the Equitainer and Equitainer II (Figures 14-3 through 14-9), Bio-Flite (Figure 14-10) (available from Animal Reproduction Systems, Chino, CA), or equine semen transporter (EST XL-SH) (Figure 14-11) (Plastilite Corp., Omaha, NE) greatly simplify transport of liquid-stored stallion semen. Disposable syringe transport systems available in the United States are the Clipper (Hamilton Research) (Figure 14-12) and Equine Express II (Exodus Breeders Supply, Ltd., York, PA) (Figure 14-13). Plastilite Corp. also supplies a disposable shipper system called the EST XL-S that is similar to the EST XL-SH, which will accommodate either syringes or bags for holding semen. Because regulations for interstate shipment of semen are not well defined, packaged semen is usually transported via air carrier throughout the United States without accompanying health certificates. Authorized shipment of semen outside the United States requires that specific regulations of the importing country be met. Health authorities responsible for importation of semen into other countries should be contacted to ensure that requirements are met before arrangement for semen transportation is made. Some countries require that extensive health screening (e.g., serologic testing, culturing of reproductive tract or semen, vaccination, and inspection of premises and animals by regulatory officials) be performed before semen is collected for preservation. Quarantine measures sometimes must be used for the stallion, farm, and mares maintained at the farm where the stallion stands to meet semen importation requirements. Cooled semen has been successfully imported into the United States from abroad for prompt insemination of mares, but considerable regulatory requirements must be met before shipments are authorized.

Of additional interest to horse owners contemplating breeding with transported, cooled equine semen is the fact that shipments transported by airlines may be subjected to x-ray security screening. One study revealed no adverse effects of x-radiation at doses up to 10 mSu (an exposure similar to that received in many airport security screening systems) on equine spermatozoal motility (either initial motility or longevity of motility), spermatozoal morphology, or fertility of irradiated semen. Mares bred with x-irradiated semen also delivered normal foals at term. However, forthcoming recommendations for screening luggage on commercial flights in the United States will result in new x-ray screening requirements that could increase the amount of radiation exposure

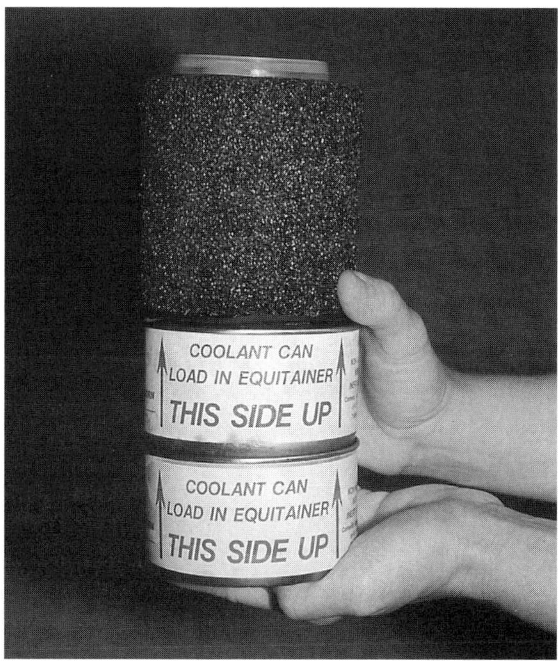

FIGURE 14-6. Placement of the loaded isothermalizer, which contains a capped semen cup with extended semen and ballast bag(s), on top of two cooling cans (frozen upside down in a freezer for 24+ hours before use).

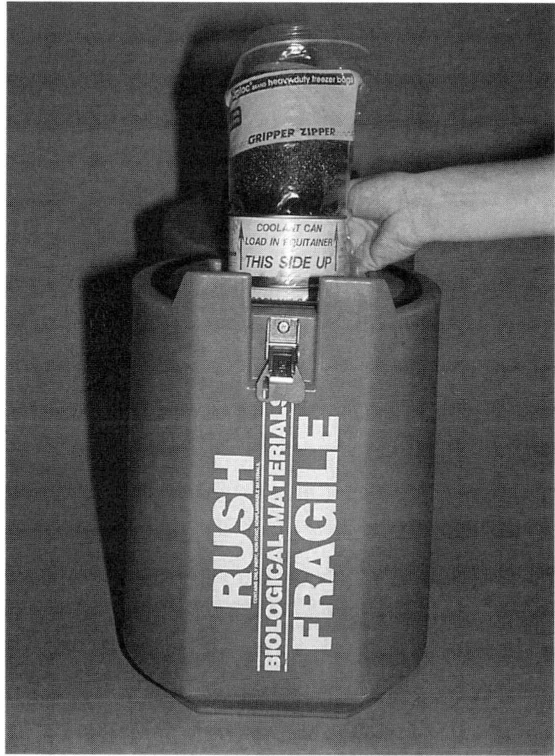

FIGURE 14-7. All components are loaded in the order shown in Figure 14-6 into a plastic bag to be inserted into the Equitainer, permitting easy removal of contents when the mare is to be bred.

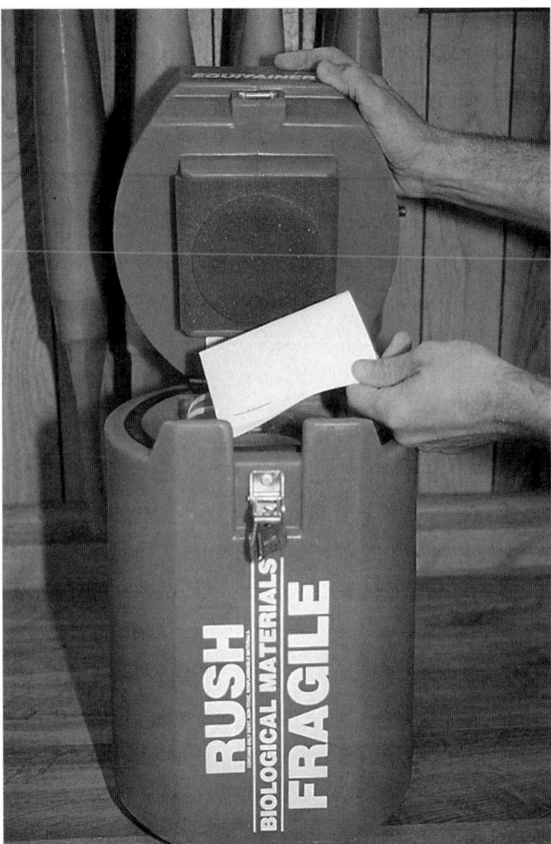

FIGURE 14-8. Placement of the record of semen shipment into the Equitainer before closing and latching the container. The latch should be secured before shipment. A record of semen shipment should be made regardless of the transport system used. Duplicate records should be maintained by the stallion owner/manager for reference if fertility or shipment problems arise. For an example of this form, refer to Figure 14-1.

300 times or more than that currently used. Effects of exposure of horse semen to this amount of radiation remain unstudied. Hamilton Thorne Research, Inc., provides a lead shield for their reusable transport systems that may protect semen from potential radiation damage; however, the shield overlies the top of the container and will not prevent radiation exposure to the sample if the transport container is exposed to radiation from the side. The container is labeled to caution airport luggage screening personnel to only allow the container to be opened for less than 2 minutes during examination. The manufacturer has found that opening the container for ≤2 minutes will not interfere with the cooling rate or holding temperature of the stored extended semen. Plastilite Corp. provides lead-foil shields for their reusable and disposable semen shipping systems.

The most accurate method for *determining the inseminate volume* required for transport for breeding is to conduct semen cooling trials for individual stallions. The semen is diluted in an appropriate extender(s) as described above and cooled for 24 hours in semen transport containers to be

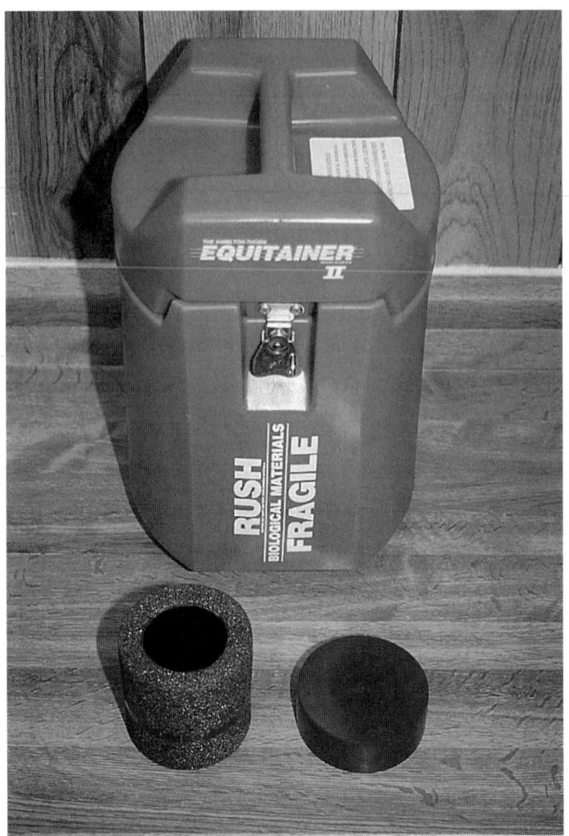

FIGURE 14-9. Components of the Equitainer II are the same as those for the Equitainer with the exception of a lead liner that encloses the isothermalizer and semen cup. The lead liner may protect the semen against radiation damage during security screening.

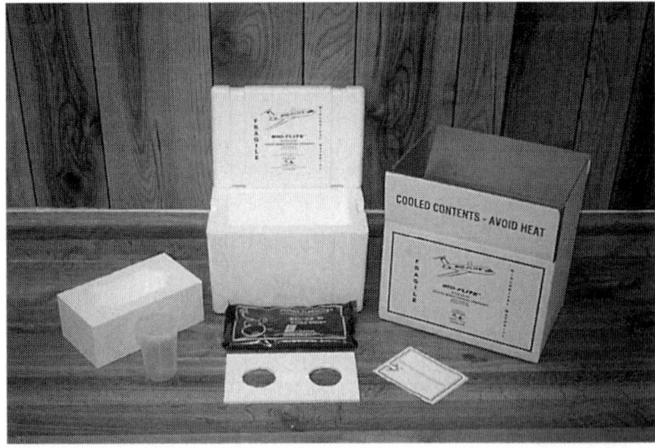

FIGURE 14-10. Components of the Bio-Flite semen cooling/transport system. *Clockwise from left:* semen cup and Styrofoam container for cup, Styrofoam shipping box and lid, outer cardboard shipping box, address label, coolant pack, and fenestrated Styrofoam plate. Extended semen is double bagged and placed in the plastic cup, and the plastic cup is capped. The plastic cup is placed within its Styrofoam container horizontally, and the Styrofoam cup container is placed within the large Styrofoam shipping box. The fenestrated Styrofoam plate is placed over the semen cup, and the coolant pack (frozen for 24+ hours) is placed on top of the fenestrated plate. The lid is placed on top of the Styrofoam shipping box, and the entire assembly is placed inside the cardboard shipping box. The cardboard box is sealed, and the address label for shipment is attached.

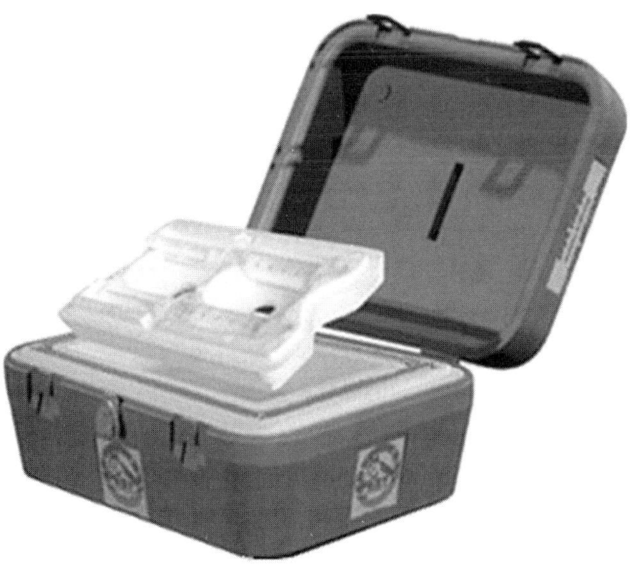

FIGURE 14-11. Components of the equine semen transporter (EST XL-SH) reusable shipper for transported semen. This container will accommodate either two polyethylene jars for bagged semen or two 50-ml Air-Tite syringes. A lead-foil shield is also available for protection against airport security radiation. Extended semen is placed in Whirl-Pak bags, the filled bags are placed in jars with cotton balls for impact protection, and the jars are placed in the tray. Syringes can be used in place of the jars for holding semen. The lid is placed on the tray, and rubber bands are placed around the tray. The coolant pack (brick) that has been frozen for at least 24 hours is placed in the bottom of the shipper, and the tray is placed (holes down) on top of the coolant pack. The lid is placed on the shipper and secured with logo labels to hold the lid tight on the base cooler. Documentation of the processed semen shipment is placed in a zipped bag and inserted into the interior lid recess. The corrugated box and luggage carrying case are then closed and secured for shipment.

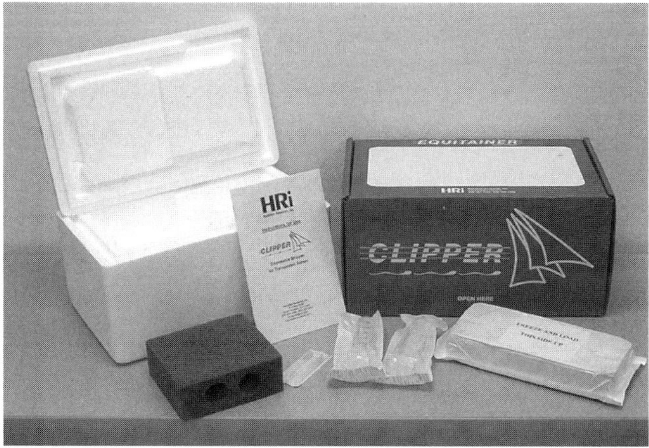

FIGURE 14-12. Components of the Clipper disposable shipper for transported semen. *Clockwise from left:* foam insulator block, Styrofoam insulated transport box and lid, cardboard shipping box, freeze pack, two sterile syringes (can be 20 or 50 ml according to preference), and two needles with plastic caps. The manufacturer recommends that the syringes be maintained at 37° C before use and that the freeze pack be frozen for at least 24 hours before use. Both syringes must be filled to capacity. If only one syringe is being filled with extended semen, the other should be filled with warm water (and labeled to indicate the contents are water). Protective caps are placed on the syringes, and labels with the stallion's name and other pertinent information are placed onto the syringes. The capped syringes are inserted fully into the foam insulator block. The frozen freezer pack is placed at the bottom of the container so that the internal Styrofoam support shelf is positioned above the freezer pack. The foam insulator block containing the syringes is place into the cut-out area of the Styrofoam support shelf. The Styrofoam lid is fitted into the top of the Styrofoam box, and the entire assembly is boxed and prepared for shipment.

used by the farm management. The cooled semen sample is gently remixed after this cooling period, and an aliquot is warmed to 37° C. Spermatozoal motility is evaluated 15 minutes after warming, and the percentage of progressively motile spermatozoa obtained is used as a guideline to ensure that future shipments will provide a minimum of 500 million progressively motile spermatozoa after 24 hours of cooling. For example, if after 24 hours of cooling the progressive spermatozoal motility is 50%, 1 billion total spermatozoa would need to be prepared for shipment to ensure that an insemination dose of 500 million progressively motile spermatozoa was available for breeding the mare. The procedure can also be performed on semen cooled for 48 hours if demand for 48-hour cooled semen is suspected.

It has become common practice for many stallion owners/managers to prepare two bags (insemination doses) of extended semen for shipment: one to be used for an initial insemination upon arrival, and one to be held for insemination again the next day. For many stallions, the longer the semen is held at a refrigerated temperature, the poorer spermatozoal motility becomes. Additionally, fertility of semen cooled for 48 hours tends to be reduced compared with that of semen cooled for only 24 hours. Except for special cases, we believe it is generally better to inseminate a mare with the transported semen as soon as practical after it arrives rather than to wait for breeding or to inseminate the mare twice with the semen in that shipment. More research must be performed before there is convincing evidence that fertility will be improved by holding a second insemination dose for breeding the day after the first insemination. Certainly, if two large doses of good-quality semen arrive, breeding the mare twice at 12- to 24-hour intervals might be advantageous. However, if sperm motility is poor when the semen arrives, it is unlikely that the second dose will survive an additional 12 to 24 hours of cooling. If the practitioner chooses to hold semen for breeding again the next day, precautions should be taken to maintain the cooled semen at 4° to 6° C until the time of the second insemination. To ensure that the temperature of the second dose of semen left in the shipping container does not increase above 10° C, causing premature spermatozoal death, the remaining semen dose can be repackaged and the container placed in a refrigerator (4° to 6° C) until it is opened for breeding the next day.

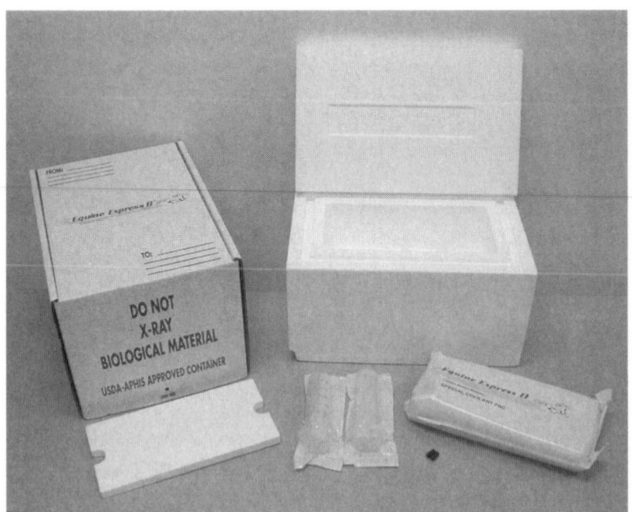

FIGURE 14-13. Components of the Equine Express II cooled semen transport system. *Clockwise from left:* cardboard shipping box, Styrofoam insulation box with lid, coolant pack, rubber caps for syringe tips, sterile syringes, and Styrofoam plank for separation of syringes from coolant pack. Two 30- or 50-ml Air-Tite syringes are filled with warm (35° to 37° C) extended semen, capped to prevent leakage, and placed into the Styrofoam box. The Styrofoam plank is placed over the semen-loaded syringes, and the frozen (24+ hours) coolant pack is placed on top of the Styrofoam plank. The Styrofoam lid is placed on top of the Styrofoam insulation box, and the entire assembly is boxed and prepared for shipment.

Breeding the Mare with Cooled Semen

When the cooled semen arrives for insemination of the mare, current recommendations are to do the following:

1. Prepare the mare for breeding (see Chapter 12).
2. Open the shipping container, carefully remove the chilled semen, gently mix it, aspirate the semen into a syringe (if the semen was not stored in a syringe during shipment), and attach an insemination pipette.
3. Inseminate the mare by infusing the semen into the mare's uterus. Uterine body breedings are adequate in most instances. There may be an advantage to deep uterine horn inseminations when semen quality is poor, or if the mare is subfertile.
4. A small aliquot of the extended semen should be warmed to 37° C, and spermatozoal motility should be assessed and recorded for quality control purposes. If spermatozoal motility is poor, inquiries can be made to determine whether this was an unexpected problem. If spermatozoal motility in additional shipments is consistently poor and the mare fails to conceive on repeated breedings, it is possible that the stallion is incapable of producing spermatozoa that survive the cooling/transportation process well. Alternatively, use of a different semen extender or dilution ratio or experimentation with centrifugation and removal of excess seminal plasma might prove beneficial for improving livability of spermatozoa harvested from that particular stallion.

Overseas workers often recommend warming the chilled semen to body temperature before insemination of the mare. In the United States, the chilled semen is usually placed directly into the uterus as soon as possible after the shipping container is opened. Because no detrimental effects on pregnancy rate have yet been determined by inseminating mares with as much as 170 ml of transported chilled semen, at present we see no reason to prewarm the chilled semen before insemination.

CRYOPRESERVATION OF SEMEN

Semen cryopreservation implies storage of spermatozoa at subzero (i.e., *frozen*) temperatures. The cryogen normally used for this task is *liquid nitrogen* (–196° C). If spermatozoa withstand the freezing and thawing process, spermatozoal integrity may be maintained almost indefinitely in liquid nitrogen, because metabolic activity of spermatozoa is considered to be negligible at this temperature.

Semen cryopreservation has the potential of adding a new dimension to the horse breeding industry by allowing long-term preservation of spermatozoa from superior stallions and permitting distribution of this semen to breeding establishments worldwide. Such a breeding policy would maximize usage of select stallions and greatly reduce mare shipping/boarding costs and transmission of contagious diseases. Geographical constraints would be abolished, and thus mare owners could select semen from a larger pool of stallions, including deceased stallions from which semen had been stored frozen.

Undesirable aspects related to the use of cryopreserved semen are also apparent. For instance, pregnancy rates are typically reduced for a high percentage of stallions, given our existing technology in this area. An increased number of progeny of popular stallions may arise if good pregnancy rates are achieved with their cryopreserved semen. Reduction in the genetic pool is also possible if all mare owners have access to semen of select sires. Opportunities for errors and corruption would also increase but could be held in check by quality control during processing steps and incorporation of improved techniques for documenting parentage.

Several features of spermatozoa are considered important for fertilization and must be retained after cryopreservation if normal fertilizing capacity is to be expected: progressive motility, normal metabolism, intact cellular membranes, the presence of acrosomal enzymes, intact surface-associated proteins responsible for sperm-egg interactions, and uninjured nucleoprotein. Cryopreserved spermatozoa undergo tremendous stresses associated with freezing, thawing, and insemination that could render them nonviable. Most spermatozoal damage results from altered membrane structure, osmotic

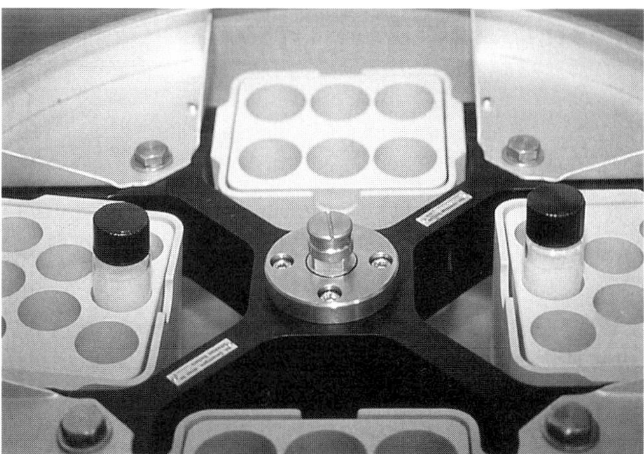

FIGURE 14-14. Equine semen, already mixed with centrifugation extender, has been placed into round-bottom tubes for centrifugation to concentrate sperm and separate seminal plasma. Tubes are placed in a centrifuge and spun for 10 minutes at 500 × *g*.

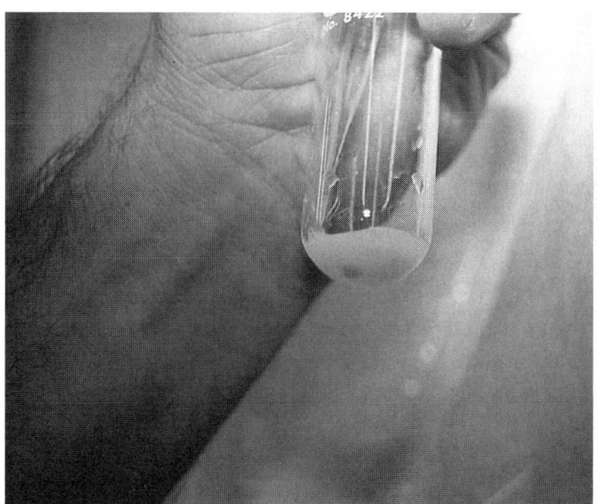

FIGURE 14-15. Aspirating seminal plasma and centrifugation extender from the spermatozoal pellet (visible in the bottom of the tube).

TABLE 14-1

German Centrifugation and Cryopreservation Media Used for Freezing Equine Spermatozoa

Centrifugation Medium (Merck I Extender)	
D-Glucose	59.98 g
Trisodium citrate dihydrate	3.70 g
Disodium ethylenediaminetetraacetic acid (EDTA)	3.70 g
Sodium bicarbonate	1.20 g
Potassium penicillin G	1,000,000 U
Amikacin sulfate	1.00 g
Deionized distilled water	qs 1000 ml
Adjust pH to 6.9 with sodium bicarbonate	
Extender can be frozen at –20° C in smaller aliquots until used.	
Cryopreservation Medium	
D-Lactose solution (11% w/v)	50.0 ml
Centrifugation medium (Merck I extender)	25.0 ml
Egg yolk	20.0 ml
Glycerol	5.0 ml
Equex STM (Nova Chemical Sales, Scituate, MA)	0.8 ml

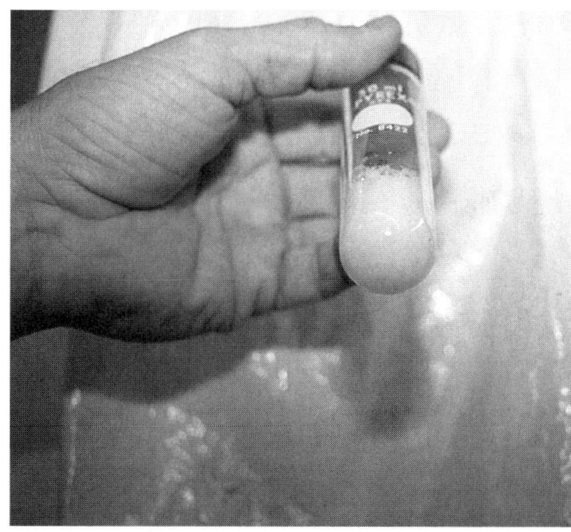

FIGURE 14-16. Freezing extender containing cryoprotectants has been added to spermatozoal pellets after centrifugation and aspiration of seminal plasma. The spermatozoa are resuspended by gently swirling the tubes after the freezing extender is added. As a result of resuspension in a freezing extender, the spermatozoal pellet is gone from the bottom of the tube. Spermatozoal concentration is then determined by counting in a hemacytometer chamber, and sufficient additional extender is added to arrive at a final concentration of 120 million sperm/ml.

shock, dehydration, salt toxicity, intracellular ice formation, fluctuations in cellular volume/surface area, or metabolic imbalance. Given the destructive forces associated with cryopreservation, it seems amazing that any spermatozoa could survive the process.

The technique for cryopreservation of stallion spermatozoa involves several steps.

Increasing Spermatozoal Concentration

This step can be accomplished by either centrifuging (Figures 14-14 through 14-16) the ejaculated semen or collecting only the sperm-rich portion of ejaculates. Either method helps remove the potentially detrimental contribution of excess seminal plasma to the ejaculate, while increasing spermatozoal concentration. If centrifugation is performed, the semen must first be mixed with an appropriate centrifugation medium (Tables 14-1 and 14-2) to minimize cellular injury. Centrifugation time and force should be adjusted to maximize spermatozoal yield while maintaining spermatozoal viability. A

TABLE 14-2

Skim Milk–Based Centrifugation and Cryopreservation Media for Freezing Equine Spermatozoa

Modified Kenney Centrifugation Medium	
Nonfat dry milk solids (e.g., Sanalac)	24.0 g
Glucose	26.5 g
Sucrose	40.0 g
Potassium penicillin G	1,000,000 U
Amikacin sulfate	1.0 g
Sodium bicarbonate (1 mEq/ml)	6.0 ml
Deionized distilled water	qs 1000 ml
This extender may be frozen at –20 °C in smaller aliquots until used.	
Cryopreservation Medium	
Centrifugation medium (listed above)	92.5 ml
Egg yolk	4.0 ml
Glycerol	3.5 ml
Once egg yolk and glycerol are added, do not refreeze.	

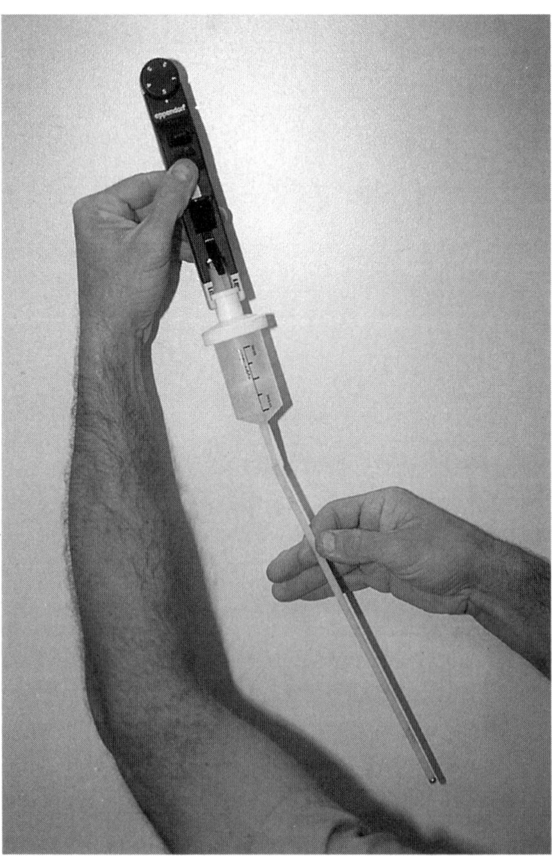

FIGURE 14-17. A 5-ml aliquot of the extended stallion spermatozoa (120 million sperm/ml) is pipetted into the plastic straws before freezing, providing a total of 600 million total spermatozoa/straw. The straws are sealed with metal or plastic balls on one end before filling and the other end after filling.

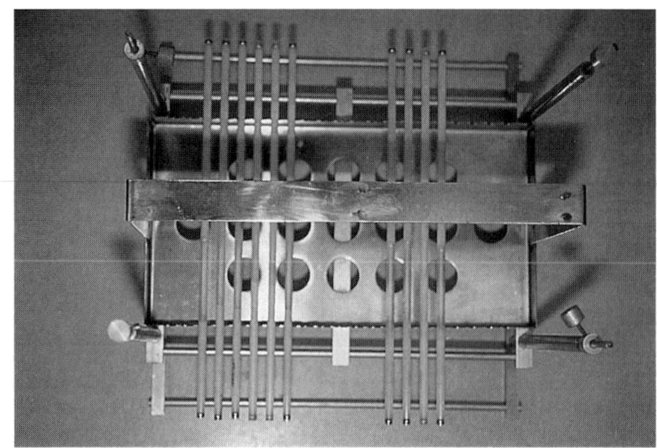

FIGURE 14-18. Semen-loaded straws are placed on a rack before being suspended in liquid nitrogen vapor. The semen freezes when placed in the vapor. It is critical to position the air bubble in the center of the straw before freezing to reduce the likelihood of a ball bursting out one end of the straw (i.e., this allows expansion and contraction of the liquid into the central air bubble during freezing and thawing). Once straws have been frozen (e.g., after 20 minutes in the liquid nitrogen vapor), the straws are plunged directly into the liquid nitrogen for several minutes before the straws are transferred to a liquid nitrogen holding tank.

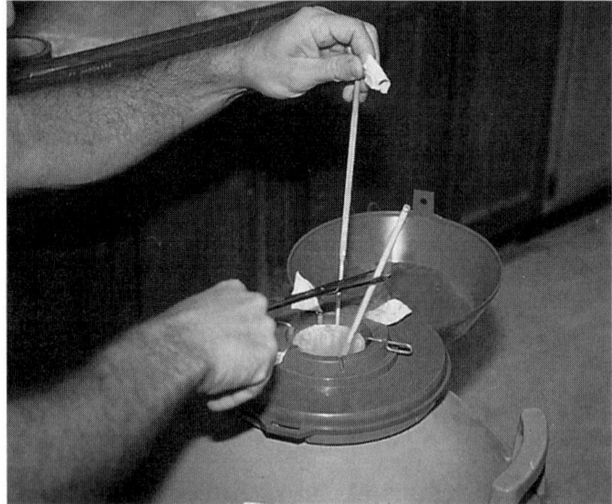

FIGURE 14-19. Transfer of straws of frozen equine semen into a liquid nitrogen holding tank for long-term storage. Straws should be transferred rapidly (e.g., within 9 seconds), one straw at a time, into canisters within the nitrogen tank. The canister is moved down into the liquid nitrogen tank between transfer of each straw to ensure that semen does not become warm enough to damage the cryopreserved spermatozoa.

Stallion Information:
Name:
Breed:
Registration #:
Age:
Present breeding status:
☐ Sexually rested ☐ Actively breeding ☐ D.S.O.
Total testicular volume (cc):
Estimated daily sperm output (x 10^9):
Additional information:

Client:

Veterinarian:

Semen Collection:
Date of collection:
Volume (cc):
[Sperm] (x 10^6/ml):
Total sperm # (x 10^9):
Initial motility (total/progressive[velocity]):
Sperm morphology (%):

Normal:	Abn heads:
Abn. Acrosomes:	Det. Heads:
Abn M/P:	Bent Midpieces:
Prox. Drop.:	Dist. Drop.:
Bent tails:	Coiled tails:
P.G.C.:	Other:

Total number of morphologically normal, progressively motile sperm (x 10^9):

Centrifugation:
Centrifugation extender used:
☐ German ☐ TAMU ☐ Other:
Antibiotic used:
☐ K^+ pen. G ☐ Amikacin sulfate ☐ Other:
Centrifugation tubes used:
☐ 50-ml plastic ☐ 50-ml glass
Centrifugation time: G-force:
Sperm number recovered in pellet (x 10^9):
Spermatozoal recovery rate:

Straw Information:
☐ Stallion name:
☐ Stallion breed:
☐ Registration number:
☐ Processing date:
☐ Processing location:
☐ Extender used:
Additional information:

Freezing Technique:
Freezing extender used:
☐ German Number of straws:
☐ TAMU Number of straws:
☐ Other Number of straws:
Antibiotic used:
Straw size: ☐ 0.5 ml ☐ 5 ml ☐ Other:
Method: ☐ Static vapor ☐ Programmable freezer
Sperm per straw (x 10^6):

Microbiological information:
Equine Viral Arteritis (EVA) test and vaccination: ☐ Test not performed ☐ Vaccination not performed
Test: Date: Results:
Vaccine used: Date:
Semen bacterial culture results (bacteria isolated): ☐ Test not performed
Pre-freeze semen:
Post-thaw semen:
Other tests performed: ☐ None
Test: Date: Results:
Test: Date: Results:

Post-thaw spermatozoal evaluation:
Number of straws evaluated:
Water bath: Temperature: °C Time: sec.

Extender		
% Motile sperm		
% Progressively motile sperm		
Spermatozoal velocity (0-4)		
Number motile sperm/straw		
Number prog. motile sperm/straw		

General assessment:

Extender:
☐ Post-thaw sperm viability appears good
☐ Post-thaw sperm viability appears marginal
☐ Post-thaw sperm viability appears poor
Extender:
☐ Post-thaw sperm viability appears good
☐ Post-thaw sperm viability appears marginal
☐ Post-thaw sperm viability appears poor

FIGURE 14-20. Equine frozen semen processing form.

centrifugation force of 500 × g for 10 minutes is generally a safe centrifugation technique for 40 to 45 ml of extended semen in 50-ml centrifuge vials. The centrifugation rotor should have a swing-basket to ensure that the spermatozoal pellet is in the bottom of the tube after centrifugation is performed. After centrifugation, most of the seminal plasma is removed from above the sperm pellet. Results of a recent experiment suggest leaving 5% seminal plasma may improve post-thaw semen quality compared to removing all of the seminal plasma.

Adding Cryopreservation Medium

The extenders for cryopreservation (Tables 14-1 and 14-2) of stallion semen consist of various mixtures of egg yolk, milk, sugars, buffers, electrolytes, antibiotics, and glycerol. The cryopreservation medium is added back to the spermatozoal pellet after step 1 (and spermatozoa are resuspended by gentle mixing) until the desired concentration of spermatozoa is achieved. The final spermatozoal concentration can vary from 100 million sperm/ml to 1.6 billion sperm/ml, depending on straw size and number of straws desired for a complete insemination dose. A breeding dose of 400 to 800 million total sperm is common when traditional insemination techniques are used.

Packaging Semen

Stallion spermatozoa most commonly are packaged in small-volume straws (0.5- or 4- to 5-ml capacity) (Figure 14-17). The 4- or 5-ml straws generally contain 600 to 800 million total spermatozoa, and one straw is used per breeding. The 0.5-ml straws usually contain considerably fewer spermatozoa, so more than one straw may have to be used to provide an adequate insemination dose (often six to eight straws).

Freezing Semen

The most common cryogen for semen cryopreservation is liquid nitrogen. Packaged semen can be placed horizontally in static nitrogen vapor at a recommended level (1 to 4 cm) above the liquid-gas interface, using a specially designed rack (Figure 14-18). Alternatively, packaged semen can be frozen in a programmable nitrogen freezer.

Storing Semen

Semen is submerged in liquid nitrogen (–196° C) contained in specially designed storage tanks to maintain spermatozoa in a dormant state (Figure 14-19). A straw of the cryopreserved semen from each freezing should be thawed (at the recommended rate) and warmed to 37° C for 10 to 15 minutes to determine postthaw spermatozoal motility. A record of this motility should be kept, and a form containing stallion and freezing information should accompany transport of each straw to be used for breeding (Figure 14-20).

Thawing Semen

Packaged semen is thawed in a water bath. Bath temperature and immersion time are designated by the company or individual responsible for freezing the semen. German straws (4 or 5 ml) are generally thawed for 42 seconds in a 50° C water bath, whereas 0.5-ml straws are generally thawed for 30 seconds in a 37° C water bath.

Insemination

Immediately after thawing, packaged semen is inseminated, using the technique prescribed by the company or individual responsible for freezing the semen. For most stallions, the best pregnancy rates will probably be achieved when mares are inseminated within 0 to 24 hours before ovulation or within 6 hours postovulation. Deep insemination near the tip of the uterine horn on the side ipsilateral to the ovulating follicle may increase pregnancy rates with frozen semen.

A variety of protocols are available for cryopreservation of stallion semen. Controlled studies that might disclose the most successful of these techniques have not been conducted. Marked variation exists among stallions with respect to "freezability" of semen, so cryopreservation protocols may need to be individualized to accommodate these idiosyncrasies. Pregnancy rates are reported to range from 0% to 70% per cycle when frozen/thawed stallion semen is used for insemination, with *pregnancy rates per cycle in the 20% to 40% range for a high percentage of stallions.* It therefore becomes obvious that much improvement is needed in the technique so that semen can be successfully frozen from a larger percentage of stallions. Intensified reproductive management of mares (e.g., repeated palpations to ensure insemination close to ovulation) may also be required to enhance pregnancy rates achieved by breeding with frozen-thawed semen because longevity of postthaw spermatozoal motility is generally reduced significantly compared with that of spermatozoa in fresh extended semen.

SUMMARY

Preservation of stallion semen in the cooled or frozen state may reduce the costs and potential health hazards incurred by transporting mares and provides easier access to genetic material that may otherwise be unavailable. Acceptable pregnancy rates are consistently obtained with cooled semen. Conversely, techniques for cryopreservation of stallion spermatozoa will require more refinement before the procedure can be considered commercially viable on a wide-scale basis.

BIBLIOGRAPHY

Brinsko SP, Varner DD: Artificial insemination and preservation of semen. In Blanchard TL, Varner DD, editors, *Stallion management. Vet Clin North Am Equine Pract* 8:205-218, 1992.

Kayser JP, Amann RP, Shideler RK et al: Effects of linear cooling rate on motion characteristics of stallion spermatozoa. *Theriogenology* 38:601-614, 1992.

Moran DM, Jasko DJ, Squires EL et al: Determination of temperature and cooling rate which induce cold shock in stallion spermatozoa. *Theriogenology* 38:999-1012, 1992.

Varner DD, Blanchard TL: Current perspectives on handling and storage of equine semen. *Proc Am Assoc Equine Pract* 40:39-40, 1994.

15

Surgery of the Mare Reproductive Tract

OBJECTIVES

While studying the information covered in this chapter, the student should attempt to:

1. Acquire a working knowledge of the conformational defects acquired through injury during parturition or that develop in aged, multiparous mares.
2. Acquire a working understanding of the surgical procedures and techniques used to correct conformational abnormalities that contribute to infertility in the mare.

STUDY QUESTIONS

1. Discuss injuries that occur during parturition and result in abnormal conformation of the genital tract of the mare.
2. Discuss conformational defects of the urogenital tract that occur in aged, pluriparous mares and contribute to infertility.
3. Describe procedures and techniques for performing a Caslick suture in the mare.
4. Describe the procedure for placing a breeding stitch in the vulva of a mare.
5. Describe the procedure for performing a perineoplasty in the mare.
6. Describe the procedure used for performing a urethral extension in the mare.
7. Describe the procedure for correcting a perineal laceration in the mare.
8. Describe the procedure for correcting a rectovaginal fistula in the mare.
9. Describe the procedure for correcting a cervical laceration in the mare.
10. List preoperative and postoperative considerations for urogenital surgeries in the mare.

Surgical procedures on the mare reproductive tract (with the exceptions of cesarean section, surgical correction of uterine torsion, and ovariectomy) are performed primarily to correct urogenital abnormalities that contribute to contamination of the reproductive tract. Contamination results from injuries that occur during parturition or conformational changes that occur with increasing age. This chapter will discuss only the more common surgical procedures performed to reconstruct vulvar, vaginal, and cervical abnormalities. For more detailed descriptions of these and other surgical procedures involving the reproductive tract, refer to veterinary medical surgical texts.

SELECTION OF CANDIDATES FOR SURGERY

Mares with conformational changes of the urogenital tract that can be corrected by surgical reconstruction are candidates for surgery, provided the results of a thorough breeding soundness examination indicate that the procedure has a good chance of restoring the mare's fertility. Exceptions to the need for a breeding soundness examination are third-degree perineal lacerations and rectovaginal fistulas, which usually arise in fertile, young mares during foaling as a result of fetal malposture during delivery. Indeed, such a mare has no reason to be infertile once contamination of the reproductive tract is prevented by surgical reconstruction. However, for other procedures used to surgically correct reproductive abnormalities, a breeding soundness examination is indicated to assess the future breeding potential of the mare. If severe and irreparable damage to the endometrium, cervix, or vagina has occurred, the owner may elect not to invest time and money into surgery and aftercare.

Before performing any surgical procedure the practitioner should make sure that the mare has been adequately immunized against tetanus.

Defects that are commonly corrected by reconstructive surgery of the reproductive tract include the following:

- Pneumovagina caused by a cranially sunken anus and tipping of the vulva (see Figure 1-8).
- Urovagina caused by cranioventral deviation of the vagina, which pulls the urethral orifice forward and results in some urine splashing into the vagina during urination (see Figure 4-16).

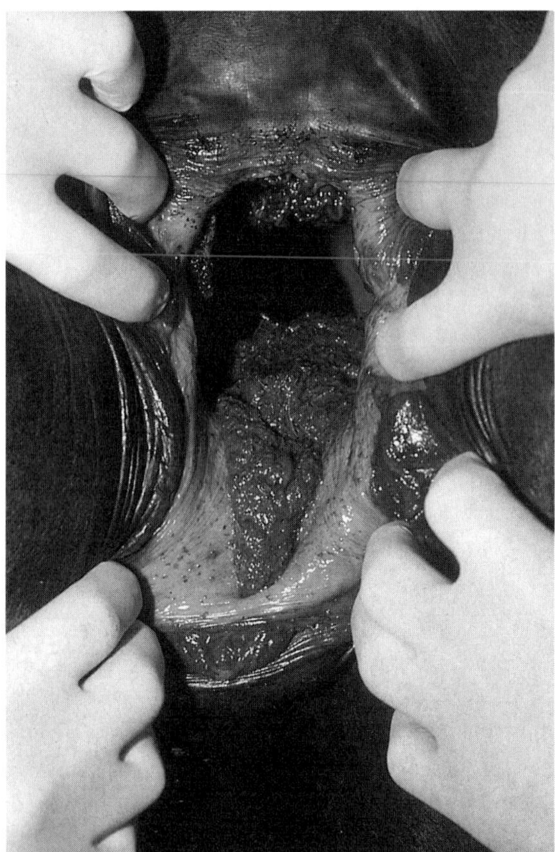

FIGURE 15-1. Third-degree perineal laceration in a mare. The perineal body and rectovaginal shelf were breached during foaling. Extensive fecal contamination is apparent.

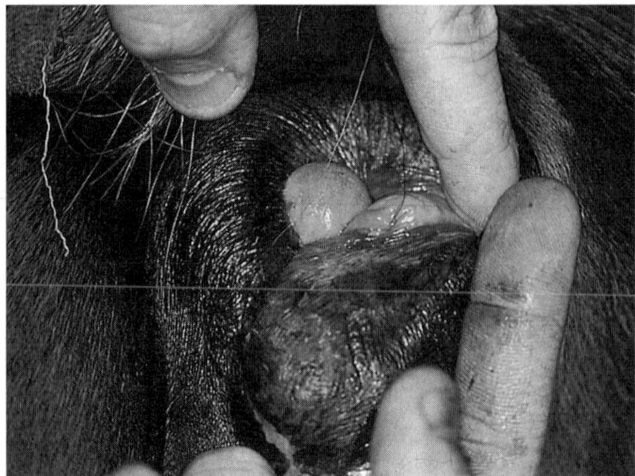

FIGURE 15-2. A rectovaginal fistula located just cranial to the anal sphincter. A finger has been passed through the fistula from the vestibule into the rectum to illustrate the location of the fistula. Fistulas may be small or large and may be located caudally, near the vestibule, or more cranially, in the vagina.

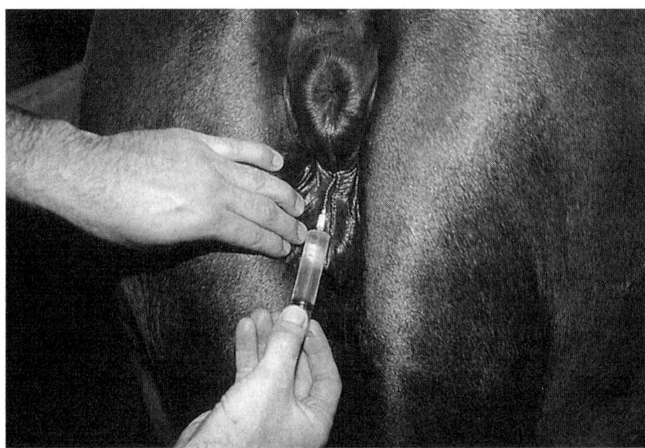

FIGURE 15-3. Caslick operation. Infiltration of the labia with a local anesthetic solution. The local anesthesia should extend from the dorsal commissure of the vulva to just below the floor of the ischium.

Perineal lacerations that occur during foaling, the most severe of which is a third-degree perineal laceration that results from complete tearing of the shelf between the rectum and vagina, including the perineal body (Figure 15-1). If a laceration through the dorsal vaginal wall perforating into the rectum does not result in formation of a third-degree perineal laceration (i.e., the perineal body is not disrupted), a rectovaginal fistula generally occurs. Fecal contamination of the vagina often follows the fistula formation, but the fistula is often not visualized by external observation (Figure 15-2).

Cervical lacerations arise from tearing of an insufficiently dilated cervix during delivery or as a result of dystocia (see Figure 4-12).

PNEUMOVAGINA

Pneumovagina is a condition wherein conformational faults predispose a mare to aspiration of air and fecal matter into the vagina. It is commonly called "wind-sucking," and the constant contamination usually culminates in ascending infection—vaginitis, cervicitis, and endometritis. Causes of pneumovagina include tearing or stretching of the vulvar seal or vulvovaginal sphincter (see Chapter 1) and a sunken perineal body that often includes the anal sphincter, resulting in tipping of the vulva forward over the pelvic brim (see Figure 1-8). The condition is quite common in underweight, aged, pluriparous mares.

The most common surgical procedure used to correct pneumovagina is the Caslick operation. To perform a Caslick operation, the mare is placed in a stock, and her tail is wrapped and tied out of the way. The perineum and vulva are scrubbed with a disinfectant soap, rinsed, and dried. To prevent the mare from moving around excessively during infiltration of local anesthetic, a sedative can be administered or a twitch can be applied to the lip. A local anesthetic such as lidocaine is injected beneath the skin at the vulvar mucocutaneous junction (Figure 15-3). Local anesthesia should extend from the dorsal commissure of the vulva to just below the floor of the ischium. The level to which the Caslick

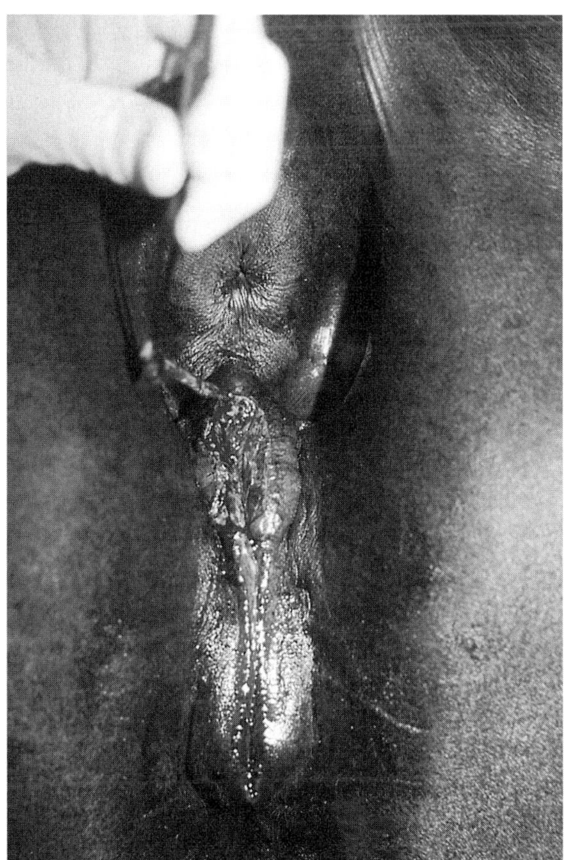

FIGURE 15-4. Caslick operation. A thin strip of skin at the mucocutaneous junction of vulvar lips is removed to prepare for suturing.

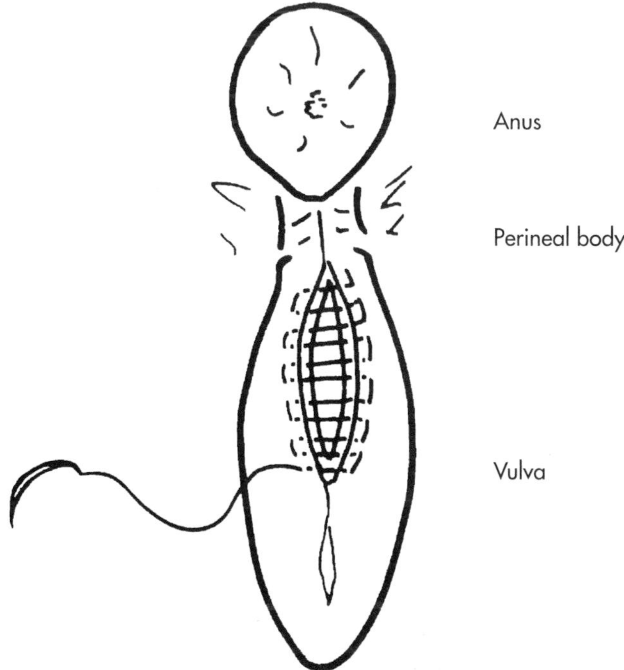

FIGURE 15-5. Caslick operation. The débrided vulvar lips are apposed intimately by suturing. A continuous horizontal mattress pattern is shown in this illustration. However, a continuous interlocking suture pattern is more commonly used.

suture line should extend ventrally can be determined by placing firm pressure with the fingers on either side of the vulva and pressing down to locate the ischium. If the Caslick suture line is not extended below this point, the vulva will bounce forward sufficiently for air to be aspirated into the vagina as the mare moves. Care should also be taken to ensure that sufficient room remains in the ventral portion of the vulva to permit penile insertion during natural cover or speculum insertion for breeding by artificial insemination and also to allow urine to escape during urination. This generally requires that four fingers can be inserted easily into the vulvar opening after completion of the operation (i.e., 10 to 12 cm of the ventral vulvar opening should be left unsutured).

After infiltration with local anesthetic, a thin strip of tissue at the mucocutaneous junction (approximately 0.5 cm wide) is removed with scissors (Figure 15-4). Care should be taken to avoid removing too much skin, as the mare will probably require several more Caslick operations over the period of the next few years. The vulvar lips are apposed intimately by suturing (Figure 15-5). Generally, no. 0 or 00 nonabsorbable suture material is used. The suture pattern used is usually not critical because little tension is exerted on the suture line (e.g., simple continuous, continuous interlocking, or continuous horizontal mattress patterns are commonly used), as long as good apposition is accomplished. Nonabsorbable suture material should be removed after healing occurs, generally in 10 to 14 days.

If the Caslick suture must be reopened for breeding or vaginal examination at a later time or to permit foaling to occur without tearing of the vulva, it can be resutured. A breeding stitch is sometimes used to preclude the need to open the Caslick suture in a mare that must be bred. This involves placement of a single simple interrupted suture at the ventral edge of the vulvar closure (Figure 15-6). Umbilical tape or heavy Vetafil is commonly used as suture material for the breeding stitch. The suture bite should extend at least 1 cm out from the vulvar lip suture line, and the deep portion of the suture should be covered by tissue to avoid abrading the stallion's penis during breeding. The suture is placed rather loosely, so it just takes up tension as the vulvar opening is stretched (to prevent tearing of the Caslick suture line). It is helpful to use a breeding roll to limit the extent of penile intromission during natural service to avoid tearing of the Caslick suture or breeding stitch (Figure 15-7).

For mares with an extremely sunken anus and perineal body, almost the entire vulva may be pulled forward into a horizontal position over the ischium. A Caslick suture may not correct pneumovagina in such mares; indeed, if the suture is carried low enough to prevent pneumovagina, the mare may not be able to expel urine through the small opening that is left. To correct such extreme instances of poor

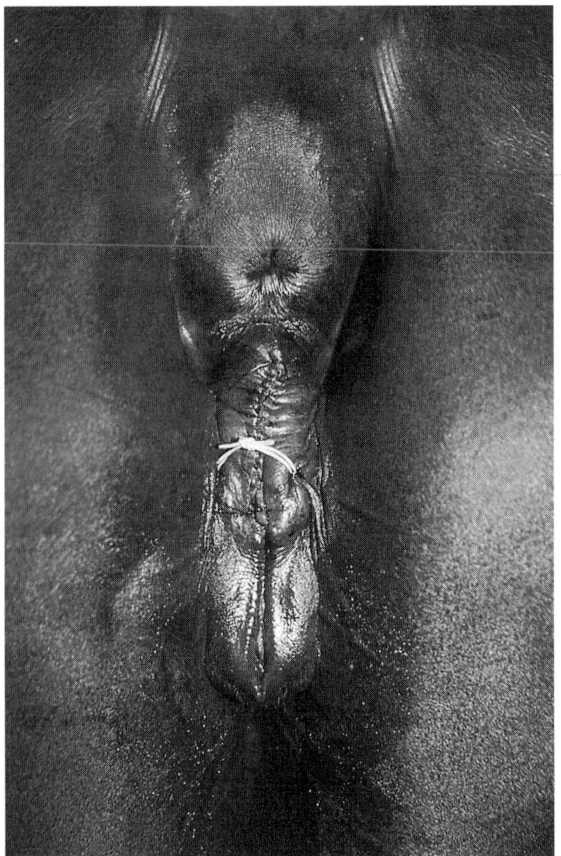

FIGURE 15-6. A breeding stitch is sometimes used to preclude the need to open the Caslick suture in a mare that must be bred by natural service. A single, simple interrupted suture is placed at the ventral edge of the Caslick operation using a large, nonabsorbable suture material such as heavy Vetafil. The suture bite should extend at least 1 cm out from the vulvar labia, and the deep portion of the suture should be covered by tissue to avoid abrading the stallion's penis during breeding. The suture is tied loosely so it just takes up tension as the vulvar opening is stretched.

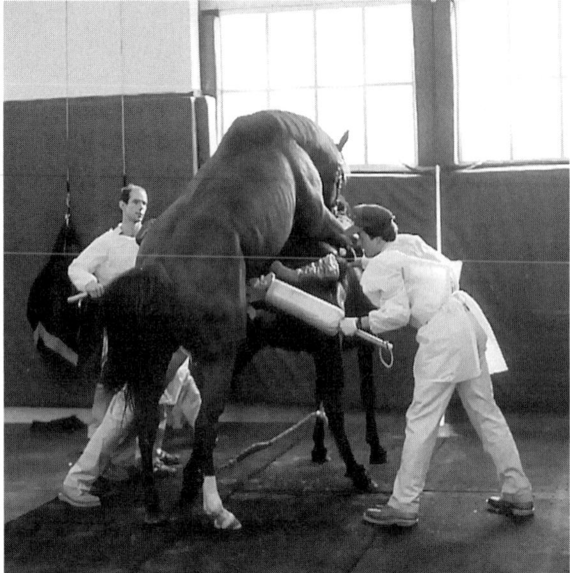

FIGURE 15-7. Use of a breeding roll to prevent full intromission of the stallion's penis into the vagina during natural service. The roll is inserted above the base of the penis, between the groin of the stallion and the rump of the mare, during breeding.

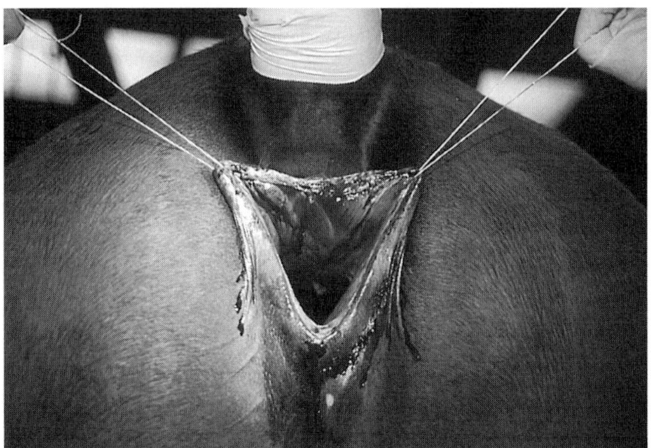

FIGURE 15-8. Modified perineoplasty (described by Dr. Steven Slusher of Oklahoma State University). After analgesia of the surgical area is attained, retraction sutures are placed to the right and left of the dorsal commissure of the vulva. The dorsal vulvar lips are retracted caudally and dorsally to expose the dorsal mucosal surface of the vulva.

conformation, a perineal body reconstruction (or perineoplasty) must be performed. We often perform a modified perineoplasty as described by Slusher (1986).

Anesthesia for perineal body reconstruction consists of systemic administration of a sedative and injection of 6 to 8 ml of local anesthetic (through an 18-gauge 1½-inch needle) into the epidural space. After analgesia is attained, retraction sutures are placed to the right and left of the dorsal commissure of the vulva, and the dorsal vulvar lips are retracted caudally and dorsally to expose the dorsal mucosal surface of the vulva (Figure 15-8). The distance from the dorsal commissure to a position ventral to the anal sphincter is measured and marked on the vulvar mucosa. This mark will serve as the apex of a triangle of mucosa to be removed. One half of this distance is measured on the dorsal vulvar mucosa to the left and also to the right of the dorsal commissure of the vulva. A line between these two points will serve as the base of the mucosal triangle to be removed (Figure 15-9). The points of the triangle are connected using a scalpel, and the superficial mucosa overlying this area is removed (Figure 15-10). Two or three stint sutures are placed horizontally in a line from the apex of the triangle to the base as shown in Figure 15-11. Small rolls of gauze work well to hold the suture material (no. 1 or 2 nonabsorbable) and prevent the suture from pulling through the skin. Just enough tension is placed to bring the triangular area into a vertical position, and stint

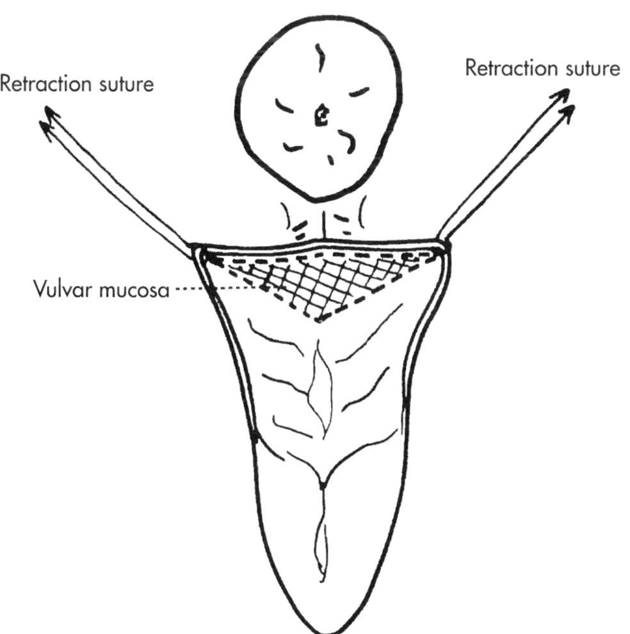

FIGURE 15-9. Modified perineoplasty. The *dotted line* indicates the area of dorsal vulvar mucosa to be removed.

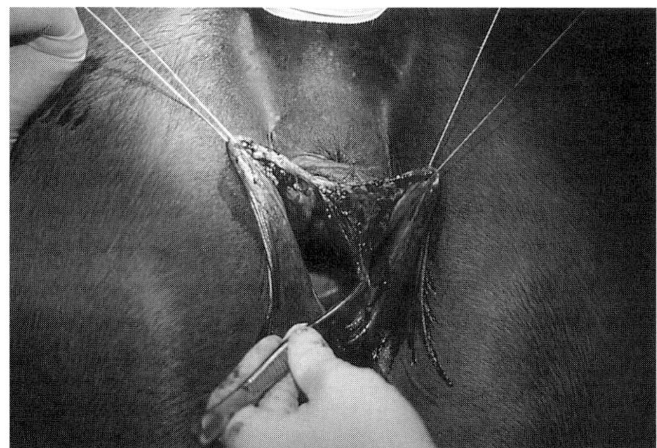

FIGURE 15-10. Modified perineoplasty. A triangular area of dorsal vulvar mucosa is removed using forceps and scissors.

sutures are removed in 5 to 10 days. If excessive tension is placed on the stints, they will cause tissue necrosis. If sutures begin to cause tissue necrosis, they can be removed one at a time at daily or alternate-day intervals to relieve pressure. Necrotic tissue generally fills in with granulation tissue within 1 to 2 weeks. This surgical procedure effectively raises the perineal body and returns the vulva to a more vertical position (Figure 15-12). The sunken position of the anus remains unchanged. If the procedure is done properly, the vulvar opening will not be appreciably shortened, and mares may subsequently be bred by natural service.

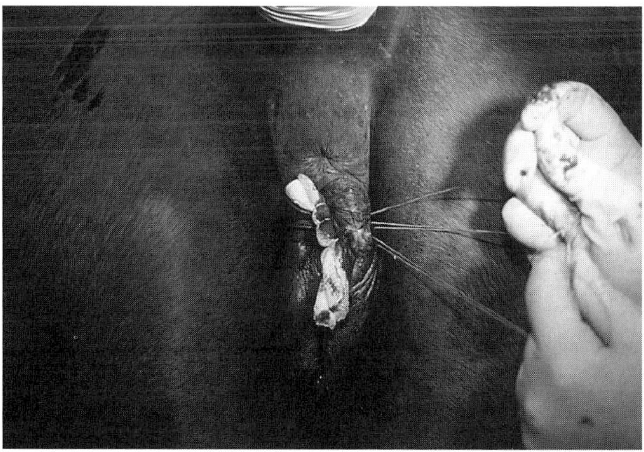

FIGURE 15-11. Modified perineoplasty. Two or three stint sutures are placed horizontally in a line from the apex to the base of the triangle shown in Figure 15-10. Small rolls of gauze or rubber tubing can be used to hold the stint sutures.

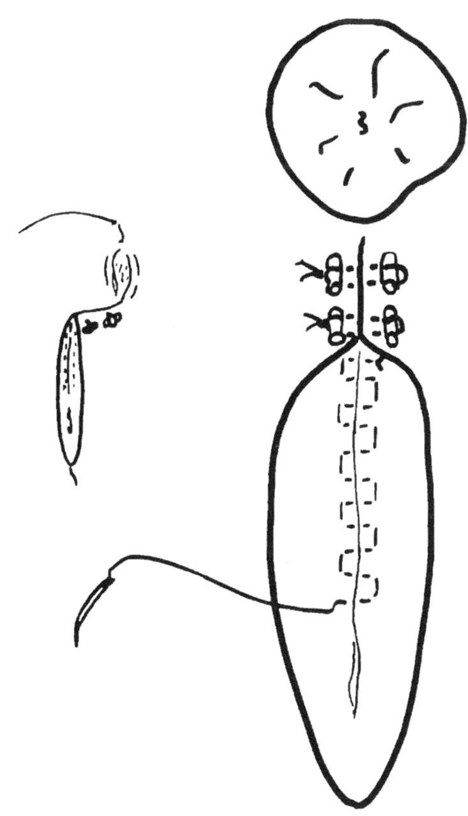

FIGURE 15-12. Modified perineoplasty. Completed placement of stint and Caslick sutures. This procedure raises the perineal body and returns the vulva to a more vertical position.

UROVAGINA

Older, pluriparous mares sometimes have reflux of urine into the vagina during urination. Reflux of urine is attributable to conformational changes that occur as a result of progressive descent of the birth canal into the abdomen from repeated stretching with pregnancy. This results in cranial displacement of the urethral opening until it is located cranial to the pelvic brim, causing the mare to "urinate uphill." The pooling of urine (urine pooling) into the vagina is termed urovagina. The constant presence of urine is irritating and contributes to infection (vaginitis, cervicitis, and endometritis) (see Figure 4-16). More severe instances culminate in chronic dribbling of urine from the vulva and between the thighs (Figure 15-13). The tail, ventral vulva, and inner thighs build exudate, and the chronically irritated skin becomes scalded. Before surgery a uterine biopsy should be procured and evaluated. If widespread and severe periglandular fibrosis is present (permanently lowering the mare's potential to conceive and carry a viable foal to term), the owner of the mare may choose not to proceed with surgery. If severe permanent changes are not present in the endometrium, the mare is a more suitable candidate for corrective surgery.

To correct urovagina, we prefer the urethral extension technique described by Brown et al (1978). This technique involves forming a tunnel from the existing urethral orifice caudally along the floor of the vestibule of sufficient length to ensure expulsion of urine from the vagina and vulva during urination. The mare is prepared for surgery by systemic administration of a sedative and injection of 6 to 8 ml of local anesthetic into the caudal epidural space. The tail is wrapped and tied dorsally, and the perineal area is scrubbed with disinfectant soap. Sterilized tissue retractors are used to pull the labia and vulva laterally to expose the urethral orifice. The transverse membranous fold (hymenal remnant) is tacked to the dorsal vaginal mucosa to avoid its interference with the surgical procedure. An elliptical incision through the mucosa is made 1 to 1.5 cm craniolateral to the urethral orifice so that it half encircles the urethral opening (Figure 15-14). Each side of the incision is continued caudolaterally so that, when sutured, the "tube" formed will get progressively wider caudally (this ensures that pressure buildup will not occur during urination, which can cause dehiscence). The incision is closed in three layers in the following order:

- A continuous horizontal mattress suture pattern, using no. 0 or 00 absorbable suture material, is used to appose and invert the inner mucosal layer (Figure 15-15).
- A simple continuous suture pattern, using no. 0 or 00 absorbable suture material, is used to appose the middle subcutaneous layer (Figure 15-16).

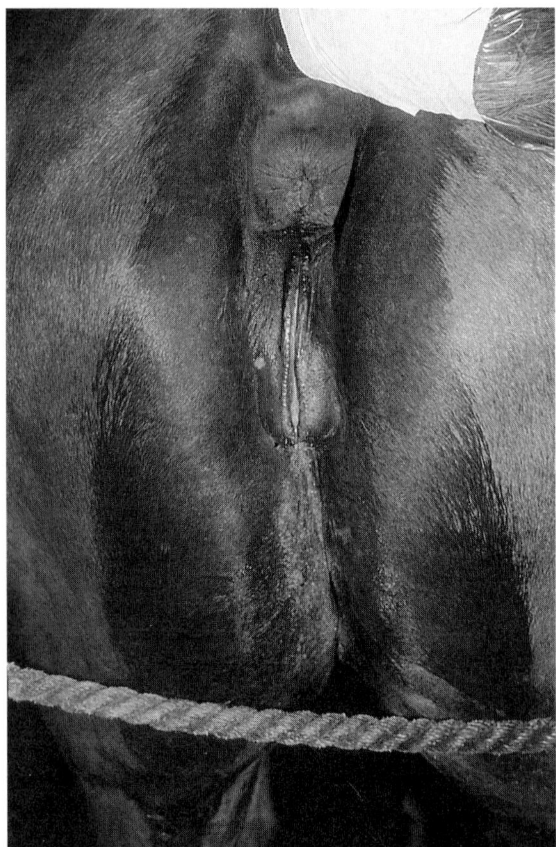

FIGURE 15-13. Urine scalding caused by constant dribbling of urine between the thighs of a mare with severe urovagina.

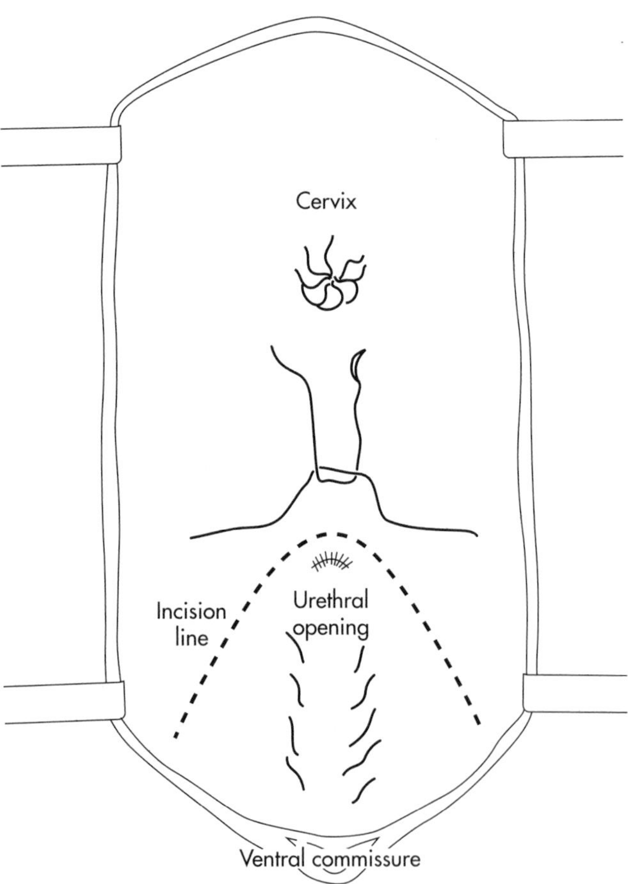

FIGURE 15-14. Urethral extension surgery. The incision line (*dotted line*) for the surgery is shown. The hymenal fold is tacked to the dorsal vagina to expose the urethral orifice and improve visualization. (Modified from Brown MP, Colahan PT, Hawkins DL: Urethral extension for treatment of urine pooling in mares. *J Am Vet Med Assoc* 173:1005, 1978.)

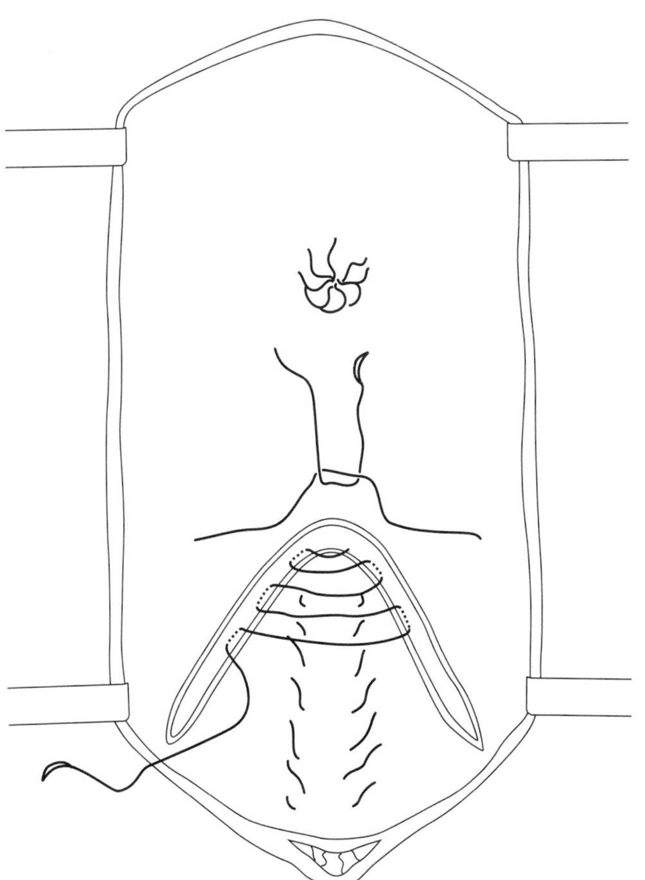

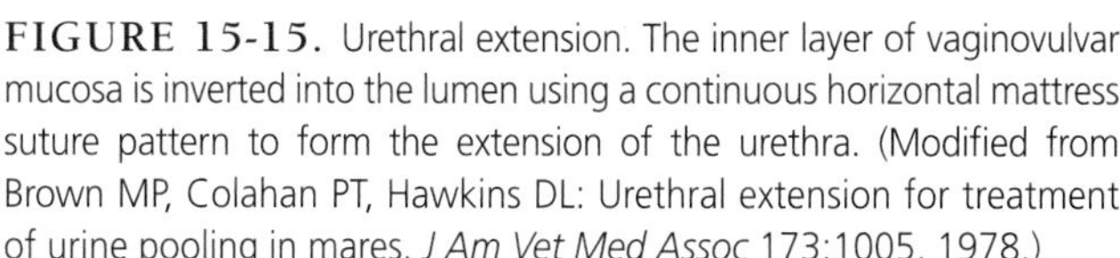

FIGURE 15-15. Urethral extension. The inner layer of vaginovulvar mucosa is inverted into the lumen using a continuous horizontal mattress suture pattern to form the extension of the urethra. (Modified from Brown MP, Colahan PT, Hawkins DL: Urethral extension for treatment of urine pooling in mares. *J Am Vet Med Assoc* 173:1005, 1978.)

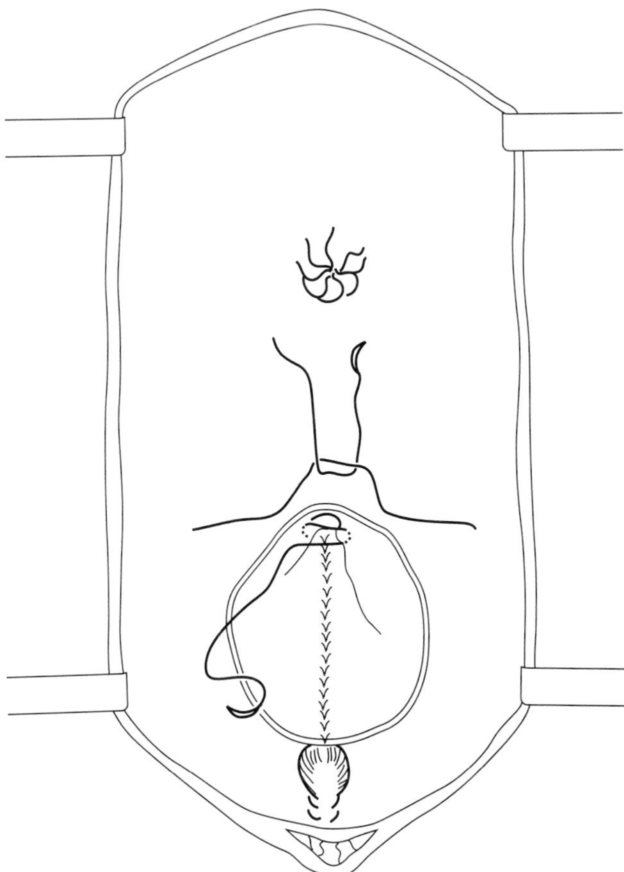

FIGURE 15-16. Urethral extension. The middle (submucosal) layer of the urethral extension is apposed in a simple continuous suture pattern. (Modified from Brown MP, Colahan PT, Hawkins DL: Urethral extension for treatment of urine pooling in mares. *J Am Vet Med Assoc* 173:1005, 1978.)

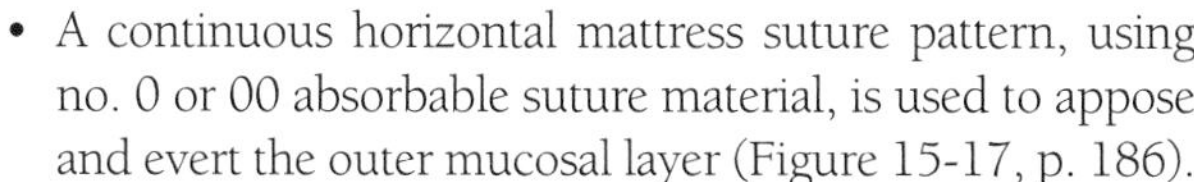

- A continuous horizontal mattress suture pattern, using no. 0 or 00 absorbable suture material, is used to appose and evert the outer mucosal layer (Figure 15-17, p. 186).

Because many mares with urovagina also have pneumovagina, a Casick's suture is placed in the vulva if necessary. Aftercare consists of administration of a broad-spectrum antibiotic for 3 to 5 days. Choosing an antibiotic eliminated through the urine (e.g., trimethoprim-sulfamethoxazole) may be beneficial. It may also be helpful to administer a nonsteroidal antiinflammatory drug, such as flunixin meglumine, for 12 to 24 hours after surgery to control postoperative pain.

PERINEAL LACERATIONS AND RECTOVAGINAL FISTULAS

Perineal lacerations occur primarily in mares delivering their first foal. They arise when the previously undilated birth canal does not safely accommodate foal passage. Third-degree perineal lacerations occur when the foal's foot is directed through the dorsal roof of the vagina (probably catching on the remnant of the hymen dorsally in the vagina) into the rectum. The strong abdominal press that ensures delivery of the foal also forces complete disruption of the vaginal roof, rectal floor, and perineal septum and body. If the malposture is corrected in time, enabling the foot to be returned to the vagina before delivery, the perineal body is spared but a rectovaginal fistula remains.

Less severe lacerations of the perineum may also occur as a result of foaling through an unopened Caslick suture, dystocia, or delivery of a large fetus. These are termed *first-* or *second-degree perineal lacerations.*

First-Degree Perineal Laceration

These lacerations only involve the skin and mucous membrane of the dorsal commissure of the vulva. They are easily corrected by suturing the edges of the torn skin.

Second-Degree Perineal Laceration

Second-degree lacerations (sometimes paired) extend deeper into the perineal body than first-degree lacerations, disrupting

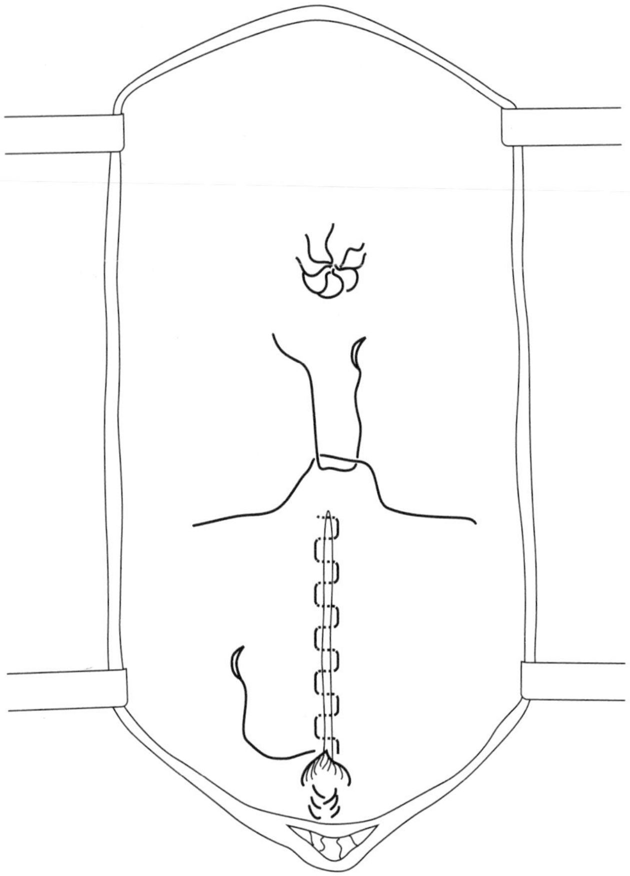

FIGURE 15-17. Urethral extension. The outer mucosal layer of the urethral extension is everted using a continuous horizontal mattress suture pattern. (Modified from Brown MP, Colahan PT, Hawkins DL: Urethral extension for treatment of urine pooling in mares. *J Am Vet Med Assoc* 173:1005, 1978.)

the musculature of the constrictor vulvae and the perineal body, compromising the ability of these muscles to constrict the vulvar opening and leading to pneumovagina. Repair is straightforward. If it is not possible to suture the wound immediately after parturition, surgery should be delayed until tissue bruising and swelling have regressed. Surgical repair is similar to that described for perineoplasty, although some "creative plastic surgery" may be required to restore normal conformation of the perineal body and vulvar labia.

The presurgical considerations for third-degree perineal lacerations and rectovaginal fistulas are the same. Surgical repair should not be attempted until swelling and healing from the acute trauma subsides. Whether antibiotic or antiinflammatory therapy in the period immediately after injury is beneficial has not been studied, but most mares do well and recover from the injury (while the anatomic defect remains) with no untoward effects. Repair should be delayed for at least 1 month after foaling. If the injury occurs near the end of the breeding season and the foal survives, some owners will elect to delay the repair of the defect until after the foal is weaned. Surprisingly, even though fecal contamination of the vagina is constant, permanent damage to the uterus usually does not occur. A major factor affecting the outcome of the surgery is softness of the stool. The stool must remain soft and pliable to avoid undue stress on the healing tissues during defecation, which leads to dehiscence. If lush, green pasture is available, simply allowing the mare to graze will keep the stool soft. If lush pasture is not available, dietary modifications are needed to ensure that the stool is soft before and for 10 days to 2 weeks after surgery. Mineral oil can be administered daily by nasogastric tube or can be mixed with grain and bran during feeding, to achieve the desired softness of the stool.

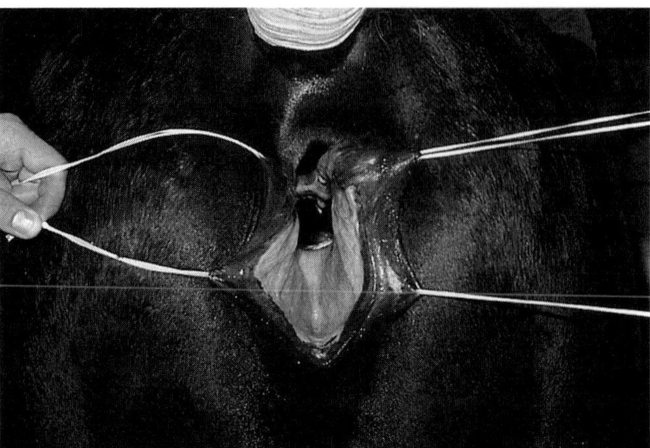

FIGURE 15-18. Surgical repair of a third-degree perineal laceration. Retention sutures are placed in the dorsolateral vulvar lips and ventrolateral anal sphincter. (Modified from Walker DF, Vaughan JT: *Bovine and equine urogenital surgery.* Philadelphia, 1980, Lea and Febiger.)

Lengthened surgical instruments are helpful in repairing deep lacerations. Surgery is performed with the mare standing in a stock. The mare is sedated, and a local anesthetic is administered into the epidural space. The tail is wrapped and tied dorsally, and the rectum is emptied of manure as far as the operator can reach. A tampon, made from a 3- or 4-inch stockinette filled with cotton, can be placed in the rectum cranial to the defect to prevent manure leakage into the surgical site during repair. The vagina and rectum are cleaned with cotton soaked in dilute povidone-iodine solution, and the perineal area is scrubbed with a disinfectant soap and dried. Retention sutures are placed in the dorsolateral vulvar lips and ventrolateral anal sphincter (Figure 15-18).

Third-Degree Perineal Lacerations

For repair of third-degree perineal lacerations (described in detail by Walker and Vaughan, 1980), a scalpel and scissors are used to dissect through the contracted scar tissue along the healed lateral borders of the defect (Figure 15-19). This dissection is continued into the rectovaginal shelf approximately 1 to $1\frac{1}{2}$ inches beyond the cranial end of the defect

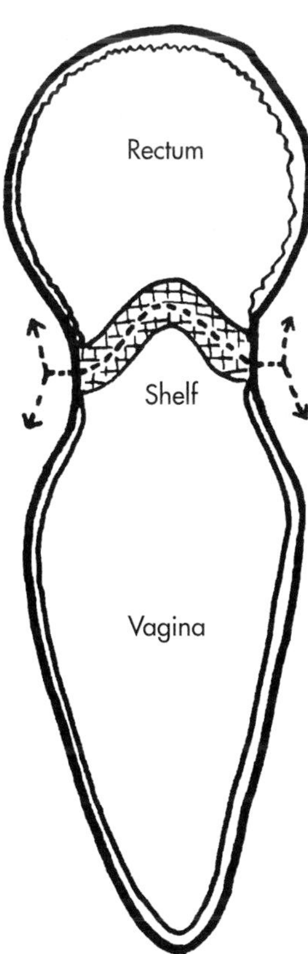

FIGURE 15-19. Surgical repair of a third-degree perineal laceration. The dissection pattern to be used lies along scar tissue from the torn rectovaginal shelf located along the cranial and lateral borders of the defect. (Modified from Walker DF, Vaughan JT: *Bovine and equine urogenital surgery.* Philadelphia, 1980, Lea and Febiger.)

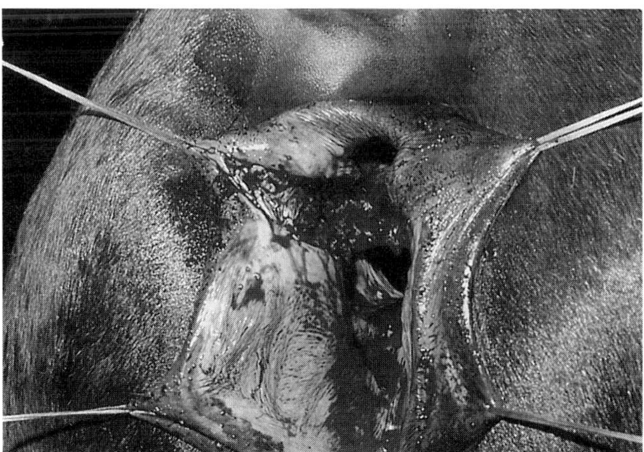

FIGURE 15-20. Surgical repair of a third-degree perineal laceration. The dissection is carried forward to separate the rectum from the vagina cranially for 1 to $1\frac{1}{2}$ inches into the remaining rectovaginal shelf. (Modified from Walker DF, Vaughan JT: *Bovine and equine urogenital surgery.* Philadelphia, 1980, Lea and Febiger.)

(i.e., dissecting between the rectal floor and vaginal roof where they are joined cranially) (Figure 15-20). The amount of dissection necessary is judged by the ease with which the lateral borders of the dissected tissue can be pulled to the midline. If this requires too much tension, further dissection will be required to provide sufficient tissue to be pulled to the center of the defect without predisposing the incision to suture dehiscence. We prefer to close the defect in two layers:

- A simple continuous suture pattern, using no. 0 absorbable suture material, is placed in the tissue just beneath the rectal mucosa (Figure 15-21). This inverts the rectal mucosal edges into the rectal lumen. Care should be taken to ensure good apposition of rectal mucosa to reduce the chances of manure leakage into the healing defect, which will cause dehiscence and formation of a rectovaginal fistula. To prevent interference with suture placement described below, the suture line is alternately extended with the six-bite pattern of closure of the perineal shelf and vaginal mucosa.
- With no. 2 or 3 absorbable suture material, interrupted six-bite sutures (placed 0.5 to 1 cm apart) are used to close the perineal shelf and vaginal mucosa (see Figure 15-21). This pattern causes the vaginal mucosa to invert

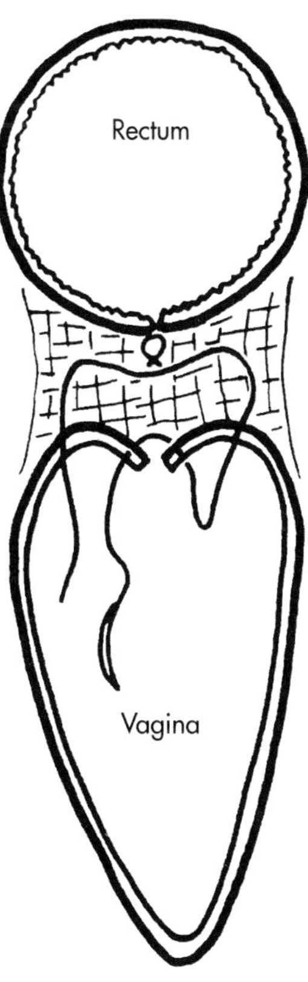

FIGURE 15-21. Surgical repair of a third-degree perineal laceration. An inverting (into rectal lumen) suture pattern is placed just beneath the rectal mucosa, ensuring that no suture material is left exposed to the rectal lumen. An interrupted six-bite suture pattern is used to close the defect in the rectovaginal shelf. (Modified from Walker DF, Vaughan JT: *Bovine and equine urogenital surgery.* Philadelphia, 1980, Lea and Febiger.)

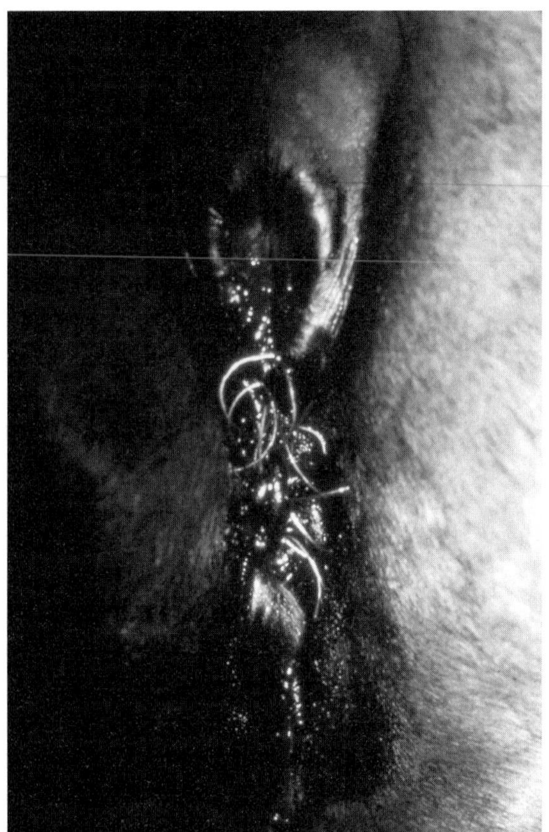

FIGURE 15-22. Surgical repair of a third-degree perineal laceration. The perineal body and vulva have been sutured, illustrating how the procedure restores the normal configuration of the anal sphincter and vulva. (Modified from Walker DF, Vaughan JT: *Bovine and equine urogenital surgery.* Philadelphia, 1980, Lea and Febiger.)

into the vaginal lumen and creates a thickly reconstructed shelf. Placement of several interrupted "six-bite" sutures is alternated with placement of several continuous sutures just beneath the rectal mucosa.

The two layers of closure are continued until the perineal shelf is rebuilt and the perineal body is reconstructed. Care must be taken to avoid gradually narrowing the rectal lumen as the suture lines progress caudally. The tampon is removed from the rectum. Nonabsorbable sutures are placed in the skin of the perineal body and the vulvar lips (Caslick suture) (Figure 15-22).

Rectovaginal Fistulas

For repair of rectovaginal fistulas (Figure 15-23) (Walker and Vaughan, 1980), a horizontal dissection line is begun in the perineal body midway between the anal sphincter and the dorsal commissure of the vulva (Figure 15-24). This horizontal line of dissection is continued cranially through the fistula and 1 to $1\frac{1}{2}$ inches beyond the defect, separating the rectal defect dorsally from the vaginal defect ventrally (Figure 15-25).

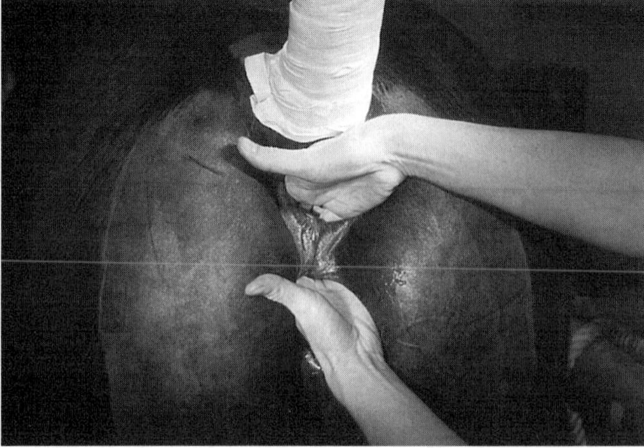

FIGURE 15-23. The rectovaginal fistula can be located by inserting fingers into the defect from both the rectal and vaginal sides.

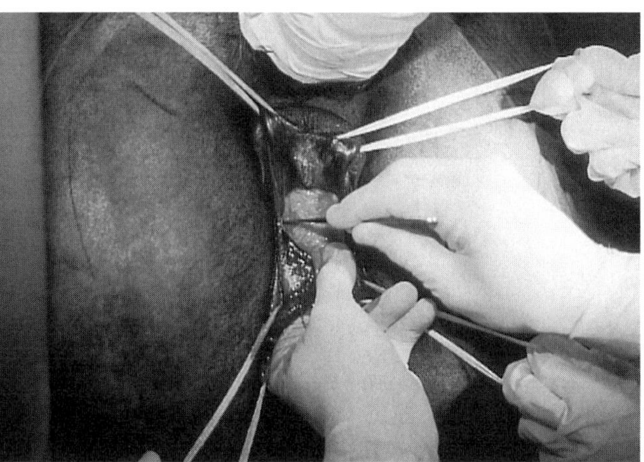

FIGURE 15-24. Surgical repair of a rectovaginal fistula. To prepare the site for reconstruction a scalpel and scissors are used to dissect horizontally through the perineal body midway between the anal sphincter and the dorsal commissure of the vulva. (Modified from Walker DF, Vaughan JT: *Bovine and equine urogenital surgery.* Philadelphia, 1980, Lea and Febiger.)

- Longitudinally oriented Halsted sutures of no. 1 absorbable suture material are placed in the submucosa of the rectal defect (Figure 15-26). This will ensure that the rectum will be closed transversely to minimize peristaltic stresses on the suture line. Walker and Vaughan (1980) recommend placing all sutures first and then tying sutures from the middle outward. Care must be taken that all sutures are placed in strong submucosal tissue to avoid tearing when sutures are tightened.
- Transversely oriented Halsted sutures of no. 0 or 1 absorbable suture material are placed in the submucosa of the vaginal defect so that the defect is closed longitudinally (Figure 15-27). This results in the openings of the rectum and vagina being closed at right angles to each other, further reducing the chance of manure leakage into the repair site (Figure 15-28).

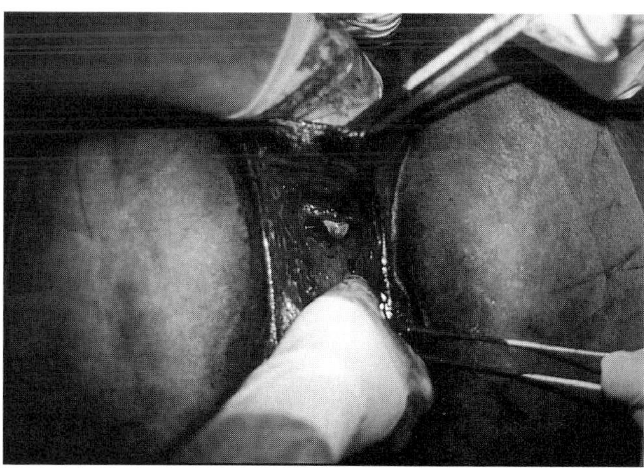

FIGURE 15-25. Surgical repair of a rectovaginal fistula. Dissection between the rectum and vagina is carefully continued cranially beyond the fistula, permitting the rectal defect to be separated dorsally from the vaginal defect ventrally. Fingers have been inserted into the rectal and vaginal openings. (Modified from Walker DR, Vaughan JT: *Bovine and equine urogenital surgery.* Philadelphia, 1980, Lea and Febiger.)

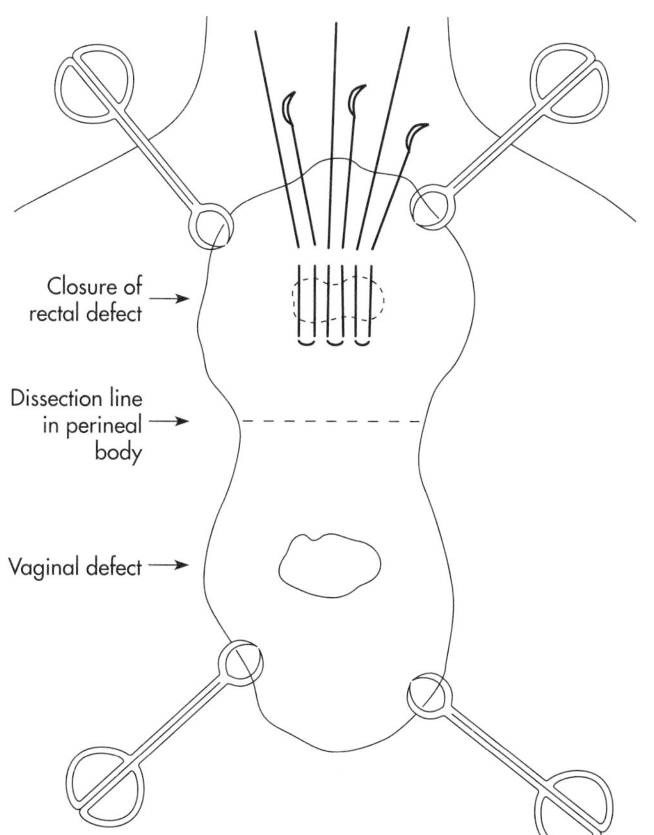

FIGURE 15-26. Surgical repair of a rectovaginal fistula. Halsted sutures are placed longitudinally in the submucosa of a rectal defect. Sutures are preplaced and then tied from the middle outward, closing the defect transversely. (Modified from Walker DR, Vaughan JT: *Bovine and equine urogenital surgery.* Philadelphia, 1980, Lea and Febiger.)

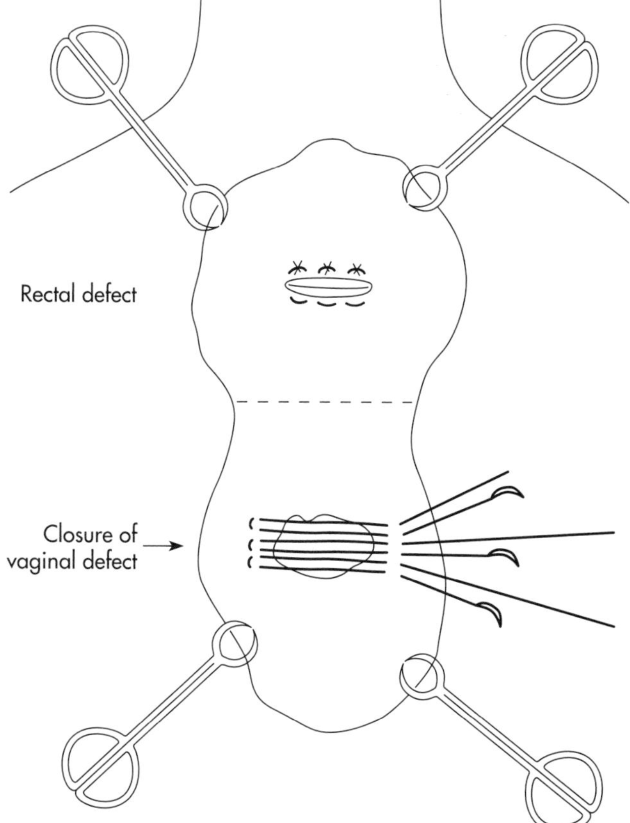

FIGURE 15-27. Surgical repair of a rectovaginal fistula. Halsted sutures are placed transversely in the submucosa of vaginal defect. Sutures are preplaced and then tied from the middle outward, closing the defect longitudinally. (Modified from Walker DR, Vaughan JT: *Bovine and equine urogenital surgery.* Philadelphia, 1980, Lea and Febiger.)

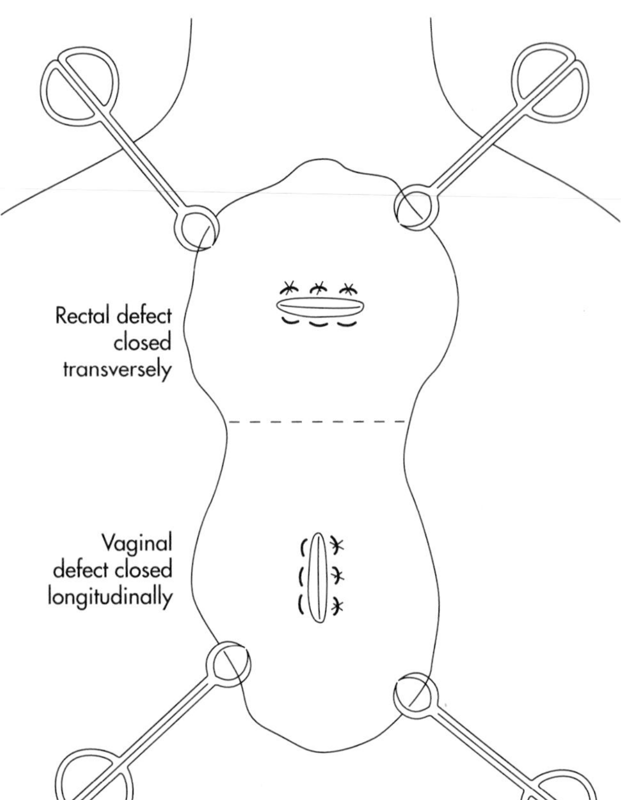

FIGURE 15-28. Surgical repair of a rectovaginal fistula. Transverse closure of a rectal defect and longitudinal closure of a vaginal defect. The dead space remaining between the rectum and vagina and the skin of the perineal body is then sutured. (Modified from Walker DR, Vaughan JT: *Bovine and equine urogenital surgery.* Philadelphia, 1980, Lea and Febiger.)

- The dead space remaining between the rectum and vagina is then closed by simple interrupted sutures of no. 0 or 1 absorbable suture material. The incised skin of the perineal body is closed with nonabsorbable suture material, which is removed 10 to 14 days later.

After repair of third-degree perineal lacerations or rectovaginal fistulas, 1 month of sexual rest is indicated to allow complete healing before breeding. Examination to ensure that healing is complete should be done before breeding.

CERVICAL LACERATIONS

Cervical tears occur during parturition. They often go undetected until they are discovered during routine postpartum examination or breeding soundness examination to determine the cause of infertility or repeated uterine infection. Cervical lacerations may be apparent as a persistently dilated very short cervix with restricting vaginal adhesions (the prognosis for correction of such lacerations is poor) or as longitudinal defects in the cervical muscle that are identified by palpation between the index finger in the cervical lumen and the thumb on the vaginal side of the cervix. The latter defects may be pie shaped and do not always extend entirely through the cervix. The presence of more than one cervical defect is possible. If the internal cervical os remains competent, cervical repair may not be required. Evaluation of cervical competency is best accomplished when the mare is in diestrus; during this time the cervix typically must be dilated to pass a finger through to the uterine lumen. Alternatively, 300 mg of progesterone in oil may be administered intramuscularly daily for 7 days to cause the cervix to close. If the cervix does not close sufficiently with progesterone administration, cervical repair will be required to restore fertility. Before cervical repair is performed, the owner should be apprised of the need to repair the cervix after each successive parturition; resultant scar tissue almost always results in tearing again because complete cervical dilation is seldom possible.

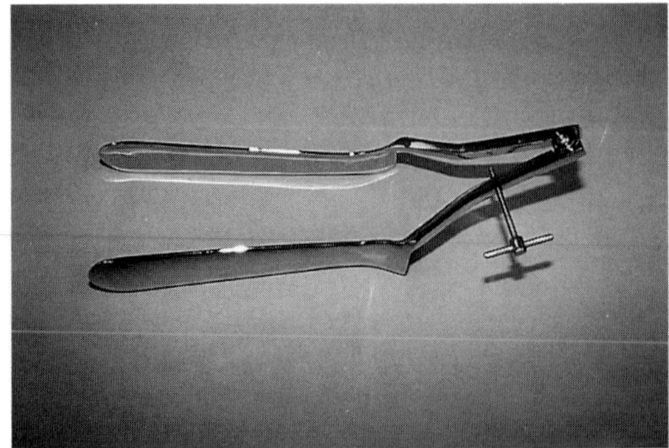

FIGURE 15-29. Two-bladed vaginal speculum used in the surgical repair of cervical lacerations.

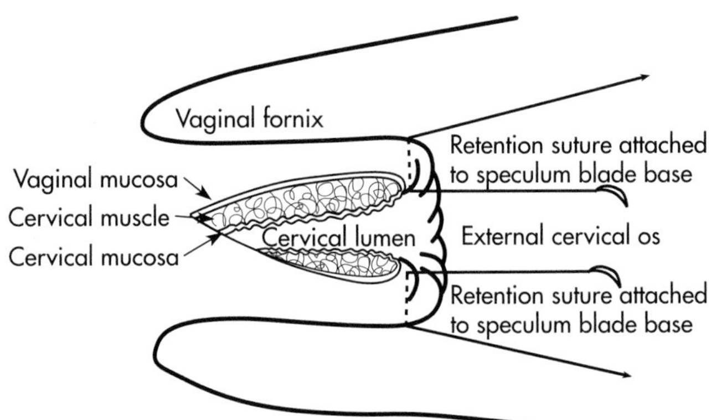

FIGURE 15-30. Surgical repair of a lacerated cervix. Retention sutures are placed in the external cervical os on either side of the cervical defect to be repaired. The retention sutures are retracted and tied around the base of each speculum blade to spread the defect and locate the tissue as near to the vulvar opening as possible. The pie-shaped cervical defect is débrided to expose the inner muscular layer. (Modified from Brown JS et al: Surgical repair of the lacerated cervix in the mare. *Theriogenology* 22:351, 1984.)

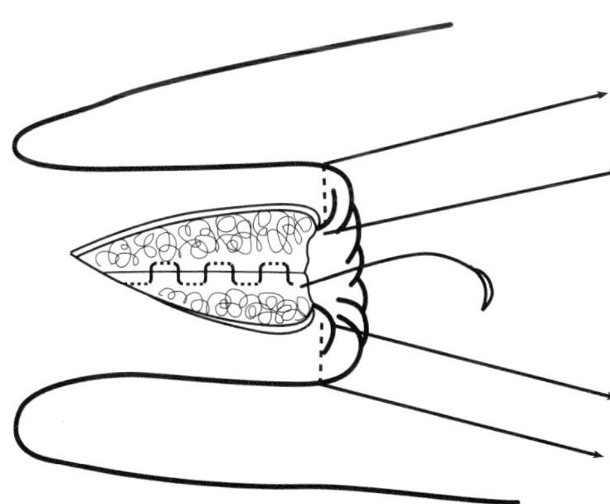

FIGURE 15-31. Surgical repair of a lacerated cervix. The inner cervical mucosal layer is sutured using a continuous horizontal mattress pattern so that it inverts into the cervical lumen. (Modified from Brown JS et al: Surgical repair of the lacerated cervix in the mare. *Theriogenology* 22:351, 1984.)

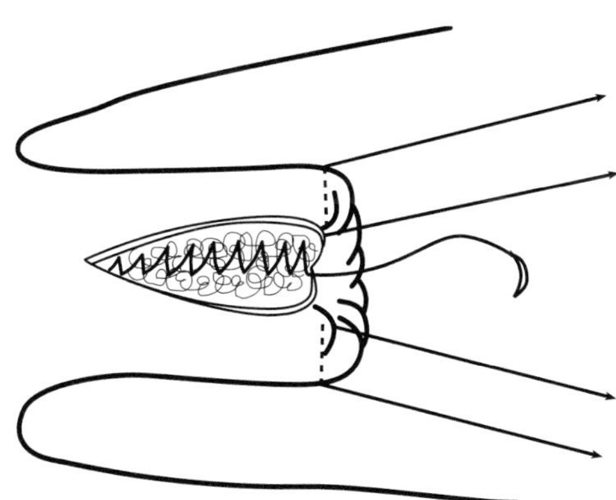

FIGURE 15-32. Surgical repair of a lacerated cervix. The middle muscular layer of the cervix is sutured using a simple continuous pattern. (Modified from Brown JS et al: Surgical repair of the lacerated cervix in the mare. *Theriogenology* 22:351, 1984.)

Preparation for surgical repair of a cervical defect (Brown et al, 1984) is similar to that for third-degree perineal laceration (i.e., sedation, epidural anesthesia, tail wrap and tie, etc.). A two-bladed speculum that opens laterally (Figure 15-29) and lengthened surgical instruments are recommended for this procedure. Retention sutures are placed in the external cervical os on either side of the cervical tear (Figure 15-30). The cervix is pulled caudally, and each retention suture is tied to one side of the speculum base. The mucosa is débrided from the pie-shaped defect until the inner muscular layer is identified (Figure 15-30). The cervical defect is closed in three layers:

- The inner mucosal layer (toward the cervical lumen) is sutured first with no. 0 or 00 absorbable suture in an inverting (into the cervical lumen) continuous horizontal mattress pattern (Figure 15-31). Suturing begins at the cranial end of the defect and continues caudally to the external os.
- The middle muscular layer is sutured with no. 0 absorbable suture in a simple continuous pattern (Figure 15-32). This is the critical layer of closure, so sufficient tissue must be procured to ensure that the layer will remain intact after healing. Thickness can be checked during progression of this suture line by inserting a finger into the cervical lumen.
- The outer mucosal layer (toward the vaginal lumen) is sutured cranially to caudally in an everting manner (into the vaginal lumen) with no. 0 or 00 absorbable suture material in a continuous horizontal mattress pattern (Figure 15-33).

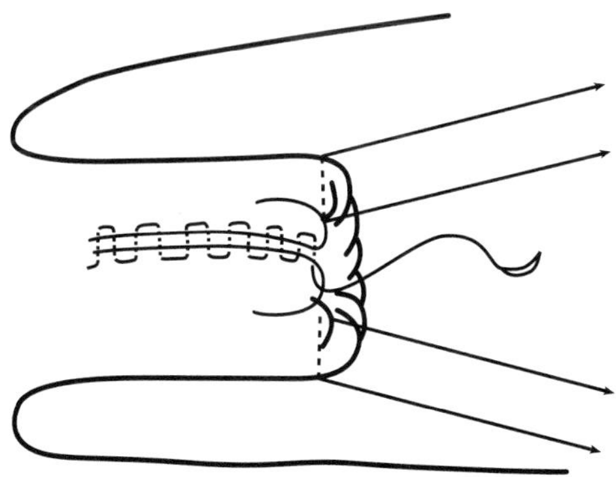

FIGURE 15-33. Surgical repair of a lacerated cervix. The outer cervical mucosal layer is sutured using a continuous horizontal mattress pattern so that it everts into the vaginal space. (Modified from Brown JS et al: Surgical repair of the lacerated cervix in the mare. *Theriogenology* 22:351, 1984.)

The retention sutures are removed and the vagina and the external cervical mucosa are covered with an oily antibiotic preparation. A Caslick suture can also be placed in the vulvar labia if necessary. A suitable broad-spectrum antibiotic can be administered for 3 to 5 days if infection is a concern. One month of sexual rest is recommended before breeding. Cervical competency and patency should also be confirmed by examination before breeding.

BIBLIOGRAPHY

Brown JS et al: Surgical repair of the lacerated cervix in the mare. *Theriogenology* 22:351, 1984.

Brown MP, Colahan PT, Hawkins DL: Urethral extension for treatment of urine pooling in mares. *J Am Vet Med Assoc* 173:1005, 1978.

Slusher S: Modified perineoplasty. Paper presented at the Western States Veterinary Conference, Las Vegas, February 17-18, 1986.

Walker DR, Vaughan JT: *Bovine and equine urogenital surgery.* Philadelphia, 1980, Lea and Febiger.

16

Surgery of the Stallion Reproductive Tract

OBJECTIVES

While studying the information covered in this chapter, the student should attempt to:

1. Acquire a working knowledge of the types of conditions in stallions that can be corrected by surgery.
2. Acquire a working understanding of the surgical procedures or treatments used for disorders of the stallion genital tract.

STUDY QUESTIONS

1. Discuss indications, techniques, and potential postoperative complications of castration of stallions.
2. Discuss methods for diagnosis and correction of cryptorchidism in stallions.
3. Describe the surgical procedures or treatments that may be used for the following:
   a. inguinal herniation.
   b. torsion of the spermatic cord.
   c. hydrocele.
   d. hematocele.
   e. testicular neoplasia.
   f. penile and preputial injuries.
   g. paraphimosis/penile prolapse.
   h. phimosis.
   i. neoplasia of the penis and prepuce.
   j. cutaneous habronemiasis.
   k. priapism.
   l. hemospermia.

CASTRATION

Orchiectomy, castration, emasculation, gelding, and *cutting* are terms for surgical removal of the testes. Castration is one of the most commonly performed equine surgical procedures, and its complications are among the most common causes of malpractice claims against veterinarians.

General Considerations

Castration prevents or decreases objectionable sexual behavior and aggressive temperament and prevents reproduction by stallions of inferior quality. Castration removes the major source of circulating androgens (and estrogens) responsible for male sexual behavior. Castration may be indicated to remove a testicular tumor or because of irreparable damage to testicular or surrounding tissue. During repair of an inguinal (or scrotal) hernia, the affected testis is usually removed.

Horses can be castrated at any age, but the age at which a horse is castrated is usually determined by managerial convenience. Most horses are castrated at 1 or 2 years of age, when objectionable sexual behavior most commonly commences. The operation may be delayed until male characteristics develop or until the owner can determine if the horse may have a future as a sire.

Before castration is performed, the scrotal region should be inspected closely to document the presence of two normal scrotal testes and the absence of an inguinal (or scrotal) hernia. The scrotal region should be palpated after the horse is sedated, if the region cannot otherwise be palpated safely. Absence of either testis or detection of intestine in the inguinal canal (or scrotum) may alter the method of anesthesia or the technique of castration.

Several different emasculators are available for equine castration. Some of the more commonly used emasculators are shown in Figure 16-1; individual preferences govern which one is used.

Castration in Lateral Recumbency

A variety of safe, short-term anesthetics can be administered intravenously, alone or in combination, to induce recumbency for the procedure. The ultra–short-acting thiobarbiturates, used alone or after administration of xylazine HCl or acetylpromazine maleate, provide a short period of general anesthesia and moderate analgesia and muscular relaxation. Recovery usually is satisfactory if only a single dose of the thiobarbiturate is given. Guaifenesin (5% to 10%) in combination with an ultra–short-acting barbiturate or ketamine HCl (with or without xylazine as a preanesthetic agent) provides good analgesia

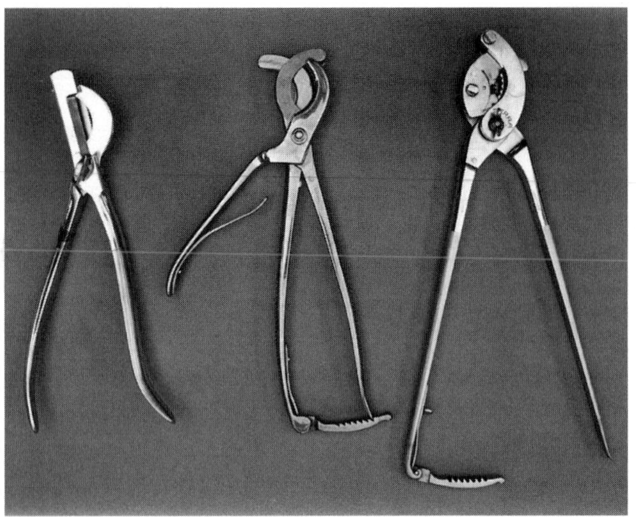

FIGURE 16-1. Emasculators commonly used for equine castrations. **A,** Improved White; **B,** Reimer; **C,** Serra. (From Varner DD, Schumacher J, Blanchard TL et al: *Diseases and management of breeding stallions.* St Louis, 1991, Mosby.)

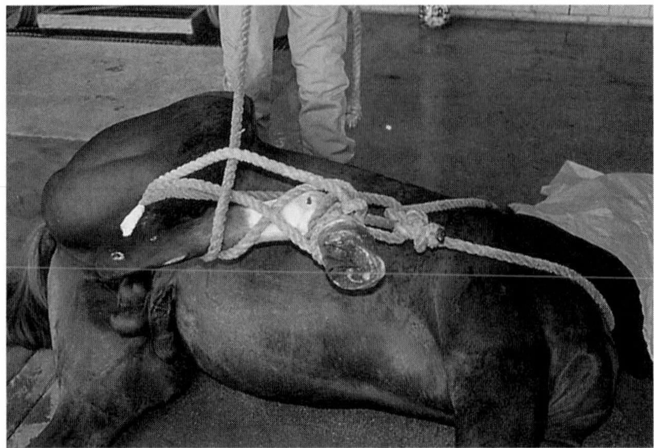

FIGURE 16-2. The horse is cast in left lateral recumbency with the right hind limb tied forward to expose the scrotum for castration.

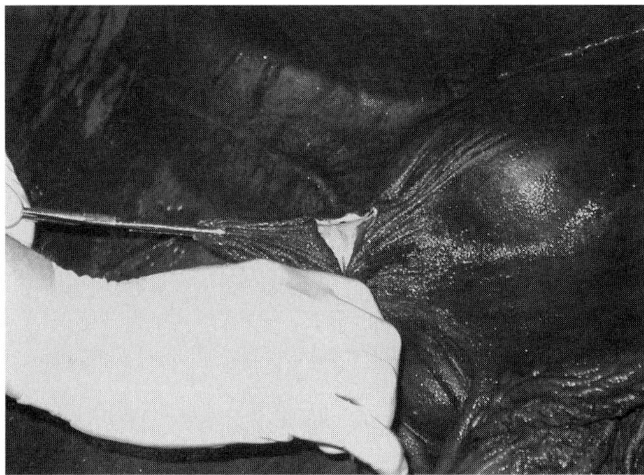

FIGURE 16-3. To remove the bottom of the scrotum, tissue forceps are attached to the midscrotal raphe, tension is exerted to "tent" the scrotum, and skin and scrotal fascia are excised with a scalpel. Care is taken to ensure that excessive tissue is not removed, and the tissue removed is in the center of the scrotum.

with smooth induction and recovery. Ketamine HCl produces general anesthesia with good analgesia for about 12 to 18 minutes if induction is preceded by sedation with xylazine HCl. The use of the neuromuscular blocking agent, succinylcholine, alone to provide restraint during castration is inhumane because the drug provides no analgesia.

After induction of general anesthesia, the horse is positioned in lateral recumbency with the upper hind limb drawn cranially toward the shoulder by a rope from the base of the neck to the pastern, and the rope is used to encircle the foot and hock to keep them in a flexed position (Figure 16-2). For the right-handed operator, the castration is most easily performed with the horse in left lateral recumbency. The following castration procedure is described for a right-handed surgeon.

The scrotum and sheath are prepared for aseptic surgery. Removing the bottom of the scrotum (Figure 16-3) to expose the testes provides better drainage, and the result is fewer complications than if the testes are exposed through an incision over each scrotal sac. To remove the bottom of the scrotum, traction is placed on the scrotal raphe, and the tented tissue is excised using a scalpel.

Alternatively, the median raphe is tensed by pulling the cranial end of the sheath forward and upward while making a longitudinal incision on each side of the median raphe (Figure 16-4). The incision is carried through the skin, tunica dartos, and underlying scrotal fascia. If an open castration technique is used, the common vaginal (parietal) tunic of each testis is also incised. The tissue between the two incisions can be excised if desired (Figure 16-5).

When an open castration technique is used, the common vaginal (parietal) tunic is incised, and the caudal ligament of the epididymis (a remnant of the gubernaculum), which affixes the common vaginal tunic to the epididymal tail and attached testis, is severed. The spermatic cord is transected close to the superficial inguinal ring with an emasculator. The common vaginal tunic is not removed when an open castration is performed.

When a closed castration technique is used, the common vaginal tunic is not incised except at the point of spermatic cord transection. The common vaginal tunic, its contents (testis, epididymis, and spermatic cord) and attached cremaster muscle are freed from the surrounding scrotal fascia by blunt dissection and removed by transection with an emasculator close to the superficial inguinal ring. The closed technique of castration can be modified (modified-closed castration) by making a longitudinal incision, 3 to 4 cm long, in the common vaginal tunic proximal to each testis (Figure 16-6). The left thumb is inserted through the incision into the vaginal cavity and ventral traction is applied while the

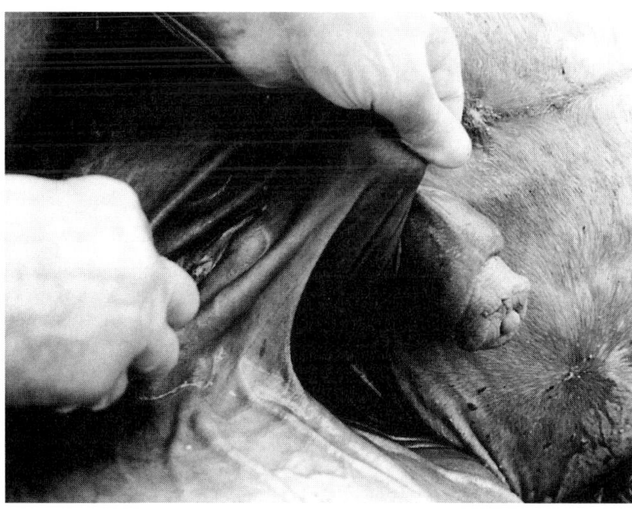

FIGURE 16-4. Two longitudinal incisions can be made in the scrotum after it is tensed by pulling the sheath craniad and upward. (From Varner DD, Schumacher J, Blanchard TL et al: *Diseases and management of breeding stallions.* St Louis, 1991, Mosby.)

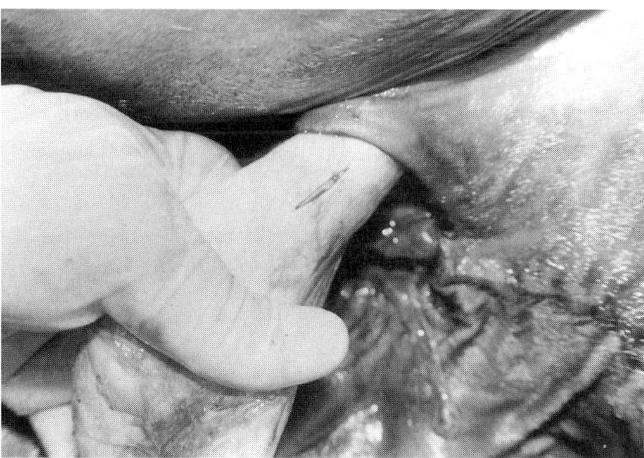

FIGURE 16-6. A small longitudinal incision is made through the parietal tunic proximal to the testis in preparation for a modified-closed castration. (From Varner DD, Schumacher J, Blanchard TL et al: *Diseases and management of breeding stallions.* St Louis, 1991, Mosby.)

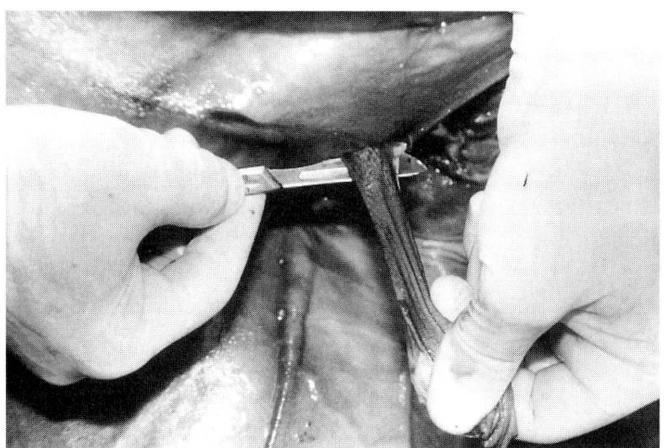

FIGURE 16-5. The skin between the two scrotal incisions may be removed for better drainage. (From Varner DD, Schumacher J, Blanchard TL et al: *Diseases and management of breeding stallions.* St Louis, 1991, Mosby.)

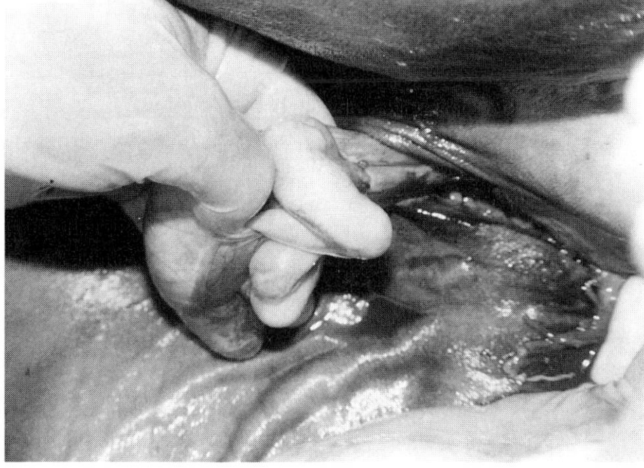

FIGURE 16-7. The surgeon's thumb is inserted through the incision of the parietal tunic and into the vaginal cavity. The incision is stretched with the thumb so the contained testis can be exteriorized. (From Varner DD, Schumacher J, Blanchard TL et al: *Diseases and management of breeding stallions.* St Louis, 1991, Mosby.)

fingers of the left hand force the epididymis and testis through the incision (Figure 16-7). Because the ligament of the tail of the epididymis affixes the fundus of the common vaginal tunic to the epididymis and attached testis, the fundus inverts and follows the testis through the incision (Figure 16-8). The left index and middle fingers are placed into the inverted fundus to maintain ventral tension on the common vaginal tunic, and the left thumb is wrapped around the spermatic cord firmly to assist in traction. The spermatic cord and attached cremaster muscle are bluntly dissected free from scrotal fascia and are transected near the superficial inguinal ring with an emasculator. By opening the common vaginal tunic, this modified-closed, or half-closed, castration technique allows observation of all enclosed structures (i.e., testes, epididymis, ductus deferens, and spermatic vessels).

Because the common vaginal tunic is removed with closed and modified-closed castrations, the likelihood of infection or hydrocele formation is decreased. If the horse has a scrotal or inguinal hernia, using the closed technique of castration and placing a ligature around the spermatic cord proximal to the site of transection prevents evisceration. The closed technique is indicated in conditions that involve the common vaginal tunic, such as neoplasia, periorchitis, or torsion of the spermatic cord.

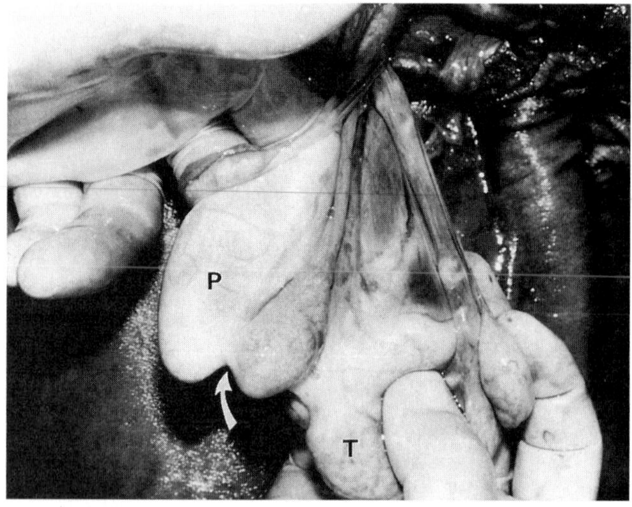

FIGURE 16-8. Exteriorizing the testis *(T)* inverts the parietal tunic *(P)* because the caudal ligament of the epididymis *(arrow)* is attached to its internal surface. Fingers are inserted into the sac produced, allowing tension to be easily maintained on the parietal tunic. (From Varner DD, Schumacher J, Blanchard TL et al: *Diseases and management of breeding stallions.* St Louis, 1991, Mosby.)

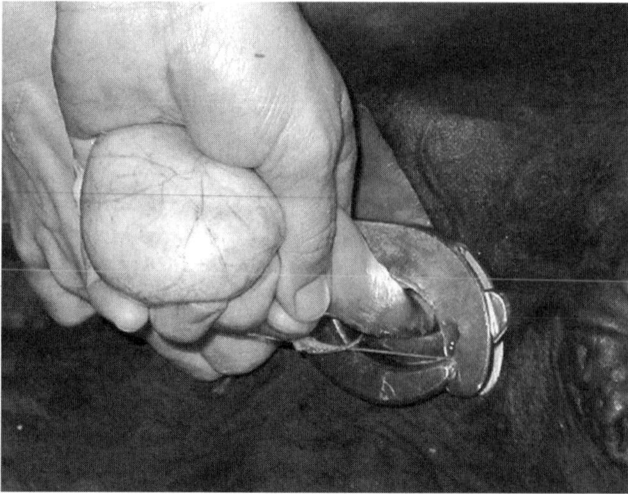

FIGURE 16-9. For a closed castration, after the scrotal fascia is stripped from the common vaginal (parietal) tunic, the emasculator is placed around the spermatic cord with the crushing portion of the instrument positioned proximally (i.e., in the "nut-to-nut" position) near the superficial inguinal ring.

Proper application of an emasculator that is in good working order is crucial to successful castration. For a closed castration, the jaws of the emasculator are placed around the distal end of the spermatic cord (Figure 16-9) (or spermatic cord contents if an open castration is performed). The jaws are closed sufficiently to prevent inclusion of skin or other tissue in the emasculator's jaws and to allow proximal movement of the emasculator to the site of transection near the superficial inguinal ring. The emasculator must be applied with the crushing portion of the instrument positioned proximal to the cutting portion. That is, the wing nut of the emasculator is positioned toward the testis ("nut-to-nut" configuration). Tension on the spermatic cord is released before transection. The spermatic cord should be divided transversely rather than tangentially because severing the vessels tangentially interferes with the natural hemostatic mechanism of segmental vasospasm. To promote satisfactory hemostasis, the emasculator should be left in place for 30 to 60 seconds, depending on the size of the cord. If the cord is large, the ductus deferens and spermatic vessels can be separated from the common vaginal tunic and cremaster muscle, and the two components are transected separately.

Fascia or tunic that may protrude from the scrotal incision sites when the horse stands should be removed using emasculators or scissors. The scrotal wound is usually left unsutured to allow drainage, but the wound can be sutured to permit healing by first intention, provided that orchiectomy has been performed aseptically. Because complete hemostasis is also required when primary closure is used, a ligature is placed around the cord proximal to the intended point of transection before the spermatic cord is transected with emasculators. The skin incision is closed with a synthetic absorbable suture material using a continuous intradermal pattern. No attempt is made to close dead space.

Castration in the Standing Position

Sedation or tranquilization for standing castration is optional but strongly recommended. Suitable drugs include chloral hydrate-magnesium sulfate preparations, xylazine HCl, butorphanol tartrate, acetylpromazine maleate, and pentozacine lactate. These drugs often are used in various combinations. The surgical site is anesthetized by infiltrating the subcutaneous tissue with 10 to 15 ml of local anesthetic, such as 2% lidocaine HCl, on each side of the scrotal raphe, followed by deposition of 10 to 15 ml into each spermatic cord. Injection directly into the spermatic cord occasionally causes hematoma formation, which may interfere with cord transection. Alternatively, 15 to 30 ml of local anesthetic can be injected into the parenchyma of each testis and allowed to diffuse proximally up the cord.

Before injection, the scrotal and inguinal areas should be scrubbed thoroughly, and the tail should be wrapped to prevent contamination of the surgical site. Even if the horse has been tranquilized or sedated, a twitch should be applied to the muzzle to prevent movement when the surgical site is infiltrated with local anesthetic. The surgeon generally works from the left side of the horse, leaning into the horse's side and avoiding the horse's kicking range. After the scrotum and spermatic cord are anesthetized, a final scrub is applied to the operative site.

Standing castration can be done using an open, closed, or modified-closed technique, as described for the recumbent horse. By performing the castration with the horse standing, the risks of general anesthesia are avoided. Drug expense is usually less, and the procedure is shorter because no recovery time from general anesthesia is required. Risks to the surgeon are greater, however, unless candidates for the procedure are selected carefully. Standing castration should be reserved for well-mannered stallions with well-developed scrotal testes and no history of recurrent scrotal swellings. If the testes cannot be palpated easily and safely and are not within the scrotum, the horse should be anesthetized and castrated in the recumbent position. Donkeys, mules, and small ponies are castrated more easily and safely when anesthetized.

Immediately before or after castration, both tetanus antitoxin and tetanus toxoid should be given to all horses not previously immunized with tetanus toxoid. A tetanus toxoid booster should be given to previously immunized horses; prophylactic antimicrobial therapy is usually not necessary.

The castrated horse should be confined to a clean stall for the first 24 hours after surgery to avoid hemorrhage from the severed spermatic vessels. Thereafter, the horse should be exercised at least 15 minutes twice daily for 10 days to prevent excessive edema in the scrotal and preputial areas. Although the ejaculate is unlikely to contain enough viable sperm after 2 days to permit impregnation, the horse should be isolated from mares for at least 2 weeks to avoid copulation. Abdominal forces during copulation could allow viscera to enter a vaginal ring.

Laparoscopic Castration

Testes of entire stallions have been removed using the laparoscopic technique with the horse sedated and standing or, if intractable, anesthetized and positioned in dorsal recumbency. To remove a scrotal testis laparoscopically, the vaginal ring is incised with scissors, and the testis is pulled into the abdomen by applying traction to the mesorchium. The ligament of the tail of the epididymis is severed, the testicular artery and vein are ligated and divided, and the testis is pulled from the abdomen. The vaginal ring is closed with staples or sutures.

A testis can also be left in situ and destroyed by disruption of its blood supply using electrocautery or ligation. The epididymis and the outer layer of the tunica albuginea remain viable, but the parenchyma of the testis undergoes avascular necrosis. Although the testis can still be palpated for up to 5 months, it is incapable of producing sperm and hormones. Failure to destroy the testicular parenchyma by disrupting the testicular blood supply has been reported. The advantages of laparoscopic castration include a rapid return of the horse to function and few complications.

Postoperative Complications of Castration

Hemorrhage. Excessive hemorrhage is the most common immediate postoperative complication of castration and is often caused by an improperly applied or malfunctioning emasculator. The spermatic vessels, especially the spermatic artery, may not be crushed sufficiently if scrotal skin is included accidentally in the jaws of the emasculator or if the spermatic cord is exceptionally large. The spermatic cords of mature and old stallions often require "double emasculation." With the technique of double emasculation, the spermatic vessels and deferent duct are isolated from the common vaginal tunic and the cremaster muscle and are transected separately.

The scrotal vessels can be lacerated when the practitioner incises the scrotum or excises the scrotal fascia. This hemorrhage usually is not serious and stops spontaneously. An excited horse, however, often has increased blood pressure that could result in excessive hemorrhage. For this reason horses caught with difficulty or after a long pursuit should be allowed to cool down before surgery. Similarly, frightened horses should be calmed before the operation. Excessive estrogens produced by grazing in some lush pastures also may interfere with hemostasis.

Severe hemorrhage occurs if the emasculator is applied upside down, because the cord is severed proximal to the crushed portion. If the blade of the emasculator is too sharp, the spermatic vessels may be severed and retract before they are properly crushed. Severe hemorrhage should be assumed to originate from the spermatic artery.

If blood flow from the spermatic cord does not diminish after the horse stands quietly for 20 to 30 minutes, the severed end of the cord can be grasped with fingers and stretched and a crushing forceps, ligature, or emasculator can be applied. If the horse was castrated while recumbent, the cord will not be anesthetized when the horse stands, and the horse is likely to resist attempts to grasp the severed spermatic cord. In this case, administration of a sedative and analgesic drug, such as xylazine HCl and butorphanol tartrate, is indicated before exploration. Intractable horses may have to be anesthetized again. Laparoscopic, intra-abdominal ligation of the testicular vasculature has been used in standing or anesthetized and recumbent horses to stop uncontrolled hemorrhage after castration.

If the end of the severed spermatic cord is inaccessible, sterile, rolled gauze can be packed tightly through the scrotal incision into the inguinal and scrotal cavities. The skin incision is then closed with closely placed sutures or towel clamps. The pack can be removed on the following day if hemostasis is achieved. If hemorrhage continues, the horse must be anesthetized and the hemorrhaging vessel(s) must be found and ligated.

Intravenous administration of 10 to 15 ml of 10% formalin in 1 liter of physiologic saline solution through an intravenous catheter may promote hemostasis. In one experiment, this dose of formalin decreased coagulation time by 67%. However, in another evaluation of the effects of intravenously administered formalin on hemostasis, no benefit was detected. Although we have noted a dramatic reduction of hemorrhage immediately after administration of formalin in our clinical practice, the safety and efficacy of this treatment have not been established.

Swelling. Swelling of the prepuce and scrotum is expected after castration and, unless excessive, is no cause for alarm. Insufficient exercise after castration results in poor drainage from the open scrotum and promotes excessive scrotal swelling. Beginning on the day after surgery, the horse should be exercised vigorously every day to promote drainage and to discourage premature closure of the scrotal wound. Turning the horse into a large clean field may be beneficial but does not ensure sufficient exercise.

The prepuce can be massaged manually to reduce swelling, provided that the horse tolerates palpation in this area. If the scrotal wound seals prematurely, it should be opened by gentle massage or dilated with a gloved finger to remove blood clots or serum from the scrotal cavity. Hydrotherapy may help prevent the wounds from resealing prematurely and decreases edema in the scrotum and prepuce.

Postoperative swelling may be caused by bacterial infection of the surgical site. Sepsis of the tissues of the scrotal cavity can occur because the open incisions expose injured tissue to the environment. Sepsis of the scrotal tissue usually resolves after systemically administered antimicrobial therapy, hydrotherapy, and establishment of proper scrotal drainage. Forced exercise promotes drainage of septic fluid from the scrotal cavity.

Infection. Clostridial infection of castration wounds is particularly catastrophic because it causes severe tissue necrosis and toxemia. Clinical signs vary with the clostridial species involved. Affected horses are usually treated by systemic administration of large doses of penicillin and nonsteroidal anti-inflammatory and analgesic agents, supportive therapy, and radical débridement of all necrotic tissue from the scrotal wound.

Infection of the spermatic cord, or septic *funiculitis,* may occur as an extension of a scrotal infection, from repeated crushing of the spermatic cord, or from bacterial contamination of the emasculator or ligature. Signs of septic funiculitis include scrotal swelling, pain, and fever. Antimicrobial treatment, drainage, and hydrotherapy may resolve the infection, but removal of the infected stump is usually necessary, especially if the cord has been ligated.

If an affected horse is not treated, the scrotum may heal, but the stump of the cord is likely to remain infected. The stump may become very large because of excessive formation of granulation tissue. This granulation tissue contains abscesses of various sizes that may drain to the exterior. A hard, chronically infected stump of the spermatic cord is sometimes called a *scirrhous cord* and can be caused by any pyogenic bacterium. Fungi also have been recovered from affected spermatic cords. Scirrhous cord caused by *Staphylococcus* species is sometimes termed *botryomycosis.* The scirrhous cord adheres to the scrotal skin, and draining tracts are usually present. The horse may display only mild or no signs of pain when the mass is palpated, and affected horses are usually afebrile. Large scirrhous cords may cause rear limb lameness and in extreme cases may be palpable per rectum.

Surgical removal of a scirrhous cord usually results in uncomplicated recovery. The operation is performed with the horse anesthetized and positioned in dorsal recumbency. An incision is made over the mass, and the affected portion of cord and a section of normal cord are exposed. Isolation of the scirrhous cord may be difficult if the infection is longstanding because of numerous large vessels that invade the mass. The spermatic cord is transected proximal to the mass with an écraseur or emasculator, and the wound is left open to heal by second intention. Postoperative management is the same as that for routine castration.

Peritonitis. Although reported rarely, septic peritonitis can occur after castration because the cavity of the vaginal process communicates with the peritoneal cavity. Extension of infection from the vaginal cavity to the peritoneal cavity (or from the peritoneal cavity to the vaginal cavity) is rare because the funicular portion of the vaginal process is collapsed as it courses obliquely through the abdominal wall. Signs of septic peritonitis include fever, depression, weight loss, tachycardia, hemoconcentration, colic, and constipation or diarrhea. Development of any of these signs after castration may warrant gross and cytologic examination of peritoneal fluid. Results of analysis of peritoneal fluid must be interpreted carefully because nonseptic peritonitis occurs in many horses as a result of castration. Nonseptic peritonitis may be related to postoperative intra-abdominal hemorrhage because free blood within the peritoneal cavity incites inflammation of the peritoneum. A nucleated cell count in the peritoneal fluid >10,000/ml indicates peritoneal inflammation. Counts >10,000/ml commonly occur for 5 or more days after uncomplicated castration, and counts >100,000/ml are occasionally noted. A diagnosis of septic peritonitis should not be based on a high peritoneal nucleated cell count alone. The presence of toxic or degenerative neutrophils or intracellular bacteria in the peritoneal fluid is more indicative of peritoneal sepsis and when accompanied by clinical signs, antimicrobial therapy and lavage of the peritoneal cavity are indicated.

Hydrocele. A hydrocele, also called a *vaginocele* or *water seed,* may appear several months after castration as a circumscribed, fluid-filled, painless swelling of the scrotum. The swelling may resemble a scrotal testis or even a scrotal hernia. If neglected, the fluid-filled vaginal tunic can become as large as a football. Sterile, clear, amber-colored fluid is obtained by needle aspiration of the scrotum. During ultrasonographic examination of the scrotum, anechoic to semiechoic fluid is seen within the vaginal tunic. The swelling is the result of a slowly increasing collection of fluid within the vaginal cavity. The condition is uncommon, and the specific cause is unknown. Hydrocele can occur in stallions as well as in castrated horses, but the highest incidence appears to be in castrated mules. Open castration predisposes the horse to the condition because the vaginal tunic is not removed during this method of castration. The vaginal tunic, therefore, should probably be removed when a mule is castrated. Removal of the vaginal tunic is the indicated treatment for castrated horses with a hydrocele.

Evisceration. Evisceration after castration of horses with normally descended testes is an uncommon but potentially fatal complication. It may occur up to 1 week after castration but usually happens within hours and may be precipitated by the horse's attempt to rise from general anesthesia. Horses that exhibit evisceration after castration probably have a preexisting, inconspicuous, inguinal hernia that a preoperative examination failed to reveal. If intestine appears in the scrotal incision after castration, the horse should be anesthetized immediately. If not, the prolapsed intestine soon becomes contaminated and damaged during the violent struggles that result from the accompanying pain. A balanced electrolyte solution should be administered intravenously in amounts adequate to combat hypotensive shock. The horse should be positioned in dorsal recumbency, and the intestine should be cleaned meticulously with copious amounts of a balanced electrolyte solution. Damaged mesentery and intestine should be repaired or resected, and the prolapsed intestine should be reduced into the abdomen as soon as possible to prevent vascular damage. Intra-abdominal traction on the intestine at the vaginal ring through a paramedian or ventral midline celiotomy may be necessary to reduce the prolapsed intestine. If the fundus of the vaginal sac has not been shredded during reduction of the prolapse, it is ligated with absorbable suture material and transfixed to the edge of the superficial inguinal ring. The superficial ring is then closed with doubled absorbable suture material (no. 2 or 3) in a continuous pattern. The superficial layers of the wound are left unsutured if the wound is grossly contaminated. As a poor alternative to suturing of the superficial inguinal ring, sterile rolled gauze can be packed into the inguinal canal. Care should be taken to avoid introducing the gauze into the abdomen. The gauze is held in position for 48 to 72 hours by suturing the scrotal incision. The vaginal ring should be palpated per rectum before the gauze packing is removed to confirm that its size has decreased so that it no longer can permit the escape of intestine and to confirm that intestine is not adhering to the pack. Antimicrobial treatment, administered parenterally, should be initiated, and if signs of septic peritonitis develop, the abdominal fluid should be evaluated. The peritoneal cavity should be lavaged if the horse develops septic peritonitis.

Prolapse. Omentum occasionally prolapses through the scrotal incision after castration. If this occurs, the vaginal ring should be palpated per rectum to determine if intestine has also exited the vaginal ring. Exposed omentum can be removed with emasculators, usually with the horse standing. Because the omentum plugs the vaginal ring, suturing of the superficial inguinal ring is usually unnecessary. The horse should not be exercised for 48 hours to prevent further prolapse.

Continued Stallion-like Behavior. Continued stallion-like behavior is a common complication of castration. Geldings displaying stallion-like behavior are sometimes called "false rigs." False rigs may display masculine behavior ranging from genital investigation and squealing to mounting and even copulation. False rigs are often said to have been "proud cut," indicating that epididymal tissue, responsible for the stallion-like behavior, was left with the horse at the time of castration. It is improbable that the epididymis would be partially excised during castration of scrotal testes because the epididymis is closely attached to the testis. In fact, very few, if any, false rigs have epididymal tissue. The epididymis is incapable of producing androgens, and geldings with epididymal tissue are endocrinologically and behaviorally indistinguishable from geldings without epididymal tissue. Spermatic cord remnants have been removed from false rigs to abolish sexual behavior, but because the cords contain no androgen-producing tissue, the efficacy of this procedure is doubtful.

The plasma concentration of luteinizing hormone is increased after castration in response to a decreasing plasma concentration of testosterone. The increase in concentration of luteinizing hormone has been postulated to stimulate production of androgens by the adrenal cortex. False rigs, however, have no higher circulating concentrations of testosterone than do normal quiet geldings, and administration of adrenocorticotropic hormone to false rigs does not increase the plasma concentration of testosterone. Therefore adrenal production of androgens is unlikely to contribute to the persistence of stallion-like behavior after castration..

Stallion-like behavior in geldings has been attributed to learned behavior, because it has been noted that some sexually experienced stallions castrated late in life continue to display masculine behavior. Many false rigs, however, have been castrated as juveniles. A retrospective survey found no difference in the prevalence of stallion-like behavior between horses castrated before or after puberty. In this study, 20% to 30% of each group displayed stallion-like behavior at least 1 year after castration, and these percentages were considered to be similar to the prevalence of stallion-like behavior in geldings. Persistent sexual behavior in geldings, therefore, may be part of the normal social interaction between horses and may be completely independent of the presence of testes. Changes in management or stricter discipline may alleviate sexual behavior or reduce it to a tolerable level.

Immunologic "Castration"

Stallion-like behavior of uncastrated or cryptorchid stallions can be alleviated temporarily by immunizing the stallion against gonadotrophin-releasing hormone (GnRH) to decrease the serum concentration of testosterone. Repeated immunization is necessary to maintain sufficient binding titer for complete neutralization of GnRH and inhibition of the reproductive endocrine axis. However, no commercial vaccine against GnRH is available.

CRYPTORCHIDISM

Cryptorchidism is a condition in which one or both testes fail to descend into the scrotum. Stallions with one or both testes in a location other than the scrotum are called *cryptorchids, rigs, ridglings, or originals.* If the testis has passed through the vaginal ring but not the superficial inguinal ring, the horse is called an *inguinal cryptorchid* or *high flanker.* Subcutaneous testes that cannot be displaced manually into the scrotum are termed *ectopic.* If the testis and epididymis are both within the abdomen, the horse is called a *complete abdominal cryptorchid.* If the testis is within the abdomen but a portion of the epididymis lies within the inguinal canal, the horse is called a *partial abdominal cryptorchid.*

Retained testes are aspermic because spermatogenesis is inhibited by temperature elevation; bilateral testicular retention, therefore, results in sterility. Because the androgen-producing Leydig cells of cryptorchid testes remain functional, cryptorchid horses develop secondary sexual characteristics and male sexual behavior.

Cryptorchidism is a sex-limited, complex developmental condition, the cause of which is not completely understood. It is the most common disorder of sexual differentiation in male horses and one of the most common congenital abnormalities in male mammals. In one retrospective study, one of every six 2- to 3-year-old colts referred to 16 North American veterinary university teaching hospitals for medical attention was cryptorchid. The condition was most prevalent in Percherons and least prevalent in Thoroughbreds. Quarter Horses ranked third, behind the Palomino, in relative risk. The mechanisms of testicular differentiation and descent in domestic animals and men are similar. The details of this process in horses have been studied but remain incompletely understood.

Causes of Cryptorchidism

Testicular descent is a complex process, and thus the causes for abnormal descent are probably varied and difficult to document. Reported mechanical causes for abnormal testicular descent in stallions include failure of the testis to regress sufficiently in size to traverse the vaginal ring; overstretching of the gubernaculum; insufficient abdominal pressure to cause expansion of the vaginal process; inadequate growth of the gubernaculum and related structures, resulting in inadequate dilation of the vaginal ring and inguinal canal for passage of the testis; and displacement of the testis into the pelvic cavity, where abdominal pressure prevents its passage through the inguinal canal.

Several reports suggest a genetic basis for cryptorchidism in horses. Some postulated methods of inheritance cited in veterinary literature include transmission by a simple autosomal recessive gene, transmission by an autosomal dominant gene, and transmission by at least two genetic factors, one of which is located on the sex chromosomes. All of the published studies dealing specifically with genetic aspects of cryptorchidism in horses suffer from the same weakness—the data presented are not adequate to support the models advocated for genetic transmission. Although cryptorchidism in many affected horses probably has a genetic basis, a definitive study dealing with a plausible genetic mechanism has yet to be performed; perhaps more than one pattern of inheritance exists. The effects of maternal environment and other factors, such as dystocia, on the development of cryptorchidism in horses have not been examined.

Retrospective studies of large numbers of cryptorchid horses indicate that retention of the right and left testis occurs nearly equally, but that unilateral retention occurs about nine times more often than does bilateral retention. Most (about 60%) retained right testes are located inguinally. Bilateral abdominal retention of testes is nearly 2.5 times as prevalent as bilateral inguinal retention, but the occurrence of both abdominal and inguinal testes in the same horse is relatively uncommon.

Diagnosis of Cryptorchidism

If no attempt has been made to castrate a horse, cryptorchidism is easily diagnosed. External palpation of the scrotum reveals the absence of one or both testes. Gonadal agenesis is extremely rare; thus if the history is reliable, the retained testis must be in an ectopic, inguinal, or abdominal position. Horses purchased as geldings but displaying stallion-like behavior pose more of a diagnostic challenge. One must determine if the horse is cryptorchid and, if so, whether one or both testes are retained.

Palpation. Examination of a suspected cryptorchid begins with palpation of scrotal contents and the superficial inguinal ring(s). The scrotum should be inspected for scars, but a scrotal scar indicates only that an incision has been made, not that a testis has been removed. If both testes cannot be palpated, a sedative should be given and the genital area should be palpated again. Sedation may relax the cremaster muscles, thereby making a subcutaneous or inguinal testis more accessible. Because the average length of the inguinal canal is about 10 cm, testes high within this canal are difficult to palpate. Inguinal testes lie in the canal with their long axis in a vertical position, and the epididymal tail precedes the testis during entry into the inguinal canal. The tail of the epididymis of a partial abdominal cryptorchid can be mistaken for a small inguinal testis during palpation.

If external palpation fails to reveal both testes, the abdomen can be palpated per rectum to locate an abdominal testis. A greater risk for a rectal tear from palpation per rectum exists in male horses than in mares because male horses are seldom palpated per rectum and may resist more violently. Most cryptorchids are seen at a young age, and young horses are more prone to a rectal tear because of their more nervous disposition, increased straining, and smaller rectum. Caudal epidural anesthesia or sedation can facilitate palpation per rectum. The risks of rectal injury must be measured against the diagnostic value of the information to be gained from examination per rectum.

During palpation per rectum, an attempt is made to trap the testis between the hand and abdominal wall just beyond the brim of the pelvis or to grasp the testis while sweeping the caudal area of the abdominal cavity. Actual palpation of an abdominal testis, however, is difficult because abdominal testes are small, flaccid, and may be mobile. Locating the vaginal ring on the side of the suspected retained testis may be informative. The lateral aspect of the wrist should be positioned on the pubic brim near the pelvic symphysis. The fingertips are pressed against the abdominal wall, and the middle finger is flexed and extended in a cranioventral direction until it enters the slit-like vaginal ring (see Figure 13-10). If the area is palpated by flexing the fingers caudally, the medial border of the ring tends to close, causing the fingers to slide over the ring. Structures converging at the vaginal ring can sometimes be identified by palpation per rectum. The ductus deferens is the most readily palpable structure, and if the testis or epididymis has descended, it can usually be felt as it exits the caudomedial aspect of the vaginal ring. In horses with complete abdominal testicular retention, the vaginal ring is usually difficult to identify by palpation per rectum. If the vaginal ring can be identified, the testis, or at least the epididymis, has probably descended into the inguinal canal. Partial abdominal cryptorchids are difficult to differentiate from horses in which both the epididymis and testis have descended through the vaginal ring.

Ultrasonography. Ultrasonography was reported to be a more useful diagnostic method than was palpation for locating retained testes in either the inguinal canal or abdominal cavity. Inguinal canals were scanned from the superficial inguinal rings outward. Transrectal scans were initiated at the pelvic brim and continued cranially using a to-and-fro scanning pattern between the midline and lateral aspect of the abdominal wall. The ultrasonic image of retained testes was found to be less dense (i.e, less echogenic) than that of normally descended testes, but retained testes were still identified easily and measured accurately in this study. A 5-MHz transrectal transducer was used for ultrasonic examinations.

Hormonal Assays. When the castration history is incomplete and external and/or internal genital examinations are inconclusive, hormonal assays have considerable diagnostic value. Testosterone and/or estrogen concentrations can be measured in the serum or plasma to help differentiate geldings from cryptorchids. A concentration of testosterone <40 pg/ml indicates absence of testicular tissue, a concentration of 40 to 100 pg/ml is nondiagnostic (i.e., equivocal), and a concentration >100 pg/ml indicates of the presence of testicular tissue.

The concentration of testosterone in the serum or plasma of young colts (<18 months of age) should be interpreted cautiously because young colts often have a testosterone concentration of <100 pg/ml. The concentration of testosterone in the serum or plasma of normal adult stallions during the winter can be as low as 200 pg/ml. To more precisely determine whether a suspected cryptorchid has testicular tissue present, an *hCG stimulation test* can be performed by administering 10,000 U of hCG intravenously. Blood samples are obtained immediately before and 2 hours after hCG administration. If testicular tissue is present, hCG causes the serum or plasma concentration of testosterone to increase (i.e., two- or threefold) above the baseline (prestimulation) concentration.

Because the testes of stallions that have reached sexual maturity produce an unusually high amount of estrogen, quantifying the concentration of total estrogen in the plasma or serum can be used to detect the presence of a retained testis in horses 3 years old and older. Horses with an estrone sulfate concentration <50 pg/ml in plasma or serum should be considered geldings, and concentrations >400 pg/ml indicate that the horse has testicular tissue. Evaluation of baseline estrone sulfate levels has been reported to be more reliable than evaluation of baseline testosterone levels for diagnosing cryptorchidism in horses. Many practitioners prefer to measure baseline estrone sulfate and testosterone concentrations, as well as testosterone concentration 2 hours after administration of hCG, to maximize the chances of endocrinologic confirmation of cryptorchidism.

Removal of Cryptorchid Testes

An abdominally retained testis can be removed through an inguinal (scrotal), parainguinal, suprapubic paramedian, or flank approach. Only the inguinal (scrotal) and parainguinal approaches allow removal of an inguinally retained testis. For all approaches except those through the flank, the horse must be anesthetized. Although immature or fractious stallions should be anesthetized for laparoscopic removal of an abdominally retained testis, abdominally retained testes of many stallions can be removed through the flank, using a laparoscopic technique, with the horse standing. Regardless of the approach, the retained testis should always be excised before the descended testis is removed.

For the inguinal approach, the horse is positioned in dorsal recumbency, and a cutaneous incision made directly over the superficial inguinal ring of the affected side. Alternatively, the bottom of the scrotum can be excised, and both the cryptorchid and scrotal testes (or two cryptorchid testes) are removed from the single scrotal incision. The superficial inguinal ring is exposed by digital dissection. An inguinal testis is readily encountered during exposure of the superficial inguinal ring.

After the superficial inguinal ring has been exposed, the vaginal process is located. The vaginal process of the partial abdominal cryptorchid lies everted within the inguinal canal and is readily encountered, whereas the vaginal process of the complete abdominal cryptorchid lies inverted within the abdominal cavity along with the epididymis and testis and must be everted into the inguinal canal.

An inverted vaginal process can be everted into the inguinal canal by exerting traction on the inguinal extension of the gubernaculum testis (IEGT), which attaches the vaginal process to the scrotum. The IEGT can be located on either the medial or lateral border of the superficial inguinal ring, at the junction of the middle and cranial third of the ring. Traction on the ligament everts the inverted process into the canal (Figure 16-10). An inverted vaginal process can also be everted into the canal by inserting a sponge forceps through the vaginal ring into the vaginal process and grasping the fornix of the vaginal process with the jaws of the forceps. Traction on the forceps everts the process into the inguinal canal.

After the vaginal process is exposed within the inguinal canal, it is incised to expose the epididymis contained within (Figure 16-11). The proper ligament of the testis, which attaches the tail of the epididymis to the testis, is located, and, by applying traction to this ligament, the testis is pulled through the vaginal ring (Figure 16-12). Often, the vaginal ring must be dilated with a finger to allow passage of the testis. The vaginal ring of immature stallions is usually more easily dilated than the vaginal ring of mature stallions. After the testis has been exteriorized, its spermatic cord is severed with an emasculator or an écraseur or the cord is ligated and transected distal to the ligature.

Taking precautions to prevent evisceration after removal of the testis is usually not necessary if the vaginal ring accommodates no more than the tips of two fingers. If the ring has been dilated beyond this diameter, the superficial inguinal ring should be sutured to prevent evisceration. The cutaneous inguinal or scrotal incision can be sutured after closure of the superficial inguinal ring or left open to heal by second intention. Activity should be restricted to hand-walking for several days before forced exercise is imposed.

To remove an abdominal testis using the parainguinal approach, a 4- to 6-cm incision, centered over the cranial aspect of the ring, is made in the skin 1 to 2 cm medial and parallel to the superficial inguinal ring. The aponeurosis of the external abdominal oblique muscle is incised in the same direction, the internal abdominal oblique muscle underlying the aponeurosis is bluntly separated, and the peritoneum is penetrated with a sharp thrust of the index and middle fingers. By sweeping the region around the vaginal ring, which is located caudolateral to the point of entry into the abdomen, the epididymis is grasped between the index and middle fingers and exteriorized. Traction on the proper ligament of the testis, which connects the tail of the epididymis to the testis, pulls the testis through the incision. After removal of the testis, the incision in the aponeurosis of the external abdominal oblique muscle is closed with heavy absorbable suture. The subcutaneous tissue and skin is sutured.

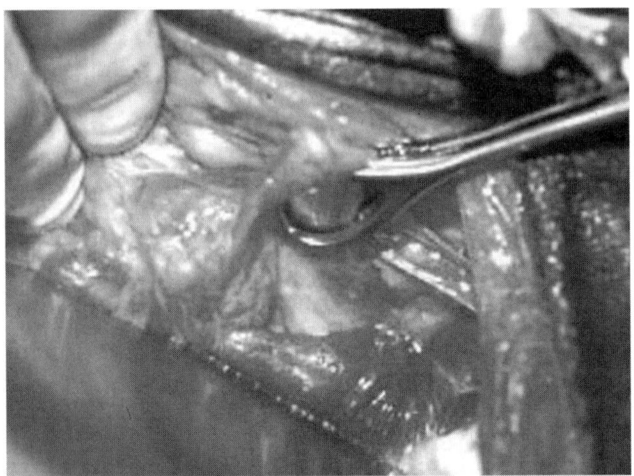

FIGURE 16-10. Using the inguinal approach for cryptorchid castration, a forceps has been applied to the inguinal extension of the gubernaculum testis and the vaginal process has been everted into the inguinal canal. (Photo courtesy Dr. Peter Rakestraw.)

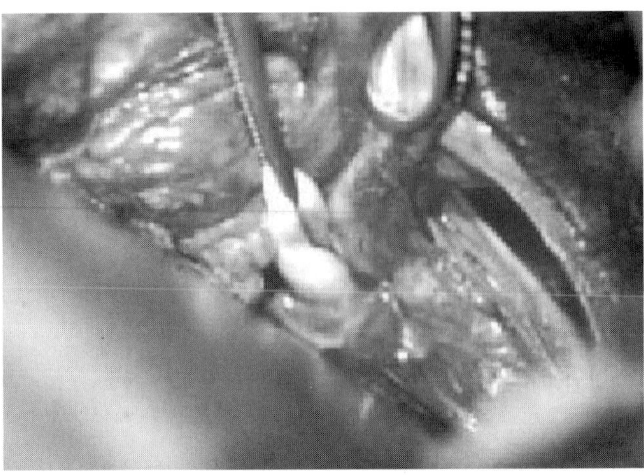

FIGURE 16-11. The everted vaginal process has been incised to expose the epididymis. (Photo courtesy Dr. Peter Rakestraw.)

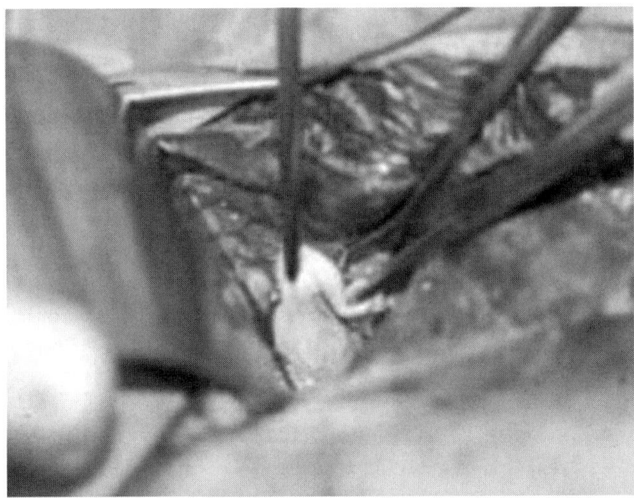

FIGURE 16-12. Traction is applied to the proper ligament of the testis (attaches the tail of the epididymis to the caudal pole of the testis) to pull the testis through the vaginal ring. (Photo courtesy Dr. Peter Rakestraw.)

Both the flank and the paramedian approaches are more invasive than the inguinal or parainguinal approaches. The inguinal and parainguinal approaches allow removal of testes through small, finger-sized abdominal perforations making surgery rapid and convalescence short. Abdominal testicular retention should be confirmed before either the paramedian or flank approach is used to remove a cryptorchid testis because retraction of an inguinal testis into the abdomen is difficult.

Laparoscopy may be useful in evaluation and castration of a horse that displays stallion-like behavior but whose history of castration is unknown and whose genital appearance is that of a gelding (Figures 16-13 and 16-14). It may also be helpful when a cryptorchid testis is removed from a horse in which the side of testicular retention is unknown. Using laparoscopy to remove an abdominal testis allows early return to exercise because the incisions into the abdomen are small. The disadvantages of laparoscopic cryptorchidectomy include the expense of the equipment and the preference for determining the location of the testis before surgery. A viscus can be penetrated if the instruments are not inserted carefully into the abdomen. If laparoscopic cryptorchidectomy is performed with the horse anesthetized, the hindquarters must be elevated to displace the viscera cranially, making positive-pressure ventilation necessary.

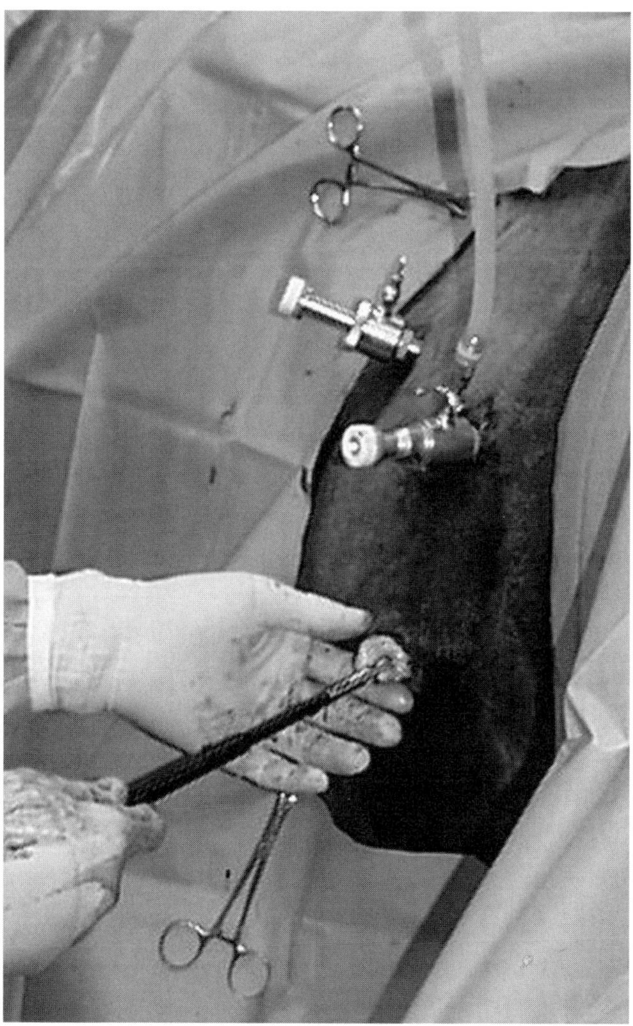

FIGURE 16-13. Three portals are required for laparoscopic cryptorchidectomy. One portal is used to insert the laparoscope, one portal to insert forceps to grasp the testicle, and one portal to insert an instrument to sever the spermatic cord. In this figure, the testis is being removed through the bottom portal. The top two portals still have the laparoscopic cannulas in place, with the more caudal cannula attached to tubing used to insufflate the abdomen. (Photo courtesy Reese Hand)

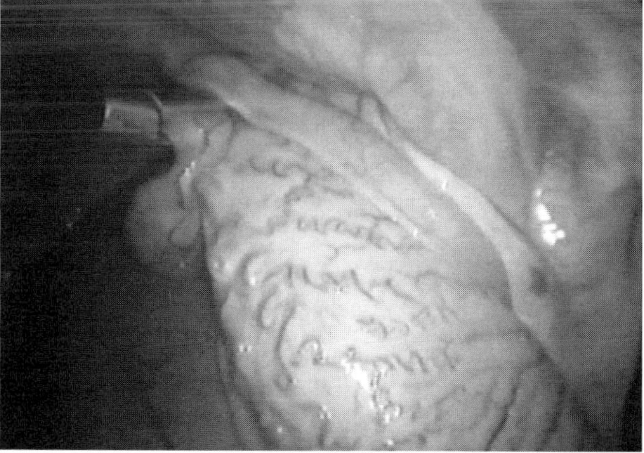

FIGURE 16-14. Laparoscopic view of abdominally located testis, with a LigaSure being applied to the spermatic cord. Application of the instrument seals the vessels in the cord. The LigaSure is then removed and laparoscopic scissors are inserted to cut the tissue. This is repeated until the entire spermatic cord is cut. A new model of the LigaSure can cut tissue as well as seal vessels, eliminating the need to insert a separate instrument to cut the tissue. (Photo courtesy Reese Hand)

INGUINAL HERNIATION

Inguinal herniation in the stallion occurs when intestine, usually the ileum or distal portion of the jejunum, enters the vaginal sac or cavity (i.e., the inguinal canal) through the vaginal ring. This hernia is sometimes referred to as scrotal rather than inguinal when the intestine extends into the scrotum. Inguinal hernias of stallions are sometimes improperly called "indirect hernias," a term used to describe a similar condition in men.

Ruptured Inguinal (Scrotal) Herniation

Ruptured inguinal (scrotal) herniation occurs when the viscera within the hernia protrude through a rent in the vaginal sac into the subcutaneous tissue of the scrotum. Inguinal rupture is protrusion of viscera into the subcutaneous tissue of the inguinal canal or scrotum through a rent in the peritoneum and musculature adjacent to the vaginal ring. Inguinal ruptures of horses are sometimes inappropriately called "direct hernias," a term borrowed from a somewhat similar condition in men. Direct hernias in men, however, are caused by weakening of the inguinal musculature and are lined by peritoneum, whereas inguinal ruptures of horses are not lined by peritoneum. Direct herniation predominates in men, whereas indirect herniation predominates in stallions.

Foals

Inguinal hernias of foals are usually congenital and are considered to be hereditary. They occur when the vaginal ring is so large that it permits viscera to enter the vaginal sac. Congenital inguinal hernias of foals may occur unilaterally (usually on the left side) or bilaterally and may occur more often in Standardbreds. Ruptured inguinal hernias occur most commonly in foals and may be caused by the high abdominal pressure generated during parturition. Inguinal hernias of adult stallions are generally considered to be acquired, but the underlying cause may be a congenitally enlarged vaginal ring. Herniation has been reported to occur during breeding or exercise, but it has also been identified in stallions being transported and or confined to a stall. The incidence of acquired inguinal herniation is reported to be higher in Standardbreds than in other breeds; the higher incidence in this breed may be caused by herniation of viscera through a congenitally enlarged vaginal ring. Inguinal ruptures of horses occur rarely and usually after a traumatic incident.

Diagnosis

Inguinal hernias (Figure 16-15), ruptured inguinal hernias, and inguinal ruptures cause a noticeable increase in the size of the scrotum. Palpation of the scrotum of an affected horse may elicit a sensation of crepitus, and peristalsis of entrapped intestine may cause movement of scrotal skin. Viscera may be identifiable during transscrotal ultrasonographic examination (Figure 16-16). Congenital inguinal hernias of foals, because of the relatively large size of the affected vaginal ring, are rarely strangulated and reduce easily. Rupture of a congenital inguinal hernia should be suspected if the viscera cannot be reduced, if the scrotum is cold and edematous, or if signs of colic accompany the hernia.

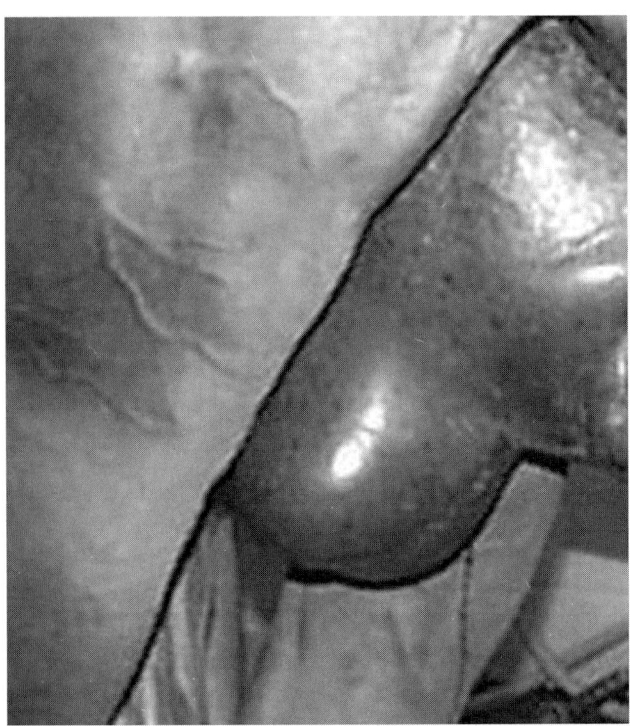

FIGURE 16-15. Inguinal hernia in the hemiscrotum of a stallion. Unilateral enlargement of the hemiscrotum is apparent.

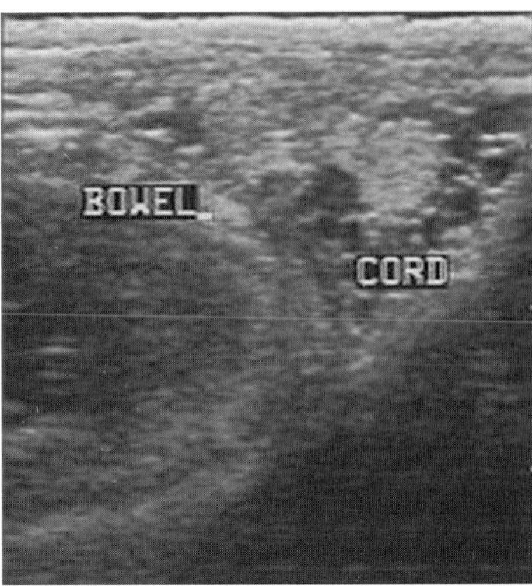

FIGURE 16-16. Ultrasonographic appearance of bowel present in the scrotum of a stallion with an inguinal hernia. Anechoic fluid is present within the vaginal space. The hyperechoic intestinal wall with anechoic fluid in the intestinal lumen is visible.

Acquired inguinal herniation is usually first recognized when the affected stallion begins to show signs of severe colic caused by strangulation of the herniated intestine. Scrotal and testicular edema usually accompany an acquired inguinal hernia because the vasculature of the spermatic cord becomes compressed. Examination of the stallion's vaginal rings by palpation per rectum reveals that intestine has entered a vaginal cavity. Omentum may also enter the vaginal cavity independently or with intestine.

Foals with a congenital inguinal hernia should be monitored regularly for signs of strangulation of the hernial contents. The hernia often resolves spontaneously by the time the foal is 6 months old, but the mechanism by which this occurs is not well understood. Application of a truss may hasten resolution. The truss is applied with the foal in dorsal recumbency after the hernia has been manually reduced (Figures 16-17 and 16-18). Care should be taken to avoid interfering with urination by compressing the penis. The truss is usually changed at 3- to 5-day intervals, and the hernia is often corrected within 1 to 2 weeks after application of the truss. Surgical correction of congenital herniation is usually not performed but becomes necessary if intestinal strangulation is detected.

Surgical Reduction

If an inguinal hernia ruptures into the subcutaneous tissue of the inguinal canal or scrotum, the entrapped viscera strangulate rapidly, necessitating immediate surgical correction. Stallions with an acquired inguinal hernia, inguinal rupture, or ruptured inguinal hernia need immediate attention because intestine within the hernia is nearly always strangulated. Reduction by external manual manipulation or

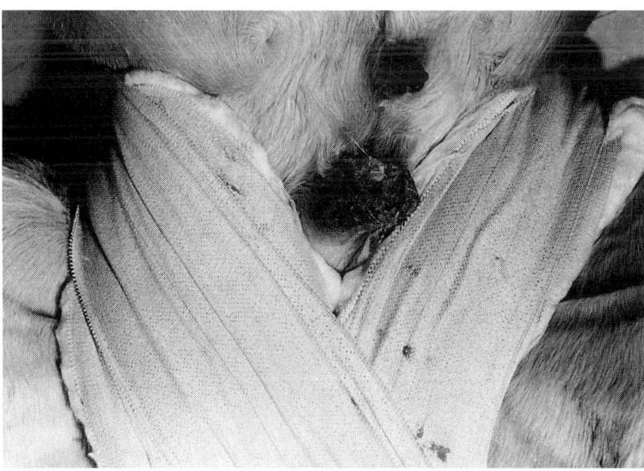

FIGURE 16-17. Ventral view of a foal with a truss ("diaper") to correct bilateral inguinal hernias. (From Varner DD, Schumacher J, Blanchard TL et al: *Diseases and management of breeding stallions.* St Louis, 1991, Mosby.)

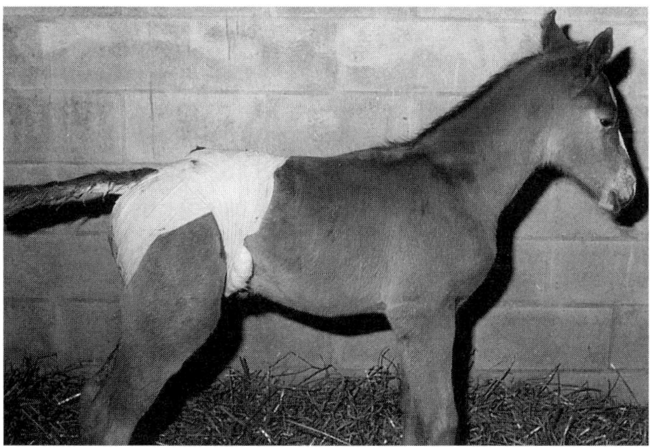

FIGURE 16-18. Standing view of a foal with a truss ("diaper") to correct bilateral inguinal hernias. (From Varner DD, Schumacher J, Blanchard TL et al: *Diseases and management of breeding stallions.* St Louis, 1991, Mosby.)

rectal traction on inguinally incarcerated intestine has been described but is difficult and rarely successful. Surgical reduction of an acquired inguinal hernia is necessary if the viability of the testis or incarcerated intestine is uncertain.

To surgically reduce inguinally incarcerated intestine, the stallion should be anesthetized, positioned in dorsal recumbency, and prepared for inguinal exploration and for celiotomy at the ventral midline. The scrotum is incised, and the parietal (common) vaginal tunic and its contents are exposed by blunt dissection, and the vaginal tunic is incised to expose the testis, its spermatic cord, and the incarcerated intestine. Attempting to save the testis is impractical unless it and the cord appear undamaged. To remove the testis, the parietal tunic and its contents are isolated, and the scrotal ligament, which attaches the tail of the epididymis to the caudal aspect of the scrotum, is severed. The spermatic cord is transected using emasculators or is ligated with heavy absorbable suture and severed distal to the ligature. The vaginal tunic can be carefully trimmed with scissors, taking care not to damage intestine.

The incarcerated intestine should be reduced through the vaginal ring into the abdomen. Reduction is most easily accomplished by placing traction on the incarcerated intestine through a small ventral midline or suprapubic paramedian celiotomy. Often the vaginal ring is so constricting that replacement of the intestine is impossible without first enlarging the ring. The ring is most easily enlarged by cutting it with a curved bistoury.

Devitalized intestine can be resected and anastomosed at the inguinal incision, but resection and anastomosis are usually more easily accomplished after the intestine is exteriorized through the celiotomy. The superficial inguinal ring is closed with a continuous or interrupted pattern using heavy absorbable suture material. Inguinal fascia and skin can be sutured or left unsutured to heal by second intention. The remaining testis often hypertrophies within a few months after removal of the affected testis, and fertility is usually maintained.

TORSION OF THE SPERMATIC CORD

Torsion of the spermatic cord occurs when the spermatic cord rotates around the vertical axis of the testis. Torsion of 180 degrees or less seems to cause no discomfort to stallions and is often considered to be an incidental finding. Torsion of 360 degrees or more causes acute venous and arterial occlusion of the testicular blood supply, and if the rotation is not corrected quickly, the testis and spermatic cord distal to the torsion become gangrenous. Torsion of the spermatic cord in the stallion apparently also occurs intravaginally. Torsion may result from an abnormally long caudal ligament of the epididymis (ligament of the tail of the epididymis) or an abnormally long proper ligament of the testis. The gubernacular attachments of the contralateral testis may also be abnormally long, making that testis prone to torsion. The spermatic cord of abdominal testes may be more prone to torsion.

Signs of torsion of the spermatic cord in stallions include scrotal swelling and signs of colic. Other diseases, such as inguinal herniation, orchitis, and epididymitis, produce similar signs, but these diseases can usually be excluded by palpation of the scrotal contents, by examination of the vaginal rings by palpation per rectum, and by ultrasonographic examination of the scrotum and its contents. Horses with gangrenous necrosis of an abdominal testis caused by torsion of the spermatic cord may display no clinical signs of torsion.

Normally, the head of the epididymis lies on the cranial pole of the testis, the tail lies at the caudal pole, and the body attaches to the dorsolateral border of the testis. With torsion of 180 degrees, the tail of the epididymis lies cranial, but with torsion of 360 degrees the testis and epididymis may

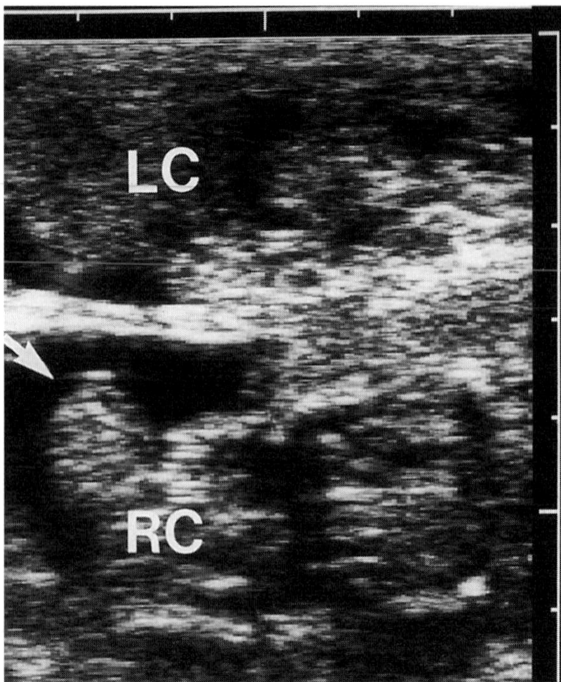

FIGURE 16-19. Transscrotal ultrasonographic image of a congested right spermatic cord *(RC)* in a stallion with right spermatic cord torsion. Anechoic fluid *(arrow)* is present around the right spermatic cord. Compare these findings with those for the left spermatic cord *(LC)*.

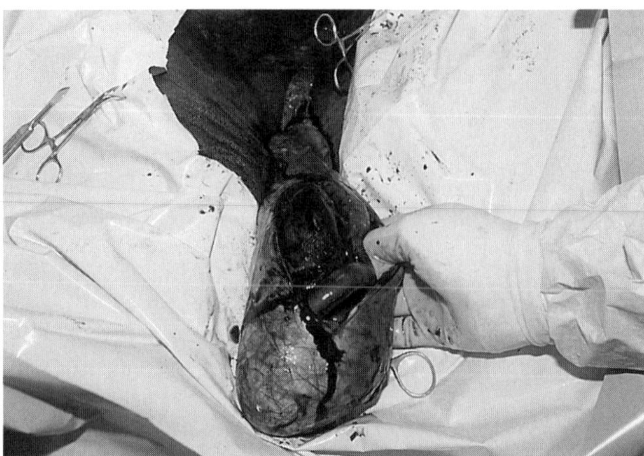

FIGURE 16-20. Infarcted testis as a result of spermatic cord torsion.

appear to be correctly positioned—with the exception being that the cranial pole of the testis is pulled more dorsally than usual (i.e., twisting shortens the cord). The affected testis and cord are enlarged and firm, and the testis may be surrounded by fluid. During ultrasonographic examination of the affected testis and cord, increased fluid density may be seen throughout the affected side of the scrotum, with testicular congestion apparent as an increase in parenchymal size and echogenicity (Figure 16-19).

A 360-degree torsion of the spermatic cord usually necessitates removal of the affected testis. If the testis is salvageable (i.e., infarction has not occurred) (Figure 16-20), orchiopexy, using nonabsorbable suture material, can be performed to permanently fix the testis in its proper position. One suture can be placed at the cranial aspect of the testis and one at its caudal aspect. The suture is passed through the adjacent dartos tissue, vaginal tunic, and tunica albuginea. A salvaged testis should be observed for atrophy caused by vascular damage at the time of torsion. The effect of transient torsion of the spermatic cord on the production of antisperm antibodies or the release of other factors that may affect fertility of stallions is unknown.

HYDROCELE

A hydrocele is a pathologic accumulation of serous fluid between the visceral and parietal layers of the vaginal tunic. Because of the insulating effect of the fluid, temperature-induced dysfunction of spermatogenesis of both testes may occur, the outcome of which can be poor semen quality with subfertility. The vaginal tunic secretes fluid, and this fluid is resorbed through the lymphatic vessels and veins of the spermatic cord. Hydrocele results when production of fluid is increased or resorption is decreased. A hydrocele may accompany testicular neoplasia or scrotal trauma, or it may be idiopathic. Idiopathic hydrocele may occur during hot weather and resolve when the ambient temperature drops. Because the vaginal cavity communicates with the peritoneal cavity, a hydrocele may form as a result of passage of abdominal fluid through the inguinal canal. Migration of parasites into the vaginal cavity and associated structures has been implicated as a cause of hydrocele.

A hydrocele appears as a painless, fluid-filled scrotal enlargement. It may occur bilaterally or unilaterally and may develop acutely or insidiously. If development is chronic, the testis within the affected tunic is usually smaller than normal as a result of atrophy (Figure 16-21). A hydrocele can usually be differentiated from other diseases that cause scrotal enlargement through examination of the scrotal contents by palpation, by transscrotal ultrasonography, and by examining the vaginal rings per rectum. Ultrasonographic examination of a hydrocele reveals anechoic to semiechoic fluid surrounding the testis (Figure 16-22). Diagnosis is verified by aseptic aspiration of a serous, amber fluid from the vaginal cavity. The fluid is characteristic of a transudate.

Exercise may cause a temporary decrease in the size of a hydrocele, and occasionally a hydrocele may resolve spontaneously. Aspiration of fluid from a hydrocele usually gives only transient relief because the fluid soon reforms. Treatment of hydrocele should be focused on removing the cause, but, because the cause can rarely be identified, the usual treatment of persistent, unilateral hydrocele is removal of the affected testis and vaginal tunic before spermatogenesis of the contralateral testis becomes affected from increased scrotal

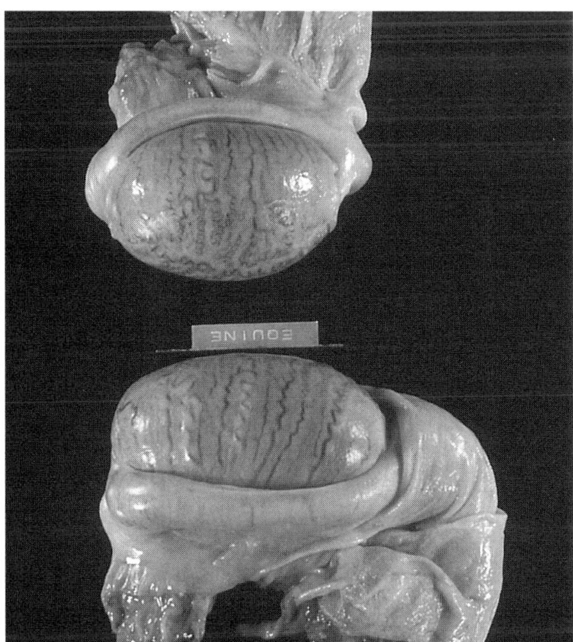

FIGURE 16-21. Normal and atrophied testes removed from a stallion with unilateral hydrocele.

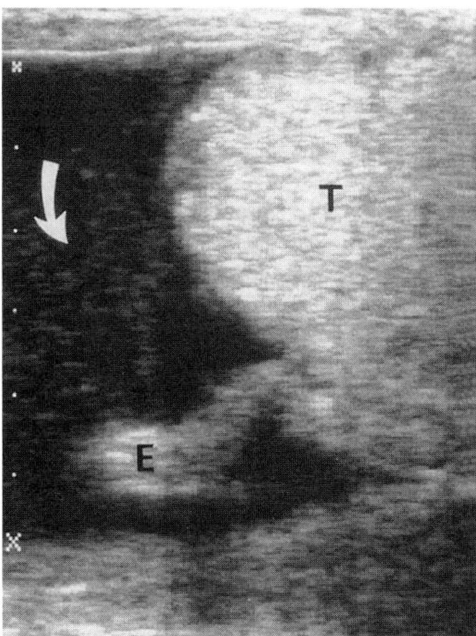

FIGURE 16-22. Ultrasonographic image of the testis *(T)*, cauda epididymis *(E)*, and vaginal space *(arrow)* in a stallion with pronounced hydrocele. (From Varner DD, Schumacher J, Blanchard TL et al: *Diseases and management of breeding stallions.* St Louis, 1991, Mosby.)

temperature. Prognosis for fertility is poor if a bilateral hydrocele persists, but reestablishment of fertility is likely if both hydroceles resolve. Sclerotherapy, using tetracycline injected into the vaginal cavity, has been used to treat men affected with hydrocele, but this treatment has not been evaluated in affected stallions.

HEMATOCELE

A hematocele resembles a hydrocele but is a collection of hemorrhagic fluid within the vaginal cavity (Figure 16-23). A hematocele is usually caused by trauma to the scrotum and its contents, but because the peritoneal and vaginal cavities of the horse communicate, a hematocele can occur as an extension of hemoperitoneum.

A hematocele caused by acute trauma to the scrotal contents is usually associated with pain. Ultrasonography may help differentiate hematocele from hydrocele and other causes of scrotal enlargement. Some causes of hematocele, such as rupture of the tunica albuginea of the testis, may be detected by ultrasonographic examination. Diagnosis is confirmed by aseptic aspiration of blood or sanguineous fluid from the vaginal cavity. Scrotal swelling associated with hematocele can be quite pronounced.

A small hematocele may cause no problem with fertility and may dissipate without treatment, but a large hematocele may insulate the testes, causing interference with spermatogenesis. Clotting and fibrin formation of blood in the hematocele may result in thick adhesions between common and proper tunics (Figure 16-24). If the hematocele is large, the hemorrhage should be evacuated from the vaginal cavity, and the testis and epididymis should be carefully inspected to identify the source of hemorrhage. If torn, the tunica albuginea should be sutured. Orchiectomy is indicated if the testis or epididymis is badly damaged. The effect of testicular trauma on formation of antisperm antibodies and secondary subfertility in stallions is unknown. Removal of the affected testis may be indicated to minimize the likelihood of such a complication and to prevent depression of spermatogenesis of the contralateral testis from increased temperature caused by inflammation of the damaged testis.

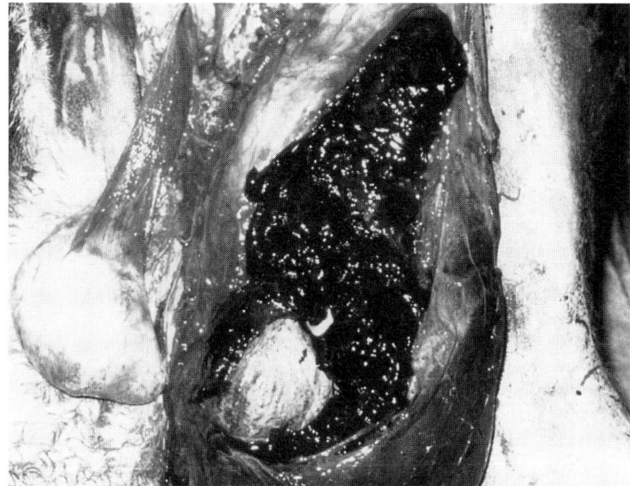

FIGURE 16-23. Massive bleeding into the vaginal space of a jack emanating from a ruptured tunica albuginea and testicular hemorrhage. (From Varner DD, Schumacher J, Blanchard TL et al: *Diseases and management of breeding stallions.* St Louis, 1991, Mosby.)

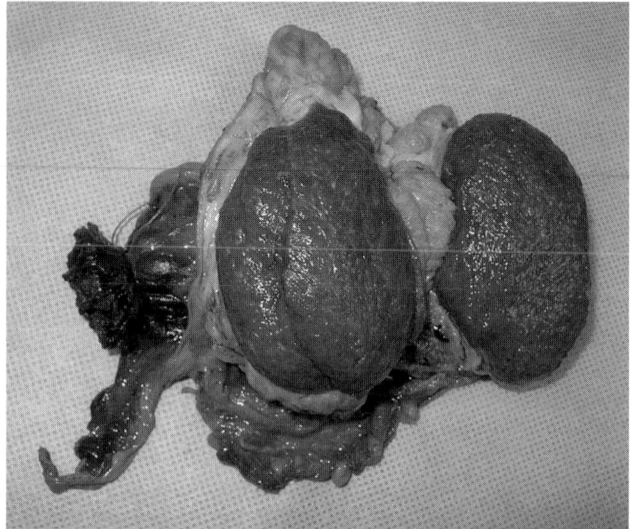

FIGURE 16-24. Chronic adhesions between common (parietal) and proper (visceral) tunics of the testis of a stallion with a history of scrotal injury and hematocele. The testicular tunics were thickened and completely adhered to each other and the epididymis. Semen quality was poor with many detached sperm heads.

VARICOCELE

A varicocele is a dilation and tortuosity of the veins of the pampiniform plexus and the cremasteric veins. Varicoceles of men and rams have been associated with testicular atrophy and decreased seminal quality, possibly caused by interference with normal exchange of heat from the testicular artery to the pampiniform plexus. Varicoceles are uncommon in stallions, and their effect on fertility is not documented. More than 50% of men with varicoceles have normal seminal quality. We have noted a varicocele in some stallions with normal seminal quality.

Most varicoceles are idiopathic, but a defect in the valves of the spermatic vein where it empties into the vena cava or renal vein or a deficiency of elastic and fibrous tissue in fascia that surrounds the spermatic vein has been postulated to cause varicocele. Varicoceles of stallions are usually unilateral and cause no pain when palpated. The affected spermatic cord appears enlarged and may have the texture of a bag of worms.

Definitive treatment of horses affected with varicocele is removal of the affected cord and testis, but treatment is unnecessary if seminal quality is unaffected. High ligation of the spermatic vein or ligation and removal of the multiple venous loops of the pampiniform plexus have been performed to treat men with varicocele. A hydrocele has formed in a small percentage of men after ligation of the spermatic vein.

TESTICULAR NEOPLASIA

Testicular neoplasms of the horse occur rarely, probably because most horses are castrated at an early age. Only primary testicular neoplasms (i.e., those that originate within the testis) have been reported, and those can be divided into germinal and nongerminal types. Germinal neoplasms arise from the germ cells of the seminiferous epithelium and are the most common type of testicular neoplasm.

Germinal testicular neoplasms reported to occur in the horse include the *seminoma, teratoma, teratocarcinoma, and embryonal carcinoma.* The seminoma is the most commonly reported testicular neoplasm of the horse. Nongerminal testicular neoplasms arise from testicular stromal cells and include the *Leydig cell tumor* and *Sertoli cell tumor.* Nongerminal testicular neoplasms of the horse are less commonly reported than are germinal testicular neoplasms. Cryptorchid testes of both men and dogs appear to be predisposed to neoplasia, but a relationship between cryptorchidism and formation of testicular neoplasia has not been established in the horse.

Diagnosis

When a horse with a suspected testicular neoplasm is examined, the contralateral testis should be used for comparison, keeping in mind that bilateral testicular neoplasia can occur. The normal testis is smooth and compliant, and a neoplastic testis is often enlarged and has either a soft or hardened texture. Neoplastic lesions located deep within the parenchyma may not be palpable. The neoplastic testis is often heavier than its normal counterpart. A neoplastic testis is usually painless when compressed and usually remains freely movable within the scrotum. Scrotal enlargement caused by neoplasia must be differentiated from other causes of scrotal enlargement, such as torsion of the spermatic cord, orchitis, hydrocele, hematocele, and inguinal herniation or rupture. Careful external palpation and ultrasonographic examination of the scrotal contents and palpation per rectum can be used to differentiate these conditions. Painless, scrotal enlargement that develops insidiously is more likely to be caused by testicular neoplasia than by inflammation or ischemia.

Ultrasonographic examination may be helpful in determining if a testis is neoplastic. Normal testicular parenchyma is homogenously echogenic, but a neoplastic testis usually contains areas of decreased echogenicity (Figure 16-25). Affected testes may contain single or multiple tumors. Testicular neoplasia can be confirmed by cytologic examination of a needle aspirate or by histologic examination of a specimen obtained with a punch or incisional biopsy of the testis. Although testicular biopsy has been performed without noticeable side effects in normal stallions, the long-term effects of testicular biopsy have not been well studied. Biopsy of neoplastic testes of men has been associated with a high incidence of neoplastic invasion of extratesticular tissue. If testicular neoplasia is strongly suspected, the affected testis should be excised. Before a neoplastic testis is removed, the sublumbar lymph nodes should be examined by palpation per rectum for enlargement caused by metastatic spread of the tumor.

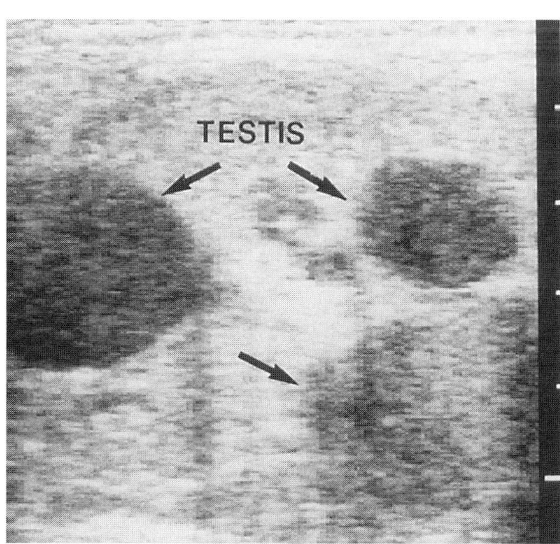

FIGURE 16-25. Transscrotal ultrasonographic image of a neoplastic stallion testis. Discrete hypoechoic areas *(arrows)* within the testicular parenchyma (testis) are typical of testicular tumors in the stallion.

Surgical Removal

When a neoplastic testis is removed, the spermatic cord should be ligated and severed as proximally as possible. The spermatic cord should be examined grossly and histologically for evidence of metastasis. The scrotal incision should be sutured to reduce postoperative inflammation, which could interfere with thermal regulation of the remaining testis, but good hemostasis is required before the scrotal incision is sutured.

PENILE AND PREPUTIAL INJURIES

Penile and preputial injuries, such as lacerations and hematomas, are usually caused by kicks, especially to the erect penis; mounting of stationary objects; masturbation; attempting to breed a mare across a fence; severe bending of the penile shaft caused by sudden movement of the mare during coitus; and improperly fitted or maintained stallion rings (Figures 16-26 and 16-27). Damage to the penile shaft, including the urethra, can be inflicted during castration performed by an inexperienced surgeon. Deep lacerations that extend into a corporeal body may result in impotence, and those that extend into the urethra may result in marked hemospermia or severe necrosis of tissue from escape of urine.

Even superficial lacerations can result in severe penile damage if left untreated (Figure 16-28). An untreated laceration to the penile epithelium may result in cellulitis and preputial edema, which, in turn, lead to prolapse of the penis and internal preputial lamina from the preputial cavity. Prolapse of the penis and prepuce may lead to penile paralysis from damage to the penile nerves or to further damage to the exposed penile and preputial epithelium. Perforations or lacerations of the glans penis may lead to vascularization with prominent hemorrhage during breeding when the corpus spongiosum becomes fully engorged (Figure 16-29).

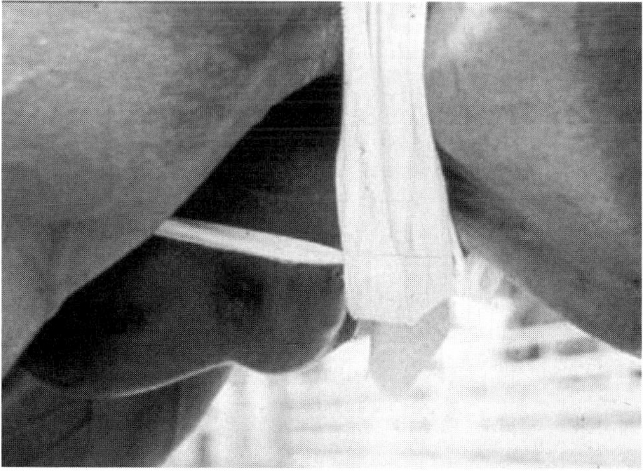

FIGURE 16-26. Swollen sheath of a stallion with an injury caused during breeding. The penis and prepuce were able to be replaced into the sheath, but would gradually fall out of the sheath. A temporary truss was used to retain the penis within the sheath.

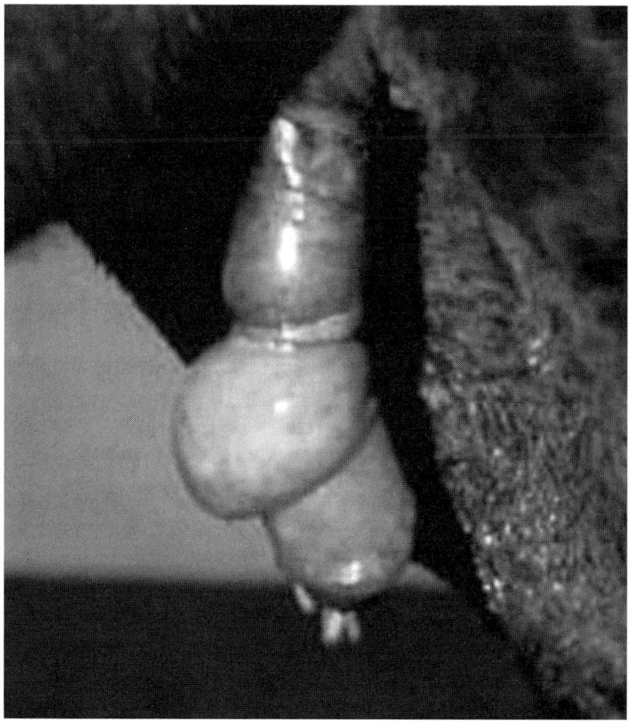

FIGURE 16-27. Prolapsed penis and prepuce of a stallion with an acute injury caused during breeding. The ring of edema around the prolapsed fornix must be reduced to return the penis to the sheath.

Fresh lacerations to the penile and preputial epithelium should be sutured with soft absorbable or nonabsorbable suture material. An infected or heavily contaminated laceration should be left open to heal by second intention, or it

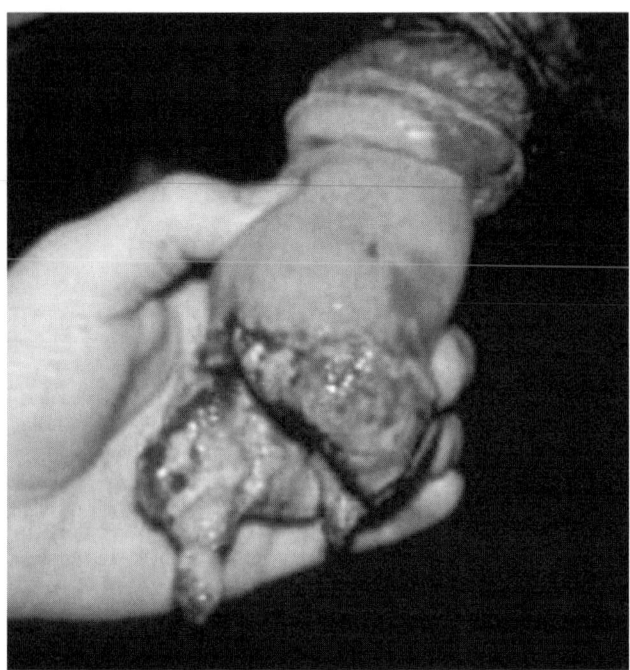

FIGURE 16-28. Chronic laceration from a kick injury to the penis. Extensive cellulitis and infection of tissues are present.

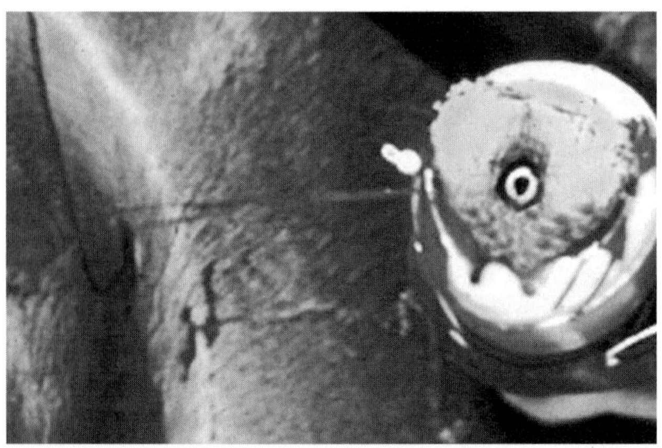

FIGURE 16-29. Perforation of the integument of the glans penis from a wire stallion brush (used to prevent masturbation) was postulated to cause a corpus spongiosal shunt that hemorrhaged during breeding in this stallion. An open-ended artificial vagina was used to permit visualization of the site of hemorrhage.

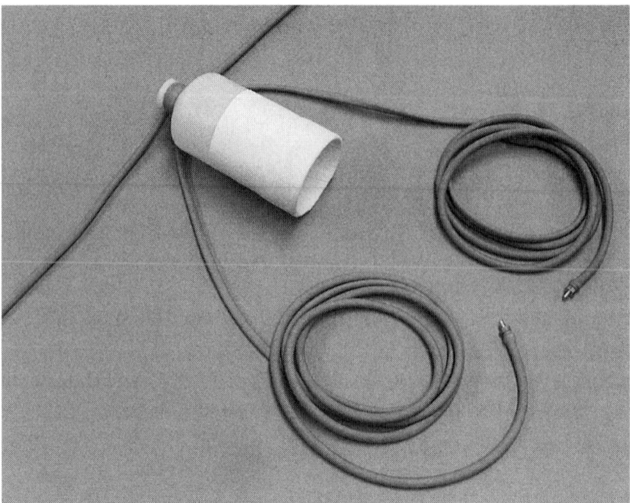

FIGURE 16-30. Device fabricated for retaining the penis within the preputial cavity of stallions with penile prolapse. (From Varner DD, Schumacher J, Blanchard TL et al: *Diseases and management of breeding stallions.* St Louis, 1991, Mosby.)

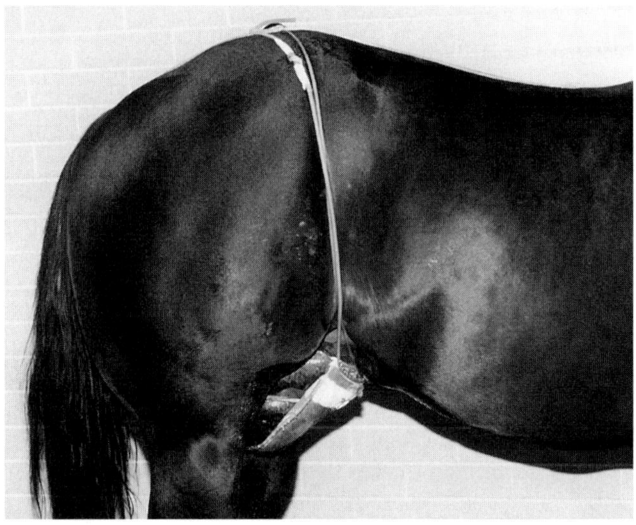

FIGURE 16-31. Nylon mesh, with attached tubing, fitted over the preputial orifice of a stallion to aid retention of the device shown in Figure 16-30 within the preputial cavity. (From Varner DD, Schumacher J, Blanchard TL et al: *Diseases and management of breeding stallions.* St Louis, 1991, Mosby.)

can be sutured at a later date when it shows no signs of inflammation. If the wound is left open, it should be dressed often with a nonirritating, antimicrobial ointment. If the laceration is accompanied by severe preputial edema, the penis and prepuce should be retained within the preputial cavity by using a retainer bottle, nylon netting, or nylon hosiery suspended at the preputial orifice with a crupper and surcingle made of rubber tubing (Figures 16-30 and 16-31). The penis can be restrained within the preputial cavity for several days with sutures placed across the preputial orifice, but sutures can exacerbate the preputial trauma. If the penis cannot be retained in the preputial cavity, an enclosing abdominal support wrap (Figure 16-32) can be used in an attempt to decrease pendent edema, with the hope of gradually reducing the swelling and edema sufficiently within a few days to allow return of the penis and prepuce to the sheath.

Penile hematomas that continue to expand should be explored to determine if the origin of the hemorrhage is a rent in the tunica albuginea. Lacerations to the tunica albuginea should be sutured. Lacerations to the urethra should also be

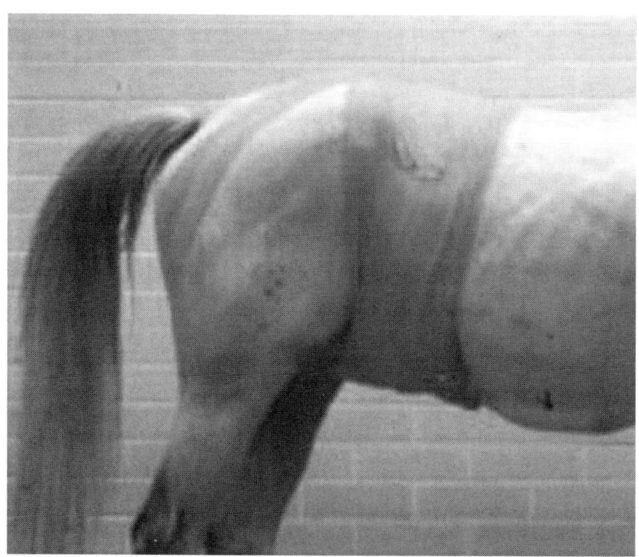

FIGURE 16-32. After the prolapsed penis and prepuce were cleansed and medicated with an emollient antibiotic salve, the swollen penis and prepuce of this stallion still could not be returned to the sheath. The swollen penis and prepuce were placed in a support wrap to elevate the organ to reduce pendent edema and allow subsequent return to the sheath after swelling was reduced.

sutured, and if the laceration is transverse, the urethra should be stented with a large-bore catheter to prevent the formation of a stenosing cicatrix. After preputial or penile trauma, the stallion should be isolated from mares until the wound is healed.

Dissection to the base of a vascular shunt of the glans penis allows ligation of the offending vessel. The penile integument is closed with interrupted sutures. Thirty days of sexual rest is indicated to permit complete healing.

PARAPHIMOSIS/PENILE PROLAPSE

Paraphimosis, or the inability of the horse to retract its penis into the preputial cavity, is usually caused by preputial edema that occurs secondary to trauma, such as preputial laceration or preputial hematoma (Figure 16-27), or by preputial edema that accompanies systemic disease such as dourine or purpura hemorrhagica. Penile prolapse can be caused by damage to the innervation of the penis, which may accompany some neurologic diseases, such as that caused by equine herpesvirus-1. Penile prolapse has been associated with severe debilitation and with administration of phenothiazine-derivative tranquilizers.

Inability of the stallion to maintain its penis and prepuce within the preputial cavity, regardless of the cause, impairs venous and lymphatic drainage of the penis and prepuce, which leads to edema of the internal preputial lamina. As the internal preputial lamina swells, the preputial ring may become constricting, causing the penis distal to the ring to swell further. The exposed penile and preputial epithelium, if not protected, becomes excoriated and infected. Eventually, the internal preputial lamina becomes fibrotic, and the prepuce loses its normal telescoping action. In addition, the pendulous weight of the prolapsed penis and prepuce may damage the internal pudendal nerves, causing penile paralysis.

The prolapsed penis should be replaced into the preputial cavity as soon as possible to protect it and the internal preputial lamina from further injury. If the penis and prepuce are so edematous that they cannot be replaced into the preputial cavity, they should be held against the ventral aspect of the body wall with a bandage. The penis and prepuce should be kept lubricated with emollient, antimicrobial dressings. The horse should receive nonsteroidal antiinflammatory drugs and daily exercise. If the preputial ring restricts penile retraction or impairs venous and lymphatic flow, it can be incised longitudinally. This incision is allowed to heal by second intention.

If paraphimosis is caused by or has caused permanent penile paralysis, the stallion is unlikely to be able to achieve erection. If a stallion with penile paralysis can ejaculate into an artificial vagina and if the stallion's breed registry permits artificial insemination, the stallion's breeding life can be extended using artificial insemination of mares. The stallion can be salvaged for uses other than breeding by amputating its penis or by permanently retracting the paralyzed penis into its prepuce. The penis can be permanently retracted into the preputial cavity with sutures placed through the annular ring (the reflection of the internal preputial lamina onto the free body of the penis) and anchored to tissue behind the scrotal area (i.e., the Bolz technique of phallopexy). The penis can also be retained within the preputial cavity by segmental posthectomy (i.e., reefing) of the entire internal lamina of the prepuce.

PHIMOSIS

Phimosis, or the inability of the horse to completely protrude its penis from the prepuce, occurs naturally in foals because the internal preputial lamina is fused to the free part of the penis for about the first month after birth. Excluding this normal physiologic condition, phimosis is usually the result of constriction of the external preputial orifice or the preputial ring caused by trauma or neoplasia (Figure 16-33). When the horse is unable to protrude its penis, it urinates within the preputial cavity, causing excoriation of the preputial epithelium, which leads to further inflammation and irritation, thereby compounding the problem (Figure 16-34).

A constricting external preputial orifice can be enlarged by removing a triangular segment of external lamina, whose base is the preputial orifice. The cut edge of the external lamina is sutured to the cut edge of the internal preputial lamina. Removing a similar triangle from the preputial fold can enlarge a constricting preputial ring, or the constricting preputial ring can be removed by segmental posthectomy after the preputial ring is incised to allow protrusion the penis and internal

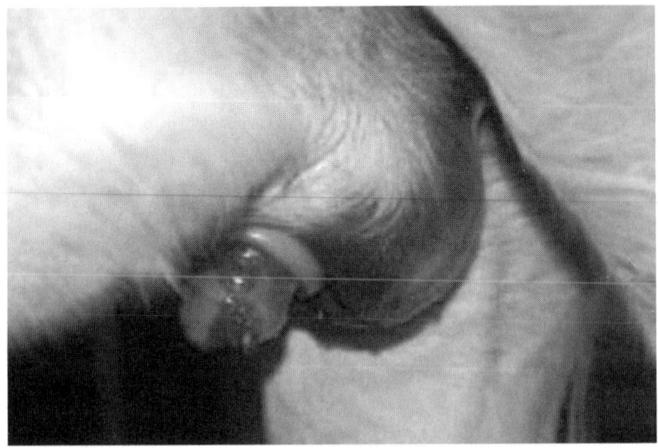

FIGURE 16-33. Phimosis due to development of extensive melanomas involving peripreputial tissues occurred in this stallion.

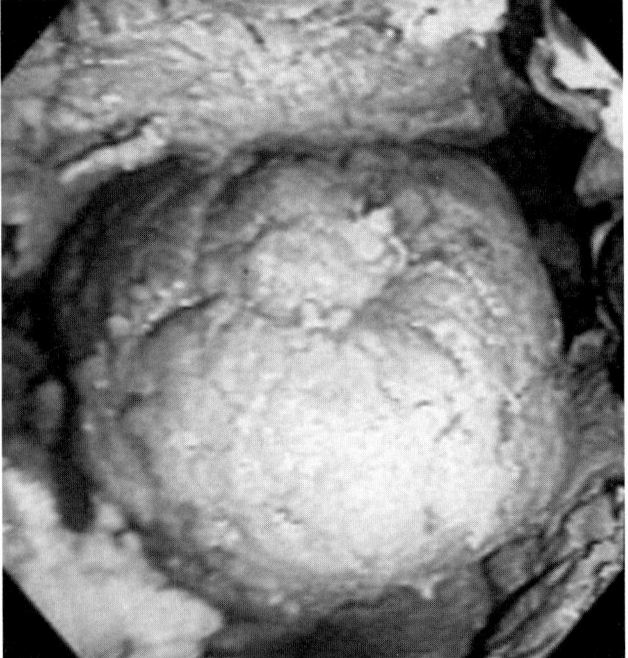

FIGURE 16-34. Endoscopic view of the preputial cavity of a stallion with phimosis. Urinary scalding contributes to the local infection and cellulitis when the horse cannot extend his penis to urinate.

lamina. (See "Neoplasia of the Penis and Prepuce" for a description of the reefing operation.)

NEOPLASIA OF THE PENIS AND PREPUCE

Any cutaneous neoplasm can affect the integument of the external genitalia, but the most common neoplasm of the penis and prepuce is *squamous cell carcinoma.* Lesions of squamous cell carcinoma are usually multiple and often involve the glans penis and the internal lamina of the prepuce (Figure 16-35). Geldings develop squamous cell carcinoma of the genitalia more often than do stallions, and horses with nonpigmented genitalia, such as Appaloosas and American Paint Horses, are most commonly affected. The malignancy of squamous cell carcinomas of the penis and prepuce of the horse is usually low, and lesions tend to remain localized; however, metastasis may occur if treatment is neglected.

Small preputial and penile neoplasms of stallions can be excised or destroyed using cryotherapy. Cryotherapy can be performed using liquid nitrogen administered as a spray or through a cryoprobe, or by using carbon dioxide administered through a cryoprobe (Figure 16-36). Lesions should be frozen to a depth of 2 to 3 mm using two or three freeze-thaw cycles. A rapid freeze and a slow thaw produce the most cellular damage. A thermocouple can be used to monitor the size and depth of the area affected by the cryogen. The penis and prepuce should be reexamined at 1- and 2-month intervals, and any recurring lesions should be frozen.

Precancerous and small lesions (i.e., 2 to 3 mm) of squamous cell carcinoma can be treated by application of 5-fluorouracil at 14-day intervals. Rubber examination gloves should be worn during application of this drug. Stallions

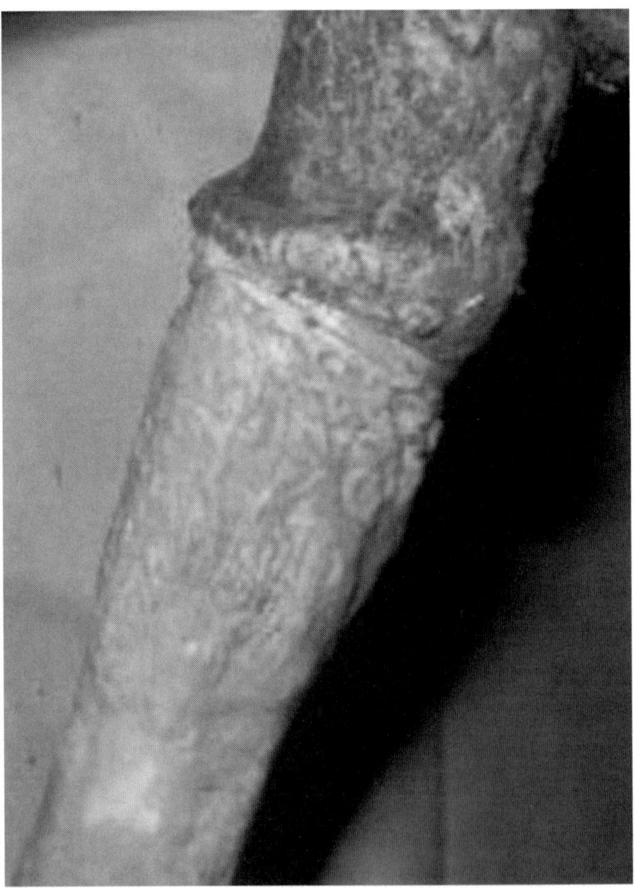

FIGURE 16-35. Multiple pale, slightly raised lesions of squamous cell carcinoma on the penis and prepuce of a stallion.

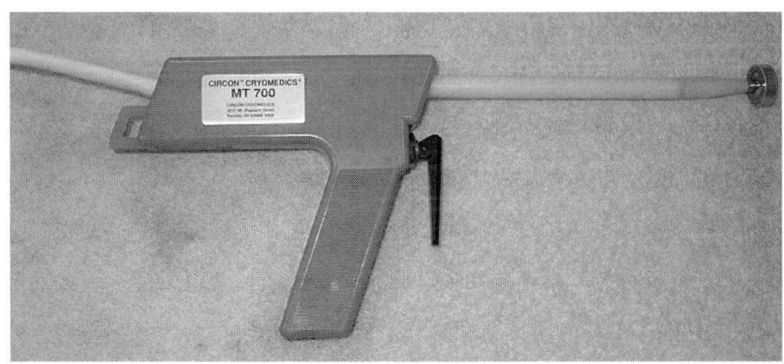

FIGURE 16-36. A 2-cm diameter cryoprobe attachment for a CO_2 cryosurgery instrument that can be used to freeze superficial squamous cell carcinomas of the penis and prepuce. Tissue should be frozen and thawed two to three times to a depth of 2 to 3 mm.

with extensive lesions of the prepuce may require segmental posthectomy (i.e., reefing).

To reef the internal lamina of the prepuce (Figure 16-37), the horse is anesthetized, positioned in dorsal or lateral recumbency, and prepared for aseptic surgery. The penis is extended by traction, and the urethra is catheterized. If desired, a tourniquet can be placed proximal to the surgical site. Parallel, circumferential, cutaneous incisions are made proximal and distal to the preputial lesion, and these incisions are connected by a longitudinal incision. The diseased segment of prepuce between the circumferential incisions is removed from the penis using scissor dissection. Bleeding vessels are ligated with absorbable sutures, and loose fascia is apposed with interrupted no. 0 or 2-0 absorbable sutures. Care must be taken to maintain the prepuce in proper alignment, and placement of a suture in the fascia at four equidistant points around the circumference of the penis may aid in orientation. The integument is apposed with interrupted no. 0 or 2-0 absorbable or nonabsorbable sutures. The amount of prepuce that can be removed without disrupting normal copulatory function is unknown. To prevent disruption of sutures caused by penile erection, the stallion should be isolated from mares for at least 2 weeks, and application of a stallion ring to the penis may be necessary. The stallion should be exercised daily to reduce postsurgical edema. Nonabsorbable sutures should be removed at 10 to 12 days.

Phallectomy (Figure 16-38) of stallions may be indicated if neoplasia has invaded the tunica albuginea, but phallectomy should be considered to be a salvage procedure. The horse should be castrated at least 2 weeks before phallectomy and separated from other horses for 2 weeks after phallectomy to decrease the likelihood of a sexually induced erection and disruption of sutures.

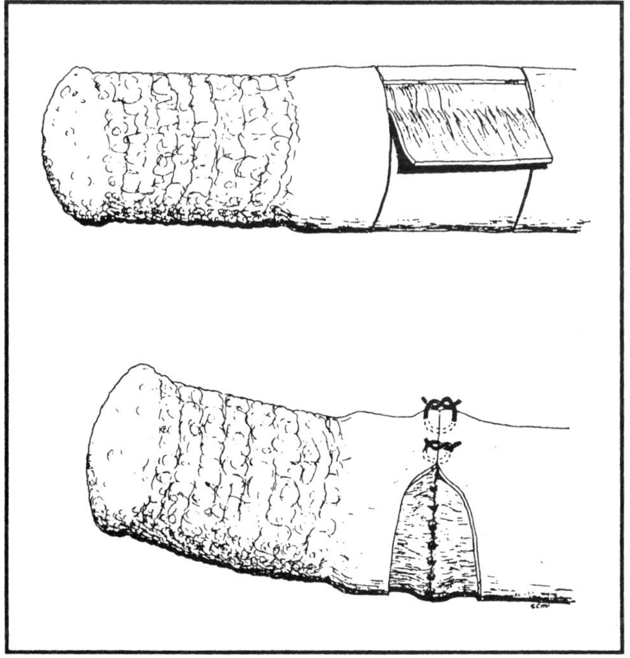

FIGURE 16-37. A reefing operation, or circumferential excision of a length of the prepuce, with subsequent closure of the preputial defect. (From Varner DD, Schumacher J, Blanchard TL et al: *Diseases and management of breeding stallions.* St Louis, 1991, Mosby.)

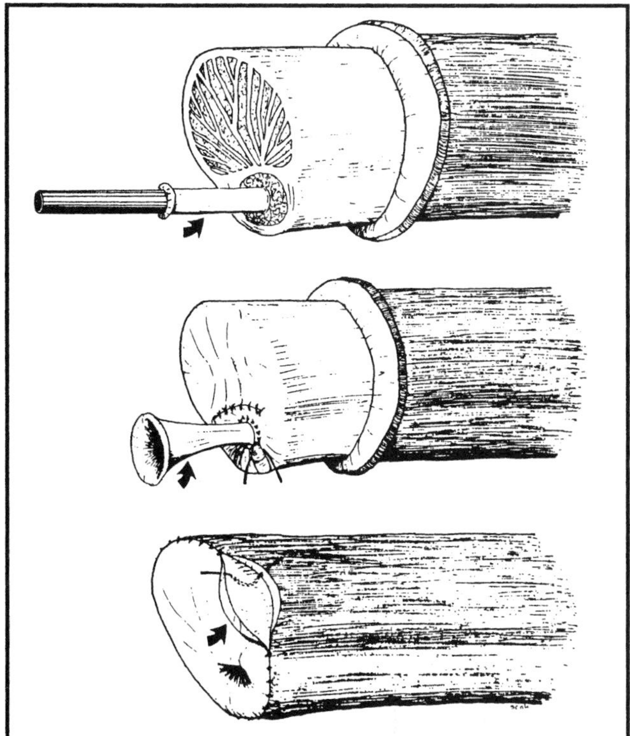

FIGURE 16-38. Amputation of the equine penis, with separate closures of the corpus cavernosum penis and corpus spongiosum penis, followed by fixation of the flared urethral mucosa *(arrows)* to the skin of the penis. (From Varner DD, Schumacher J, Blanchard TL et al: *Diseases and management of breeding stallions.* St Louis, 1991, Mosby.)

CUTANEOUS HABRONEMIASIS

Summer sores (i.e., *cutaneous habronemiasis*) are pruritic, pyogranulomatous lesions caused by aberrant cutaneous migration of the larvae of the equine stomach worm *Habronema*. Summer sores can be found anywhere on the integument, and when the genitalia are involved, the urethral process and preputial ring are the most common sites of infestation (Figure 16-39). Summer sores appear in the warm months of the year when flies, which are the nematode's intermediate host, are prevalent. Summer sores of the genitalia may disappear with the advent of cold weather. Horses that are prone to exposing their penis are particularly vulnerable to cutaneous habronemiasis of the genitalia. Migration and encystment of *Habronema* larvae cause formation of exuberant granulation tissue characterized by small, yellow, caseous granules. Skin surrounding the granulation tissue may be depigmented. Lesions of the preputial ring interfere with the normal telescoping action of the prepuce, and lesions of the urethral process may involve the corpus spongiosum penis, causing hematuria or hemospermia.

Summer sores may resemble lesions of pythiosis, carcinoma, the fibroblastic form of sarcoid, or exuberant granulation tissue caused by trauma. The presence of small granules in the lesion usually enables the condition to be differentiated from other diseases with similar appearance. When the lesion is squeezed, larvae can occasionally be extruded onto a slide and identified microscopically. Histologic characteristics of lesions are granulation tissue infiltrated with eosinophils, granules, and larvae; affected horses often have a marked eosinophilia.

Administration of ivermectin (administered systemically) or an organophosphate (administered systemically or topically) has been effective in resolving lesions by eliminating the migrating larvae. Systemic administration of corticosteroids or diethylcarbamazine has been successful in resolving lesions by eliminating the horse's response to the larvae.

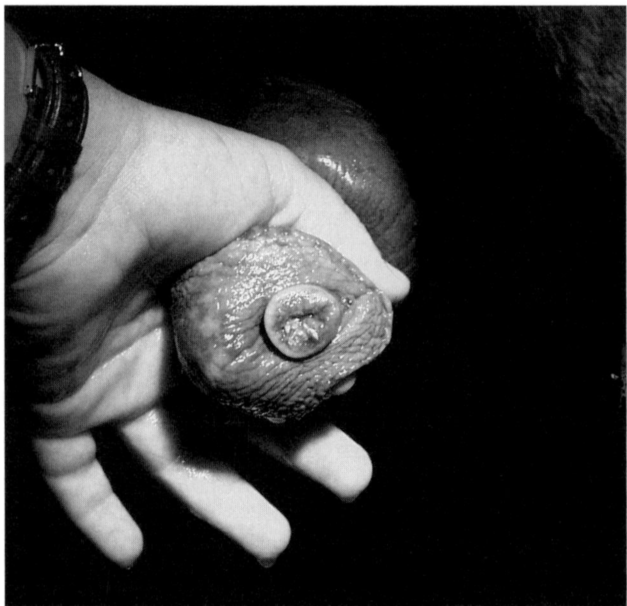

FIGURE 16-39. *Habronema* granuloma of urethral process of a stallion.

Lesions of the internal lamina of the prepuce can be surgically excised. Small lesions can be removed by elliptical excision, but large or multiple lesions are often best removed by reefing. Lesions of the urethral process may necessitate amputation (Figures 16-40 and 16-41). The urethral process can be amputated with the horse anesthetized or with the

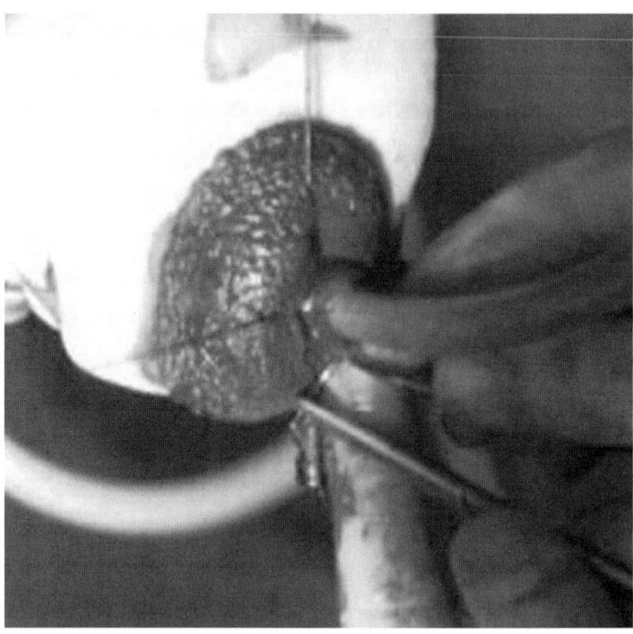

FIGURE 16-40. To surgically remove a large urethral granuloma unresponsive to medical therapy, the penis and prepuce are scrubbed with a disinfectant and dried. A sterile stallion catheter is passed into the urethra and held in place by retention needles passed through the proximal portion of the urethral process behind the lesion.

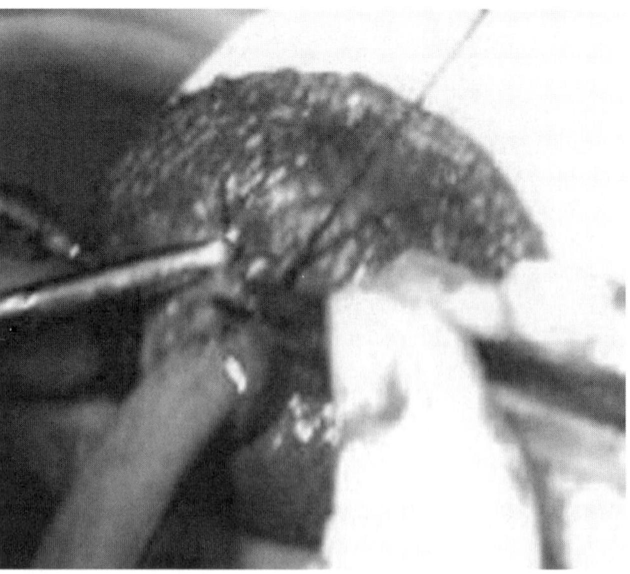

FIGURE 16-41. The urethral granuloma is excised, and the inner urethral mucosa is sutured to the outer integument of the urethral process in an interrupted pattern.

horse standing and sedated. A male urinary catheter is passed into the urethra, and if surgery is performed with the horse standing, the base of the urethral process is infiltrated with local anesthetic. The urethral process is circumferentially excised proximal to the lesion, and the epithelium of the stump is rolled inward and sutured to the urethral mucosa, using 2-0 or 3-0 absorbable suture material, to close the exposed corpus spongiosum penis. Fibrous tissue at the suture site may tear during subsequent breeding, causing hemospermia. Cauterization of these sites with silver nitrate sticks usually results in adequate healing.

PRIAPISM

Priapism, or persistent erection without sexual arousal, occurs when detumescence of the engorged corpus cavernosum penis (CCP) fails because of disturbances of arterial inflow or venous outflow (Figure 16-42). Priapism occurs uncommonly in horses but is economically devastating when a valuable breeding stallion is affected; impotence is the usual outcome, and phallectomy may be required.

In stallions, priapism is primarily caused by administration of phenothiazine-derivative tranquilizers, which block the sympathetic impulses that initiate detumescence. When detumescence does not occur, blood in the CCP stagnates and partial pressure of CO_2 in the stagnant blood rises, causing erythrocytes to sickle. The sickled erythrocytes obstruct venous outflow from the CCP, and the collecting veins eventually become irreversibly occluded. Arterial supply to the CCP is still patent in the early stages of priapism, but if priapism persists, it too becomes irreversibly occluded. Eventually the trabeculae of the cavernosal tissue become fibrotic and lose the expansile capacity necessary for normal erection (Figure 16-43). In addition to damaging erectile tissue, prolonged erection may also result in penile paralysis by damaging the pudendal nerves, which is perhaps caused by compression of the nerves against the ischium or retractor penis muscles due to the pendant penis.

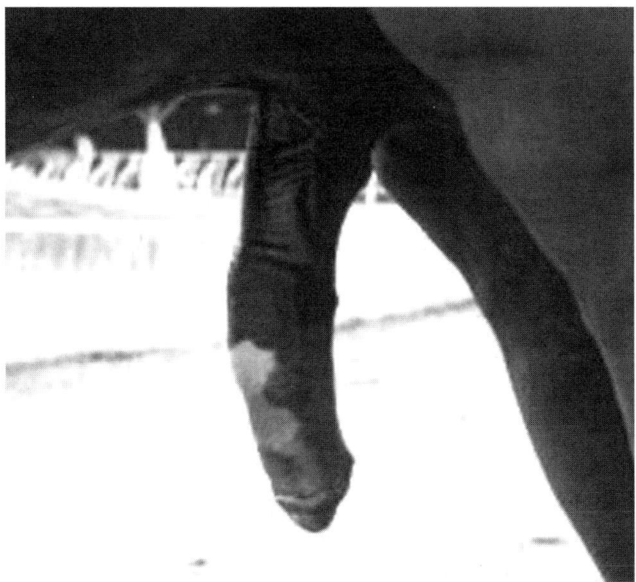

FIGURE 16-42. Persistent erection (priapism) in a stallion after administration of acepromazine.

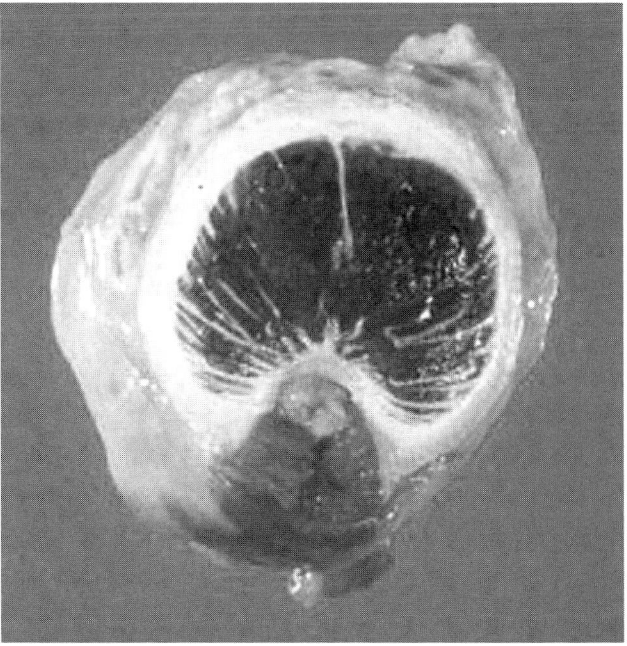

FIGURE 16-43. Cross-section of amputated penis from a stallion with chronic priapism unresponsive to treatment. Blood within the CCP was clotted, and cavernosal trabeculae are thickened and fibrotic.

Horses with priapism have been treated empirically with administration of diuretics and corticosteroids, general and regional anesthesia, penile and preputial massage, emollient dressings, and slings. Although such treatments usually fail to resolve priapism, some are beneficial because they prevent damage to the exposed organ. Benztropine mesylate (Cogentin, Merck and Company, Inc., West Point, PA), a cholinergic blocker administered systemically (8 mg by slow intravenous injection), and 1% phenylephrine HCl (GensiaSicor Pharmaceuticals, Inc., Irvine, CA), a sympathomimetic drug aseptically injected directly into the CCP (2 to 10 mg), have been used successfully to bring about detumescence in horses affected with priapism. These drugs should not be given if ventricular tachycardia or high blood pressure is present, and heart rate should be monitored after administration.

When priapism is recognized but does not respond to medical treatment, the horse should be treated by irrigation of the CCP to evacuate sludged blood. Heparinized saline (10 U/ml of saline) is injected through a 12-gauge needle inserted into the erect CCP proximal to the glans penis. Sludged blood and saline are released 10 to 15 cm caudal to the scrotum through a small stab incision in the tunica albuginea of the CCP or through one or two 12-gauge needles inserted into the CCP. The CCP is irrigated until fresh hemorrhage appears in the efflux (Figure 16-44). If a stab incision is made in the tunica

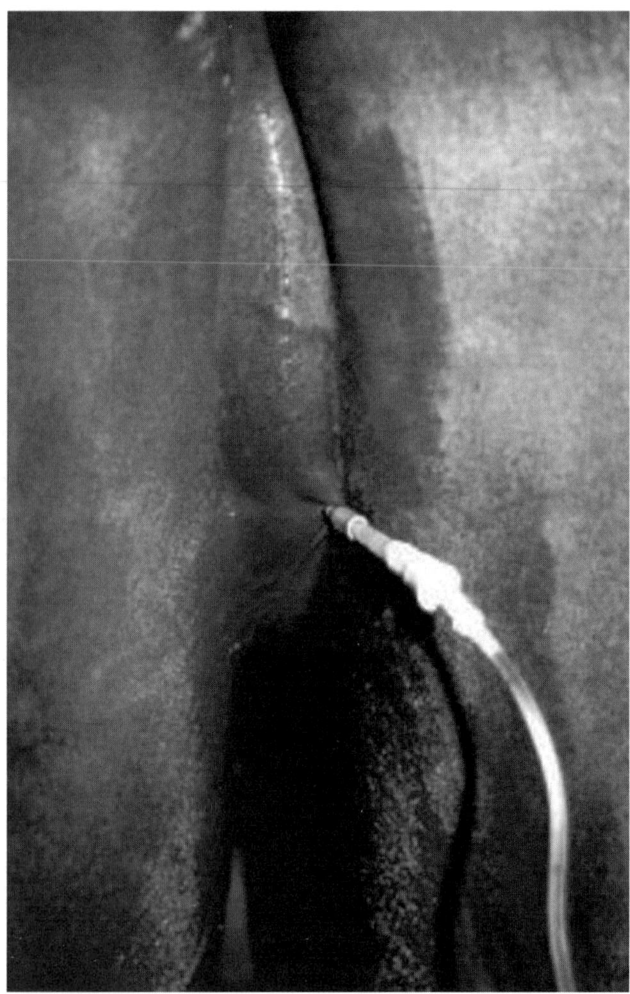

FIGURE 16-44. Placement of large-bore needles into the erect CCP (caudal to the scrotum and just proximal to the glans penis) of a stallion with priapism for irrigation of the cavernosal tissue with heparinized saline.

albuginea of the CCP, it should be sutured after irrigation. If arterial blood fails to appear after irrigation, the arteriolar supply to the CCP is probably permanently damaged and impotence is likely. Failure of erection to subside after irrigation indicates that arteriolar inflow is patent and that venous outflow is occluded. If erection recurs after irrigation of the CCP, the CCP can be anastomosed to the corpus spongiosum penis (CSP) to create a shunt for blood trapped within the CCP (Figure 16-45). This shunt is unlikely to interfere with subsequent erection and ejaculation.

HEMOSPERMIA

Hemospermia, a cause of infertility in stallions, has been attributed to bacterial and viral urethritis; improperly applied stallion rings; habronemiasis of the urethral process; and wounds to the glans penis. Hemospermia is also commonly caused by urethral defects, the cause of which is unknown. Regardless of the cause of hemospermia, the source of hemorrhage is

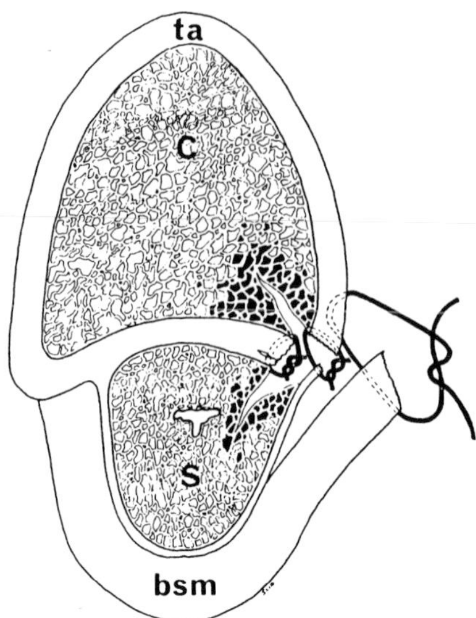

FIGURE 16-45. Creation of a vascular shunt between the CCP *(C)* and the CSP *(S)* as a surgical treatment for priapism in stallions. After incision of the CCP and CSP, the incised tunica albuginea of the CSP is sutured to the incised tunica albuginea overlying the lateral aspect of the CCP. The incised bulbospongiosus muscle *(bsm)* is then resutured to the tunica albuginea of the CCP. (From Varner DD, Schumacher J, Blanchard TL et al: *Diseases and management of breeding stallions.* St Louis, 1991, Mosby.)

probably the CSP. Hemorrhage occurs at the end of ejaculation, when contraction of the bulbospongiosus muscles causes pressure within the CSP to increase from 17 to 1000 mm Hg. Blood in the ejaculate, even in amounts than cannot be detected grossly, can contribute to infertility.

Hemospermia may occur more commonly in stallions bred often. Affected stallions are sometimes slow to ejaculate, and ejaculation often appears to cause pain. Hemospermia is usually diagnosed by gross examination of semen that has been collected with an artificial vagina. The site of hemorrhage can often be determined by examining the urethra with a sterilized, flexible endoscope that is at least 100 cm long. Endoscopic examination of the urethra of stallions affected with hemospermia often reveals a longitudinal defect, 5 to 10 mm long, on the caudal surface of the urethra at the level of the ischial arch (Figure 16-46); no gross signs of inflammation surround the defect.

Horses affected with hemospermia have been treated nonsurgically by sexual abstinence and by systemic administration of formalin, methenamine, or antimicrobial drugs. Enforcing sexual abstinence for a protracted time (e.g., many months) is often unsuccessful in resolving hemospermia. Horses with hemospermia seem to be most effectively treated by temporary urethrotomy performed at the level of the ischial arch (Figure 16-47). Urethrotomy is performed with the horse standing, using sedation and epidural anesthesia. To facilitate identification of the urethra during dissection, a urethral catheter or small foal stomach tube is inserted into the urethra and advanced until it is proximal to

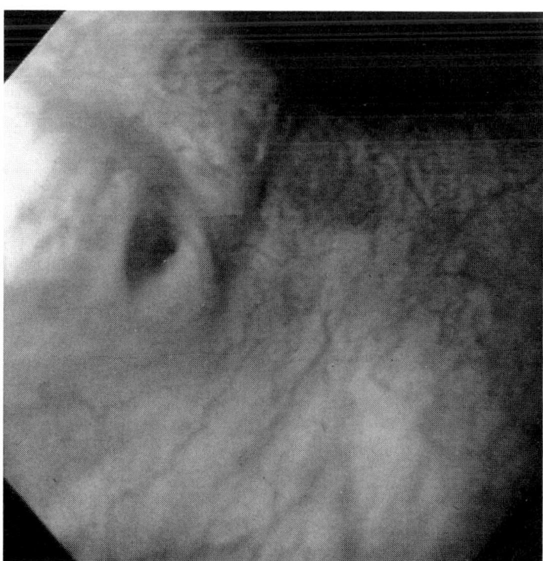

FIGURE 16-46. Endoscopic image of a longitudinal rent in the caudal urethral mucosa at the level of the ischial arch of a stallion with hemospermia.

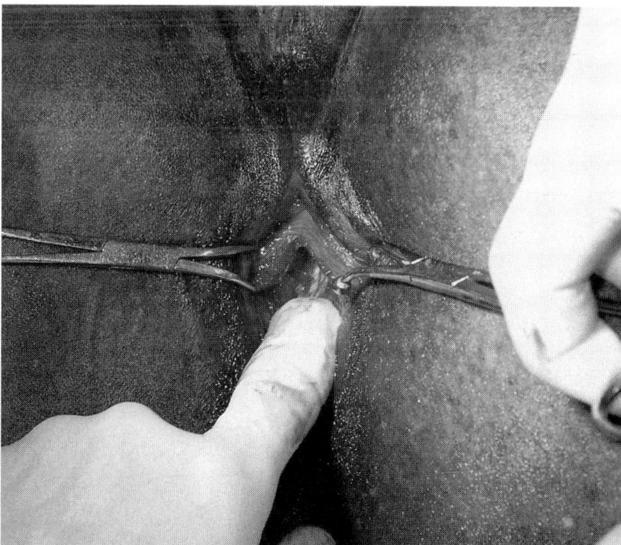

FIGURE 16-47. Perineal urethrostomy performed in a stallion as treatment for hemospermia due to urethral tear. Caudal epidural anesthesia is used for analgesia. After the penis is scrubbed with disinfectant, a sterile urethral catheter is passed to the level of the ischium to aid in identifying urethra for location of incision to be made.

the ischial arch. A longitudinal incision, 8 to 10 cm long, centered on the ischial arch, is made on the perineal raphe. The incision extends through skin, retractor penis and bulbospongiosus muscles, CSP, and urethral mucosa. Incising the urethral mucosa may be unnecessary for resolution of hemospermia. Opening the CSP without entering the urethra may reduce the risk of complications associated with urethrotomy, such as urethral fistula or stricture. The wound is allowed to heal by second intention. Daily installation of suppositories composed of an antimicrobial drug and a corticosteroid into the urethral lumen has been advocated but is probably unnecessary. Stallions should receive sexual rest for at least 3 months after surgery. Horses may bleed at the urethrotomy for more than a week after surgery, especially at the end of urination when the bulbospongiosus muscles contract. The ischial wound generally heals within 3 to 4 weeks.

Incising the CSP at the level of the ischium may decrease cavernosal pressure at the end of urination, and this decreased pressure in the CSP may be responsible for the apparent success of temporary urethrotomy in eliminating hemospermia. When the bladder has emptied, the bulbospongiosus muscles contract to expel urine that remains in the urethra, and these contractions increase pressure within the CSP and may prevent healing of a urethral lesion that communicates with the CSP. The incision into the CSP converts this semiclosed vascular space into an open space, and during urination, blood flow is diverted from the urethral lesion to the urethrotomy, thus permitting the lesion to heal.

Because the urethral defects are typically located at the posterior surface of the urethra near the ischial arch and are accessible through ischial urethrotomy, primary closure of the defect may be indicated. Urethral endoscopy aids the surgeon in identifying the exact location of the defect. To confirm the location of the defect, a hypodermic needle can be inserted percutaneously into the lumen of the urethra at the level of the ischial arch during endoscopic examination. The urethral mucosal tear is sutured in an interrupted pattern using 3-0 Vicryl. The remaining layers of tissue are not sutured but are left to heal by second intention.

HEMATURIA

A urethral defect of geldings, identical to the urethral defect at the ischial arch of stallions that causes hemospermia, also causes hematuria in geldings. Hematuria occurs typically at the end of urination when the bulbospongiosus muscles contract to expel urine. Occasionally, the affected horse shows sign of pain at the end of urination. Geldings with hematuria caused by a urethral rent are treated by temporary urethrotomy, the same treatment received by stallions with hemospermia caused by the identical urethral lesion. The ischial incision may need to penetrate only into the CSP to be effective. By incision of the CSP, vascular pressure at the end of urination is reduced and with the reduction in pressure, blood no longer flows through the defect at the end of urination. This allows the defect to heal.

BIBLIOGRAPHY

Fortier AL, Mac Harg MA: Topical use of 5-fluorouracil for treatment of squamous cell carcinoma of the external genitalia of horses: 11 cases (1988-1992). *J Am Vet Med Assoc* 205:1183-1185, 1994.

McKinnon AO, Voss JL: Hemospermia and urospermia. In McKinnon AO, Voss JL, editors, *Equine reproduction,* Philadelphia, 1993, Lea and Febiger.

Schumacher J, Varner DD, Schmitz DG et al: Urethral defects in geldings with hematuria and stallions with hemospermia. *Vet Surg* 24:250-254, 1995.

Varner DD, Schumacher J, Blanchard TL et al: *Diseases and management of breeding stallions,* St Louis, 1991, Mosby, pp 140-340.

Walker DF, Vaughan JT: *Bovine and equine urogenital surgery,* Philadelphia, 1980, Lea and Febiger, pp 115-176.

Wilson DV, Nickels FA, Williams MA: Pharmacologic treatment of priapism in two horses. *J Am Vet Med Assoc* 199:1183-1184, 1991.

17

An Overview of Embryo Transfer in Horses

OBJECTIVES

While studying the information covered in this chapter, the student should attempt to:

1. Acquire a working knowledge of reasons for performing embryo transfer in horses, and the breed associations that permit use of this procedure.
2. Acquire a working knowledge of the methods for synchronizing ovulation in donor and recipient mares to be used in an embryo-transfer program.
3. Acquire a working understanding of nonsurgical and surgical techniques used to perform embryo transfer in horses.

STUDY QUESTIONS

1. Discuss the reasons behind selection of mares as embryo donors.
2. Discuss considerations used when selecting mares as embryo recipients.
3. Discuss the methods used to synchronize ovulation in a group of donor and recipient mares in an embryo-transfer program.
4. Discuss the advantages and disadvantages of using ovariectomized mares as embryo recipients in an embryo-transfer program.
5. Discuss the techniques used to recover embryos from a donor mare.
6. Discuss the methods used for transfer of embryos to a recipient mare.

BACKGROUND

Embryo transfer refers to the procedure for collecting a fertilized ovum (embryo) from a donor mare and transferring it to the reproductive tract of a recipient mare with synchronized ovulation. Nowadays, the embryo is removed from the uterus of a donor mare and transferred to the uterus of a recipient mare; however, as technologies continue to develop, it may become feasible to collect oviductal embryos commercially for transfer to recipient mares.

The first embryo transfer (involving rabbits) was reported more than a century ago; however, this means of assisted reproduction was not developed for use in the horse until the early 1970s and did not become popular among horse enthusiasts until the late1980s. Currently, most equine breed associations in the United States permit embryo transfer. Notable exceptions include the Jockey Club (Thoroughbreds), the United States Trotting Association (Standardbreds), and the American Miniature Horse Association. It is important to contact a breed association before implementing embryo transfer because of changing regulations regarding its acceptance or specific policies regarding its use.

TECHNIQUE

The customary procedure for performing embryo transfer begins with synchronization of ovulation between a donor mare and the recipient mares, followed by insemination of the donor mare (Figure 17-1). The uterus of the donor mare is usually flushed 7 or 8 days after ovulation, and the retrieved embryo is transferred into the uterus of a recipient mare. This transfer can be accomplished either nonsurgically (via transcervical deposition of the embryo) or surgically (via laparotomy/uterotomy, laparoscopy-guided needle puncture, or transvaginal needle puncture). Under ideal conditions (i.e., experienced personnel, fertile donor and recipient mares, and fertile stallions), one can expect an embryo recovery rate of 50% to 70% and an embryo-transfer success rate of 50% to 70% (i.e., percentage of transferred embryos that maintain pregnancy) resulting in an overall pregnancy rate of 25% to 50% per cycle. If the ovulations of the donor mare and recipient mare are not well synchronized, personnel are inexperienced, or subfertile donors, recipients, or stallions are used, the success rate will be reduced accordingly. This reduced success rate can be quite dramatic and extremely disappointing.

It is imperative that donor mares be in good condition for breeding. These mares should have normal reproductive cycles. If one is unsure of the fertility of a donor mare, a thorough breeding soundness examination should be conducted to

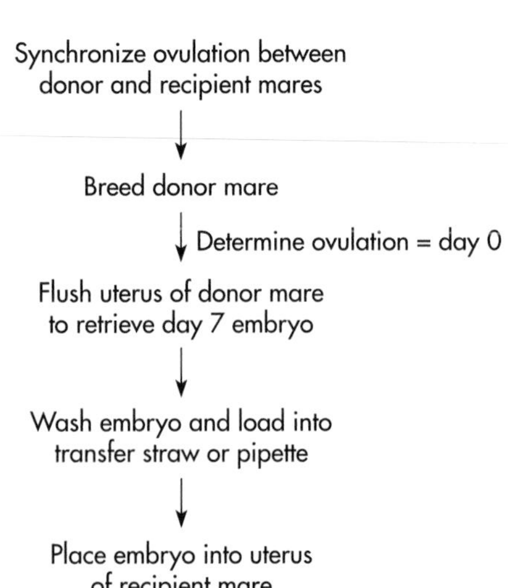

FIGURE 17-1. Flowchart illustrating the typical nonsurgical embryo transfer procedure in the mare.

detect any problems that might affect the mare's reproductive performance. Before embryo transfer is initiated with a given mare, the value of the mare and any offspring should be critically assessed because of the high costs of embryo transfer.

SELECTION AND MANAGEMENT OF DONOR MARES

There are numerous motives for commercial use of embryo transfer.

Management of Subfertile Mares

Many subfertile mares may be good candidates for embryo transfer. For instance, embryo transfer may be used as a therapeutic alternative for mares that become pregnant but repeatedly experience early embryonic death. Other good candidates are mares with widespread endometrial periglandular fibrosis, cystic glandular distention, or endometrial cysts; mares with irreparable cervical disease; or mares that experience unexplained habitual abortion. The value of the donor mare's offspring should be the primary consideration in any decision to perform an embryo transfer. The procedure can be very expensive and typically costs more for subfertile mares because of suboptimal embryo recovery rates and the poorer quality of embryos recovered. Furthermore, embryo transfer is not the answer to restoration of fertility for all subfertile mares. As shown by recent research, subfertility in some older mares may be due to reduced intrinsic viability of oocytes, innate embryonic defects, or oviductal dysfunction leading to interruption of early embryonic development. Embryo transfer would not correct such factors.

Exploitation of Superior Mares

Under usual circumstances, a mare is capable of producing a maximum of one foal per year, whereas a stallion may sire dozens to hundreds of foals per year. As a result, the stallion typically has much greater genetic influence on the breed than the dam. Although embryo transfer is unlikely to alter this imbalance, some breed associations will permit more than one foal to be registered per year from a dam, thereby increasing the mare's contribution to the gene pool. Even in those breed associations that permit the birth of only one foal per dam per year, one may be able to produce foals from mares at an earlier age than would otherwise be advisable (e.g., at 2 years of age). Furthermore, it may be possible to register more than one embryo-transfer foal during the same calendar year if the mare is bred to stallions of different breed registries. For example, an embryo-transfer foal could be produced by a Quarter Horse mare bred to a Paint stallion and be eligible for registration by the American Paint Horse Association, even if another embryo-transfer foal was obtained when the same mare was bred to an American Quarter Horse stallion and was registered by the American Quarter Horse Association in the same year. Embryo transfer may also be a viable option for use in mares that foal late in the breeding season. Embryo transfer offers the advantage of allowing these mares to be rebred early in the next breeding season, while at the same time producing a foal after being bred late in the current breeding season.

Reproductive Management of Performance Mares

Embryo transfer allows a mare to be taken out of competition for only 1 or 2 weeks to produce a foal. The mare is bred at the appropriate time; then an embryo is collected at day 7 or 8 postovulation for transfer to a synchronized recipient mare. The donor mare can then return to a performance career. Hence, the previous requirement of extended delays in training and competition to allow for production of a foal is eliminated.

Assessment of Fertility

Embryo transfer is occasionally used as an indirect means to assess fertility of either mares or stallions. It can be especially useful to rapidly ascertain potential pregnancy rates of processed semen (e.g., to test whether the semen of a given stallion retains a high level of fertility when it is stored at 5° C for 24 hours or is subjected to cryopreservation).

SELECTION OF RECIPIENT MARES

Recipient mares should be relatively young (i.e., 3 to 10 years of age), exhibit normal reproductive cycles, and have no history of reproductive problems. A complete breeding soundness examination should be conducted to ensure that recipient mares have no abnormalities, which could reduce their ability to carry a foal to term. Ideally, recipient mares should be at least as large or slightly larger than the donor mare. It is also important that the mares are easy to handle. If possible, mares with a history of good lactation and mothering ability should be chosen. Mares selected as recipients should be identified permanently (e.g., by freeze-branding) to facilitate accurate record keeping.

SUPEROVULATION

The hormonal preparations and schedules currently used to induce superovulation in other animals are not successful in the horse. Injections of equine chorionic gonadotropin (eCG) or porcine follicle-stimulating hormone (FSH-P) or a combination of FSH-P and porcine luteinizing hormone have yielded excellent results in other species but decidedly poor results in mares. The reason that mares are nonresponsive to eCG probably stems from the fact that this hormone binds exclusively with luteinizing hormone (LH) receptors in the mare, whereas it has both follicle-stimulation hormone (FSH) and LH activity in the other species. Although mares appear to be relatively refractory to FSH-P, repeated administration of high doses of this preparation can slightly increase the rate of double ovulations in mares. However, this slight increase in ovulation rate probably does not justify the high cost of treatment.

French and U.S. workers have reported that the number of ovulations increased to an average of 2 to 3 per cycle in mares treated with crude equine pituitary extract (EPE) or an FSH-enriched fraction from the same extract. In a recent study, it was found that twice-daily administration of EPE resulted in an average of 7.1 ovulations per mare compared to 2.3 ovulations when mares were treated once per day. Embryo production in mares treated with these hormonal preparations can be increased accordingly, with the embryo recovery rate being approximately half of the ovulation rate. At this time, preparations such as EPE are not available commercially.

Passive immunization of mares against the α subunit fragment of inhibin is reported to result in a slight increase in ovulation rate in mares (on average <2 ovulations), but the increased ovulation rate can persist over several cycles. This treatment regimen resulted in some undesirable side effects at the injection site.

Because of current restrictions in many breed associations regarding the number of foals that can be registered by embryo transfer per year from a given mare, the need to devise methods to superovulate mares is less of a priority than it is in other species. Nonetheless, superovulation of mares could reduce embryo-transfer costs and increase embryo yield in mares whose breed associations permit registration of numerous foals per year.

SYNCHRONIZATION OF OVULATION

Considerable attention should be given to synchronizing ovulation between the donor and recipient mares to maximize the chance of success of the embryo-transfer procedure (Figure 17-2). The greater individual variation in the length of estrus in mares as well as the effect of season on ovulation makes this feat more difficult to accomplish in mares than in cows. *Ideally, the recipient mare should ovulate from 1 day before to 2 days after the donor mare.*

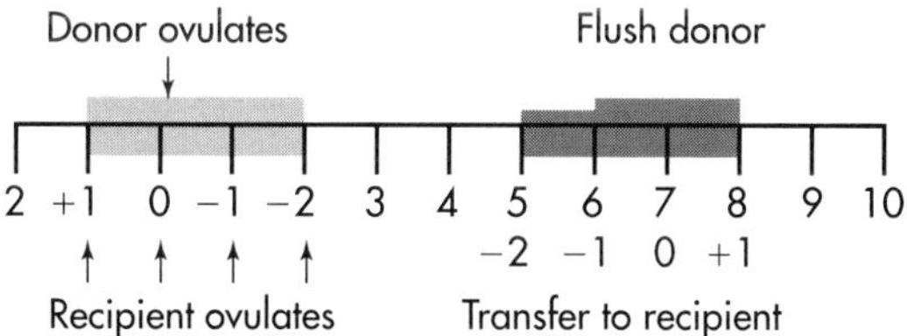

FIGURE 17-2. Schematic representation of synchrony between donors and recipients for successful embryo transfer.

Unless one has a large recipient herd from which to select mares in natural ovulatory synchrony with the donor mare, it will be necessary to use hormonal protocols to induce synchronous ovulation. Prostaglandins and progestins have been used independently to attempt synchronization of ovulation in mares; however, neither preparation reliably induces the tight synchrony of ovulation that is required for embryo transfer. To help increase the likelihood of acceptable synchronization, the products should be administered to recipient mares 1 day after they are given to the donor mare. Human chorionic gonadotropin (hCG) can be administered to mares, or deslorelin implants (Ovuplant) can also be used to accelerate ovulation and improve the degree of synchrony between the donor and recipient mares. To help ensure that a recipient mare with well-synchronized ovulation will be available at the time of embryo transfer, it is advisable to attempt to *synchronize ovulation of the donor mare with at least two recipient mares.* This protocol also may also provide multiple suitable recipient mares if more than one embryo is recovered from the donor mare.

Prostaglandins

Prostaglandins are typically administered twice, 14 days apart, with the injections given to the recipient mares 1 day after the injections are given to the donor mare. Because prostaglandins only induce luteolysis when a mature corpus luteum is present, it may be possible to administer only one injection each to the donor mare and recipient mares if all mares are confirmed to be in mid-diestrus at the time of treatment. Preferably, mares receiving injections should have ovarian follicles of similar size at the time of treatment to help assure similar rates of follicular development after prostaglandin injection.

Progestins

To synchronize estrus, progestins can be given to mares to artificially lengthen the luteal phase of the cycle. The progestins are typically administered to all mares for 14 to 15 days, with prostaglandins being administered concurrently on the last day of progestin treatment to induce regression of any functional corpora lutea that remain on the ovaries. The orally active progestin, altrenogest (Regu-Mate), is oftentimes used for regulating synchronization of estrus. A drawback of the use of progestin treatment alone is that ovarian follicles of mares are not uniformly regulated. Therefore, although the onset of estrus is relatively synchronous, the intervals from termination of treatment to ovulation are more variable among mares treated in this manner.

Progesterone and Estradiol-17β

Synchronization of ovulation is most effectively accomplished using a combination of the hormones progesterone and estradiol-17β, because this treatment inhibits follicular development more uniformly than does administration of progesterone alone. The result is less variation in synchrony of ovulations in treated mares. Incorporation of estradiol-17β in the treatment regimen may also promote better expression of posttreatment estrus behavior. Progesterone (150 mg) and estradiol-17β (10 mg) in oil are administered intramuscularly, daily for 10 days, with prostaglandin given on the last day of steroid treatment. If hCG is administered when a 35-mm follicle is detected, approximately 70% to 75% of mares ovulate on days 10 to 12 after the last day of steroid treatment. Use of deslorelin has been purported to reduce variability in the interval to ovulation compared with the use of hCG; however, to avoid follicular suppression and delayed return to estrus in deslorelin-treated mares, removal of the implant 2 days after administration has been recommended. Progesterone-estradiol preparations have not yet been approved in the United States for use in horses; however, they are readily compounded and commercial sources are available.

If a recipient mare ovulates more than 3 days *after* the donor mare, progesterone in oil (300 mg/day) should be administered to the recipient mare, beginning on the day on which ovulation occurs. Although not ideal, this treatment may allow one to salvage the use of a recipient mare for a given cycle if another recipient mare did not ovulate in suitable synchrony with the donor mare (e.g., perhaps when ovulation occurs as much as 5 to 6 days after that in the donor mare). The recipient mare should be given the progesterone supplementation for a minimum of 5 days or until her corpus luteum has become fully functional. Progesterone supplementation may be necessary until 100 to 150 days of gestation. No treatment is currently effective if the recipient mare ovulates far in advance (>2 days) of the donor mare.

Ovariectomized, Progesterone-Treated Mares as Embryo Recipients

One way to avoid the difficulties associated with synchronizing ovulation in mares is to use ovariectomized, progesterone-treated mares as embryo recipients. Progesterone in oil (300 mg) is administered intramuscularly once daily to recipient mares 2 days after the donor mare has ovulated. Thus the recipient mares are primed with progesterone treatment for 5 to 6 days before transfer of the embryo. If an embryo transfer is performed, the progesterone treatment is continued daily until days 100 to 150 of gestation. Thereafter, placental progestin production is sufficient to maintain the pregnancy to term. If an embryo is not transferred or a pregnancy is not detected in the recipient mare by transrectal ultrasonography 14 to 16 days after the donor mare ovulated, progesterone treatment is discontinued. Progesterone use should be discontinued for at least 1 week before supplementation is reinitiated for a subsequent transfer. Embryo-transfer pregnancies in ovariectomized mares have a normal gestational length. Additionally, these recipients appear to undergo normal parturition, lactation, and postpartum uterine involution and can be used repeatedly as embryo-transfer recipients.

Altrenogest has been used successfully by some workers as the sole progestin supplement in ovariectomized recipient mares. One study suggests that this product, when used at the label dosage, may be less reliable in maintaining the pregnancy than progesterone in oil during the initial stage of pregnancy; however, some practitioners switch from injectable progesterone to oral altrenogest supplementation after supplementary corpora lutea formation (i.e., after days 40 to 45 of gestation).

EMBRYO RECOVERY

Suppliers of media and equipment for embryo recovery and transfer are provided in Table 17-1.

A nonsurgical transcervical procedure is used to retrieve the embryo from the uterine lumen of the donor mare. This is usually attempted on day 7 or day 8 postovulation. Embryo recovery rates are lower when attempted at earlier times, and when recoveries are attempted later than day 8, embryos tend to be more easily damaged. Although embryos are easier to identify on day 8, recovery on day 7 has historically been preferred because the smaller day 7 embryos are less susceptible to trauma induced during the collection and transfer procedures. However, more recently, a number of practitioners have reported that routine embryo retrieval from donor mares on day 8 results in a higher recovery rate and excellent posttransfer pregnancy rates.

To prepare for an embryo recovery, the donor mare is first placed in a set of stocks, and her tail is wrapped and elevated. The hindquarters and perineum are prepared aseptically. Before continuing with the embryo recovery, it is important to rinse all soap or disinfectant scrub from the hindquarters (including the vulvar opening and vestibular lumen) to avoid embryotoxic effects of soap or disinfectant residues.

For embryo recovery, a uterine flushing catheter and sterile examination sleeve are required. We recommend use of an 80- or 150-cm-long balloon-tipped silicone catheter (Bivona, Inc.; Table 17-1) for embryo retrieval (Figure 17-3, p. 225). Using a sterile plastic sleeve to cover the hand and arm, the operator gently passes the catheter tip through the cervical opening and into the posterior uterine body. A small amount of sterile, nontoxic water-soluble lubricant should be applied to the outside of the sleeve and catheter before the operator attempts

TABLE 17-1

Supplies and Sources for Embryo Transfer Equipment

Item	Supplier	Telephone
Silicone equine embryo flush catheters	Cook Veterinary Products	800-826-2380
	Bivona, Inc.	800-348-6064
Y-junction tubing for embryo flush	American Embryo Systems	800-272-8338
	Fisher Scientific	800-766-7000
	Reproductive Resources	800-331-0195
Tubing connectors	VWR Scientific	800-932-5000
Tubing with stainless spike for Bivona catheter	Bivona, Inc.	800-348-6064
Silastic laboratory tubing (0.215-inch ID; 0.375-inch OD)	VWR Scientific	800-932-5000
Flow-control tubing clamps	Fisher Scientific	800-766-7000
Embryo filters	Minitube of America	800-646-4882
Minitube filter	Reproductive Resources	800-331-0195
EmCon filter	American Embryo Systems	800-272-8338
Large-volume VCI filter	Reproductive Resources	800-331-0195
	American Embryo Systems	800-272-8338
Modified Dulbecco's PBS (1-liter bags)	American Embryo Systems	800-272-8338
	Reproductive Resources	800-331-0195
Modified Dulbecco's PBS (powdered media)	Sigma Chemical Company	800-325-3010
Emcare embryo flushing and holding solutions	Professional Embryo Transfer Supply, Inc	800-735-9215
Vigro flushing and holding media	AB Technology, Inc.	800-335-8595
20-liter polyethylene carboy with spigot	Sigma Chemical Company	800-325-3010
Fetal calf serum with penicillin/streptomycin	Reproductive Resources	800-331-0195
Fetal bovine serum	Equitech-Bio	800-259-0591
Newborn calf serum (heat inactivated)	American Embryo Systems	800-272-8338
	Life Technologies	800-828-6686
Bovine calf serum	HyClone Laboratories	800-492-5663
Penicillin-streptomycin	American Embryo Systems	800-272-8338
	Sigma Chemical Company	800-325-3010
Round grid Petri dish (100 × 15 mm)	American Embryo Systems	800-272-8338
	Fisher Scientific	800-766-7000
	Reproductive Resources	800-331-0195
Small Petri dishes (with or without grid)	Fisher Scientific	800-766-7000
Embryo holding dishes (35 × 10 or 60 × 15 mm)	Fisher Scientific	800-766-7000
4-well embryo wash dishes	American Embryo Systems	800-272-8338
	Reproductive Resources	800-331-0195
Ureteral catheter connector	Cook Veterinary Products	800-826-2380
0.25- or 0.5-ml French straws	American Embryo Systems	800-272-8338
0.25- or 0.5-ml French straws	Reproductive Resources	800-331-0195
	Minitube of America	800-646-4882
	I.M.V.	800-342-5468
	Veterinary Concepts	800-826-6948
Disposable 0.25-ml 21-inch insemination gun	American Embryo Systems	800-272-8338
	Reproductive Resources	800-331-0195
	Veterinary Concepts	800-826-6948
Disposable 0.5-ml 25-inch insemination gun	American Embryo Systems	800-272-8338
	Reproductive Resources	800-331-0195
Micropipettor for French straws	I.M.V.	800-342-5468
Pipette protector (8 inch)	Veterinary Concepts	800-826-6948
Syringe filter (0.2 µm)	Fisher Scientific	800-776-7000
Embryo transport tubes	Fisher Scientific	800-776-7000
Small snap-cap (5ml)		
Large screw cap (50 ml)		
Parafilm sealing film (2 inch width)	Fisher Scientific	800-776-7000
Drummond microdispenser with glass bores	Fisher Scientific	800-776-7000
Equine embryo flush kit	American Embryo Systems	800-272-8338
	Reproductive Resources	800-331-0195

TABLE 17-1

(continued)

Full Line of Embryo Transfer Products and Supplies

Veterinary Concepts, Inc. P.O. Box 39 Spring Valley, WI 54767 800-826-6948; fax 800-227-1324	IMV International 6870 Shingle Creek Minneapolis, MN 55430 800-341-5468 www.imv-technologies.com
Professional Embryo Transfer Supply, Inc. P.O. Box 188 Canton, TX 75103-0188 800-735-9215; fax 903-567-4927 www.pets-inc.com	Har-Vet P.O. Box 39 Spring Valley, WI. 54767 800-872-7741; fax 800-227-1324 www.har-vet.com
AB Technology, Inc. NE 1335 Terre View Dr Pullman, WA 99613 800-335-8595; fax 509-335-4047 www.abtechnology.com	

General Laboratory and Chemical Suppliers

Fisher Scientific 711 Forbes Ave Pittsburgh, PA 15219 800-766-7000 www.fisherscientific.com	Sigma Chemical Co. P.O. Box 14508 St. Louis, MO 63178-9916 800-325-3010; fax 800-325-5052 www.sigma-aldrich.com
VWR Scientific P.O. Box 7900 San Francisco, CA 94120 800-932-5000 www.vwrsp.com	

to place the catheter in the uterus. The balloon cuff of the catheter is then filled with 60 to 80 ml of air or sterile saline and pulled posteriorly to establish a good seal at the junction of the uterine body and internal cervical os (Figure 17-4).

Although some practitioners report acceptable results for embryo transfer using lactated Ringer's solution, Dulbecco's phosphate-buffered saline containing 1% (v/v) neonatal calf serum (NCS) or fetal calf serum (FCS) and penicillin-streptomycin has traditionally been the medium of choice for the embryo recovery. Complete flushing media and media components are available commercially (Table 17-1). Although the practitioner can prepare the media after the proper components are acquired, purchase of prepared products from commercial sources ensures proper measurements of solutes and ideal water quality.

Volumes of 1000 to 1500 ml (30° to 37° C) are typically used for each flush, and the procedure is repeated three to four times. In mares with large pendulous uteri, larger fluid volumes and massaging the uterus per rectum may be beneficial in suspending the embryo in the flush media and improving the recovery of the fluid and embryo. The container of flush solution is connected to the uterine catheter by tubing, and the fluid is allowed to enter the uterine lumen by gravity flow (Figure 17-5). The fluid is either collected in 1000-ml graduated cylinders or, preferably, allowed to pass through a specially designed (70- to 75-μm pore size) embryo filter to permit escape of fluid and retention of any collected embryos. The filter device must always contain a small amount of fluid, so that any collected embryos are continually bathed in the fluid and not subjected to desiccation. At least 90% of the infused fluid should be retrieved; if it is not, the mare can be given 20 IU of oxytocin intravenously and/or the uterus can be manipulated per rectum to help aid evacuation of the fluid. If an in-line filter was not used to collect the embryos, the retrieved fluid in the graduated cylinders should be allowed to stand undisturbed for 10 to 15 minutes, thereby allowing time for any embryos contained in the fluid to sink to the bottom of the cylinder. Then all but 50 ml of fluid is siphoned carefully from the top of each cylinder and subsequently passed through an embryo filter to retrieve any embryos that may have been accidentally siphoned with the fluid.

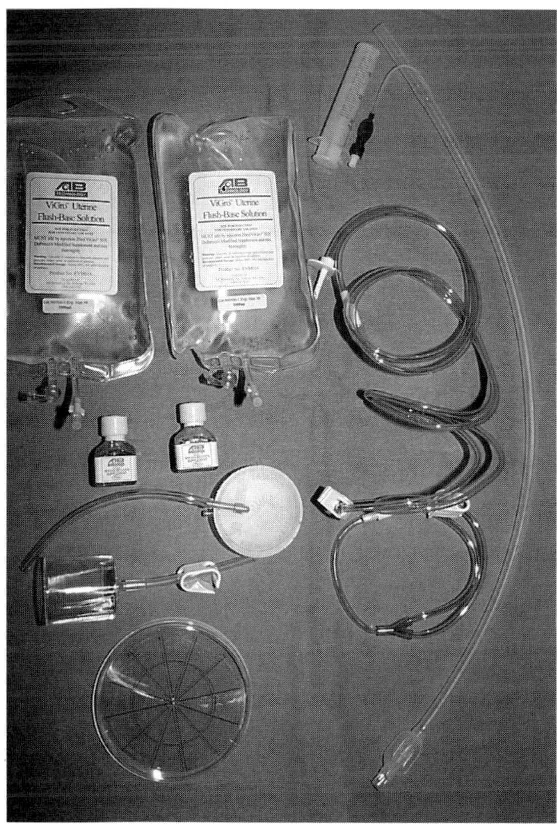

FIGURE 17-3. Equipment used for nonsurgical uterine flushing to retrieve embryos in the mare. *Clockwise from upper left:* bags of commercially prepared flush media; syringe for inflating the balloon of the flushing catheter; the flushing catheter and tubing with a Y connector; search dish; two types of commercially available flush filters to catch the embryo; and commercially available neonatal calf serum to be added to flush media.

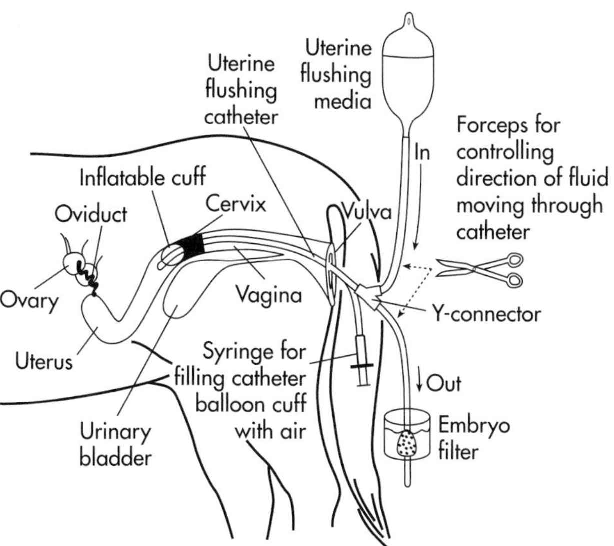

FIGURE 17-4. Illustration of catheter placement in the uterus of a mare before the flushing procedure. After insertion of the catheter through the cervix, the balloon is distended with air and the catheter is pulled gently backward to seal the balloon at the internal cervical os.

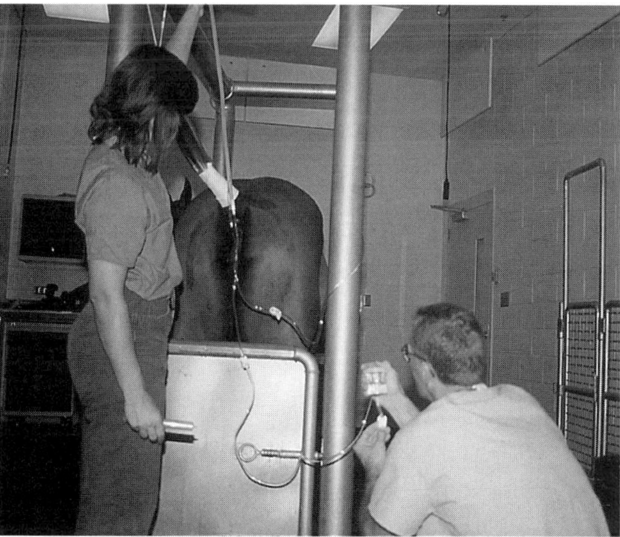

FIGURE 17-5. Nonsurgical uterine flushing procedure to recover embryos from a donor mare.

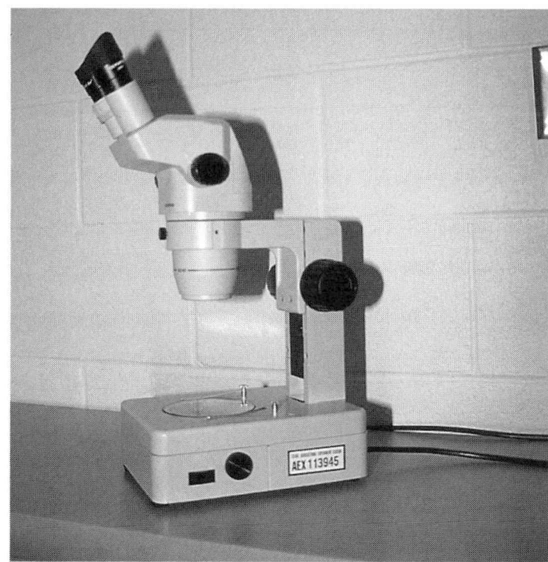

FIGURE 17-6. Stereoscope used to examine aliquots of fluid (in Petri dishes) recovered from the uterus of a donor mare to locate and evaluate embryo(s).

Fluid remaining on the filter is rinsed into sterile plastic Petri dishes (± grid; typically 100-mm diameter and 15-mm depth) and is examined using a dissecting microscope (10 to 40× magnification) to identify any embryos (Figure 17-6). Day 8 embryos are often visible with the naked eye. Embryos identified are aspirated into a sterile 3 French tomcat catheter, a sterile 25-μl glass capillary pipette, or a 0.25- to 0.5-ml French straw attached to a syringe (Figure 17-7) and transferred into small embryo wash plates containing filter-sterilized flush medium with 10% (v/v) NCS or FCS. Whenever embryos are aspirated into a handling device, air and medium should be on either side of the medium

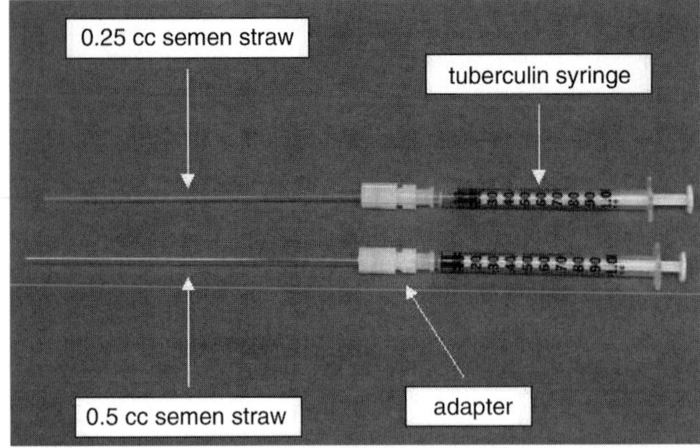

FIGURE 17-7. Embryo handling equipment consisting of tuberculin syringes with 0.25 or 0.5-ml semen freezing straws and adapter. (From Vanderwall DK: Current equine embryo transfer techniques. In Ball BA, editor, *Recent advances in equine reproduction,* pp A0204-0400. Ithaca, NY, 2000, International Veterinary Information Service.)

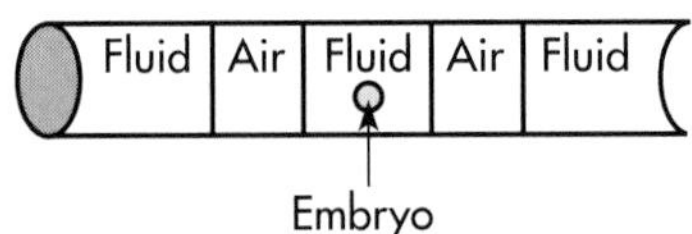

FIGURE 17-8. Drawing of an embryo in a transfer straw positioned between air and fluid columns. (From Vanderwall DK: Current equine embryo transfer techniques. In Ball BA, editor, *Recent advances in equine reproduction,* p A0204.0400. Ithaca, NY, 2000, International Veterinary Information Service.)

containing the embryo (Figure 17-8). This helps prevent loss of the embryo during handling. The embryo is washed at least 3 to 6 times by transferring it sequentially into the different fluid droplets or wells of the wash plate. After the washing procedure, the embryo is examined at higher magnification (40 to 80×) and graded as excellent to poor on an ordinal scale of 1 to 4 (Table 17-2). It is then ready for transfer into a recipient mare. Although embryos may be held in a covered wash plate for 2 to 4 hours at room temperature (20° to 25° C) before transfer or packaging for shipment, it is recommended that the transfer or packaging be performed within 1 hour after collection.

EMBRYO TRANSFER

Embryos can be transferred either surgically or nonsurgically into the recipient mare. Although surgical transfer of embryos is still preferred by some laboratories, the majority of embryo transfers are now performed nonsurgically.

Surgical embryo transfer is typically performed by exteriorizing one of the mare's uterine horns via a standing flank laparotomy. A stab incision is made through the uterine wall at an avascular location with a surgeon's needle. The embryo (in 0.25 ml of medium) is transferred into the uterine lumen using a fire-polished glass pipette, plastic tom-cat catheter, or 0.25- to 0.5-ml French straw via the puncture site. The puncture wound is not sutured, and the uterine horn is replaced into the peritoneal cavity followed by closure of the flank incision in a routine fashion. The recipient mare is held in a stall for 5 to 7 days to monitor healing of the flank incision as well as general health. Systemic antibiotics are generally administered for 5 to 7 days, but administration of exogenous progesterone or antiinflammatory drugs is usually not considered to be necessary. Phenylbutazone can be administered for 2 to 3 days to control postoperative pain. At 5 to 7 days after transfer, the mare is examined for pregnancy and can be returned to a small paddock or pasture if no postsurgical complications arise. Skin sutures can be removed in 10 to 14 days.

TABLE 17-2

Ordinal Scale for Grading and Description of Embryos

Grade	Category	Appearance	Characteristics
1	Excellent	Spherical	Uniform cell size, color, and texture
2	Good	Minor imperfections	Few extruded blastomeres; irregular shape; trophoblastic separation
3	Fair	Obvious problems	Extruded blastomeres; degenerate cells; collapsed blastocoele
4	Poor	Severe problems Oblong or irregular	Collapsed blastocoele; many extruded blastomeres; degenerate cells

The nonsurgical approach involves transcervical deposition of the embryo into the uterine body. To perform this procedure, prepare the hindquarters of the recipient mare as described above. Load the embryo into either (1) an insemination pipette or (2) a 0.5-ml capacity straw used for frozen semen. If the embryo is loaded into the insemination pipette, a 10- to 12-ml syringe containing approximately 5 to 6 ml of air should first be secured to the appropriate end of the pipette, then the medium and embryo should be loaded into the pipette in 0.25- to 0.5-ml (0.5- to 1-inch) increments using the following sequence: medium, air, medium containing embryo, air, medium, air (similar to the drawing in Figure 17-8). This loading procedure minimizes movement of the embryo within the pipette and helps ensure that it will be discharged into the uterus at the appropriate time. Using a sterile lubricated sleeve to cover the hand and arm, the operator places the tip of the loaded pipette in a cupped palm and carefully guides the tip of the pipette to the anterior of the vagina. The index finger is used to identify the external cervical os, and the tip of the pipette is inserted through the cervical lumen into the uterine body. When resistance is met, the pipette is pulled posteriorly (approximately 1 to 2 cm) and the embryo and medium are deposited into the uterine body. In one study, the pregnancy rate in mares was improved when the insemination pipette was placed in a guarded sheath before embryo transfer. The pipette is pushed through the sheath at the cervical os, and only the pipette is passed into the uterus.

If a 0.5-ml semen straw is used to load the embryo, flexible tubing attached to a 3- to 6-ml syringe is first fitted to the end of the straw, which contains a plug of cotton and polyvinyl chloride (PVC) powder. Load the embryo and medium into the straw by aspiration with the syringe similarly to the way it is loaded into a handling device (see Figure 17-8). Wetting the PVC powder creates a seal on the end of the straw attached to the tubing and syringe. The embryo is deposited into the uterus as described above, except that the straw containing the embryo is first placed in a disposable, 21-inch insemination gun that is designed for insemination with 0.5-ml straws (Figure 17-9).

Some operators prefer to elevate the uterus per rectum with one hand while transferring the embryo to minimize resistance to the pipette as it is passed into the uterus. The value of this procedure is unknown. Studies to date suggest that administration of antibiotics or antiinflammatory drugs to the recipient mare at the time of transfer have no benefit. Exogenous progestins also have questionable value, unless the recipient mare requires supplementation because of ovariectomy or asynchronous ovulation, as described above.

The pregnancy rate achieved with the surgical approach is reported to be higher by some laboratories; however, other workers have reported pregnancy rates after nonsurgical transfer to be similar to or better than those achieved with surgical transfer (i.e., ≥70%). Technician variation probably contributes greatly to the differences noted among laboratories for pregnancy rates after nonsurgical embryo transfer. The advantages of the nonsurgical technique over the surgical technique are simplicity, reduced expense, reduced posttransfer complications, and more efficient use of recipients.

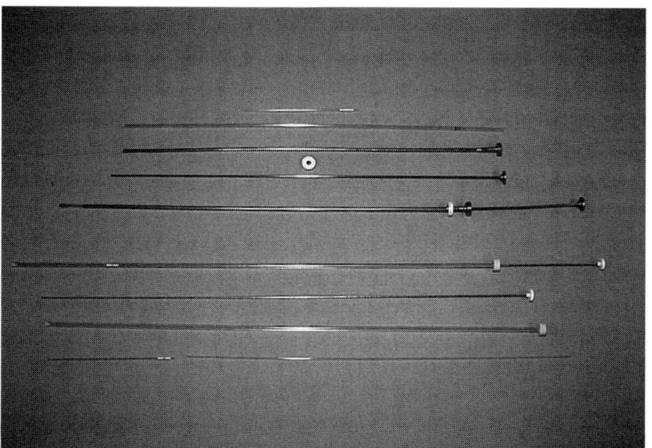

FIGURE 17-9. Two types of insemination guns used for nonsurgical transfer of embryos. From *top:* 0.5-ml straw, protective sheath, metal cannula, O-ring for holding the protective sheath on the metal cannula, metal plunger for pushing the fluid and embryo through the straw, and assembled unit; assembled disposable unit, inner metal plunger for pushing the fluid and embryo through the straw, outer plastic cannula, 0.25-ml straw *(bottom left)* and inner plastic guide *(bottom right)* to be placed behind the straw when it is loaded into the outer plastic cannula.

TRANSPORT OF EMBRYOS

The availability of suitable recipients is often a limiting factor in performing embryo transfer. The ability to transport embryos to facilities with large numbers of recipient mares and experienced personnel has greatly expanded the use of equine embryo transfer.

The transport medium most commonly used is Ham's F-10, supplemented with 10% (v/v) FCS or NCS, penicillin (100 U/ml), and streptomycin (100 µg/ml). Before supplements are added, this medium must be buffered by bubbling a gas mixture of 90% N2, 5% O_2, and 5% CO_2 through it for 3 to 5 minutes. The color of the medium will change from pink to pale orange when the correct pH range has been achieved. After preparation, the medium should be filter-sterilized before use. Some embryo transfer facilities will provide the prepared, sterilized medium so that the practitioner can avoid the tedious preparation steps. The shelf life of the prepared medium is approximately 72 to 96 hours. Therefore this shipping medium cannot be stored and must be prepared and shipped to the collection facility within 24 to 48 hours of embryo collection.

Recently, alternative media have become available (Emcare embryo holding solution or Vigro Holding plus media; Table 17-1), which does not require the gas bubbling procedure or additional supplementation. This complete medium contains a zwitterion buffer, bovine serum albumin, and antibiotics. The shelf life of this medium is 18 months from the date of manufacture. Similarly composed embryo flushing media are also available from these sources.

Approximately 4.5 ml of shipping medium is placed in a 5-ml snap-cap tube so that a small air space remains at the top of the tube. The embryo is carefully transferred to this tube, and the cap is securely snapped in place and wrapped in Parafilm. The 5-ml tube containing the embryo and medium is then placed in a 50-ml conical centrifuge tube that is then filled with Ham's F-10, capped, and wrapped in Parafilm. These tubes are then packaged in an Equitainer (Hamilton Thorne Research; Table 17-1), following procedures similar to those used for transported, cooled semen. When packaged correctly, the embryo is passively cooled to approximately 5° C and should remain viable for at least 24 hours, thus allowing air or ground transport to distant commercial embryo transfer facilities. Pregnancy rates for embryos transferred after transport when this system is used are similar to those obtained when embryos are transferred fresh.

STORAGE OF EMBRYOS

Cryopreservation of equine embryos has not been very successful. In general, equine embryos (Figures 17-10 and

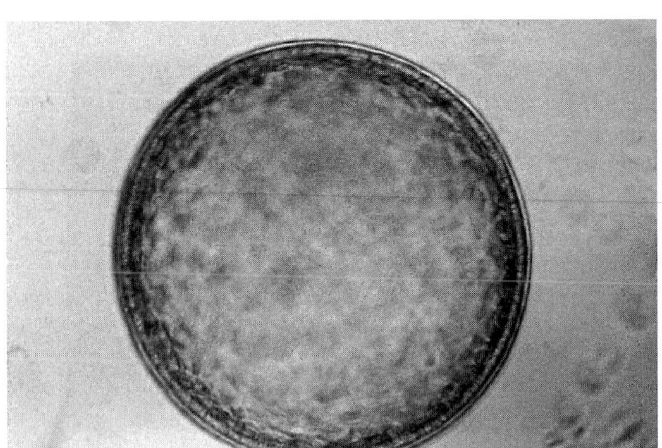

FIGURE 17-10. A viable equine embryo in the expanded blastocyst stage with its surrounding zona pellucida. The majority of equine embryos apparently pass from the oviduct into the uterus as late morulae or early blastocysts. (Courtesy Dr. Duane Kraemer.)

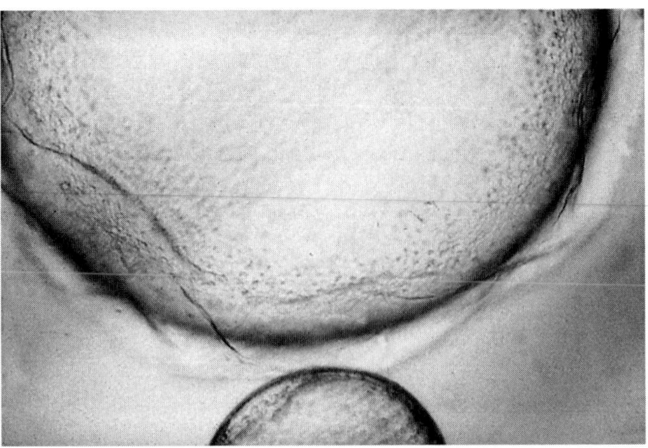

FIGURE 17-11. Twin equine embryos recovered during a uterine flushing procedure. The smaller embryo is approximately one-fourth the size of the larger, indicating that it probably arose from an asynchronous ovulation 3 to 4 days after the initial ovulation. (Courtesy Dr. Duane Kraemer.)

17-11) seem to better tolerate the freezing/thawing process when in a morula/early blastocyst stage and ≤200 μm in diameter. Although embryos recovered at days 5 to 6 are in the acceptable size range for freezing, embryo recovery rates are extremely low on day 5 and are lower on day 6 than on days 7 to 8. Unfortunately, embryos recovered at day 7 or 8 of gestation are 400 to 1200 mm in diameter, and these larger embryos are less tolerant of current freezing and thawing processes. Development of newer cryopreservation techniques or methods to accelerate oviductal transit of embryos may increase the commercial feasibility of embryo cryopreservation.

BIBLIOGRAPHY

Hinrichs K: Embryo transfer. In Robinson NE, editor, *Current therapy in equine medicine,* ed 3, Philadelphia, 1992, WB Saunders.

McKinnon AO, Squires EL, Voss JL et al: Equine embryo transfer. *Comp Cont Educ Pract Vet* 10:343, 1988.

Squires EL: Embryo transfer. In McKinnon AO, Voss JL, editors, *Equine reproduction,* Philadelphia, 1993, Lea and Febiger.

Vanderwall DK: Current equine embryo transfer techniques. In Ball BA, editor, *Recent advances in equine reproduction,* Ithaca, NY, 2000, International Veterinary Information Service.

18

Evaluation of Breeding Records

OBJECTIVES

While studying the information covered in this chapter, the student should attempt to:

1. Understand how to gather relevant information from breeding farm records.
2. Understand how to evaluate data garnered from breeding farm records.
3. Understand how to interpret the results of the breeding farm record evaluation.

STUDY QUESTIONS

1. Define the term *seasonal pregnancy rate*, and explain its use and limitations for assessing fertility.
2. Define the term *cycles/pregnancy*, and explain how it is used to assess fertility.
3. Explain the makeup of a stallion's book of mares, and discuss how it influences pregnancy rates.
4. Discuss factors that influence whether a mare becomes pregnant when bred to a given stallion.

Evaluation of breeding farm records is integral to obtaining an accurate history for evaluating the reproductive performance of a stallion. A challenging aspect of taking a history is determining which information is most relevant. Often, especially if a stallion has produced unsatisfactory pregnancy rates, the stallion owner/manager and mare owner have differing opinions as to the cause of the poor fertility. The veterinarian should provide advice based only on accurate information. He or she must be familiar with the breeding farm procedures to glean objective data that will support a meaningful assessment of the fertility problem. Breeding records should be the most detailed, objective historical information that the clinician can obtain.

Breeding records exist in many forms that range from poorly organized handwritten papers to highly organized computerized spreadsheets listing numerous mathematical parameters. However, even computerized record-keeping programs usually remain inadequate for summarizing and measuring relevant fertility endpoints and require further collation and analysis to accurately assess breeding performance.

The clinician should not hesitate to request breeding records from previous breeding seasons as well as the current breeding season to facilitate determination of whether the fertility of a stallion has changed. A stallion's fertility can change from year to year simply because of the reproductive quality of the mares in his book. A decrease in the quality of mares bred commonly follows a decline in the stallion's popularity. As the stallion's stud fee drops, the owner/manager must accept mares of lesser reproductive quality to fill the stallion's book.

LEARNING TO EVALUATE BREEDING FARM RECORDS

This exercise is intended to introduce the reader to the breeding records that may be available on breeding farms that have stallions standing at stud. Keep in mind that the stallion owner/manager may not keep data regarding each mating, leaving a conclusion to be drawn about a stallion's "subfertile" condition solely from results of semen evaluation. Analysis of the breeding records should be considered as much a part of the breeding soundness evaluation as other components of the examination.

Table 18-1 provides an example of a typical breeding record. Records may also be provided as day-to-day worksheets that have not been tabulated. The information that is commonly recorded is listed across the top of the table and includes the following:

- *Mare*—Identification of the mare.
- *Begin status*—The reproductive status of the mare before the current breeding season.

Mares are classified as the following:

Maiden—Usually a young mare that has not been bred in previous years and thus has not produced a foal.

Barren—A mare that was bred the previous year but is not pregnant. Several reasons besides reproductive unsoundness exist for mares to be classified as barren. For example, late-foaling mares may have only had

TABLE 18-1

Mares Bred Summary

Mare	Begin Status	Date Foaled	Dates Bred	Days Since	Status after Last Exam
Betty	Slipped		2/26/00	258	In-foal
Suzy	Maiden		2/29/00	255	In-foal
Kelly	In-foal	2/14/00	3/20/00 2/24/00 2/22/00	235	Barren
Konnie	In-foal	3/12/00	4/20/00 4/1/00		In-foal

one chance to become pregnant before the end of the breeding season.

Slipped—A mare in which pregnancy was diagnosed in the previous breeding season, but that failed to carry the pregnancy to term due to embryonic loss or abortion.

In-foal—A mare that became pregnant the previous breeding season and is assumed to still be pregnant or has recently delivered a term foal at the time she is booked to be bred to the stallion.

Not bred—A mare that was not bred the previous year, which is the owner's choice sometimes when the mare foals late in the year. Skipping breeding that summer allows early rebreeding the next year with the hope of producing an early-born foal in the following year. Some managers include "not bred" mares in the barren category.

- *Date foaled*—The date the mare foaled.
- *Dates bred*—The dates on which the mare was bred.
- *Days since*—The difference between the date the report was printed and the last breeding date. For those mares found to be "in-foal," this number can be considered their current gestation length.
- *Status after last exam*—The current pregnancy status: either *in-foal, barren, or slipped.*

The following list includes endpoints that should be measured (also summarized in Table 18-2). Although this is not a complete list, the endpoints listed should be considered first. Computerized programs sometimes measure certain endpoints differently, and in some cases incorrectly, so do not assume that a farm summary sheet of these measures is accurate. Instead, perform the calculations yourself to ensure accuracy.

- *Total number of mares bred*—Count the number of mares in the "Mare" column.
- *Total number of mares pregnant*—Count the number of mares identified as in-foal in the "Status after Last Exam" column.
- *Seasonal pregnancy rate*—Divide the total number of mares bred by the total number of mares in foal and multiply this figure by 100 to provide the seasonal pregnancy rate as a percentage.
- *Cycles per pregnancy*—Count the number of cycles a mare was bred in the "Dates Bred" column. The dates bred number assumes that each mare was in normal estrus and was bred at the appropriate time relative to ovulation. Some mares are *doubled,* which means that they are bred more than once during a given estrous cycle, usually because the mare did not ovulate as planned. In general, if two dates are within one week of each other, assume they are the same estrous cycle. Do not count doubles as separate estrous cycles (see discussion later in this chapter).

TABLE 18-2

Summary of Reproductive Endpoints To Be Assessed from Stallion Breeding Records

Reproductive Endpoint
Total number of mares bred in book
Number of mares pregnant
Seasonal pregnancy rate (%)
Overall cycles/pregnancy
Mare Status
Barren
Total no. mares
% of book
No. pregnant
% barren mares pregnant
Maiden
No. of mares
% of book
No. pregnant
% maiden mares pregnant
In-foal
No. of mares
% of book
No. pregnant
% in-foal mares pregnant

- *Number of mares that are classified as barren, in-foal, or maiden before the breeding season*—Count the individual classifications in the "Begin Status" column. Mares in the *slipped* category are usually included in the barren mare group. If the number of slipped mares is high, a separate group identifying this number should be included. After the number of mares in each group is assessed, the *percentage* of each category in the stallion's book should be determined.
- *Pregnancy status of mares in each classification*—Assess the pregnancy status of mares in each classification, and determine the *percentage* pregnant in each classification (Table 18-3). This is important because a stallion may achieve acceptable pregnancy rates in mares expected to have normal fertility (i.e., in-foal and maiden mares) but poor pregnancy rates in mares with breeding problems (i.e., barren mares). The overall pregnancy rate achieved by such a stallion could appear to be unacceptable, but it could be entirely due to breeding a predominant percentage of mares with breeding problems.

TABLE 18-3

Pregnancy Status for Stallion 4 Based on Mare Status (Barren, Foaling, Maiden, Not Bred, or Slipped)

Mare type	No. of Mares	No. of Mares Pregnant	% Pregnant
No. barren total	24	16	67
No. foaling total	43	32	74
No. maiden total	14	8	57
Total	81	56	69

INTERPRETATION

Total Number of Mares Bred

This value determines the total number of *different* mares in a stallion's book and is used in the denominator when the clinician determines a seasonal pregnancy rate. The clinician should recognize that the inherent fertility and management of all mares in the book are not equal. One goal of evaluating a stallion's book is to describe these differences. Maiden and barren mares are generally bred earlier in the breeding season and therefore should have more opportunities (more estrous cycles) to become pregnant. Foaling mares, because they cannot be bred until after parturition, are generally bred later in the breeding season and therefore will have fewer opportunities to become pregnant. If the total number of mares becomes too great for a given stallion, the overall seasonal pregnancy rate may decrease with a concomitant increase in cycles/pregnancy (because the stallion is being "overbred," meaning he is bred so often that insufficient numbers of sperm are being produced in ejaculates to result in good pregnancy rates). On some well-managed farms, as the number of mares in the book increases, so does a stallion's fertility. This paradoxical increase in fertility is due to the stallion's popularity (usually associated with a higher stud fee), which results in the stallion owner/manager being able to pick and choose the highest quality mares for breeding. A secondary reason for the increased fertility with increasing book size is that the overall value of (and investment in) the mare is generally higher, resulting in more intense management to prepare the mare for breeding. The combination of mares with high reproductive quality and intense management of mares can dramatically improve the pregnancy rate achieved by a given stallion.

Total Number of Mares Pregnant

This parameter can be defined in different ways depending on (1) when pregnancy examinations occur and (2) how data are entered for mares that become pregnant yet later suffer embryonic death or abortion. We recommend that, for initial evaluation, the clinician consider the mare pregnant regardless of whether she maintains the pregnancy. The number of mares losing pregnancies tends to be low; however, there are some rare stallions that may contribute to production of abnormal embryos that culminate in embryonic loss. To identify such a stallion, determining the number (and percentage) of mares that lose their pregnancy after a positive pregnancy diagnosis is warranted.

The clinician should also be aware of an economic fact in the Thoroughbred industry: the stud fee (guaranteed live foal) is contractually transferable from the mare owner to the stallion owner when the foal stands and suckles after it is born. Therefore, a seasonal pregnancy rate based on pregnancy diagnosed ultrasonographically 14 days after ovulation will virtually always be greater than the *actual foaling rate* upon which the economic status of the farm will depend. The 14-day pregnancy rate and the foaling rate can differ by 10% to 20%. The payment of stud fees for some breeds may be contractually due before the breeding season. In this case and particularly if no live foal guarantee is offered, in theory less incentive exists for the stallion owner/manager to get the mare pregnant. In the Thoroughbred industry, stallions at stud with no contractually guaranteed live foal usually achieve high pregnancy rates (per cycle and per season) because only highly fertile mares are booked to these stallions with high stud fees.

Seasonal Pregnancy Rate

This parameter is based on the number of mares in which pregnancy is diagnosed at a particular point in gestation divided by the total number of mares in a stallion's book. This endpoint is very important economically, but it is not a sensitive indicator of a stallion's fertility because it does not reflect the total number of cycles that a mare is bred to achieve the pregnancy. A stallion can achieve a relatively low pregnancy rate per cycle but end the season with a seasonal pregnancy rate similar to that of a stallion achieving a relatively high pregnancy rate per cycle. The only difference is that the stallion with a relatively low pregnancy rate per cycle must breed the mares in his book more times during the season to reach the same seasonal pregnancy rate.

Several factors that can alter seasonal pregnancy rate include the following:

1. *The point at which the seasonal pregnancy rate is determined* (i.e., during the breeding season, shortly after the breeding season, or many months after the breeding season). When this value is calculated near the start of the next breeding season, it will more closely approximate the *foaling rate.*
2. *The number of estrous cycles that a mare was bred.* It is common for the stallion manager/owner to *add mares on to a stallion's book* as the end of the breeding season approaches. Adding mares on to a stallion's book is often done when mares are switched from one stallion to another for a variety of reasons. These mares are included in the total number of mares that the stallion breeds, but in reality are given fewer opportunities to become pregnant (usually only one cycle) than other mares in the stallion's book. If mares added on to a

stallion's book near the end of the breeding season do not become pregnant, the seasonal pregnancy rate for that stallion will be lowered but will not truly represent the actual rate for the stallion. Therefore, if a stallion is presented because of a *low seasonal pregnancy rate,* it is important to determine that all mares were bred during an adequate number of estrous cycles to have a reasonable chance of becoming pregnant (see discussion later in this chapter).

3. *Inclusion or exclusion of mares that exhibit early embryonic death.* The assumption can be made that the majority of embryonic deaths are due to mare and not stallion factors. If an accurate seasonal pregnancy rate figure is to be created to describe the stallion's inherent fertility, all diagnosed pregnancies (which indicate that the stallion was able to accomplish fertilization in those mares) should be included in calculating the rate. However, keep in mind that counting an embryonic death as a pregnancy when figuring seasonal pregnancy rate is of no economic relevance (i.e., stud fees will not be transferred). If embryonic deaths are included as pregnancies in calculating seasonal pregnancy rate, an inflated economic value for the seasonal pregnancy rate is created.

Cycles/Pregnancy (Pregnancy Rate/Cycle)

This measure is a more sensitive indication of a stallion's fertility because it measures how *efficient* a stallion is in establishing pregnancies. To determine this value, count the number of cycles a mare was bred in the "Dates Bred" column. The assumption is made that all entries into the Dates Bred column were for mares in normal estrus, and mares were being bred near to the time of ovulation. This assumption is not always correct, especially for breedings by artificial insemination on some farms where mares bred artificially are either not in estrus or not near ovulation. Whenever it is typical for a high number of breedings per estrus period to occur, pregnancy rates may not reflect truly the fertility of either the stallion or the mares. This situation is unlikely to occur when breeding occurs by natural service because the mare must actually stand for breeding by the stallion (the best indicator of estrus).

Some mares are *doubled,* which means that they are bred more than once during an estrus period. Doubles occur because the mare does not ovulate as predicted, so another breeding is provided to ensure that the mare is bred near to the time of ovulation. The incidence of doubles is a reflection of the overall managerial (broodmare manager and veterinarian) ability to detect and breed mares at the proper time to maximize pregnancy rates. On well-managed farms, the *double rate* may range from 0% to 10%. A double does not count as a cycle. If two breeding dates are within 7 days of each other, breeding during only one estrous cycle is included in the calculation of cycles/pregnancy. An example of a double is the mare Kelly, the third mare listed in Table 18-1. She was bred on February 22 and February 24. Both matings occurred during only one estrus period and thus would count for breeding on only one cycle. In rare instances for mating by natural service, but more commonly for mating by artificial insemination, breeding more than twice (e.g., triples or quadruples) during one estrus period may occur. Again, multiple matings in one estrus period should only be counted as one mating for that estrous cycle. The *total number of cycles* can be determined by counting all dates bred excluding multiple matings during single estrous periods (usually doubles). To calculate the cycles/pregnancy, divide the total number of mated cycles in all mares bred by the total number of mares becoming pregnant (*not* by the total number of mares in the book).

Cycles/Pregnancy (Pregnancy Rate/Cycle) for Cycles 1 Through 6

This parameter evaluates the per cycle pregnancy rate of the first through sixth cycles that mares were bred. All mares in the book are bred on at least one estrous cycle; therefore the number of mares in this category should equal the total number of mares in the stallion's book. Ideally, if all mares are of equal and high fertility, the pregnancy rate achieved in mares bred during the last estrous cycle should be the same as that in the first estrous cycle, and these pregnancy rates would accurately reflect the stallion's fertility. However, because fertility of individual mares varies, actual pregnancy rates for each successive estrous cycle of breeding are seldom the same. Mares that are subfertile tend to take more estrous cycles to become detectably pregnant. Table 18-4 reveals that pregnancy rates achieved during the first three estrous cycles are similar (for the stallion used) but dramatically decrease for breedings on the fourth estrous cycle (i.e., only one of seven mares bred on the fourth estrous cycle became pregnant). This decline in pregnancy rate per cycle as mares in the stallion's book are bred over successive estrous cycles indicates that those mares are themselves subfertile.

Whether all mares that do not become pregnant after breeding on a particular estrous cycle get rebred on the following estrous cycle can also be determined from this type of table. In Table 18-4, 32 of 81 mares became pregnant on the first cycle; therefore 49 should have returned for a second cycle breeding, yet only 44 were bred a second time. Therefore 5 mares were only bred one time, yet did not return to estrus; thus the mares were not given adequate opportunity to become pregnant.

Barren, Foaling, and Maiden Mares

Barren. This group contains nonpregnant mares coming into the breeding season of interest. Mares in this group will usually have lower fertility than the other groups. Several reasons why a mare might be barren are discussed in the following paragraphs.

Not bred the previous season. This can occur because the owner simply decided not to breed the mare, or the mare

TABLE 18-4

Pregnancy Rate for Stallion 4 Based on Cycle Number

Cycle No.	No. of Cycles	No. of Mares Pregnant	% Pregnant/Cycle
1st cycle	81	32	40
2nd cycle	44	15	34
3rd cycle	18	7	39
4th cycle	7	1	0
5th cycle	3	1	0
6th cycle	0	0	0
Total	153	56	37

may have foaled late in the previous season and did not have ample opportunity to become pregnant. Mares classified as barren for these reasons have normal fertility.

Subfertile. These mares have intrinsic fertility problems that contributed to their failure to become pregnant during the previous breeding season and are commonly older than the rest of the mare population. In most cases, the subfertile mares will account for the majority of the mares classified as barren.

Aborted. These mares have aborted since the previous breeding season. Some managers and computer programs use the term "slipped" instead of the term "aborted" and include these mares in a separate category from the barren mares. Once they recover, they tend to have fertility similar to the Not Bred group.

Foaling. These mares have produced a foal in the current breeding season and will be rebred during the same season. One should expect high fertility in this group of mares because they recently conceived and carried a foal to term. Reduced fertility may be seen in this group if a predominant proportion of the mares foaled late in the breeding season, thus having only one to two estrous cycles available for rebreeding. Fertility in this group may also be reduced if some event (injury/illness to the stallion) prematurely shortens the breeding season.

Maiden. Mares that have never been bred. Mares in this group are generally young; however, occasional maiden mares are older because their owner has elected not to breed them when young (usually due to a continuing performance career). Older maiden mares are generally less fertile than young maiden mares, which typically have high fertility. Mares that have been recently retired from strenuous performance careers may not be cycling regularly when they first become available for mating (typically in February) and thus may require more breedings to become pregnant. However, because maiden mares are generally available for breeding early in the season, their chances of becoming pregnant are high.

Pregnancy Status for Each Mare Class

The pregnancy status can reveal important information about stallion fertility. As a general rule, breeding of maiden and foaling mares should result in the highest fertility achievable by a stallion and represents a stallion's intrinsic fertility. Breeding of barren mares may result in similar or lesser fertility. If a large proportion of the barren mares in a stallion's book are nonpregnant because of intrinsically lower individual mare fertility, measures of stallion fertility that reflect the entire mare group will be lower than that achieved in the foaling and maiden mare groups. Conversely, mares may be barren because they were not bred the previous year, in which case their fertility may be similar to that of foaling and maiden mare groups, resulting in the stallion achieving high fertility measures for the entire mare book.

In some cases, foaling mares may represent the group of lowest fertility. This may be due to a large proportion of foaling mares delivering their foals late in the season, leaving an insufficient number of estrous cycles available in the remainder of the season to truly test their fertility (i.e., perhaps only one to two estrous cycles before the breeding season ended). In this case, neither the stallion nor the foaling mares are at fault.

Number of Covers or Breedings (Matings) in a Cycle

The number of matings in a cycle (i.e., usually is the double rate, unless mares are being bred more than twice during estrus) refers to the average number of natural covers or inseminations performed per estrus. This value is a reflection of management ability to time breeding near to ovulation. Excessive covers or inseminations per cycle can result in overuse of a stallion (i.e., semen is essentially being wasted). Intense mare management to minimize the number of covers or inseminations per cycle will result in more ejaculates (semen) being available to breed more mares.

MATHEMATICS OF HORSE BREEDING

Although there are many factors involved in the breeding process, perhaps the most critical is realizing that mares need adequate exposure to the stallion for high fertility to be achieved (i.e., a 100% pregnancy rate per cycle is not achievable, so mares not becoming pregnant on the first service must be bred a sufficient number of times to afford a realistic opportunity to become pregnant during the season). To illustrate this principle, if a stallion achieves a 50% pregnancy rate per cycle, mares must on average be bred at least two estrous cycles to yield a 75% seasonal pregnancy rate. Yet, a 75% seasonal pregnancy rate would be considered to be low on well-managed breeding farms. Evaluation of breeding records will reveal whether the low seasonal pregnancy rate is simply due to insufficient exposure to the stallion, or if other factors explain the low seasonal pregnancy rate.

Evaluating the Effect of Breeding Frequency on Fertility

One factor that will modulate fertility during the breeding season is how often stallions are used. For a farm that is using natural cover, the *breeding frequency* represents the

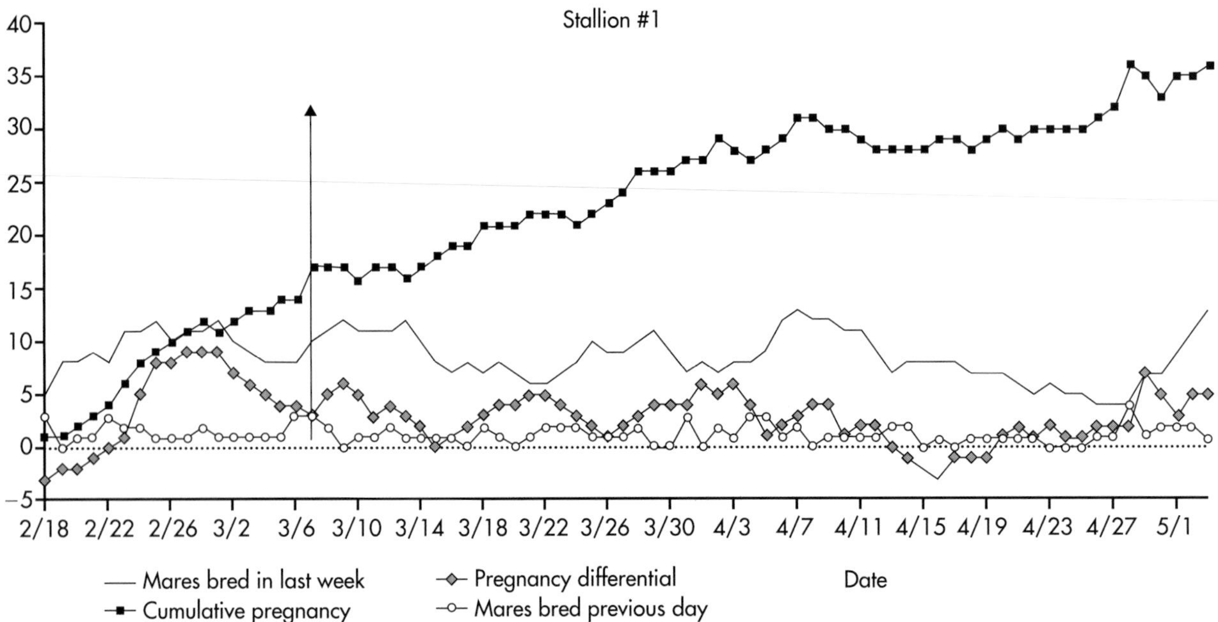

FIGURE 18-1. Stallion 1. This figure graphically represents an example of a highly fertile Thoroughbred stallion bred by natural cover. Note that the cumulative pregnancy value continues to climb regardless of preceding breeding frequencies. There is no indication that a threshold breeding frequency, above which fertility declines, has been reached. Although there are peaks and valleys in the pregnancy differential, they are probably related to nonstallion factors. This stallion would be expected to achieve a 90% seasonal pregnancy rate, requiring less than an average of 1.5 estrous cycles per pregnancy, in a book of 100 mares bred by natural service.

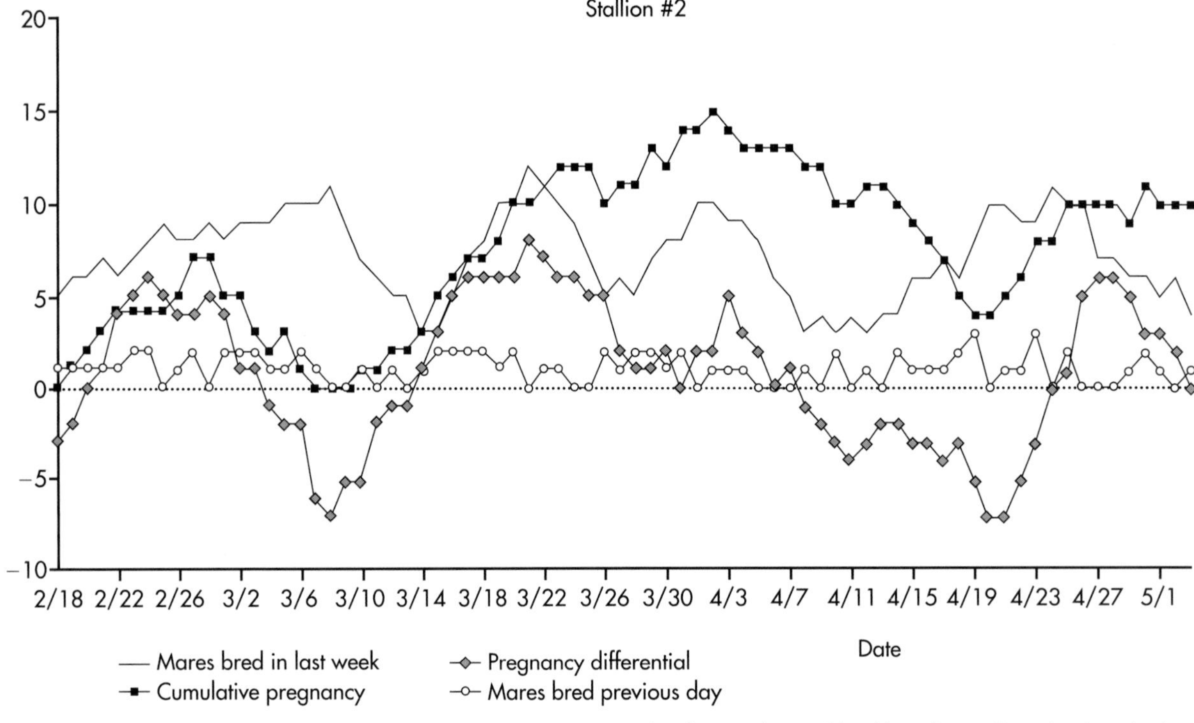

FIGURE 18-2. Stallion 2. This figure graphically represents an example of many Thoroughbred breeding stallions that breed a large book of mares. Note that a steep decline in pregnancy differential occurs from February 28 to March 8, which probably corresponds to the increase in breeding frequency during the previous week to 11 mares. There are times later in the season when breeding frequency again rises to this level, but it is not maintained for as long a period as that from February 6 to March 8. Other declines in pregnancy differential and cumulative pregnancy value occur during the breeding season, but the declines are more gradual and are not associated with peaks in breeding frequency. This figure is representative of most breeding stallions that do reach threshold levels of breeding frequencies at times in the breeding season. Such stallions typically achieve an 80% to 90% seasonal pregnancy rate, requiring 1.5 to 2.2 estrous cycles per pregnancy in a book of 80 to 90 mares if bred by natural cover.

number of times a stallion is bred in a given time period (i.e., the number of times bred in a day or week). On farms where artificial breeding is used, the *breeding frequency* represents the number of mares bred with an individual ejaculate. No stallion will have mares presented for breeding at even intervals throughout the breeding season. Therefore, pregnancy rates achieved by the stallion when used for different breeding frequencies can be used to evaluate whether overuse of the stallion has occurred (i.e., whether he has been bred too frequently for ejaculates to contain sufficient numbers of sperm to effect good fertility). Use of breeding frequencies to evaluate this phenomenon is presented in Figures 18-1 thorough 18-4; and this method relies on the following parameters:

1. *Number of mares bred in last week*—This identifies the number of mares bred in the week before the day in question. This parameter is an evaluation of the long-term effect of frequent breedings, with the intent to determine whether there is a threshold breeding frequency above which fertility of the stallion declines. This phenomenon occurs in many stallions; if periods of too high breeding frequency are numerous during the season, reduced fertility becomes apparent.
2. *Number of mares bred the previous day*—This identifies the number of mares bred (either by natural or artificial breeding) on that day.
3. *Pregnancy differential*—For each date every mare is bred, a pregnancy score is given (+1 if pregnancy results, –1 if no pregnancy results or a zero for all double dates except for the last one of the cycle). The scores are summed for the week previous to a particular date and graphically indicate the fertility of a stallion for the previous week.
4. *Cumulative pregnancy value*—This value represents the summed pregnancy scores (+1 or –1) for the entire breeding season leading up to the date of interest. The zero line represents a 50% pregnancy rate per cycle.

To illustrate the effects of breeding frequency, the reader is referred to Figure 18-1. The arrow (March 7th) represents the date for recording the following breeding frequency values: number of mares bred in last week = 10; number of mares bred previous day = 3; pregnancy differential = 3; and cumulative pregnancy value = 17. Interpretation of these data reveals that on March 7th: there were 10 mares bred in the previous week, 3 more mares became pregnant than were nonpregnant (pregnancy differential), and for the breeding season on this date there are 17 more mares pregnant than nonpregnant. Using this approach, the reader should study Figures 18-1 through 18-4, while referring to the following interpretations.

For breeds that use artificial insemination there are additional factors that influence overall fertility. For example, mares may be inseminated with *fresh semen immediately* after collection, with stallions and mares being managed on the same farm. Assuming good management, this method of artificial breeding is expected to result in high fertility. *Tailgate breeding* may also occur, in which case the mare is moved to the farm by trailer, is inseminated in the trailer, and is immediately returned to the farm of origin. Because with tailgate breeding mares and stallions are under different management, pregnancy rates achieved in mares bred in this manner is sometimes lower than that achieved for mares managed at the farm where the stallion stands at stud. For mares bred with *transported, cooled semen,* each mare is again under different management than those maintained on the farm where the stallion stands at stud. Additional factors that may adversely affect pregnancy rates when mares are bred with transported, cooled semen are that insemination timing in relation to ovulation can be more variable and that for some stallions the same level of fertility is not achieved with cooled semen as with fresh semen. Pregnancy rates achieved with *frozen semen* tend to be substantially lower for most stallions than those achieved with fresh or cooled semen. Therefore, in addition to those factors outlined for evaluation of the Thoroughbred breeding operation, additional parameters must be considered when one evaluates the fertility achieved by a stallion used for artificial insemination. An example of one such evaluation is given using Figure 18-4 and Tables 18-3 through 18-6.

Figure 18-4 demonstrates several points regarding a stallion's lower-than-expected fertility when used in an artificial insemination breeding program. This stallion did not begin the breeding season until March 8 instead of February 15. The loss of almost a month of breeding season resulted in lost opportunities for barren and maiden mares to become pregnant. During March 10 through April 10, this stallion was bred infrequently, yet only achieved approximately a 50% pregnancy rate per cycle. When the number of inseminations per week exceeded 10 (March 11), the pregnancy rate declined. This is a typical graphic presentation of the effect of overbreeding, in that pregnancy rates decline when the stallion is bred to too many mares; however, there are other factors contributing to the reduced fertility (Tables 18-3 through 18-6).

Table 18-3 lists the fertility of differing mare groups bred to this stallion. The reader should note that the lower fertility in maiden than in barren mares is not typical. The overall seasonal pregnancy rate is low (69%). Evaluation of Table 18-5 reveals extreme variation in fertility achieved by different methods of breeding for this same stallion. Mares inseminated as soon as possible with semen that was *picked up* at the stud farm had a 91% pregnancy rate per season, whereas other methods of breeding resulted in pregnancy rates per season of only 54% to 67%. This finding suggests that, under the *right conditions* (i.e., intense mare management for prompt insemination at a time near to ovulation—the method used for breeding with transported, cooled semen), this stallion has the potential to be very fertile and raises the question of whether the low pregnancy rates were primarily due to inadequate breeding management.

Table 18-6 summarizes this stallion's fertility endpoints. The value for *cycles per pregnancy* was high, whereas that for *cycles per mare* was low, indicating that mares were not bred

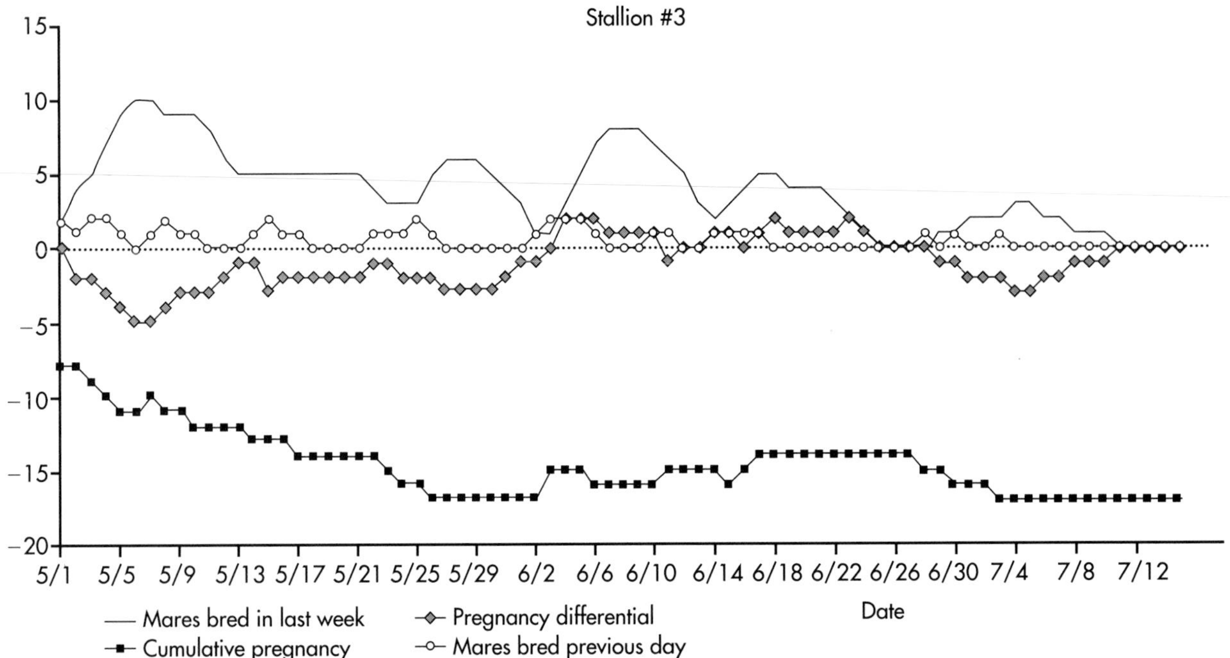

FIGURE 18-3. Stallion 3. This figure graphically represents an example of a Thoroughbred stallion with low fertility. Even though breeding frequency remains low (zero to two mares per day), the pregnancy differential remains below the zero line (zero line = 50% pregnancy rate per cycle) and his cumulative pregnancy value is very low.

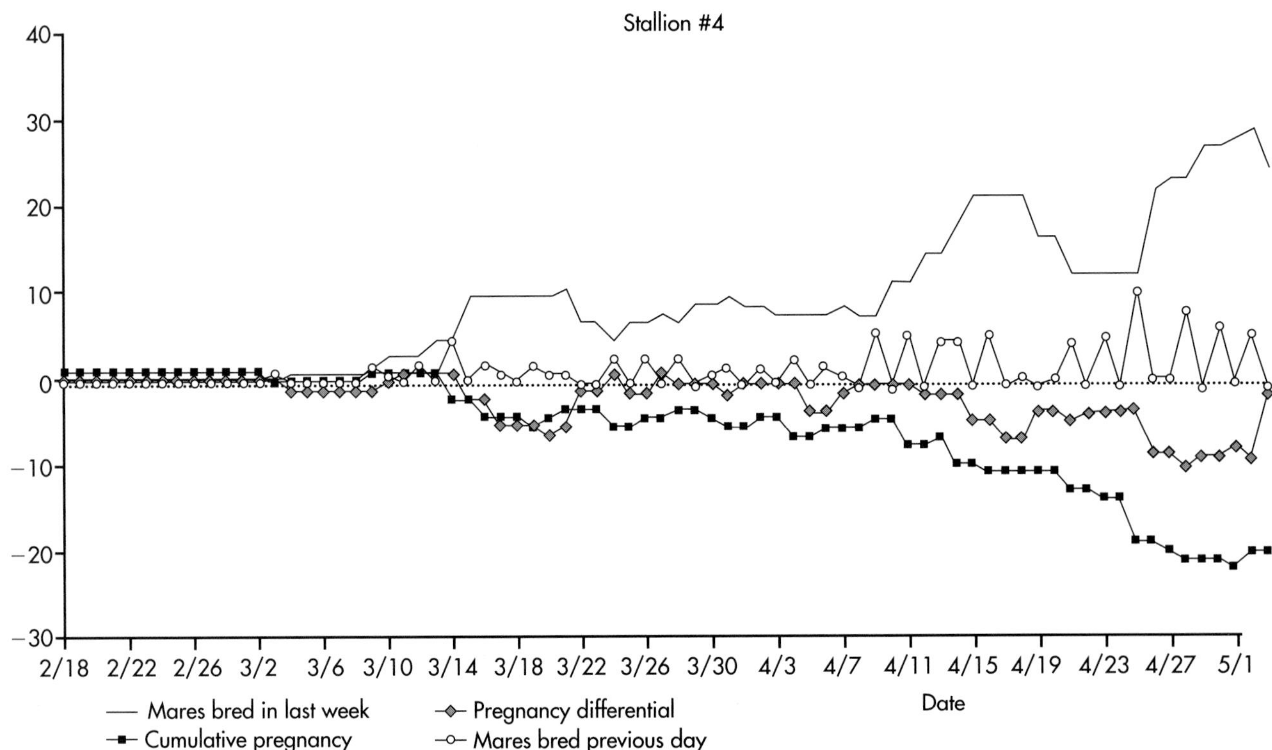

FIGURE 18-4. Stallion 4. This figure graphically represents an example of a Quarter Horse stallion with low fertility. The stallion was bred artificially to mares on the same farm, mares hauled to the farm (tailgate breeding), and mares at outside farms with transported, cooled semen (semen mailed overnight for breeding the next day or semen picked up at the farm for breeding the same day).

TABLE 18-5

Pregnancy Status of Mares Based on Location (on-Farm with Fresh Semen or off-Farm with Shipped Semen) for Stallion 4

	Barren			Foaling			Maiden			
Location of Mare	No. Pregnant	No. Bred	Percent Pregnant	No. Pregnant	No. Bred	Percent Pregnant	No. Pregnant	No. Bred	Percent Pregnant	Pregnant Overall
Mare and stallion on farm	3	11	27	14	21	67	7	10	70	24/42 (57%)
Overnight	2	2	100	4	6	67	0	1	0	6/9 (67%)
Pick-up	10	10	100	9	10	90	2	3	67	21/23 (91%)
Trailer-bred	1	4	25	5	6	83	1	3	33	7/13 (54%)
Total	16	27	59	33	43	77	10	17	59	58/87 (67%)

TABLE 18-6

Summary of Stallion 4 Fertility Parameters

Cycles/Pregnancy	Cycles/Mare	Covers/Cycle
2.73	1.89	1.79

often enough when the pregnancy rate per cycle was so low. The number of *covers per cycle* was also quite high, which indicates that mares were often being bred too soon during the estrus period, long before ovulation occurred. Because the stallion's pregnancy rate declined dramatically when 10 or more mares were bred in the previous week, intensive mare management to constrain breeding to near the time of ovulation should increase pregnancy rates per cycle.

Index

Page numbers followed by f indicate figures; t, tables; and b, boxes.

C

F

G

H

T

U